J. Ring B. Przybilla (Eds.)

New Trends in Allergy III

Foreword by O. Braun-Falco

With 168 Figures and 152 Tables

Springer-Verlag
Berlin Heidelberg New York
London Paris Tokyo
Hong Kong Barcelona
Budapest

Prof. Dr. med. Dr. phil. JOHANNES RING
Hautklinik und Allergie-Abteilung
Universitäts-Krankenhaus Eppendorf
Martinistrasse 52, 2000 Hamburg 20
Federal Republic of Germany

Priv.-Doz. Dr. med. BERNHARD PRZYBILLA
Dermatologische Klinik und Poliklinik
Ludwig-Maximilians-Universität
Frauenlobstrasse 9–11, 8000 München 2
Federal Republic of Germany

ISBN-13: 978-3-642-46719-6 e-ISBN-13: 978-3-642-46717-2
DOI: 10.1007/978-3-642-46717-2

Library of Congress Cataloging-in-Publication Data
New trends in allergy III / Johannes Ring, Bernhard Przybilla (eds.); foreword by O. Braun-Falco. p. cm. Contains papers presented at a symposium, held July 13–15, 1990 in Munich. Includes bibliographical references and indexes.
(alk. paper) 1. Allergy – Congresses. [1. Hypersensitivity – congresses.] I. Ring, Johannes, 1945–. II. Przybilla, Bernhard, 1949–. III. Title: New trends in allergy three. [DNLM: WD 300 N5321 1990] RC583.2.N483 1991 616.97–dc20 DNLM/DLC

Softcover reprint of the hardcover 1st edition 1991

Production Editor: Isolde Scherich
Reproduction of the figures: Gustav Dreher GmbH, Stuttgart
Typesetting: K+V Fotosatz GmbH, Beerfelden

27/3145-543210 – Printed on acid-free paper

Foreword

The international symposium "New Trends in Allergy", held in Munich from July 13 to 15, 1990, brought together for the third time since 1980 some of the most experienced researchers working in the field of allergy. This volume comprises the papers presented at this meeting.

All over the world, and not merely in the industrialized countries, allergy is becoming a cause of evermore serious diseases. In recent years, research in the field of allergy has provided numerous important and fascinating results extending our knowledge considerably. Despite the new insights into basic mechanisms of allergic reactions, improved diagnostic methods, and new therapeutic approaches, however, many questions remain to be answered, including:

Are allergies really increasing in frequency?

If so, what are the reasons? Especially, does environmental pollution play a role?

Which factors influence IgE synthesis? Can the IgE immune response be switched off?

Does the nervous system interact with allergic reactions? If so, what are the mechanisms?

Are new approaches in allergy prophylaxis and allergy therapy efficient? What measures have proven useful and deserve to be employed in daily practice?

In this volume, these questions and other current topics are dealt with. As each issue is covered by authors competent in the respective fields, the result is an extensive and critical review of the state of the art. Going through these papers, one comes to the conviction that allergy research is a multifacetted, explosively expanding, most stimulating field of work.

I would like to express my gratitude to all those at the Department of Dermatology of the University of Munich who worked hard to insure the success of the symposium. Furthermore, I am very grateful to Springer-Verlag for publishing this volume so splendidly. May it find a wide distribution and thus improve the understanding of allergic diseases to the benefit of our patients.

Munich, March 1991 O. BRAUN-FALCO

Contents

Drug Reactions

Hyposensitization

Autoimmune Diseases

Contact Dermatitis

Mite Allergy

Environmental Pollution and Allergy

Prophylaxis and Therapy

List of Senior Authors

BAUR, X., Professor Dr.
Berufsgenossenschaftliches Forschungsinstitut für Arbeitsmedizin an der Ruhr-Universität Bochum, Gilsingstrasse 14, W-4630 Bochum 1, FRG

BEHRENDT, Heidrun, Professor Dr.
Medizinisches Institut für Umwelthygiene an der Heinrich-Heine-Universität, Auf'm Hennekamp 50, W-4000 Düsseldorf, FRG

BIEBER, T., Priv.-Doz. Dr.
Dermatologische Klinik und Poliklinik der Ludwig-Maximilians-Universität, Frauenlobstrasse 9–11, W-8000 München 2, FRG

BIENENSTOCK, J., M.D.
Department of Pathology and Intestinal Diseases Research Unit, McMaster University, Health Science Centre, 1200 Main Street West, Hamilton, Ontario L8N 3Z5, Canada

BINDSLEV-JENSEN, C., M.D., Ph.D.
Food Allergy Unit TTA 7523, National University Hospital, 20 Tagensvej, 2200 Copenhagen N, Denmark

BISCHOFF, S. C., Dr.
Institut für Klinische Immunologie, Inselspital Bern, 3010 Bern, Switzerland

BOUSQUET, J., M.D., Ph.D.
Clinique des Maladies Respiratoires, CHU, Hôpital l'Aiguelongue, Avenue du Majour Flandre, 34059 Montpellier Cedex, France

BRAUN-FALCO, O., Professor Dr. med. Dr. h.c. mult.
Dermatologische Klinik und Poliklinik der Ludwig-Maximilians-Universität, Frauenlobstrasse 9–11, W-8000 München 2, FRG

BREITENEDER, H., Dr.
Institut für allgemeine und experimentelle Pathologie, Neubau AKH, Erweiterungsbau Ost, Ebene 3, Währinger Gürtel 18–20, 1090 Wien, Austria

BREWCZYŃSKI, P. Z., Dr.
IInd Clinic of Internal Diseases of Silesian School of Medicine, Rozdzienskiego 86/125, 40-203 Katowice, Poland

BRUIJNZEEL-KOOMEN, Carla A. F. M., Dr.
Swiss Institute of Allergy and Asthma Research, Obere Strasse 22, 7270 Davos, Switzerland

CHURCH, M. K., M. Pharm., Ph.D., D.Sc.
Immunopharmacology Group, Clinical Pharmacology, Centre Block, Southampton General Hospital, Southampton SO9 4XY, United Kingdom

CZECH, W., Dr.
Funktionsbereich Allergologie/Immundiagnostik, Universitäts-Hautklinik, Hauptstrasse 7, W-7800 Freiburg i. Br., FRG

DAHINDEN, C. A., Priv.-Doz. Dr.
Institut für Klinische Immunologie, Inselspital Bern, 3010 Bern, Switzerland

DIEPGEN, T. L., Priv.-Doz. Dr.
Dermatologische Klinik und Poliklinik, Universität Erlangen, Hartmannstrasse 14, W-8520 Erlangen, FRG

DORSCH, W., Professor Dr.
Kinderklinik, Johannes Gutenberg Universität, Allergologie und Pneumologie, Langenbeckstrasse 1, W-6500 Mainz, FRG

ENDERS, F., Dr.
Dermatologische Klinik und Poliklinik der Ludwig-Maximilians-Universität, Frauenlobstrasse 9–11, W-8000 München 2, FRG

FROSCH, P. J., Professor Dr.
Hautklinik, Städtische Kliniken Dortmund, Beurhausstrasse 40, W-4600 Dortmund 1, FRG

FUCHS, T., Dr.
Abteilung Dermatovenerologie I, Hautklinik, Georg-August-Universität, von-Siebold-Strasse 3, W-3400 Göttingen, FRG

GOLLHAUSEN, R., Dr.
Dermatologische Klinik und Poliklinik der Ludwig-Maximilians-Universität, Frauenlobstrasse 9–11, W-8000 München 2, FRG

HAEN, E., Dr.
Walther-Straub-Institut für Pharmakologie und Toxikologie, Universität München, Nußbaumstrasse 26, W-8000 München 2, FRG

HERMANN, K., Dr.
Hautklinik und Allergie-Abteilung, Universitäts-Krankenhaus Eppendorf, Martinistrasse 52, W-2000 Hamburg 20

HÖLZLE, E., Professor Dr.
Hautklinik der Heinrich-Heine-Universität Düsseldorf, Moorenstrasse 5, W-4000 Düsseldorf 1, FRG

HULTSCH, T., M.D.
Allergic Diseases Section, Laboratory of Clinical Investigation, National Institute of Allergy and Infectious Diseases, National Institute of Health, Rockville Pike 9000, Bethesda, MD 20892, USA

IKAI, K., M.D.
Department of Dermatology, Kyoto University Faculty of Medicine, Shogoin, Sakyo-ku, Kyoto 606, Japan

ISHIZAKA, K., M.D., Ph.D.
La Jolla Institute for Allergy and Immunology, 11149 North Torrey Pines Road, La Jolla, CA 92037, USA

ISHIZAKA, Teruko, M.D.
Division of Allergy, La Jolla Institute for Allergy and Immunology, 11149 North Torrey Pines Road, La Jolla, CA 92037, USA

JÄGER, L., Professor Dr.
Institut für Klinische Immunologie, Medizinische Fakultät, Friedrich-Schiller-Universität, Humboldtstrasse 3, O-6900 Jena, FRG

JENSEN-JAROLIM, Erika, Dr.
Institut für Klinische Immunologie, Inselspital Bern, 3010 Bern, Switzerland

JOHANSSON, S. G. O., Professor
Department of Clinical Immunology, Karolinska Hospital, 10401 Stockholm, Sweden

KALVERAM, C. M., Dipl.-Chem.
Küperweg 8, W-4400 Münster, FRG

KÁRPÁTI, S., Priv.-Doz. Dr.
Dermatologische Klinik und Poliklinik der Ludwig-Maximilians-Universität, Frauenlobstrasse 9–11, W-8000 München 2, FRG

KARVONEN, J., Professor Dr.
Department of Dermatology, University of Oulu, 90220 Oulu 22, Finland

KLEINE-TEBBE, J., Dr.
Abteilung für Klinische Immunologie und Asthma OPD, Universitätsklinikum Rudolf-Virchow, Augustenburger Platz 1, W-1000 Berlin 65, FRG

KUNZ, Barbara, Dr.
Hôpital Necker Enfants malades, Service de Dermatologie, 149 rue de Sevres, 75743 Paris Cedex 15, France

KUREK, M., Dr.
Bahnstrasse 31/12, 7000 Eisenstadt, Austria

LAU-SCHADENDORF, Susanne, Dr.
Kinderklinik- und Poliklinik (KAVH), Universitätsklinikum Rudolf Virchow, Standort Charlottenburg, Heubnerweg 6, W-1000 Berlin 19, FRG

LEHR, H.-A., Dr.
Abteilung für Experimentelle Chirurgie, Universität Heidelberg, Im Neuenheimer Feld 347, W-6900 Heidelberg, FRG

LEVI-SCHAFFER, Francesca, Dr.
Department of Pharmacology, School of Pharmacy, Hadassah Medical School, The Hebrew University, P.O. Box 1172, 91010 Jerusalem, Israel

LUGER, T.A., Professor Dr.
Klinik und Poliklinik für Hautkrankheiten, Universität Münster, Von-Esmarch-Strasse 56, W-4400 Münster, FRG

MERK, H.F., Professor Dr.
Hautklinik, Universität zu Köln, Joseph-Stelzmann-Strasse 9, W-5000 Köln 41, FRG

MEURER, M., Professor Dr.
Dermatologische Klinik und Poliklinik der Ludwig-Maximilians-Universität, Frauenlobstrasse 9–11, W-8000 München 2, FRG

MIYAMOTO, T., M.D.
Department of Medicine and Physical Therapy, University of Tokyo, 18-1 Sakurodai, Sagamihara-shi, Kanagawa-kan 228, Japan

ORANJE, A. P., M.D., Ph.D.
Department of Dermatology and Venereology,
Division of Paediatric Dermatology,
Sophia Children's Hospital, Gordelweg 160, 3038 GE Rotterdam,
The Netherlands

POULSEN, L. K., Ph.D.
Laboratory of Medical Allergology, National University Hospital,
Department TTA 7542, 20 Tagensvej, 2200 Copenhagen N,
Denmark

PRINZ, J. C., Dr.
Dermatologische Klinik und Poliklinik der Ludwig-Maximilians-Universität, Frauenlobstrasse 9–11, W-8000 München 2, FRG

PRZYBILLA, B., Priv.-Doz. Dr.
Dermatologische Klinik und Poliklinik der Ludwig-Maximilians-Universität, Frauenlobstrasse 9–11, W-8000 München 2, FRG

RAKOSKI, J., Professor Dr.
Dermatologische Klinik und Poliklinik der Technischen Universität München, Biedersteiner Strasse 29, W-8000 München 40, FRG

RAULF, Monika, Dr.
Berufsgenossenschaftliches Forschungsinstitut für Arbeitsmedizin,
Institut an der Ruhr-Universität Bochum, Gilsingstrasse 14,
W-4630 Bochum 1, FRG

REYES-LÓPEZ, P. A., M.D.
Instituto Nacional de Cardiologia "Ignacio Chávez", Juan
Badiano 1, Secc. XVI Tlalpan, 14080 México, D.F., Mexico

RIEBER, E. P., Professor Dr.
Institut für Immunologie, Universität München, Goethestrasse 31,
W-8000 München 2, FRG

RING, J., Professor Dr. Dr.
Hautklinik und Allergie-Abteilung, Universitäts-Krankenhaus
Eppendorf, Martinistrasse 52, W-2000 Hamburg 20

ROSENDAHL LASSEN, A., Ph.D.
ALK Laboratories, Bøge Allé 10–12, 2970 Hørsholm, Denmark

ROTHE, A., Dr.
Zentralinstitut für Arbeitsmedizin, Abteilung Spezielle Noxen,
Nöldnerstrasse 40–42, O-1134 Berlin, FRG

RUZICKA, T., Priv.-Doz. Dr.
Dermatologische Klinik und Poliklinik der Ludwig-Maximilians-Universität, Frauenlobstrasse 9–11, W-8000 München 2, FRG

SCHAUDER, Sylvia, Priv.-Doz. Dr.
Hautklinik, Georg-August-Universität Göttingen, von-Siebold-Strasse 3, W-3400 Göttingen, FRG

SCHULTZE-WERNINGHAUS, G., Professor Dr.
Zentrum der Inneren Medizin, Abteilung für Pneumologie, Klinikum der Johann-Wolfgang-Goethe-Universität, Theodor-Stern-Kai 7, W-6000 Frankfurt/Main 70, FRG

STICHERLING, M., Dr.
Abteilung Dermatologie und Venerologie, Hautklinik, Universität zu Kiel, Schittenhelmstrasse 7, W-2300 Kiel, FRG

TAGAMI, H., M.D.
Department of Dermatology, Tohoku University School of Medicine, 1–1 Seiryomachi, Aoba-ku, Sendai 980, Japan

TAIEB, A., Professor
Service de Dermatologie et Laboratoire de Biochimie, Hôpital des Enfants, CHU de Bordeaux, 33077 Bordeaux Cédex, France

TAN, E.M., M.D., Ph.D.
W.M. Keck Autoimmune Disease Center, Scripps Clinic and Research Foundation, 10666 North Torrey Pines Road, La Jolla, CA 92037, USA

TAUER, Iva, Dr.
Abteilung für Pneumologie, Medizinische Klinik I, Klinikum Grosshadern, Ludwig-Maximilians-Universität, Marchioninistrasse 15, W-8000 München 70, FRG

THOMAS, P., Dr.
Dermatologische Klinik und Poliklinik der Ludwig-Maximilians-Universität, Frauenlobstrasse 9–11, W-8000 München 2, FRG

VARGA, J.M., Dr.
Universitätsklinik für Dermatologie und Venerologie, Anichstrasse 35, 6020 Innsbruck, Austria

VERVLOET, D., Professor
Service de Pneumologie – Allergologie, Département des Maladies Respiratoires, Hôpital Sainte-Marguerite, 13009 Marseille, France

VIELUF, D., Dr.
Hautklinik und Allergie-Abteilung, Universitäts-Krankenhaus Eppendorf, Martinistrasse 52, W-2000 Hamburg 20, FRG

VOCKS, E., Dr.
Dermatologische Klinik und Poliklinik der Technischen Universität, Biedersteiner Strasse 29, W-8000 München 40, FRG

WAHN, U., Professor Dr.
Kinderklinik, Freie Universität Berlin, Heubnerweg 6, W-1000 Berlin 19, FRG

DE WECK, A. L., Professor Dr.
Institut für Klinische Immunologie, Inselspital Bern, 3010 Bern, Switzerland

WILHELM, K.-P., Dr.
Klinik für Dermatologie, Medizinische Universität zu Lübeck, Ratzeburger Allee 160, W-2400 Lübeck, FRG

List of Chairmen

BLASER, K., Professor Dr. med.
Institut für Allergie- und Asthmaforschung SIAF, Obere Strasse 22, 7270 Davos, Switzerland

BORELLI, S., Professor Dr. med. Dr. phil.
Dermatologische Klinik und Poliklinik der Technischen Universität München, Biedersteiner Strasse 29, W-8000 München 40, FRG

BRAUN-FALCO, O., Professor Dr. med. Dr. h.c. mult.
Dermatologische Klinik und Poliklinik der Ludwig-Maximilians-Universität München, Frauenlobstrasse 9–11, W-8000 München 2, FRG

BREIT, R., Professor Dr. med.
Städtisches Krankenhaus München-Schwabing,
Dermatologische und Allergologische Abteilung, Kölner Platz 1, W-8000 München 40, FRG

BURG, G., Professor Dr. med.
Klinik und Poliklinik für Hautkrankheiten, Universität Zürich, Zürich, Switzerland

CHRISTOPHERS, E., Professor Dr. med.
Dermatologische Klinik der Christian-Albrechts-Universität, Schittenhelmstrasse 7, W-2300 Kiel, FRG

CZARNETZKI, B.U., Professor Dr. med.
Hautklinik der freien Universität Berlin, Klinikum Rudolf Virchow, Augustenburger Platz 1, W-1000 Berlin 65, FRG

DUKOR, P., Professor Dr. med.
Sandoz-Forschungsinstitut, Brunner Strasse 59, 1235 Wien, Austria

FRUHMANN, G., Professor Dr. med.
Institut und Poliklinik für Arbeitsmedizin, Ziemssenstrasse 1, W-8000 München 2, FRG

FUCHS, E., Professor Dr. med.
Pfitznerstrasse 5, W-6200 Wiesbaden, FRG

GIANNETTI, A., Professor Dr. med.
Department of Dermatology, Universita di Modena,
Via del Pozzo, 41100 Modena, Italy

HORNSTEIN, O.P., Professor Dr. med.
Dermatologische Universitätsklinik, Hartmannstrasse 1,
W-8520 Erlangen, FRG

IKAI, K., Professor Dr. med.
Department of Dermatology, Kyoto University, Faculty of
Medicine, 54 Kawara-cho, Shogoi, Sakyo-ku, Kyoto 606, Japan

IPPEN, H., Professor Dr. med. Dipl.-Chem.
Hautklinik der Georg-August-Universität, Von-Siebold-Strasse 3,
W-3400 Göttingen, FRG

KLASCHKA, F., Professor Dr. med.
Hautklinik im Klinikum Steglitz der Freien Universität Berlin,
Hindenburgdamm 30, W-1000 Berlin 45, FRG

KOWNATZKI, E., Professor Dr. med.
Universitäts-Hautklinik der Albert-Ludwigs-Universität,
Hauptstrasse 7, W-7800 Freiburg, FRG

LÖWENSTEIN, H., Professor Dr. med.
ALK Laboratories, Boge Allee 10–12, 2970 Horsholm, Denmark

MARGHESCU, S., Professor Dr. med.
Hautklinik Linden der Medizinischen Hochschule,
Ricklinger Strasse 5, W-3000 Hannover 91, FRG

MESSMER, K., Professor Dr. med.
Klinikum Heidelberg, Abteilung für Experimentelle Chirurgie,
Im Neuenheimer Feld 347, W-6900 Heidelberg, FRG

NASEMANN, Th., Professor Dr. med.
Buchenstrasse 3, W-8139 Bernried/Obb., FRG

PLEWIG, G., Professor Dr. med.
Hautklinik der Heinrich-Heine-Universität, Moorenstrasse 5,
W-4000 Düsseldorf, FRG

RAJKA, G., Professor Dr. med.
Rikshospital et Universitetsklinik, Hudavdelingen, Pilestredet 32,
Oslo 1, Norway

RIETHMÜLLER, G., Professor Dr. med.
Institut für Immunologie der Ludwig-Maximilians-Universität München, Goethestrasse 31, W-8000 München 2, FRG

RÖLLINGHOFF, M., Professor Dr. med.
Institut für klinische Mikrobiologie und Infektionshygiene, Wasserturmstrasse 3, W-8520 Erlangen, FRG

SCHILL, W.-B., Professor Dr. med.
Hautklinik der Justus-Liebig-Universität Giessen, Gaffkystrasse 14, W-6300 Giessen, FRG

SCHMUTZLER, W., Professor Dr. med.
Abteilung Pharmakologie RWTH, Schneebergweg, W-5100 Aachen, FRG

SCHÖPF, E., Professor Dr. med.
Universitäts-Hautklinik der Albert-Ludwigs-Universität, Hauptstrasse 7, W-7800 Freiburg, FRG

SCHULZ, K.-H., Professor Dr. med.
Björnsonweg 16a, W-2000 Hamburg 55, FRG

STEIGLEDER, G.K., Professor Dr. med.
Universitäts-Hautklinik, Joseph-Stelzmann-Strasse 9, W-5000 Köln 41, FRG

STINGL, G., Professor Dr. med.
1. Universitäts-Hautklinik, Alser Strasse 4, 1090 Wien, Austria

WAGNER, H., Professor Dr. med.
Institut für Mikrobiologie der Technischen Universität München, Ismaninger Strasse 2, W-8000 München 80, FRG

WOLFF, H.H., Professor Dr. med.
Klinik für Dermatologie und Venerologie, Universität Lübeck, Ratzeburger Allee 160, W-2400 Lübeck 1, FRG

WOLFF, K., Professor Dr. med.
1. Universitäts-Hautklinik, Alser Strasse 4, 1090 Wien, Austria

Epidemiology

Are Allergies Increasing?

B. Kunz[1] and J. Ring[2]

[1] Dermatologische Klinik und Poliklinik der Ludwig-Maximilians-Universität, Frauenlobstrasse 9–11, W-8000 München 2, Federal Republic of Germany
[2] Universitätshautklinik und Allergie-Abteilung, Universitätskrankenhaus Eppendorf, Martinistrasse 52, W-2000 Hamburg 20, Federal Republic of Germany

Abstract

A presumed rise in the prevalence of atopic diseases in industrialized countries is currently subject to extensive discussion. Due to a lack of epidemiological long-term studies, the controversy between experts was for some time basically confined to speculation.

Only recently, data from various European countries have confirmed an increase of atopic diseases. Studies from Sweden, Switzerland and Denmark showed a clear-cut multiplication of hay fever, bronchical asthma and atopic eczema, respectively. Japanese investigators have aimed at the putative role of air pollutants in this development. They were able to show a relationship between the exposure to particulate air pollutants (diesel exhaust) and the prevelance of mountain cedar pollinosis. The lack of baseline data has hampered up to now the evaluation of epidemiologic trends in Germany. We performed a pilot survey study involving more than 1000 pre-school children that yielded preliminary insights into an unexpectedly high prevalence of allergic conditions in Bavaria. The comparison to actual epidemiologic data from other European countries suggests an increase of allergies in Germany similar to that observed elsewhere. Longitudinal epidemiologic studies and a closer monitoring of environmental hazards are required to allow an objective evaluation of trends in the prevalence of allergic diseases and their putative triggering factors.

Introduction

There is no doubt that allergy is indeed an increasingly frequent diagnosis in clinical medicine. This is not only a subjective impression of many physicians in different specialities but also clearly results from practice and hospital statistics [13, 37, 63]. It is doubtful, however, that these figures really reflect an actual increase in prevalence of allergic diseases.

Increase or Pseudo-Increase?

A critical evaluation has to take into account the following factors [48]:

- Frequent news media reports about an "unexplained rise" of allergic diseases have alerted the public awareness concerning these problems [34]. The topic has been so extensively discussed that it has almost become fashionable to be "allergic".
- A higher information level among patients in combination with an easily accessible public health care system in western countries might prompt people to consult doctors even for minor health problems (such as sneezing or red eyes).
- New insights into the pathophysiology of immediate type allergies have improved diagnostic capacities and enlarged specialized knowledge. In consequence, nowadays, allergy is more commonly diagnosed because it is both more frequently suspected and more reliably recognized.
- In public discussion, there is some confusion about the definition of allergic diseases. The term "allergy" is readily used for a variety of symptoms that may originate from different pathophysiological mechanisms. True allergies should be distinguished form pseudo-allergic reactions – that is, intolerance due to nonimmunological phenomena – by proof of immunological sensitization.

An objective evaluation of a putative increase of allergic diseases can only be performed on the basis of repeated investigations of a representative population sample, focusing on well-defined disease entities and providing evidence for immunological reactions explaining the reported symptoms.

Evidence for an Increasing Prevalence of Allergic Diseases

Several factors are hampering a clear analysis of the question [32]:

1. There is a lack of good epidemiologic investigations in the general population. Most of the studies performed up to now have concerned preselected population subgroups.
2. Comparisons of study results are difficult because of:
   - Heterogeneity of the groups investigated regarding age, sex, living conditions, occupational exposition, and others.
   - Differences of methodology which quite frequently lacks proof for the allergic nature of the reported symptoms.
   - Prevalence differences of poorly understood origin (genetic background?) between countries.
   - "Natural" background variability of prevalence rates that may differ from one point in time to another.

Nevertheless, there are some quite conclusive studies on the increase of atopic and other allergic diseases in industrialized as well as in developing countries.

Respiratory Allergies

The most extensive studies were done in Switzerland. In 1958, a population survey yielded an overall prevalence of hay fever in Zürich of only 4.8% [5]. In 1986, 28 years later, a much higher prevalence rate (10.02%) was found [66]. A similar trend has been observed by Japanese investigators, who report a rise in hay fever prevalence from 2%–3% in the 1950s to 10%–15% in 1987 [18].

Methodologically more convincing are repeated studies by the same investigator such as that performed by Varonier in 1968 and 1981 in schoolchildren in Geneva [60]. He found a significant increase in hay fever and asthma in different age groups. The same trend was observed in a longitudinal study carried out in Swedish conscripts by Aberg [1] (see Tables 1, 2). Moreover a study from the United Kingdom showed a significant increase in childhood asthma between 1956/1957 (1.8%) and 1968/1969 (2.3%) [36]. In most of these epidemiologic investigations, the diagnosis has been established by a physician; however, it has to be mentioned that the allergic nature of the respiratory diseases has not been confirmed, since no skin prick or in vitro allergy tests have been performed.

Atopic Eczema

Even if atopic eczema by some authors is not considered an allergic disease in the proper sense of the term, it is by many characteristics closely related to classical IgE-mediated disorders [46, 51, 52] such as allergic asthma and hay fever and

Table 1. Prevalence of hay fever in children and young adults.

Region	Age (years)	Prevalence (%)		Author
		1st study	2nd study	
Geneva (Switzerland)	4–6	0.5 (1968)	1.1 (1981)	Varonier et al. [60]
	15	4.4 (1968)	6.1 (1981)	Varonier et al. [60]
Sweden	17–20	4.4 (1971)	8.4 (1981)	Aberg [1]

Table 2. Prevalence of bronchial asthma in children and young adults.

Region	Age (years)	Prevalence (%)		Author
		1st study	2nd study	
Great Britain	5–15	1.8 (1956/1957)	2.3 (1968/1969)	Morrison-Smith et al. [36]
Geneva (Switzerland)	4–6	1.7* (1968)	2.0* (1981)	Varonier et al. [60]
	15	1.9 (1968)	2.8 (1981)	Varonier et al. [60]
Sweden	17–20	1.9 (1971)	2.8 (1981)	Aberg [1]

* Not significant.

Table 3. Prevalence of atopic eczema in children and young adults.

Region	Age (years)	Prevalence (%)		Author
		1st study	2nd study	
Denmark	0–7	3.2 (1960–1964)	10.2 (1970–1974)	Schultz Larsen et al. [55]
Geneva (Switzerland)	4–6	2.2* (1968)	2.8* (1981)	Varonier et al. [60]
	15	2.3* (1968)	1.5* (1981)	Varonier et al. [60]
Japan	0–15	2.8 (1981)	4.0 (1988)	Ueda et al. [59]

* Not significant.

therefore will be discussed here. There are considerable differences in the prevalence of atopic eczema among European countries.

While Varonier in Switzerland found only a slight rise in atopic eczema prevalence in young children [60], an epidemiologic study performed by Schultz Larsen showed that the cumulative incidence rate of atopic eczema in a twin population of Fyn, Denmark, has tripled within 10 years [55] (Table 3). A significant increase of atopic eczema in children is also reported from Japan. Between 1981 and 1988, the prevalence rose from 2.81% to 4.00% [59].

Allergic Contact Eczema and Sensitization

Very few data are available on the frequency of allergic contact eczema and contact sensitization among the general population. In 1975, the contact sensitization to nickel in a Finnish population sample over the age of 10 years was found to be 4.5%; in this study, only 1 of 90 schoolgirls was sensitized [42]. Twelve years later, a study by the same investigators reports 16% of nickel-sensitized schoolgirls in the same area, indicating a significant increase of the condition within the last decade [43].

Taking together the results of these repeated epidemiological studies, a real increase of certain allergic conditions can be stated for several European countries. No such longitudinal studies are available for West Germany.

Results of Own Investigations in the Federal Republic of Germany

Apart from clinical statistics, epidemiologic data on allergic diseases are sparse. A recent interview-based investigation in 8771 grammar school pupils (with skin testing and nasal provocation in a part of the sample) found a prevalence of allergic rhinitis of 16.7% [53].

In 1988/1989, we performed an epidemiologic pilot study concerning a variety of allergic diseases in 1083 Bavarian children (for details see [26]).

Briefly, questionnaires were mailed to the parents prior to a routine pre-school physical examination. On the examination day, in particular the questions concerning a history of atopic diseases and those concerning allergic reactions were carefully reviewed with the parents. The study protocol included dermatological evaluation, a modified skin prick test (Stallerkit, Merieux, Fresnes, France) with six aero- and food allergens, and a ready-for-use patch test (True test, Pharmacia Uppsala, Sweden) comprising 23 standard allergens. The possible interference of air pollutants with the prevalence of atopic diseases was studied using surface active monitors to measure the SO_2/NO_x concentrations in the childrens' bedrooms.

Immediate Type Sensitization and Atopy

Some 36% of the children reacted to at least one allergen in the skin prick test. Reactions to airborne allergens (seasonal as well as perennial) were more frequently observed than those to food allergens [22, 26] (Table 4). These findings fit quite well to what we know to be relevant sensitizing agents in that age group.

Some 22.8% of the parents reported that their child had a present or past history of one of the classical atopic diseases; this was most frequently allergic rhinoconjunctivitis (11.8%). Atopic eczema (separately evaluated from cradle cap) was reported in 8.6% and bronchial asthma in 4.6% (for more details see [26]).

Type IV Reactions and Contact Dermatitis

The patch test standard showed at least one positive reaction for 15.8% of the children tested. The allergen list was headed by merthiolate (8.8%), nickel sulfate (7.1%), potassium dichromate (4.1%), and cobalt chloride (2%).

According to the questionnaire, 6.2% of the children had experienced symptoms of contact eczema.

Other Possible Allergic Reactions

Table 5 summarizes other reactions perceived by the parents as being allergic in origin. Food and drugs are the most frequently incriminated triggers, urticaria being the most common disease.

Dermatological Evaluation

The actual prevalence of eczema at the day of examination was 10.3%. An etiological differentiation of the skin lesions was not undertaken. With respect to the correlation between the wearing of fashion jewelry and nickel sensitization, ear piercing was noted: 34.1% of the children had pierced ear lobes (girls 71.3%, boys 1.9%). There was a significantly higher rate of nickel contact allergy among persons *with* pierced ears compared to those *without*.

In conclusion, this epidemiologic pilot study showed an unexpectedly high prevalence of allergic sensitization and allergic diseases already in childhood, even

Table 4. Prevalence of allergic sensitization in Bavarian children ($n = 902$).

	Prevalence (%)
Pollen allergens (birch, grass)	21.7
Indoor allergens (cat, Dermatophagoides pteronyssinus)	19.2
Food allergens (egg, cow's milk)	9.1

Table 5. History for "allergic" reactions in Bavarian children ($n = 960$).

	Prevalence (%)
Urticaria	3.4
Angioedema	1.7
Migraine	2.9
Drug reactions	7.0
Food reactions	7.0
Insect sting reactions	3.1

if, as expected, reported symptoms and skin test results do not yield complete concordance [26]. Despite missing baseline figures that would allow a statistical evaluation of epidemiological trends in West Germany, a comparison of our data to those of other industrialized countries [1, 2, 10, 12, 15, 17, 18, 20, 43, 55, 59, 60, 66] suggests a parallel increase of allergic diseases, also in Germany.

Possible Explanations for an Increase in Atopic Diseases

A number of factors influencing the development of atopic diseases have been described [31, 50, 52]. Changes in those predisposing variables might account for the observed increase.

Genetics

A genetic predisposition to atopy is well established. The capacity to enhanced IgE production has been described as an autosomal recessive characteristic; the production of specific IgE to environmental allergens seems in part to be linked to the human leucocyte antigen (HLA) system [30, 31]. This hereditary factor might play a role in differences of the prevalence of atopic diseases between different regions or countries, but is very unlikely to interfere in the actual epidemiologic trend, considering that genetic changes in a population need a much longer time period to develop. Twin studies have pointed out that monozygotic twins are in more than 50% not concordant with respect to the development of respiratory allergy, thus demonstrating the importance of "environmental realization factors" for allergy [14].

Allergen Exposure

There is in fact a huge body of evidence that the risk for both sensitization to allergens and manifestation of an atopic disorder in predisposed individuals is largely influenced by allergen exposure. Dependence on dose, nature of the allergen, intensity and modalities of contact and time of first exposure in life has been reported [7, 8, 18, 35, 44, 54, 64, 67]. Changes in lifestyle may result in altered allergen exposure. In prospering industrialized countries, nutritional habits have been influenced by the importation of formerly unknown tropical fruits and crustacea, some of them (e.g., kiwi) being common sensitizers.

In the northern part of Europe, energy-saving measures prompted by the oil crisis had considerable consequences on the indoor climate and subsequently on mould and house dust mite colonization [28]. A similar rise in house dust mite populations has been observed in the highlands of Papua New Guinea after the introduction of sleeping blankets and changes of housing conditions [58]. In both cases, the rise of indoor allergens was accompanied by increased prevalence of allergic asthma.

Another source of potently sensitizing indoor allergens are furred pets, nowadays present in more than 50% of German and Swedish households [27].

Air Pollutants as Adjuvants

The rising prevalence of allergic (especially atopic) diseases in industrialized countries has been paralleled by an increase in atmospheric pollution. Many substances released into indoor or outdoor air by combustion processes such as cigarette smoke, sulfur dioxide, oxides of nitrogen, or vehicle exhaust fumes exert a well-known irritating effect on the respiratory epithelium [38, 49, 61]. Besides a local impairment of defense mechanisms and subsequently enhanced susceptibility to respiratory tract infections (secondary mucosal damage) [11, 56, 61] this may lead to direct mucosal damage and thus facilitate allergen penetration [65, 67]. A number of recent investigations have therefore focused on the putative role of air pollutants as adjuvant factors in the allergic process, yielding the following results:

- Various pollutants can promote IgE production to natural allergens SO_2 alone or in combination with O_3 or NO_x [41, 47], diesel exhaust particles [33, 39, 57], tobacco smoke by active or passive smoking [4, 9, 16, 62, 68], and mercuric chloride [45].
  The pathogenetic mechanisms underlying this process are unknown. Particles present in polluted air can bind to pollen surface and promote as allergen carriers their absorption by alveolar macrophages [39]. Moreover, direct interactions between pollen and air pollutants can result in alterations of allergenicity [6].
- The degree of atmospheric pollution by motor vehicle exhaust in combination with pollen exposition has been found to be positively correlated to the prevalence of allergic rhinitis [18, 21]. A similar relation was reported between

industrial pollution (SO_2/NO_x, suspended particles) and allergic respiratory diseases [3] or sensitization to house dust extract [19] and pollen allergens [40], respectively.

In our study, a multivariate analysis (CART procedure) did not show any significant correlation between the indoor air levels of SO_2/NO_x and the prevalence of atopic diseases [24], possibly due to rather low pollutant concentrations during the investigation period (for details see [25]). The CART analysis of the 1988 data, on the other hand, established another highly significant correlation: children whose mother had been smoking during pregnancy had a 2.6-fold higher risk for atopic diseases than had children of nonsmoking mothers [23]. Similar findings have been reported by Magnusson [29].

Conclusion

Long-term epidemiological studies in several countries have demonstrated a significant rise of allergic, especially atopic diseases during the last 20 years. Although longitudinal studies are not available for our country, actual prevalence data suggest a similar trend in West Germany. The reasons for this development are still unknown, but two main hypotheses are to be retained: an increase in allergen exposure by changes in lifestyle and an adjuvant effect of environmental pollutants in the manifestation of atopic diseases. The exact nature of the latter is still very poorly understood. Appropriate basic research as well as careful environmental monitoring are necessary to cast some more light onto the causalities of the actual development. On the other hand, it is just as important to do what can be done right now to prevent and diminish atopic manifestations: allergen avoidance in predisposed individuals (especially breast feeding of infants, house dust mite reduction, and abstention from pets) and general reduction of potentially harmful substances in our environment (cigarette smoke, motor vehicle exhausts, industrial pollution, etc.) Waiting until we have discovered the last clue to the complex interactions that determine the dynamics of allergic diseases would be a dangerous waste of time. If our aim is prevention, it seems essential to get down to the problem of environmental pollution right now.

References

1. Aberg N (1989) Asthma and allergic rhinitis in Swedish conscripts. Clin Exp Allergy 19:59–63
2. Aberg N, Engström I, Lindberg U (1989) Allergic diseases in Swedish school children. Acta Paediatr Scand 78:246–252
3. Andrae S, Axelson O, Björksten B, Fredrikson M, Kjellman N (1988) Symptoms of bronchial hyperreactivity and asthma in relation to environmental factors. Arch Dis Child 63:473–478
4. Bahna SL, Heiner DC, Myhre BA (1983) Immunoglobulin E pattern in cigarette smokers. Allergy 38:57–64
5. Batschelet E, Klunker W, Schnyder UW, Storck H (1958) Die Häufigkeit atopischer Erkrankungen in Zürich. Schweiz Med Wochenschr 40:1109–1113

6. Behrendt H, Friedrichs KH, Kainka-Stänicke F, Darsow U, Becker W, Tomingas R (1990) Allergens and pollutants in the air – a complex interaction. Allergologie 13:257
7. Björksten F (1986) Early allergen contacts. J Allergy Clin Immunol 78:1010–1012
8. Björksten F, Suoniemi I, Koski V (1980) Neonatal birch pollen contact and subsequent allergy to birch pollen. Clin Allergy 10:585–591
9. Burrows B, Halonen M, Lebowitz MD, Knudson RJ, Barbee RA (1982) The relationship of serum immunoglobulin E, allergy skin tests, and smoking to respiratory disorders. J Allergy Clin Immunol 70:199–204
10. Charpin D, Kleisbauer JP, Lanteaume A, Vervloet D, Lagier F, Charpin J (1988) Existe-t-il un facteur urbain dans l'asthme et l'allergie? Rev Mal Respir 5:109–114
11. Dodge R, Solomon P, Moyers J, Hayer C (1985) A longitudinal study of children exposed to sulfur oxides. Am J Epidemiol 121:720–736
12. Dupal HD, Horak F, Türk R (1982) Häufigkeit der Inhalationsallergie bei Schulkindern im ländlichen Raum im Vergleich zum Großstadtgebiet. Laryngol Rhinol Otol 61:648–650
13. Eaton KK (1982) The incidence of allergy – has it changed? Clin Allergy 12:107–110
14. Erdford-Lubs ML (1971) Allergy in 7000 twin pairs. Acta Allergy 26:249–285
15. Gassner-Bachmann M (1989) Allergie und Umwelt. Erkrankungen und Sensibilisierungen bei Schulkindern einer Landbevölkerung und ihre regionalen Umweltbedingungen. Allergologie 12:492–502
16. Gerrard JW, Heiner DC, Ko CG, Mink J, Meyers A, Dosman JA (1980) Immunoglobulin levels in smokers and non-smokers. Ann Allergy 44:261–262
17. Holmgren D, Aberg N, Lindberg U, Engström I (1989) Childhood asthma in a rural county. Allergy 44:256–259
18. Ishizaki I, Koizumi K, Ikemori R, Ishiyama Y, Kushibiki E (1987) Studies of prevalence of Japanese cedar pollinosis among the residents in a densely cultivated area. Ann Allergy 58:265–270
19. Kagamimori S, Katoh T, Naruse Y, Watanabe M, Kasuya M, Shinkai J, Kawana S (1986) The changing prevalence of respiratory symptoms in atopic children in response to air pollution. Clin Allergy 16:299–308
20. Kajosaari M (1982) Food allergy in finnish children aged 1 to 6 years. Acta Paediatr Scand 71:815–819
21. Kaneko S, Shimada K, Horiuchi H, Endo À, Kodama M, Shinoda N, Imai T, Takiguchi K (1980) Nasal allergy and air pollution. Oto-Rhino-Laryngology Tokyo 23 [Suppl 4]:270
22. Kunz B, Ring J (1990) Nehmen Allergien zu? Allergologie 13:297
23. Kunz B, Ring J, Dirschedl P (1989) Effect of maternal smoking during pregnancy on the development of atopic diseases in the child. J Invest Dermatol 92:465
24. Kunz B, Ring J, Gries A, Überla K (1989) Correlation between indoor air concentration of SO_2 and NO_x and prevalence of atopic diseases in children. Proceedings of the 5th International Conference of Indoor Air Quality and Climate, 29 July – 3 Aug 1990, Toronto
25. Kunz B, Dirschedl P, Ring J, Greif A, Gries A, Huber H, Letzel H, Schotten K, Stickl H, Überla K (to be published) Environmental monitoring: epidemiological tools for the evaluation of indoor air pollution, allergic diseases and tonsillar microbial colonization.
26. Kunz B, Ring J, Überla K (to be published) Epidemiology of allergic diseases in preschool children
27. Lowenstein H, Gravesen S, Larsen L, Lind P, Schwartz B (1986) Indoor allergens. J. Allergy Clin Immunol 78:1035–1038
28. Luoma R (1984) Environmental allergens and morbidity in atopic and non-atopic families. Acta Paediatr Scand 73:448–453
29. Magnusson CGM (1986) Maternal smoking influences cord serum IgE and IgD levels and increases the risk for subsequent infant allergy. J Allergy Clin Immunol 78:898–904
30. Marsh DG (1975) Allergens and the genetics of allergy. Academic, New York
31. Marsh DG, Meyers DA (1981) The epidemiology and genetics of atopic allergy. N Engl J Med 305:1551–1558
32. Massicot JG, Cohen SG (1986) Epidemiologic and socioeconomic aspects of allergic diseases. J Allergy Clin Immunol 78:954–958
33. Miyamoto T, Takafuji S (1990) Environmental pollution and allergy. Allergologie 13:257
34. Mizrahi A, Mizrahi A (1985) Poids et évolution des maladies allergiques dans la population. Allerg Immunol (Paris) 17:170–174

35. Morrison Smith J, Springett VH (1979) Atopic disease and month of birth. Clin Allergy 9:153–157
36. Morrison Smith J, Harding LK, Cumming G (1971) The changing prevalence of asthma in school children. Clin Allergy 1:57–61
37. Moshkevich VS (1985) Epidemiology of allergic diseases of the respiratory passages in the Kazakh SSR. J Hyg Epidemiol Microbiol Immunol 29:47–58
38. Mücke W (1988) Zur umwelthygienischen Beurteilung von Dieselabgasen. Off Gesundheitswes 50:147–150
39. Muranaka M, Suzuki S, Koizumi K, Takafuji S, Miyamoto T, Ikemori R, Tokiwa H (1986) Adjuvant activity of diesel exhaust particulates for the production of IgE antibody in mice. J Allergy Clin Immunol 77:616–623
40. Oberbarnscheidt J, Stiller-Winckler R, Krämer U, Dolgner R, Behrend H (1990) Untersuchungen zum Einfluß von Luftschadstoffen auf die Sensibilisierung und den Immunstatus 6jähriger Kinder. Allergologie 13:316–317
41. Osebold JW, Gershwin LJ, Zee YC (1980) Studies on the enhancement of allergic lung sensitization by inhalation of ozone and sulfuric acid aerosol. J Environ Pathol Toxicol Oncol 3:221–234
42. Peltonen L (1979) Nickel sensitivity in the general population. Contact Dermatitis 5:27–32
43. Peltonen L (1989) Nickel sensitivity in schoolchildren in Finland. In: Frosch PJ, Dooms-Goosens A, Lachapelle JM, Rycroft RJG, Scheper RJ (eds) Current topics in contact dermatitis. Springer, Berlin Heidelberg New York, pp 184–187
44. Platt-Mills TAE, Heyman PW, Chapman MD, Smith TF, Wilkin SR (1985) Mites of the genus Dermatophagoides in dust from the houses of asthmatic and other allergic patients in North America: development of a radioimmunoassay for allergen produced by D. farinae and D. pteronyssinus. Int Arch Allergy Appl Immunol 77:163–165
45. Provost-Danon A, Abadie A, Sapin C, Bazin H, Druet P (1981) Induction of IgE synthesis and potentiation of anti-ovalbumin-IgE antibody response by $HgCl_2$ in the rat. J Immunol 126:699–702
46. Przybilla B, Ring J (1990) Food allergy and atopic eczema. Semin Dermatol 9:220–225
47. Riedel F, Krämer M, Scheibenbogen C, Rieger CHL (1988) Effects of SO_2 exposure on allergic sensitization in the guinea pig. J Allergy Clin Immunol 82:527–534
48. Ring J (1986) Nehmen Allergien wirklich zu? Fortschr Med 17:343–344
49. Ring J (1987) Luftverschmutzung und allergische Erkrankungen. Münch Med Wochenschr 129:182–185
50. Ring J, Burg G (eds) (1986) New trends in allergy II. Springer, Berlin Heidelberg New York
51. Ring J, Dorsch W (1985) Altered releasability of vasoactive mediator secreting cells in atopic eczema. Acta Derm Venereol Suppl [Stockh] 114:9–23
52. Ruzicka T, Ring J, Pryzbilla B (eds) (1991) Handbook of atopic eczema. Springer, Berlin Heidelberg New York (to be published)
53. Schata M, Jorde W, Hartenstein W (1988) Ergebnisse epidemiologischer Untersuchungen bei allergischen Erkrankungen. Schweiz Rundsch Med Prax 77:884–888
54. Schultze-Werninghaus G, Merget R (1990) Platinum salt asthma. Allergologie 13:257–258
55. Schultz Larsen F, Holm NV, Henningsen K (1986) Atopic dermatitis. A genetic-epidemiologic study in a population-based twin sample. J Am Acad Dermatol 15:487–494
56. Spinaci S, Arossa W, Bugiani M, Natale P, Bucca C, de Candussio G (1985) The effects of air pollution on respiratory health of children: a cross sectional study. Pediatr Pulmonol 1:262–266
57. Takafuji S, Suzuki S, Koizumi K (1987) Diesel exhaust particulates inoculated by the intranasal route have an adjuvant activity for IgE production in mice. J Allergy Clin Immunol 79:639–645
58. Turner KJ, Dowse GK, Steward GA, Alpers MP, Woolcock AJ (1985) Prevalence of asthma in the South Fore People of the Okapa District of Papua New Guinea. Int Arch Allergy Appl Immunol 77:158–162
59. Ueda H, Fujisawa Y, Inasaka H (1989) Epidemiology of atopic dermatitis in Japan. Abstract 5th International Congress of Pediatric Dermatology, 11–15 July 1989, Milan
60. Varonier HS, De Haller J, Schopfer C (1984) Prevalence de l'allergie chez les enfants et les adolescents. Helv Paediatr Acta 39:129–136
61. Ware JH, Ferris BG Jr, Dockery DW, Spengler JD, Stram DO, Speizer FE (1986) Effects of ambient sulfur oxide and suspended particles on respiratory health of preadolescent children. Am Rev Respir Dis 133:834–842

62. Warren CPW, Holford-Strevens V, Wong C, Manfreda J (1982) The relationship between smoking and total immunoglobin E levels. J Allergy Clin Immunol 69:370–375
63. Weeke ER (1987) Epidemiology of hay fever and perennial allergic rhinitis. Monogr Allergy 21:1–20
64. Wittig HJ, McLaughlin ET, Leifer KL, Belliot JD (1978) Risk factors for the development of allergic disease: analysis of 2190 patient records. Ann Allergy 41:84–88
65. Wüthrich B (1989) Epidemiology of the allergic diseases: are they really on the increase? Int Arch Allergy Appl Immunol 90:3–10
66. Wüthrich B, Schnyder UW, Henauer SA, Heller A (1986) Häufigkeit der Pollinosis in der Schweiz. Ergebnisse einer repräsentativen demoskopischen Umfrage unter Berücksichtigung anderer allergischer Erkrankungen. Schweiz Med Wochenschr 116:909–917
67. Zetterström O (1985) The importance of air pollution for the development of respiratory allergy and bronchical hyperreactivity. Annual Meeting of the European Academy of Allergology and Clinical Immunology, 2–5 June 1985
68. Zetterström O, Osterman K, Machedo L, Johannson SGO (1981) Another smoking hazard: raised IgE concentration and increased risk of occupational allergy. Br Med J 283:1215–1217

Epidemiology of Various Allergic Reactions

D. Vervloet and D. Charpin

Service de Pneumo-Allergologie, Département des Maladies Respiratoires, Hôpital Sainte-Marguerite, 13009 Marseille, France

Abstract

In a study group including 2067 adults 20–60 years old who volunteered to get a check up examination in the Public Health Care in Marseille, France, we wanted to evaluate the prevalence of atopy, the prevalence of allergic reactions to hymenoptera venoms and the prevalence of systemic reactions to drugs.

Identification of atopy usually relies on answers to a standardized questionnaire including questions on hay fever, perennial rhinitis and bronchial asthma. However, these questions lack specificity if atopy is defined also by the presence of specific IgE antibodies against major common aero-allergens. The presence of IgE against major common aero-allergens (Phadiatop®), was found in 20% of the total group. The percentage of positive Phadiatop® tests was 42% in patients with history of hay fever, 27% in patients with history of perennial rhinitis, 52% in patients with history of asthma and 15% in people without any clinical history of atopic symptoms. Symptoms identified by a standardized questionnaire cannot by themselves reliably predict atopy and depend of some extraneous variables as sex and age.

In the same group, we evaluated the prevalence of allergic reactions to hymenoptera venoms by a standardized questionnaire and skin tests to venoms in subjects reporting a history of allergic reactions. According to the questionnaire, 1.2% of the study population has a history of systemic reactions and 0.85% has both such history and positive skin tests to venoms. Local reactions were found in 7% of the total group.

In the same study group 14.7% including 66% women reported reliable histories of systemic reactions (SR) to drugs. The cumulate prevalence of asthma, hay fever and childhood dermatitis was higher in the SR group. By contrast, the percentage of people with presence of IgE antibodies to common aero-allergens (Phadiatop®) was similar in subjects with or without a history of SR. Thus, atopy defined by an objective criteria i.e. the presence of specific IgE against aero-allergens is not associated with the occurrence of SR to drugs. Such a history should not be included as part of the atopic status.

Prediction of Atopy from the Response to a Respiratory Symptoms Standardized Questionnaire

Epidemiologic studies on atopic diseases usually rely on answers to standardized questionnaires about hay fever, perennial rhinitis and bronchial asthma. This method is simple but such questionnaires lack specificity. Atopy may also be identified by demonstrating serum specific IgE. This approach is more difficult to implement in a large series and the relationship between atopy, defined as the presence of specific IgEs against common aeroallergens, and symptoms is not straigthforward. A factor that must be kept in mind when interpreting data obtained by either approach is the influence of criteria such as sex and age. The goal of this study was to first evaluate the prevalence of atopy in a large population and then assess the predictive value of symptoms suggestive of atopy in relation to some extraneous variables.

This study includes 2067 adults, 20–60 years old, who volunteered for examination in the Bouches-du-Rhone Public Health Care Center in Marseille. In France, all subjects eligible for social security (i.e. 95% of the total population) are entitled to 5-year checkups. We studied subjects attending the center from January to July of 1987. They included 1164 men and 903 women whose mean age ($\pm$SD) was 39.3$\pm$9.2 years (40.1$\pm$9.4 years or men and 38.5$\pm$8.9 years for women; not statistically different).

The study protocol included an interview and blood test. A standardized questionnaire was administered by a medical doctor. In addition to demographic characteristics, questions on symptoms considered to be suggestive of an atopic diathesis (atopic symptoms), namely hay fever, perennial rhinitis and bronchial asthma were included. Subjects were also asked about their smoking habits. A 10 ml blood sample was taken. In addition to routine biochemical tests, we checked for specific IgEs against common airborne allergens using the Phadiatop test which has been shown [1–3] to be a much more reliable test than total serum IgE level in the identification of atopic symptoms. It includes testing for major aeroallergens such as house dust mites, animal dander, grass pollens and molds [1]. Unlike skin tests, this in vitro test does not involve the introduction of antigenic materials. It provides clearly positive or negative results. The Phadiatop test was performed on 2005 subjects.

Phadiatop Testing

Overall, 20% of the study population had positive Phadiatop tests. This result varied widely according to age and sex. The percentage of positive tests was significantly ($p<0.0001$) higher in males 22% than in females (17%). As shown in Fig. 1, this difference lessened with age. Although the percentage of positive Phadiatop tests was much higher in subjects complaining of atopic symptoms, no symptom was very closely linked to a positive test (Table 1). In women no relation was observed between positive Phadiatop tests and smoking habits; however, men who never smoked exhibited a statistically higher percentage ($p<0.005$) of positive Phadiatop tests (28.5%) than current smokers (21.7%). Education was

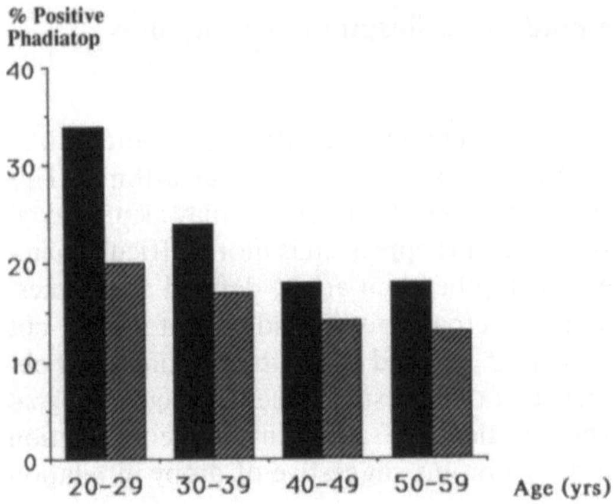

Fig.1. Percentage of positive Phadiatop tests according to age range and sex (*black columns*, male subjects; *hatched columns*, female subjects)

Table 1. Percentage of positive Phadiotop tests according to symptoms.

Symptoms	Percentage (%)
History of hay fever	41.8
History of perennial rhinitis	27.3
History of asthma	51.8
No history of atopic symptoms	14.8

not correlated with the results of the Phadiatop test. The percentage of positive tests was 19.3% in subjects who attended primary school only, 20.2% in those who attended secondary school and 21.9% in those who attended university.

Relative Value of Predictors of Atopy

As shown in Table 2, three variables displayed significant correlation with positive Phadiatop tests, namely atopic symptoms, male sex and young age (subjects between 40 and 59 years had fewer positive tests). No correlation was observed with either smoking habits or education.

Predictive Value of Atopic Symptoms (Table 3)

The predictive value of each symptom decreased with age, especially between the first and second age group (Table 3). This drop was more obvious in males than in females. The age-related decrease in predictive value was sharper in males. In all age groups, apart from the first, the predictive value of perennial rhinitis was very low. The percentage of positive Phadiatop tests ranged from 12% to 25%

Table 2. Linear logistic regression analysis relating presence of serum specific IgE (Phadiatop test) to several independent variables.

Independent variable	p value	OR	95% C.I.
Atopic symptoms	<0.0001	1.54	1.37 – 1.72
Sex (M/F)	<0.001	1.24	1.11 – 1.40
Age (years)[a]	<0.004		
2/1		1.11	0.92 – 1.29
3/1		0.81	0.67 – 0.98
4/1		0.75	0.60 – 0.95
Smoking habits		1.05	0.93 – 1.18
Education[b]			
2/1		0.80	0.70 – 0.94
3/1		1.09	0.93 – 1.27

[a] For age range, category 1 includes subjects 20 – 29 years old; category 2, 30 – 39; category 3, 40 – 49 and category 4, 50 – 59.
[b] For education, category 1 includes subjects who attended only primary school, category 2 secondary school and category 3 university.
OR, ODDS ratio; C.I., confidence interval.

Table 3. Predictive value of atopic symptoms.

Symptom	Age (years)							
	20 – 29		30 – 39		40 – 49		50 – 59	
	M (%)	F (%)	M (%)	F (%)	M (%)	F (%)	M (%)	F (%)
Hay fever	66	35	47	34	37	27	28	32
Perennial rhinitis	54	30	25	22	21	12	12	21
Asthma	75	45	54	16	45	31	57	40

in men and from 12% to 22% in women as compared to 22% and 17%, respectively, in the population as a whole.

This study shows that a standardized questionnaire cannot by itself reliably predict atopy. It is also necessary to demonstrate the presence of specific IgEs against common aeroallergens. Failure to use this combined approach can give misleading results.

Prevalence of Allergy to Hymenoptera Stings

In the literature, there are few studies devoted to assessing the prevalence of hymenoptera stings [4 – 9]. The figures derived from these studies range from as low as 0.15% or as high as 4.0%. None of these studies considered a nonselected group originating from a general population. Thus we decided to carry out such a study in an health care center performing checkups on the same population as above.

For all subjects, a standardized questionnaire was administered by an allergologist. Apart from demographic characteristics, this questionnaire asked about history of previous hymenoptera stings, history of local and general reactions (i.e. Quincke oedema, giant urticaria, wheezing, breathlessness, malaise and loss of consciousness) immediately following the sting, time of the last sting and whether or not the subjects visited a doctor for the reactions following the sting.

All subjects reporting a general reaction immediately following the sting were asked to be skin tested with venom allergens. These tests were performed on the volar surface of the forearm using intradermal injections of serial ten-fold dilutions of honeybee, yellow jacket, wasp and *Vespa crabro* venoms (Laboratories Dome, Paris, France). The starting dilution used was 10:5. Each intradermal injection included 0.05 ml of the diluted venom. At the same time a positive control test using 9% codeine phosphate and a negative control test using coca solution were performed. The tests were read 15–20 min later and were considered positive if the negative control test was negative and if the wheal induced by the venom injection was at least of the same diameter as the positive control from the positive control test.

All subjects reporting severe local reactions of a general type and a random sample of 82 subjects with a history of previous sting without any reaction had a blood sampling for RAST determinations to honeybee, yellow jacket and wasp (Laboratoire Pharmacia, Paris, France) using the method described in the kit and all the kit reagents. However, among the studied population, some subjects had no blood sample taken and some sera tubes were broken or held a too small amount of serum. Thus only 21 out of 24 sera in the systemic reaction group and 101 out of 153 in the local reaction group were evaluated.

Three-quarters of the interviewees acknowledged a history of previous sting. Among those previously stung, 10% had had a severe local reaction (i.e. 7.4% of the total study group).

Some 24 subjects, i.e. 1.16% of the study group, reported a history of at least one type of general reaction following the sting. These reactions were as follows: malaise 18 times, Quincke's oedema 11 times, breathlessness 10 times, giant urticaria 7 times, loss of consciousness 6 times (some subjects reported several types of reactions). Three times out of four stings responsible for these reactions had occurred in the last 3 years. A general reaction following the sting had occurred only once in 15 subjects, twice in 4 subjects and more than twice in 5 subjects.

Among the 24 subjects reporting systemic reactions following the sting, 15 agreed to skin test to venoms. These tests were positive in 11 subjects. All subjects had no reaction to the negative control test. Thus, 1.12×11, i.e. 0.85%, can be considered to have a history of true systemic reaction. In the four subjects who had negative skin tests the systemic reaction occurred 9.2 ± 4.3 years before the study time, whereas this interval was only 3.6 ± 3.7 years for subjects with positive skin tests. The type of systemic reaction reported by these 24 subjects was Quincke's oedema (in association with breathlessness and giant urticaria twice, and malaise without loss of consciousness twice.

Table 4. Prevalence of insect sting allergy in adults (surveys performed in southeast France).

Year of survey publication	Population	Diagnostic criteria	Prevalence (%)
1987	1465 subjects, 18–65 years, general population (national poll survey)	Standardized questionnaire (national computer network)	3.4
1987	8221 subjects, 18–65 years, general population	Standardized questionnaire Door-to-door	2.0
1989	2067 subjects, 18–65 years, health care center patients	Standardized questionnaire and positive skin tests to venoms Health care center	0.9

In the group of 24 subjects with a history of systemic reaction, 21 had a RAST evaluation. The Rast to honeybee, wasp and yellow jacket were negative in 7 subjects, grade 1 in 2, grade 2 in 11, grade 3 in 1. Among the 14 subjects who received both skin tests and a RAST evaluation, only 2 responded negativly to both.

In the group of subjects with a history of severe local reaction, 15.8% had a RAST of grade 2 or more. A positive RAST to yellow jacket accounted for the majority of these.

In the group of control subjects ($n=82$), only 6% had a RAST of grade 2 or more. In addition, in this group yellow jacket antigen accounted for almost all the positive RAST (4 out of 5).

This study and some others done in southeast France (Table 4) show that systemic reactions are not uncommon in the general population. RAST are not sensitive or specific enough to be considered as diagnostic of allergy to venoms in an epidemiological study.

Atopy and Systemic Reactions to Drugs

It is often stated that atopic status is a risk factor for the occurrence of systemic reactions (SR) to common drugs. More specifically, it has been suggested that reactions to anaesthetic drugs could be more frequent in atopics. The relevance of atopic status as a risk factor for SR to drugs has even been put forward in IgE-mediated drug reactions, such as reactions to penicillin [10] or muscle relaxants [11, 12]. Thus, in epidemiological standardized questionnaires, drug allergy has sometimes been included as one of the possible signs of the atopic status [13]. However, in most of these studies, atopy was only defined on the basis of responses to questions related to the occurrence of asthma, seasonal or perennial rhinitis and childhood dermatitis, without measuring any laboratory parameter such as specific IgE. In this survey, our goal was to determine whether subjects reporting SR to drugs had a higher prevalence of atopy, as defined by clinical and biological criteria.

In the same group as above the protocol included a standardized questionnaire and a Phadiatop test. The questionnaire related to: (1) demographic characteris-

Table 5. Characteristics of subjects from the SR or no SR groups.

	SR group	Control group
Number of subjects	303 (14.7%)	1764
Men	34%	57%
Women	66%	43%
Mean age (±SD)	39.3±9.0	39.5±9.2

tics, sex, age and education all of which can influence the prevalence of atopy; (2) symptoms suggestive of atopy (i.e. asthma, hay fever, perennial rhinitis, history of childhood dermatitis); (3) drugs (which drug?, which type of SR?). The Phadiatop test was performed on a blood sample for detection of specific IgEs against major aeroallergens. The test has been shown to be much more reliable than the IgE level identifying respiratory allergy. Sensitivity of this serological test has been shown to be 85% relative to skin tests and 94.5% relative to RAST to common allergens. Its specificity was 100% in the former study and 96.9% in the latter. This test was performed in 2005 subjects with positive test considered as indicative of atopy. It provides a yes or no response.

Overall, 303 subjects (i.e. 14.7% of the study group) reported reliable histories of SR to drugs. The characteristics of subjects from the SR or the no SR group are listed in Table 5. The age range was very similar in both groups. In contrast, the percentage of women was almost twice as high in the SR group ($p<0.001$), whereas there were more men in the no SR group.

The drug involved in these SR could not be identified in 27 instances. Among the remaining 276 subjects (Table 6), antibiotics accounted for 45% of the reactions, aspirin or nonsteroidal antiinflammatory drugs for 17%, intravascular radiological contrast media for 6% and miscellaneous other drugs for 31%. Among the 124 subjects who reported antibiotics as the responsible drug, 54 reported penicillin, 13 a drug from the ampicillin subgroup, 10 a sulfamide, 8 a macrolide, 6 a cycline and the remaining 32 an unspecified antibiotic. There were 31 subjects who reported aspirin, 17 nonsteroidal antiinflammatory drugs, 5 glafenine and 3 others paracetamol. Nine subjects stated that the responsible drug was a corticosteroid. Five subjects reported a SR following anti-tetanus serotherapy.

The SR consisted of giant urticaria in 129 subject (63%), angio-oedema in 99 (33%), malaise in 71 (23%), tightness of breath in 55 (18%) and loss of consciousness in 25 (8%). Many subjects reported several types of SR following drug intake.

Table 6. Drug involved in systemic reactions.

	Number of cases	Percentage
Antibiotics	124	45
Aspirin or NSAID	48	17
Iodine	18	6
Others	86	31

Table 7. Prevalence of symptoms suggestive of atopy in the SR or no SR group.

	SR (%)	No SR (%)
Asthma	9.2	5.2
Hay fever	24.7	16.5
Childhood dermatitis	12.2	5.1

Table 8. Percentage of positive Phadiatop tests in the no SR group, overall and according to the drug involved.

No SR (%)	SR		
	Overall (%)	Penicillin (%)	Aspirin (%)
19.5	17.6	19	17

The prevalence of any symptoms suggestive of atopy (Table 7) was significantly higher in the SR group ($p<0.01$). This was especially true for asthma and childhood dermatitis, whose prevalence was twice as high in the SR group. In contrast, the percentage of positive Phadiatop tests was very similar in the SR group (17.6%) and the no SR group (19.5%). Within the SR group, the prevalence of positive Phadiatop tests (Table 8) was similar regardless of the drug involved, for example, penicillin (19%) and aspirin (17%). The linear logistic regression analysis showed that, among the independant variables considered, several had a significant relationship to occurrence of drug reaction: sex ($p<0.001$), symptoms of atopy ($p<0.01$) and age. There was a significant trend ($p<0.001$) towards a higher prevalence of SR in younger subjects. Taking as the reference category the younger subjects (20–29 years old), those in the age range of 40–49 and 50–59 had a lower risk of SR to drug. By contrast, the relationship between education and occurrence of SR was not straightforward. It should be noted that a positive Phadiatop test was not associated with the occurrence of SR to drugs.

References

1. Merrett J, Merrett TG (1988) Phadiatop - a novel IgE antibody scrrening test. Clin Allergy 17:409–416
2. Birnbaum J, Vervloet D, de Luca H, Charpin D, Segalen C, David B, Charpin J (1987) Evaluation of a new test for predicting atopy. J Allergy Clin Immunol 79:157
3. Matricardi PM, Fattorossi A, Nisini R, Le Moli S, Castaglinolo PP, d'Amelio R (1989) A new test for specific IgE to inhalant allergens (Phadiatop TM) in the screening of immediate respiratory hypersensitivity states. Ann Allergy 63:532–535
4. Chaffe FH (1970) The prevalence of bee sting allergy in an allergic population. Acta Allergol (Copenh) 25:292–293
5. Settipane GA, Boyd GK (1970) Prevalence of bee sting allergy in 4992 boy scouts. Acta Allergol 25:286

6. Settipane, Newstead GJ, Boyd GK (1972) Frequency of hymenoptera allergy in an atopic and normal population. J Allergy Clin Immunol 50:146–150
7. Golden DBW, Valentine MD, Kagey-Sobotka A, Lichtenstein LM (1982) Prevalence of hymenoptera venom allergy. J Allergy Clin Immunol 69:A124
8. Herbet FA, Salkie ML (1982) Sensitivity to hymenoptera in adult males. Ann Allergy 48:12–13
9. Bousquet J, Ménardo JL, Aznar R, Robinet-Lévy M, Michel FB (1984) Clinical and immunologic survey in beekeepers in relation to their sensitization. J Allergy Clin Immunol 73:332–340
10. Smith JW, Johnson, JE Cluff LE (1966) Studies on the epidemiology of adverse drug reactions. II. An evaluation of penicillin allergy. N Engl J Med 274:998–1002
11. Fisher M, Munro IM (1983) Life-threatening anaphylactoid reactions to muscle relaxants. Anesth Analg 62:559–564
12. Moneret-Vautrin DA, Laxenaire MC, Boileau S, Grilliat JP (1985) Facteurs de risque des réactions anaphylactoïdes aux myorelaxants. Etude rétrospecitive à partir de 103 chocs. Ann Fr Anesth Reanim 4:152–157
13. Nelson, HS (1985) The atopic diseases. Ann Allergy 55:441–447

Epidemiology of Contact Allergy

P. J. Frosch[1] and J. Zimmermann[2]

[1] Department of Dermatology, Staedtische Kliniken Dortmund, Beurhausstrasse 40, W-4600 Dortmund, Federal Republic of Germany
[2] Department of Dermatology, University of Heidelberg, Vossstrasse 2, W-6900 Heidelberg, Federal Republic of Germany

Abstract

Contact dermatitis is not a rare disease, it represents 2% – 6% of all skin diseases. Localization, sex, age, and occupation may vary greatly according to the source population studied. A prospective study in Heidelberg, West Germany, in which 1155 patients were examined during a 2 year period (1986 – 1988) provided these results: (1) women outnumber men by 2:1; (2) the hands and face are primarily affected in young women, in older patients the legs are another important localization; (3) occupational contact dermatitis was found in 10% of patients; (4) high risk professions were hairdressers, nurses, metalworkers, cleaning personnel, and housewives; (5) major allergens were nickel, fragrance mix, balsam of Peru, octhilinone neomycin, formaldehyde, potassium dichromate, and various medications (heparin ointments, bufexamac).

Exact data on the prevalence and incidence of contact dermatitis are still rare. Observational studies have to improve in quality with regard to definition of source population, proof of diagnosis, and exposure period to allergens and irritants. Data on the prevalence of contact dermatitis in the general and working populations are still poorly documented.

Introduction

Reliable data on the epidemiology of contact allergies are a basic requirement for effective preventive measures instituted by both industry and state authorities. However, good epidemiological studies in the field of contact dermatitis are rare due to the complex and multifactorial nature of the disease. In many reports no clear definition was given; allergic contact dermatitis was not verified by appropriate patch testing; irritant contact dermatitis and atopic dermatitis were not differentiated; the information was based on questionnaires only ("have you had a rash on your hands other than common warts?"). The data are even "softer" regarding the prevalence of contact dermatitis in the general population. In light of these shortcomings, some important figures derived from the literature and based on our own clinical experience in Heidelberg and Dortmund will be given.

Prevalence of Contact Dermatitis in the General Population

Contact dermatitis is not a rare disease as every dermatologist knows. Based on several studies the frequency in the general population ranges between 2.3% and 6.2% (Table 1). The data of Johnson and Roberts [10] and Coenraads et al. [3], in which a clinical examination was performed on every subject rather than relying on information supplied by a questionnaire, are the most reliable. Menné et al. [16] questioned and examined 2552 Danish women regarding the presence of hand eczema now or in the past. A remarkably high figure of 22% was found. This indicates that a short-term cross-sectional study may underestimate the prevalence of contact dermatitis compared to a long-term study in which data collected over several years are analyzed. In many patients contact dermatitis is short-lived, if it is of the acute irritant type or if the allergen is quickly found and eliminated. Unfortunately, the data shown in Table 1 do not permit a clear distinction between allergic and irritant contact dermatitis.

Eczema is more prevalent in females than in males. Depending on the source population the difference may reach a factor of up to 2.5 [12,15]. Only in one study, from the UK, were males affected nearly twice as frequently as women [17]. Apart from industrial influences these differences my be due to age.

The severity of contact dermatitis is usually slight; but it can lead to hospital admission in severe cases. In the Netherlands the National Medical Registry supplies accurate figures for 1987. Nine out of 100000 inhabitants per year were hospitalized because of contact dermatitis, which was 6% of all skin diseases and 1% of all hospital admissions [13]. At the Department of Dermatology of the Staed-

Table 1. The prevalence of contact dermatitis in the general population.

Author	Number of cases investigated	Contact dermatitis (%)
Johnson and Roberts [10]	20749 (USA)	5.4
Weismann et al. [19]	584 (Denmark)	3.8
Agrup [1]	14100 (Sweden) (hand only)	2.3
Menné et al. [16]	2552 (Denmark) (hand, earlier or present)	22.0
Coenraads et al. [3]	3140 (Netherlands)	6.2

Table 2. Diagnoses (ICD code) of 2148 inpatients at the Department of Dermatology, Städtische Kliniken, Dortmund (January to December 1989).

ICD	Diagnosis	Patients (*n*)	%
692	Contact dermatitis	73	3.4
691	Atopic dermatitis	216	10.1
696	Psoriasis	184	8.6
708	Urticaria	133	6.2
172	Melanoma	94	4.4
053	Zoster	82	3.8
035	Erysipelas	64	3.0

ICD, International Coding of Diagnoses.

tische Kliniken in Dortmund, 73 of 2148 inpatients (3.4%) in 1989 suffered from contact dermatitis as the major complaint leading to admission (Table 2). The population served by the hospital is about 3 millions. Characterized earlier by heavy steel industry and coal mining the occupational scene has recently changed to more or less "clean jobs".

Incidence in the Working Population

Few data exist on the actual incidence of contact dermatitis in the working population exposed to both irritants and allergens. Table 3 shows the comparison of two countries and a breakdown of occupational skin diseases by division of industry per 1000 workers per year. The average is very similar in both countries; however, workers in the health services are affected most frequently in Germany. Leather and metal processing are other high risk professions. The overall incidence of 0.5–2.8 per 1000 workers seems very low, but not all cases of mild disease are included in these figures. Therefore, the actual incidence in the working population will be higher. In Germany the data of the *Hauptverband der Gewerblichen Berufsgenossenschaften* are very interesting and the best documentation we have so far. The *Berufsgenossenschaften* are nonprofit organizations insuring the employee for disability by disease or trauma due to occupational factors and are divided by industrial division (construction, food production, health care, metal industry, etc.). The reports of suspected cases of occupational skin diseases have steadily climbed over recent years and, in 1987, passed the 15000 mark. In 1988 33% of all reported cases of occupational disease were due to skin diseases.

The number of sick leaves of more than 3 days due to occupational dermatoses reached 4453 in 1984, which was nearly half of all occupational diseases

Table 3. Incidence of occupational diseases by industry per 1000 workers per year. [From [14].

USA	Incidence (per 1000)	FRG	Incidence (per 1000)
Construction	0.7	Construction	0.7
Manufacturing	1.2		
Leather	2.7		
Metal production	1.8	Iron/steel	0.6
Machinery	1.4		
Electricity production	1.4		
Rubber	1.9		
Chemical	1.3	Chemical	0.6
Food	1.7	Food	0.6
Miscellaneous	2.6		
Health service	0.8	Health service	2.8
Agriculture	2.8		

The total incidence of occupational disease in the USA is 0.6 per 1000 and in the FRG 0.5 per 1000.

Table 4. Occupational skin diseases in the FRG based on the yearly reports of nonprofit insurance institutions (*Berufsgenossenschaften*). [From 2].

	Reported cases		Compensated cases	
	Number	Percent	Number	Percent
Total	31442	100	853	100
Industry				
Metal		15		13
Mechanics/electrical engineering		9		8
Food production/restaurant		7		3
Construction		12		38
Health service		32		11
Various		24		26

Shown are the data for 3 years (1978 – 1980) based both on reported cases where the suspicion was sufficient and the recognized and compensated ones.

(10959). These figures clearly demonstrate the growing socioeconomical significance of occupational skin diseases and call for additional measures of prevention [11].

Table 4 shows the major industrial divisions related to occupational skin diseases. A comparison of reported and compensated cases is very instructive. There is a large number of compensated cases in the construction industry in contrast to a relatively low one in the health services. Masons suffer primarily from chronic allergic contact eczema due to the presence of potassium dichromate in cement. This is an allergen virtually impossible to avoid unless it is complexed with ferrous sulfate, a measure still not introduced in Germany. The dermatitis of many nurses is not recognized because the hand eczema is slight and does not lead to a complete loss of occupational abilities. Furthermore, atopic or irritant eczema of nonoccupational origin is often subsequently after a careful workup by an acknowledged specialist.

The data of the *Berufsgenossenschaften* on verified cases of occupational eczema (BK Nr. 5101) permit the distinction between allergic and irritant contact dermatitis to be made with confidence because they are based on dermatological examinations, including patch and prick testing in most cases. For 1982 the figures are shown in Table 5. The leading diagnosis was allergic contact eczema of

Table 5. Diagnosis and localization of 2004 recognized cases of occupational dermatitis.

Diagnosis (localization)	Cases (n)	%
Allergic contact dermatitis (hands)	1006	50.0
Irritant contact dermatitis (hands)	366	18.2
Allergic contact dermatitis (various locations)	198	9.9
Irritant contact dermatitis (various locations)	86	4.3
Other dermatoses	348	27.6

Based on the 1982 figures of the *Berufsgenossenschaften*. A total of 9778 cases were reported.

the hands followed by irritant hand dermatitis. Unfortunately, no further data regarding the involved substances are available.

Prospective Studies in West Germany

The lack of precise information on various aspects of contact dermatitis has recently led to two prospective studies in West Germany.

At the Department of Dermatology, University of Heidelberg, a prospective study, with the aid of a personal computer, was carried out for 2 years (1986 to 1988). A total of 1155 patients were evaluated using detailed codes for personal data, diagnoses, localization, occupation, results of patch testing (standard series and various supplementary occupational trays), history clinical criteria and prick tests for atopy, the use of gloves and barrier creams, etc. A complete history regarding occupational and nonoccupational contactants was taken from every patient and careful patch testing with these substances was performed if they were suspected of causing contact dermatitis. The results of this study are published in detail elsewhere [21]. The major results are as follows:

1. Women were more frequently affected than men (2:1)
2. Those most often affected were from 30–35 years of age
3. 30% of the patients had hand eczema
4. An occupational cause was identified in 10% of the series

The different types of eczema were differentiated in the following way: Allergic hand eczema 147/1155 (12.7%), dyshidrotic hand eczema 101(8.7%), facial eczema 103 (8.9%), stasis dermatitis of the leg 54 (4.7%), irritant hand eczema 44 (3.8%), atopic hand eczema 24 (2.1%), atopic eczema over the remaining body 80 (6.9%).

According to Wilkinson and Wilkinson [20] the MOAHL index is a useful parameter for characterizating the studied population. In this study it was found to be 35–10–9–30–5 (male, occupational, atopic eczema, hand eczema, leg dermatitis). If a population consisting primarily of males who work in an industrial setting is studied, the allergen spectrum and pattern of diagnoses will be different from a population consisting primarily of older females. In the former group hand eczema of occupational origin will be found more frequently and, as described by Wilkinson and Wilkinson [20], potassium dichromate might be the leading allergen. In the latter group iatrogenic sensitizations due to intensive use of medications for the treatment of leg ulcers and dermatitis will be found. The rank order of positive reactions to allergens of the standard series is given in Table 6. Nickel sulphate is the leading allergen, affecting an overwhelming predominance of females (90% of the positive reactions). In patients with atopic eczema the sensitization rate to nickel was 24.1% when compared to 14.1% in the total population the difference was highly significant. Women were more frequently sensitized to fragrance mix (75.2%) and to the preservative kathon CG (75.8%). Only potassium dichromate affected males more often (46% vs 34.5).

Table 6. Frequency of positive test reactions in 1155 patients seen at the Contact Clinic of the Department of Dermatology, University of Heidelberg (1986–1988).

Allergen	%
Nickel sulphate	14.0
Balsam of Peru	8.2
Fragrance mix	8.1
Cobalt chloride	5.5
Kathon CG	5.4
Neomycin sulphate	4.9
Formaldehyde	4.6
Potassium dichromate	3.6
Rosin	2.9
Wool alcohols	2.8
Thiram mix	2.5
Paraben mix	2.3

Table 7. High risk occupations and major allergens. [From 21].

Metal workers	Potassium dichromate, formaldehyde, balsam of Peru
Hairdressers	Glyceryl monothioglycolate (acid permanents), *p*-phenylenediamine (hair colors), nickel sulphate
Nurses	Thiuram compounds (rubber gloves), chloromethylisothiazolinone (liquid detergents), scented lotions (hand lotions)
Cleaning staff	Thiuram compounds (rubber gloves), chloromethylisothiazolinone (liquid detergents), lanolin creams (hand care lotions)
Housewives	Nickel sulphate (fashion jewelry, other sources?), scented lotions (hand lotions), chloromethylisothiazolone (liquid detergents), thiuram compounds (rubber gloves)

High risk occupations and major allergens identified are listed in Table 7. Relatively new but very significant allergens are kathon CG and glyceryl monothioglycolate. The preservative kathon CG (chloromethylisothiazolinone and methylisothiazolinone) is found primarily in liquid detergents and various cosmetics (shampoos, hand and skin lotions, etc.) [7]. The active ingredient of acid hair permanents, glyceryl monothioglycolate, is today the leading cause of allergic contact dermatitis in hairdressers [9]. In a multicenter trial of the German Contact Dermatitis Research Group 30.9% of 178 hairdressers investigated because of hand dermatitis reacted to glyceryl monothioglycolate. Preventive measures like gloves were frequently not used.

Among the nonoccupational allergens medical ointments (heparin, bufexamac), eyedrops (beta blockers, gentamicin), plants, and sunscreens were found. This confirms other reports [4, 6, 8, 18].

The second prospective study, funded by the *Bundesministerium für Forschung und Technologie* (BMFT) in West Germany, is the IVDK (*Informationsverbund Dermatologischer Kliniken – Epidemiologie von Kontaktallergien*) (project). In this multicenter study eight dermatology departments use the same hardware and software (Alldat-IVDK) for documenting various aspects of contact dermatitis. Special emphasis is placed on standardized epicutaneous testing (recommendations of the German Contact Dermatitis Research Group) as well as type and toxicity of occupational substances. So far about 1500 patients have been evaluated. The initial data will be analyzed by the end of 1990. After a total evaluation period of 4 years a solid data base, derived from approximately 5000 patients, will be available.

Conclusions and Methodological Considerations

Although we do have some figures on contact dermatitis regarding frequency, severity, localization, age, sex, major and minor allergens, risk professions, etc., many questions remain to be answered. Contact dermatitis is multifactorial and is often a combination of allergic and irritant of irritant and atopic dermatitis. Contact dermatitis may be short-lived if it is of the irritant type or if the allergen is avoided after its recognition. This type of contact dermatitis may be missed in a cross-sectional short-term study and may be identified only by a longitudinal long-term study. Allergens change considerably over time and are only identified if new ones are tested. Furthermore, testing techniques and particularly test interpretation need further standardization. In observational studies a selection bias may result from intentional discontinuance of a known allergen (e.g., fragrances, nickel). A patient may not show up as a "new case" or may be lost in a follow-up study. Too little is known about the incidence of contact dermatitis in the general and working populations. The induction period of contact sensitization varies with the allergen and depends on various factors (genetics, type and duration of exposure, skin condition, etc.). It is relatively short with nickel or glyceryl monothioglycolate and relatively long with potassium dichromate or wool alcohols. The data on sensitization risk can therefore only be judged appropriately after long follow-ups and experimental studies on dose response relationships.

Improvement of the quality of epidemiological studies on contact dermatitis will be undoubtedly followed by increased public interest. This in turn should lead to effective preventive measures and lower the incidence of contact dermatitis. Based on the extraordinary frequency of nickel sensitization among young females, the Danish parliament recently passed a law which prohibits the sale of fashion jewelry containing enough nickel to produce a positive dimethyl glyoxime test. As many youngsters and even parents are not aware of the high risk of nickel sensitization due to jewelry, particularly earrings, a warning statement should at least be mandatory. The long-term danger of a nickel allergy is the development of a vesicular hand eczema in workers with increased nickel exposure.

References

1. Agrup G (1969) Hand eczema. Acta Derm Venereol [Suppl 61] (Stockh) 49
2. Butz M, Drexel G, Emmerich N, Plinske W, Schönberger A, Wohlberedt F (1985) Das Berufskrankheitengeschehen. Eine exemplarische Darstellung ausgewählter Berufskrankheiten. Hauptverband der gewerblichen Berufsgenossenschaften, Bonn, pp 1–117

3. Coenraads PJ, Nater JP, van der Lende R (1983) Prevalence of eczema and other dermatoses of the hands and arms in the Netherlands. Clin Exp Dermatol 8:495–503
4. Ducombs G, Benezra C, Talaga P, Andersen KE, Burrows D, Camarasa JG, Dooms-Goossens A, Frosch PJ, Lachapelle JM, Menné T, Rycroft RJG, White IR, Wilkinson JD (1990) Patch testing with the "sesquiterpene lactone mix": a marker for contact allergy to Compositae and other sesquiterpene-lactone-containing plants. Contact Dermatitis 22:249–252
5. Fabry H (1981) Statistik der Berufskrankheiten der Hautgefährdungskataster. Dermatosen 29:42–44
6. Frosch PJ, Raulin C (1987) Kontaktallergie auf Bufexamac. Hautarzt 38:331–334
7. Frosch JP, Schulze Dirks A (1987) Kontaktallergie auf Kathon CG. Hautarzt 38:422–425
8. Frosch PJ, Weickel R, Schmitt T, Krastel H (1988) Nebenwirkungen von ophthalmologischen Externa. Z Hautkr 63:126–136
9. Frosch PJ, Kleinhans D, Fuchs T (1989) Formaldehyde and glyceryl monothioglycolate: results of the German Contact Dermatitis Research Group. Frosch PJ, Lachapelle JM, Rycroft RJG, Scheper RJ (eds) In: Current topics in contact dermatitis. Springer, Berlin Heidelberg New York, pp 274–280
10. Johnson MLT Roberts J (1978) Skin conditions and related need for medical care for persons 1–74 years, United States 1971–1974. Vital and Health statistics. US Department of health, Education and Welfare, Washington (National Health Survey, ser 11, no 212)
11. Johnson MLT, Burdick AE, Johnson KG, Klarman HE, Krasmer M, McDowell AJ, Roberts J (1979) Prevalence, morbidity and cost of dermatological diseases. J Invest Dermatol 73:395–401
12. Kavli G, Förde OH (1984) Hand dermatoses in Tromsö. Contact Dermatitis 10:174–179
13. LMR (1987) National Medical Registration. LMR Yearbook 1987. SIG, Utrecht
14. Mathias CGT, Morrison JH (1988) Occupational skin diseases, United States results from Bureau of Labor Statistics annual survey of occupational injuries and illnesses, 1973 through 1984. Arch Dermatol 124:1519–1524
15. Meding BE, Swanbeck G (1987) Prevalence of hand eczema in an industrial city. Br J Dermatol 116:627–634
16. Menné T, Borgan Ö, Green A (1982) Nickel allergy and hand dermatitis in a stratified sample of the Danish female population, an epidemiological study including a statistic appendix. Acta Derm Venereol (Stockh) 62:35–41
17. Rea JN, Newhouse ML, Halil T (1976) Skin diseases in Lambeth. A community study of prevalence and use of medical care. Br J Prev Soc Med 30:107–114
18. Schauder S, Ippen H (1988) Photoallergisches and allergisches Kontaktekzem durch Dibenzoylmethan-Verbindungen und andere Lichtschutzmittel. Hautarzt 39:435–440
19. Weismann K, Krakauer R, Wanscher B (1980) Prevalence of skin diseases in old age: Acta Derm Vernereol (Stockh) 60:352–353
20. Wilkinson DS, Wilkinson JD (1979) Comparison of patch test result in two adjacent areas of England. I. Industrial allergens. Acta Derm Venereol [Suppl 85] (Stockh) 59:189–192
21. Zimmermann J (1990) Epidemiologie von Kontaktallergien. Thesis, University of Heidelberg

Allergens

Epitopes on Allergens

L. Jäger, C. Diener, W.-D. Müller, and G. Schlenvoigt

Department of Clinical Immunology, Friedrich Schiller University, Bachstrasse 18, O-6900 Jena, Federal Republic of Germany

Abstract

By conventional immunological and physicochemical techniques natural allergens have been separated into antigenic and allergenic fractions. During the last years new methodological developments enabled to investigate their structures in detail. The first step was the identification of antigenic and allergenic (IgE-binding) epitopes on these molecules. This has been done for several major allergens from pollen, insect, fungal and epidermal allergens e.g. Usually 2–6 antigenic and 1–3 allergenic sites have been found. In some cases the primary structure of such epitopes or even the complete allergen has been uncovered. In a few of them (Der p I, Chi t I e.g.) even the three-dimensional structure could be disclosed. Obviously sequential epitopes dominante - at least in grass pollen allergens. The methods which have been applied are monoclonal antibodies, improved techniques of peptide analysis and synthesis and above all cloning procedures.

These developments are very important both from practical and theoretical points of view. They will improve diagnostic procedures and disclose the basis of often surprising cross-reactivities. More important is the fact that B-cell-epitopes (being active during the manifestation of the allergic reaction) are obviously not identical with T-cell epitopes (important during sensitization). This fact could open new ways for a scientific-based approach to immuntherapy. Other prospective developments concern the presentation of these epitopes together with MHC-structures, the identification of possibly individual-specific patterns of sensitization and an reevaluation of the exact mechanisms of the initial step of IgE-mediated reactions. The dogma that bridging of membrance-bound IgE antibodies is induced by identical epitopes obviously has to be modified.

Introduction

Allergens are substances that cause allergic reactions – especially those mediated by IgE. In clinical practice they are defined by their binding to such antibodies. This thinking is correct as long as it is part of a diagnostic analysis. It is not possible, however, to equate this definition with the practice of immunotherapy, as more and more information is becoming available suggesting that B cell epitopes are not necessarily identical to those of T cells. This is one of the reasons why identification of epitopes is, at present, one of the main fields in allergologic research.

Structure of Allergens

Allergens usually have a molecular mass ranging between 10 and 70 kDa. The lower limit is obviously determined by immunogenicity, the upper by the permeability of mucosal membranes. The situation, however, is actually more complicated, as natural allergens consist of a mixture of antigens. Only some of them are able to bind IgE antibodies. Major allergens are those which bind IgE in more than 50% of the patients, minor allergens act in the same way in less then 10%. As will be shown later on, this estimate of heterogeneity is probably too high, as different structures may bear identical, or at least similar, epitopes. This is another point which underlines the importance of epitope analysis.

Functional Aspects of Antigen Binding Sites

There are two opposing views of the mechanisms of antigen recognition. According to the lock and key model, the binding sites of antibody molecules simply recognize patches at the surface of antigens that are complementary to them in shape and chemical properties. This model stresses the fact that antibodies must have access to an antigenic site in order to bind. It has led to the view that antibody accessibility is the primary intrinsic determinant of antigenicity.

In contrast, the induced fit model proposes that the mechanism of binding occurs by induced complementarity involving significant side chain movements of the antigen and possibly minor movements of the backbone conformation [55]. This second model explains the correlation between antigenicity and local mobility of the peptide main chain and has been described by the analogy of the adaptation between glove and hand. These different interpretations are not only of academic interest, they directly influence the experimental approach to investigating epitopes.

Due to the restricted area of the antibody binding site (70 nm^2), only a few amino acids (AA) or other structures can be recognized. One could infer that a binding site would be able to bind to a certain sequence of AA from epitope peptide chain, i.e., *sequential or continuous epitope binding.* The existence of such antigens has been shown by mutation of similar polypeptides. Additional evidence comes from the persistence of antigen binding sites after treatment of allergens, which should interfere with conformation stabilizing covalent or non-covalent bonds.

Antibodies can also recognize a distinct patch primarily or secondarily accessible on the surface of the antigen. They bind to a set of residues that are not continuos in the sequence , but are brought together by the folding of the peptide chain or by the juxtaposition of two separate chains. Such an epitope is usually referred to as *discontinuous or conformational.*

Number of Epitopes per Antigen

The antigen binding site of the antibody recognizes only a restricted part of the total surface. There are various concepts concerning the number of epitopes present. On one extreme is a model in which continuous or discontinuous epitopes can, in principle, be formed by any part of the molecule. The number of epitopes is therefore virtually unlimited. According to other models, the antigen bears only a restricted number of epitopes. At present it is impossible to find a definite answer because of technical limitations. Analysis of polyclonal sera is hampered, especially by the inadequate sensitivity of present techniques. Investigations by means of monoclonal antibodies (mabs) are restricted by the limited number of clones. Nevertheless, the data available indicate the existence of a limited number of *immunodominant* structures. Investigations of grass pollen allergens, e.g., Phl p VII, Lol p IV, and Amb a I, and of the mite allergen Der p I have clearly shown that 60%–95% of the mabs bind to one site [29].

These investigations were initiated in order to determine whether allergic disease is elicited by a limited number of epitopes or allergens or could it be possible that any part of the allergen, even the hitherto "nonallergenic" antigens, can induce allergic reactions? Such information is indispensible to any attempt to improve diagnostic of therapeutic procedures.

Methods for Analyzing Allergens and Epitopes

Epitopes are defined by their binding to antibodies or to the analogous structures of the T cell receptor (TCR). They can, therefore, only be identified by immunological methods. Nevertheless, additional information concerning structure, localization, etc., is necessary (Fig. 1). This can be derived from:

- Defined cleavage
- Identification of the sequence of the AA and synthesis of appropriate peptides
- Genetic methods (identification of mRNA, sequencing, cloning, and synthesis)
- Interference of mono- and polyclonal antibodies

The ultimate goal would be to identify the total three-dimensional structure, including the location and structure of epitopes.

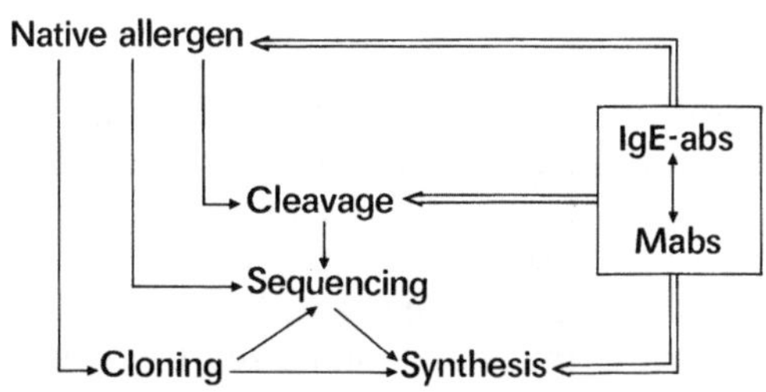

Fig. 1. Methods for identification of epitopes on allergens

Cleavage and Peptide Synthesis

The oldest methods of cleavage and synthesis are those conventionally used in peptide chemistry. More or less defined fragments can be recovered by cyanogen bromide (CNBr) or tryptic cleavage for example. This has been done with Lol p IV and cod allergen M [19, 28]. The allergenic activity of the fragments has to be evaluated by conventional means – either by polyclonal human sera or the appropriate mabs. In principle, these and similar techniques can be used to identify sequential epitopes. Conformational epitopes are usually destroyed and cannot be localized. On Lol p IV this holds true for binding site B [28]. By a combination of cleavage and identification of the AA in the fragments, the AA sequence of ragweed antigen E (Amb a III [31]), Lol p II [2] as well as of the major allergen from codfish (Gal d I [18]) could be identified. A more recent variant is the identification of the sequence of the N-terminal AA by automatic Edman degradation or similar procedures. Sequences of AA of the major allergens from hazel and birch pollen [19], for example, have been analyzed in this way.

Another approach is to analyze the effect of deglycosylation. This is very interesting as most natural allergens are glycoproteins. Generally, however, there are no significant effects after periodate oxidation, treatment with glycosidases, etc. This holds true for most pollen allergens and has been investigated in detail, e.g., for group I allergens from grasses [40] and timothy [23] (own results), and for Bet v I [30] and Cla h II [54]. Nonetheless, loss of activity has been reported for phospholipase A2 [57] and for certain food allergens. However, such results from deglycosylation procedures do not prove that the carbohydrate is part of the epitope itself. It could well be of indirect importance, e.g., by stabilizing the conformation.

The identification of the complete AA sequence also gives no definite information concerning epitopes. Instead, this information can be obtained from:

- Inhibition by a series of overlapping oligopeptides. The application of modern automatic peptide synthesizers has made this a feasible procedure.
- Prediction on the basis of physicochemical properties. In most cases, the tertiary structure is reduced to a linear scale of AA sequence, and an attempt is made to correlate the location of continuous epitopes with structural properties such as accessibility, protrusion, mobility, and hydrophilicity [55]. Although it is generally recognized that most protein epitopes are discontinuous, the emphasis on continuous epitopes in such studies is due to the potential usefulness of predicting which linear peptide fragments are likely to cross-react with the native protein.

Such predictions give very interesting results and may be improved by trial and error procedures. Confirmation by application of antibodies is always needed, however. Mazur et al. [45], using a computer analysis of the X-ray defined Chir t I component III and derived peptides, predicted correctly the sequence of residues 91–101. However, discrepancies existed at the N-terminal. Using the oligopeptide technique, Lowenstein and Schou [38] identified epitopes which are obviously hidden in the intact solubilized Der f/m I molecule.

Genetic Techniques

The development of genetic techniques has opened new doors for the analysis of allergens. The starting point is usually the preparation of the mRNA, which is used to prime the synthesis of single stranded complementary DNA (cDNA) using reverse transcriptase. Single stranded cDNA can then be converted into double stranded cDNA. This cDNA can be used to generate the nucleotide base sequence and thereby the putative AA sequence of the allergenic protein. The cDNA can also be ligated into a suitable vector; the protein encoded can then be produced in an appropiate host [8].

By means of these techniques, several major allergens from mites, midges, and grass and tree pollen have been cloned and synthesized. A modification which will be very important in the near future for the identification of epitopes is to selectively induce point mutations and to analyze the modified allergens (see Kraft et al., this volume). It should be mentioned, however, that these techniques have to be supplemented by adequate immunological tools.

Application of Mabs

Mabs are valuable tools for identifying epitopes comprising nearly all important major allergens. For example, they have been used in purification and standardization methods [11, 27]. One of their advantages is the identity of all antibody molecules. From the different lines of investigation two, the identification of IgE binding sites and the analysis of cross-reactivity, will be discussed here. The limitation of mabs is that they usually cannot provide topographical information.

IgE Binding Sites

Information on IgE binding sites on allergens is important for both research and clinical practice. It could improve our knowledge of basic mechanisms in sensitization and answer questions concerning mechanisms underlying immunotherapy. Furthermore, such information offers opportunities to synthesize antigens for diagnosis and therapy. Unfortunately, interpretation of the information available is difficult, particularly due to methodological problems.

The binding interference between mabs and IgE is usually analyzed by sandwich assays, the allergen being bound to the solid phase either directly or by means of an allergen specific mab (mab I). The solid phase prepared in this way is incubated with a mixture of the second mab (mab II) to be evaluated and the IgE containing sera. Their binding can be determined by labelled antisera (Fig. 2). The disadvantage of this procedure is the possible interference of IgG usually existing in patients. The direct binding of the allergen to the solid phase, moreover, can induce conformational changes.

After initially disappointing experiences, more and more interfering mabs have now been described. Antigenicity in mice and binding to human IgE are not necessarily identical. Usually there is more diverse array of antigenic epitopes

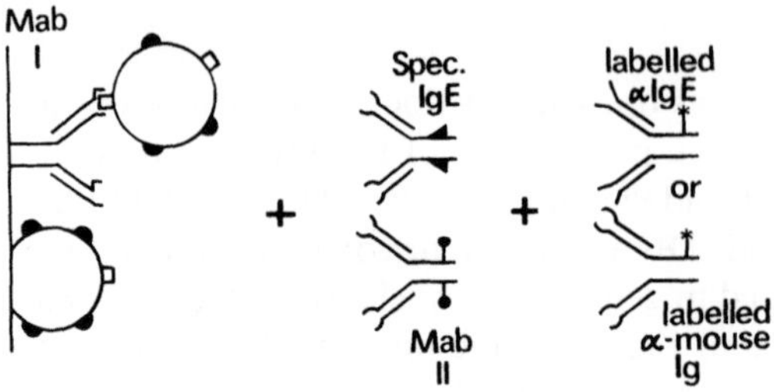

Fig. 2. Evaluation of IgE binding epitopes

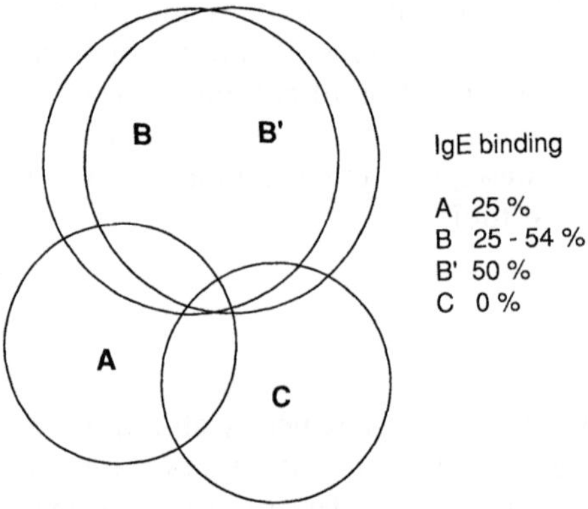

Fig. 3. *Left*, epitopes on phospholipase A2 defined by murine mabs; *right*, interference of pooled serum from bee venom allergics with the binding of the mabs

than IgE binding ones. The interpretation of negative results, however, must be done cautiously as concentrations and affinities of the different populations play an important role. Moreover, one binding site for polyclonal IgE could possibly be blocked by the mab whilst those with different structures remain accessible. The reverse evalution therefore is more conclusive.

By criss-cross evaluation we identified three epitopes on phospholipase A2: A and C by one mab each, B by four, and slightly different B′ by a single one (Fig. 3). Epitope A is related to the active center of the enzyme. On mellitin we identified one epitope by means of two mabs. It is close to the IgE binding site as patients' sera block the binding of the mabs by 60% and 70% respectively.

Several laboratories have produced mabs to both groups of major allergens from house dust mites. They have been used for purification, development of specific immunoassays, and epitope mapping. By their means, a very high degree of cross-reactivity within both groups has been identified. A summary of the results, using 19 mabs from four labs, is given in Fig. 4. It could be shown that Der p I obviously bears four partially overlapping epitopes. Between Der f I and Der m I there is a higher degree of cross-reactivity than between Der f I and Der p I [36]. This corresponds to the taxonomic relationship. Within the N-terminal 30 AA, there are only two inhomologies between Der f I and Der m I, whereas there are seven between Der f I and Der p I. Similar results have been published by Chapmans's group (whose mabs were included in the study already mentioned) identifying four nonoverlapping, nonrepeated epitopes on Der p I, one epitope on Der f I, and one cross-reacting epitope. The IgE-binding site is outside the thus

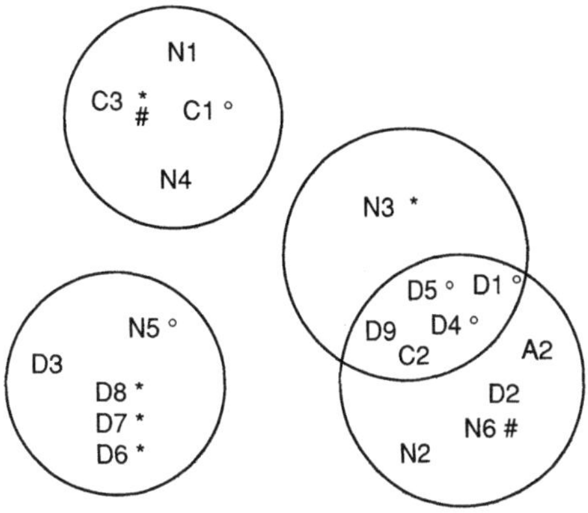

Fig. 4. Cluster of epitopes on Der p I defined by murine mabs. *Letters* characterize mabs from different laboratories; individual *circles* represent overlapping epitopes. Additional signs for varying cross-reactivities. [From 36]

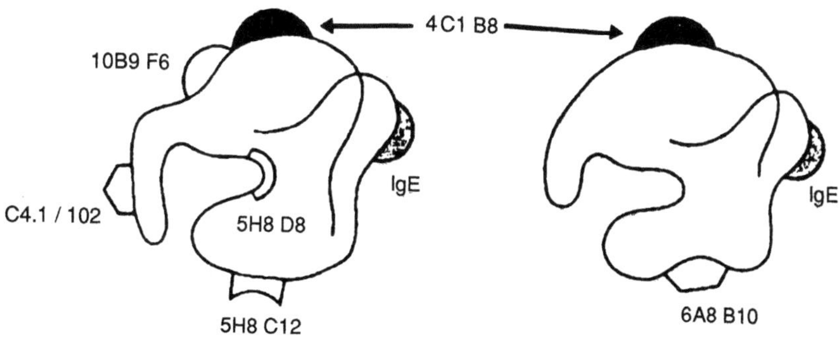

Fig. 5. Epitope mapping in Der p I (*left*) and Der f I (*right*). [From 14]

defined epitopes (Fig. 5). IgE binding, however, was inhibited up to 80% by a polyclonal cross-reacting antiserum from rabbits (anti-P1Eq). The differences between murine, rabbit and human antibody response could reflect genetic differences. Another possibility is that differences in allergenic exposure and immunization in mice and allergic patients, respectively, result in altered processing of the allergens [14].

According to Chapman et al. [12] human IgE is almost fully cross-reactive between species. The results of Lind et al. [36] are somewhat different, as they also identified species specific sensitizations in allergics and were able to block them by up to 45% by murine mabs. Ley et al. [34] reported murine mab inhibition of IgE binding by between 6% and 50%.

An overview of the information which is available at present is shown in Table 1. The data given are minimal and should be interpreted cautiously, as usually not all mabs available are used in the same investigation.

Most investigators conclude that they could identify only "nonrepetitive" epitopes [13, 29, 51]. It must, however, be stressed that the techniques applied usually cannot differentiate between inhibition by a single epitope and that by several identical or similar ones. Nevertheless, there is increasing evidence to suggest that the classical bridging of membrane IgE by identical epitopes does not seem to be the typical situation.

Table 1. Epitopes on allergens from grasses and other sources. [From 11].

Allergen	Epitopes	
	Antigenic	Allergenic
Grasses		
Dac g I	4	2?
Lol p I	>6	2 (−4)
Poa p I	4	1 [a]
Fes e I	4	2
Poa p IV	4	3
Lol p IV	4	2
Phl p V	3	2
Phl p VII	6−8	1 [a]
Lol p X	4?	1−2?
Par j I	2	1 [a]
Par o I	1	1 [a]
Other sources		
Amb a I	3	2
Amb a III	4	4
Bet v I	6?	1 [a]
Der p I	5	1
Der f I	2−3	2?
Der p II	1	1 [a]
Der f II	>3	1 [a]
Chi t I	5	3
Bla g I	2	1 [a]
Api m I	3	2
Api m III	3	1 [a]
Dol m V	5	1 [a]
Fel d I	4	1 [a]
Gad c I	4	3?

[a] Molecule clearly binds IgE, but the number of binding sites are unknown.

Cross-Reacting Epitopes

Cross-reactivity is a well-known phenomenon in allergology and is based on identical or similar epitopes on different molecules. Within a given species this is very common. By a single mab we were able to identify three different allergens in timothy pollen by crossed radioimmunoelectrophoresis (CRIE) and more than seven by immunoblotting. Similar results have been reported for other grass pollen [22], *Parietaria* [17], and chironomides [43].

There are, however, cross-reactivities beyond species barriers too. They have been described between the group I and group IV allergens of different grass pollens [20]. Among our mabs there is one which binds to structures in extracts from all grass pollens analyzed up to now. The data on cross-reactivity in mites have already been mentioned. According to some authors, cross-reactivity is a general phenomenon in allergy [8].

MHC Structures, T Cell Epitopes

Analysis of allergens was, for a long time, exclusively oriented toward the identification of IgE binding, that is, B cell epitopes. This is adequate as long as the aim is the identification of an already existing sensitization, i.e., the diagnosis. It, however, is not necessarily adequate for trying to analyze pathogenetic or even therapeutic mechanisms.

From experimental immunology it is known that the initial steps of sensitization are the presentation of antigen together with major histocompatibility complex (MHC) class II structures and the activation of T helper cells with appropriate receptors. These interactions are usually dissected into analysis of interactions of MHC structures and epitopes and identification of T cell binding epitopes. In most experiments, however, the two components cannot be separated.

Interactions Between MHC Structures and Epitopes

For MHC class I the structure of the antigen presenting site is known; that of class II seems to be similar [53]. It is possible to imagine that, in the "groove", a sequence of 10–13 AA can be presented as a sequential or continuous epitope. It is much more complicated to envisage the presentation of conformational or discontinuous epitopes within the dimensions given. The importance of native structures for certain allergens, however, is well known.

One typical procedure for gaining insight into these interactions in allergology is the analysis of associations with MHC structures, which has been done by Marsh et al. [41]. These investigations, not only include an analysis of the binding of epitopes to the MHC structures, but also the availability of appropriate T cell receptors.

T Cell Binding Structures

Identification of the influence of T cell binding structures has been attempted by repeating former proliferation studies and by establishing specific T cell clones. Both were performed with highly purified allergens or fragments of them.

Even within these strict conditions, the results of proliferation studies remain controversial. A recent study by Phillips et al. [52] was unable to find differences between T cell proliferation in response to Amb a I in atopic patients and controls after 7 days of allergen stimulation. However, after restimulating with allergen and culturing the cells for a further 7 days, proliferation was only obtained from the atopic donors' cells.

The isolation of allergen specific T cell clones from allergic patients is another recent achievement. For example, trials using mite allergens have been successful. O'Hehir et al. [48–50] generated a panel of stable T cell clones from a single mite allergic donor by stimulation with *D. farinae* extract. Interestingly, although IgG and IgE antibodies to *Dermatophagoides* allergens are highly cross-reactive, most of the clones were *D. farinae* specific. They have subsequently been shown to recognize either Der f I or Der f II. Some Der f I/Der p I cross-reactive clones have also been isolated. Patients with asthma or atopic dermatitis had much better proliferative responses than skin test positive patients with rhinitis.

The identification of T cell epitopes follows the principles outlined for B cells. This information is only just becoming available. The first step is to identify the molecules binding to or stimulating T cells. The next step is to identify the binding sites themselves by using fragments or synthesized peptides or by the interference of mabs with known specificity. Amphipathic regions in particular are considered to contain T cell binding sites.

For Lol p I, II, and III, similar HLA-D binding aggretopes have been located in the C-terminal regions. At least for Lol p II and III a special sequence of DNA (EYSTS) could be identified in the first hypervariable region of the DRβI chain [4]. This development could be a scientific approach to improving immunotherapy. Besides epitopes which stimulate T helper cells, there seem to be others which either block them or induce suppressor mechanisms. Ishizaka et al. [26] for example, identified such effects by denaturing ragweed antigen E. Other investigators reported analogous results using distinct cleavage products or conjugates (e.g., rye grass pollen extracts conjugated with polysarcolysine [58]. One general limitation of these investigations is usually the lack of information concerning the epitopes involved, but such techniques provide a better basis for the development of modified allergens. Inhibitory epitopes can be derived from quite different sources. O'Hehir and Lamb [47] competitively blocked both the response of DRw52 restricted, CD4+T cell clones reactive with house dust mite and the polyclonal response to the mite allergen by means of peptides derived from the C-terminal of the HA-1 molecule of influenzae hemagglutinins. The effect has been localized at the level of antigen presenting cells.

Relationships Between B and T Cell Epitopes

Information concerning the relationship between B and T cell epitopes is still very limited. Obviously, they can be identical, but in principle they seem to be different. Atassi [7] analyzed the proliferative effects using the strategy of overlapping peptides in immunized mice. Five T-sites were localized in four high responder strains. Three of them coincided with the antigenic sites recognized by antibodies from outbred mice. However, there was at least one site which was only recognized by T cells. Ansari et al. [3], using predictive methods, were unable to identify identical B and T cell epitopes on Lol p II. There was, however, one B cell site on Lol p I homologous to the presumed T cell site on Lol p II. On Chir t II the T sites seem to be distinct from the three known B sites [44]. The same has been shown for the vespid venom allergen 5 (Dol m V [32]). The existence of cross-reactive idiotypes on B and T cells from patients sensitized by *Phleum* antigen B suggests identical or similar epitopes [39].

Heterogeneity of Sensitization

The primary aim of these sophisticated investigations is to improve our knowledge of immune mechanisms, from the sensitization to the manifestation of IgE mediated reactions, as well as diagnostic and therapeutic procedures.

The practical value of this knowledge, however, depends on whether or not the thus identified epitopes are representative of all relevant allergic patients or at least most of them. At this point, the crucial question of the heterogeneity of sensitization occurs. As sensitization very much depends on genetic makeup, a high degree of heterogeneity in human beings is to be expected. Nevertheless, investigations into Amb a III seem to show that the antigenic site is independent of the species immunized (mouse, rabbit, and human IgE and IgG [7]).

The different patterns of sensitization in allergic patients with major, intermediate, and minor allergens seem to confirm the expected heterogeneity (e.g., grass pollen, fungi, flour), but a few allergens generally dominate. Our own investigations into grass pollen, moreover, demonstrated that heterogeneity on the epitope level could well be less than that on the molecular level.

On the epitope level, only a few detailed investigations have been published so far. There are enormous technical limitations because of the polyclonal immune response of patients. The usual procedure is to evaluate the interference of patients' sera with mabs of defined specificities – usually with a restricted number of individual sera. It must be made sure that IgE is involved, as IgG antibodies can also be found in healthy persons [29]. In mite allergy, Chapman et al. [14] reported a predominance of those epitope(s) which could be blocked by P1Eq. More detailed investigations have been made by Bose et al. [9, 10] in *Lolium.* By means of murine mabs they identified five epitopes on Lol p I. Four of the mabs blocked binding of IgE. The interpretation of their results is hampered by the fact that maximal inhibition was only 35.1%. Even though it cannot be concluded that their A-E sites correspond to distinct IgE epitopes, a certain degree of heterogeneity is obvious. From investigations in Lol p IV they reported similar results. Nevertheless, certain epitopes dominate. This immunodominance is still more obvious from the investigations of Mourad et al. [46] in Lol p I.

We obtained similar results from investigations in patients with bee venom allergy (Fig. 6). The major allergen is phospholipase A2. As already mentioned two of the three epitopes bind IgE. The patients presented similar patterns of sensitization with only quantitative differences. The interference in site C is within the background range expected from the method.

A quite new aspect has come from results recently published by Marsh et al. [41]. They confirmed the humoral heterogeneity to Amb V from different species of ragweed and to Lol p I, II, and III. However, they also identified common MHC binding structures on both groups of allergens. The humoral heterogeneity therefore could well be induced by identical T cell epitopes – very important information for future approaches to immunotherapy.

Although it is premature to draw any final conclusions, the present situation can be summarized as follows: First, epitopes are the decisive structures on allergens, and natural allergens bear a limited number of such immunodominant structures. Second, repeated identical structures are not the rule; IgE bridging on mast

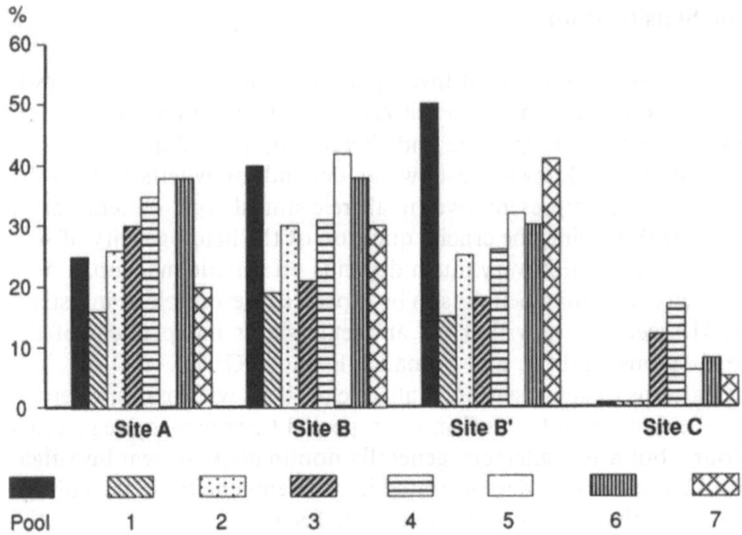

Fig. 6. Percent interference of pooled and individual sera (from patients with bee venom allergy) with the binding of murine mabs to phospholipase A2

cells/basophils can be induced by different epitopes. Third, in spite of patient heterogeneity, a similar pattern of sensitization seems to dominate. Its further identification is important both from a practical and a scientific point of view. Finally, IgE and T cell epitopes, that is, sensitizing and eliciting epitopes, are not necessarily identical. Moreover, T cell heterogeneity seems to be less than that of B cells. A detailed analysis is important for future approaches to immunotherapy.

References

1. Adorini L, Apella E, Dona G, Nagy ZA (1989) Mechanisms influencing the immunodominance of T cell determinants. J Exp Med 168:2091–2104
2. Ansari AA, Shenbagamurthi P, Marsh DG (1989) Complete amino acid sequence of a *Lolium perenne* (perennial rye grass) pollen allergen, Lol p II. J Biol Chem 264:1181–1185
3. Ansari AA, Shenbagamurthi P, Kihara T, et al. (1989) Molecular studies of human response to grass allergens (Abstr). Allergologie [Suppl] 12:35
4. Ansari AA, Shenbagamurthi P, Shinomiya N, Zwollo P, Marsh DG (1990) HLA-D sequence analysis in relation to immune responsiveness to grass allergens, Lol p II and III (Abstr). J Allergy Clin Immunol 85:201
5. Atassi H, Atassi ZM (1985) Localization of the continous allergenic sites of ragweed allergen Ra3 by a comprehensive synthetic strategy. FEBS Lett 188:96–100
6. Atassi H, Atassi ZM (1986) Antibody recognition of ragweed Ra3: localization of the full profile of the continuous antigenic sites by synthetic overlapping peptides representing the entire protein chain. Eur J Immunol 16:229–235
7. Atassi ZM (1989) Mapping of the antibody and T-cell recognition profiles of ragweed allergen Ra3 (Abstr). Allergologie [Suppl] 12:33
8. Baldo BA, Donovan GR (1988) The structural basis of allergenicity: recombinant DNA based strategies for the study of allergens. Allergy 43:81–97

9. Bose R, Rector ES, Fischer J, Tarono R, Delespesse G (1986) Production and characterization of mouse monoclonal antibodies to allergic epitopes on Lol p I. Immunology 59:309
10. Bose R, Ekramoddoullah AK, Kisil FT, Sehon AH (1988) Human and murine antibodies to rye grass pollen allergen Lol p IV share a common idiotype. Immunology 63:579–584
11. Chapman MD (1989) Purification of allergens. Curr Opin Immunol 1:647–653
12. Chapman MD, Sutherland WM, Platts-Mills TAE (1984) Recognition of two Dermatophagoides pteronyssinus-specific epitopes on antigen P1 using monoclonal antibodies: binding to each epitope can be inhibited by serum from dust mite-allergic patients. J Immunol 133:2483–2494
13. Chapman MD, Heymann PW, Platts-Mills TAE (1987) Epitope mapping of two major inhalant allergens, Der p I and Der f I, from mites of the genus *Dermatophagoides*. J Immunol 139:1479–1484
14. Chapman MD, Heymann PW, Platts-Mills TAE (1988) Epitope mapping of major dust mite *(Dermatophagoides)* allergens using monoclonal antibodies. In: Todt A (ed) Mite allergy. UCB Institute of Allergy, Brussels, pp 27–29
15. Chapman MD, Heymann PW, Aalberse R, et al. (1989) Monoclonal antibodies as probes of the structure of dust mite, cat and cockroach allergens (Abstr). Allergologie [Suppl] 12:32
16. Corbi AL, Ley V, Sanchez-Madrid F, Carreira J (1985) Isolation of the major IgE-binding protein from *Parietaria judaica* pollen using monoclonal antibodies. Mol Immunol 22:1081–1089
17. Corbi AL, Ayuso R, Carreira J (1986) Identification of IgE binding polypeptides cross-reactive with the *Parietaria judaica* main allergenic polypeptide. Mol Immunol 23:1357–1363
18. Elsayed S, Apold A (1983) Immunochemical analysis of cod fish allergen M: locations of the immunoglobin binding sites as demonstrated by the native and synthetic peptides. Allergy 38:449–459
19. Elsayed S, Holen E, Dybendal T (1989) Synthetic allergenic epitopes from the amino-terminal region of the major allergens of hazel and birch pollen. Int Arch Allergy Appl Immunol 89:410–415
20. Esch RE, Klapper DG (1987) Cross-reactive and unique grass group I antigen determinants defined by monoclonal antibodies. J Allergy Clin Immunol 79:489–495
21. Esch RE, Klapper DG (1989) Identification and localization of allergenic determinants on grass group I antigens using monoclonal antibodies. J Immunol 142:179–184
22. Haas H, Becker WM, Maasch HJ, Schlaak M (1986) Analysis of allergen components in grass pollen extracts using immunoblotting. Int Arch Allergy Appl Immunol 79:434–440
23. Haavik S, Paulsen BS, Wold J (1987) Glycoprotein allergens in pollen of timothy. Int Arch Allergy Appl Immunol 83:231–237
24. Heymann PW, Chapman MD, Platts-Mills TAE (1986) Antigen Der f I from the dust mite Dermatophagoides farinae: structural comparison with Der p I from Dermatophagoides pteronyssinus and epitope specificity of murine IgG and human IgE antibodies. J Immunol 137:2841–2847
25. Heymann PW, Chapman MD, Aalberse RC, et al. (1989) Antigenic and structural analysis of group II allergens (Der p II and Der f II) from house dust mites (*Dermatophagoides* spp.) J Allergy Clin Immunol 83:1055–1067
26. Ishizaka K, Kishimoto T, Delespesse G, King TP (1974) Immunogenic properties of modified antigen E. I. Pressence of specific determinants for T-cells in denatured antigen and polypeptide chain. J Immunol 113:70
27. Jäger L, Diener C, Müller W-D, Schlenvoigt G (1989) Monoclonal antibodies in identification and standardization of allergens. In: Pichler WJ (ed) Progress in Allergy and Clincal Immunology. Hogrefe & Huber, Toronto, pp 410–414
28. Jaggi KS, Ekramoddoullah AK, Kisil FT (1989) Allergenic fragments of rye grass (*Lolium perenne*) pollen allergen Lol p IV. Int Arch Allergy Appl Immunol 89:342–349
29. Jaggi KS, Ekramoddoullah AK, Kisil FT, et al.(1989) Identification of two distinct allergenic sites on rye grass pollen allergen, Lol p IV. J Allergy Clin Immunol 83:845–852
30. Jarolim E, Tejkl M, Rohac M, et al. (1989) Monoclonal antibodies against birch pollen allergens: characterization by immunoblotting use for single-step affinity purification of the major allergen Bet v I. Int Arch Allergy Appl Immunol 90.54–61
31. King TP (1976) Chemical and biological properties of some atopic allergens. Adv Immunol 23:77
32. King TP (1990) T cell epitope of a vespid venom allergen Ag 5 (Abstr). J Allergy Clin Immunol 85:213

33. King TP, Kochoumian L, Joslyn A (1984) Mellitin-specific monoclonal and polyclonal IgE and IgG1 antibodies from mice. J Immunol 133:2668–2673
34. Ley V, Saiz JC, Carreira J (1986) Isolation and characterization of the main allergen of *Dermatophagoides farinae* by monoclonal antibodies that recognize IgE related epitopes. Mol Immunol 23:1311–1318
35. Lind P, Hansen OC, Horn N (1988) The binding of mouse hybridoma and human IgE to the major fecal allergen, Der p I, of *Dermatophagoides pteronyssinus:* relative binding site location and species specificity studies by solid-phase inhibition assays. J Immunol 140:4256–4262
36. Lind P, Horn N (1988) Extensive analogy between the epitope specificty of mouse hybridoma and human IgE response to *D. pteronyssinus* major allergen, Der p I. In: Todt A (ed) Mite allergy. UCB Institute of Allergy, Brussels, pp 30–34
37. Lind P, Lowenstein H (1988) Characterization of asthma-associated allergens. Baillieres Clin Immunol Allergy 2:67–89
38. Lowenstein H, Schou C (1990) Monoclonal antibodies to a synthetic peptide derived from Der f I and Der m I (Abstr). J Allergy Clin Immunol 85:278
39. Malley A (1989) Characterization of T- and B-cell epitopes of timothy grass pollen antigen B (AgB) (Abstr). Allergologie [Suppl] 12:33
40. Marsh DG, Milner FH, Johnson P (1966) The allergenic activity and stability of purified allergens from the pollen of common rye grass (*Lolium perenne).* Int Arch Allergy Appl Immunol 29:521–535
41. Marsh DG, Zwollo P, Huang SK, et al. (1989) Molecular genetics of human immune responsiveness to allergens. In: Chadwick D, et al. (eds) IgE, Mast cells and the allergic response. Wiley, Chichester, pp 171–187
42. Mazur G, Becker W-M, Baur X (1987) Epitope mapping of major insect allergens (chironomid hemoglobins) with monoclonal antibodies. J Allergy Clin Immunol 80:876–883
43. Mazur G, Baur X, Modrow S, Becker W-M (1988) A common epitope on major allergens from non-biting midges (Chironomidae). Mol Immunol 25:1005–1010
44. Mazur G, Steigemann W, Modrow S, et al. (1989) Chironomid allergens: location of B-cell and T-cell epitopes in the 3-D structure (Abstr). Allergologie [Suppl] 12:33
45. Mazur G, Baur X, Hoffmann H, Liebers V (1990) Chironomid allergens (Chi t I): identified and predicted B cell and T cell epitopes. J Allergy Clin Immunol 85:200
46. Mourad W, Mecheri S, Peltre G, David B, Hebert J (1988) Study of the epitope structure of purified Dac g I and Lol p I, the major allergens of *Dactylis glomerata* and *Lolium perenne* pollens, using monoclonal antibodies. J Immunol 141:3486–3491
47. O'Hehir RE, Lamb JR (1990) Immunomodulation of cellular responses to house dust mite using nonstimulatory peptides (Abstr). J Allergy Clin Immunol 85:200
48. O'Hehir RE, Young DB, Kay AB, Lamb JR (1987) Cloned human lymphocytes-T reactive with *Dermatophagoides farinae* (house dust mite) – a comparison of T-cell and B-cell antigen recognition. Immunology 82:635–640
49. O'Hehir RE, Echels DD, Frew AJ, et al. (1988) MHC class-II restriction specificity of cloned human lymphocytes-T reactive with *Dermatophagoides farinae* (house dust mite). Immunology 64:627–632
50. O'Hehir O, Young D, Kay AB, Lamb J (1989) Clonal analysis of the cellular immune response to the house dust mite *Dermatophagoides farinae.* Int Arch Allergy Appl Immunol 88:170–173
51. Olson JR, Klapper DG (1986) Two major human allergenic sites on ragweed pollen allergen antigen E identified by using monoclonal antibodies. J Immunol 136:2109–2115
52. Phillips L, Chambers C, Underwood BJ, et al. (1987) Lymphocyte proliferation to antigen E: demonstration of the restriction of antigen E-specific T-cells to ragweed-allergic donors. J Allergy Clin Immunol 79:933–940
53. Rothbardt JB (1989) Major histocompatibility complex-peptide interaction. Curr Opin Immunol 2:99–105
54. Swärd-Nordmo M, Paulsen BS, Wold JK (1989) Immunological studies of the glycoprotein allergen AG-54 (Cla h II) in *Cladosporium herbarum* with special attention to the carbohydrate and protein moieties. Int Arch Allergy Appl Immunol 90:155–162
55. Van Regenmortel MHV (1989) Structural and functional approaches to the study of protein antigenicity. Immunol Today 10:266–272

56. Von Grüningen R, Schneider CH (1989) Antigenic structure of the hexacosapeptide mellitin – evidence for three determinants with a helical conformation. Immunology 66:339–343
57. Weber A, Schröder H, Thalberg K et al. (1987) Specific interaction of IgE antibodies with a carbohydrate epitope form honey bee venom phospholipase A2. Allergy 42:464–470
58. Wheeler AW, Johansson SGO (1989) Demonstration of human, rye grass pollen extract-specific, helper and suppressor stimulating activities of modified allergens by effects on in vitro hapten-specific antibody production. Int Arch Allergy Appl Immunol 90:320–325

Cloning of Birch Pollen Allergens

H. Breiteneder[1], O. Scheiner[1], K. Pettenburger[1], R. Valenta[1], M. Tejkl[1], K. Hoffmann-Sommergruber[1], M. Duchêne[1], H. Rumpold[2], M. Breitenbach[3], and D. Kraft[1]

[1]Institute of General and Experimental Pathology, Neubau AKH, Erweiterungsbau Ost, Ebene 3, Währinger Gürtel 18–20, 1090 Vienna, Austria
[2]Institute of Clinical Chemistry and Laboratory Diagnostics, Lazarettgasse 14, 1090 Vienna, Austria
[3]Institute of Microbiology and Genetics, University of Vienna, Althanstrasse 14, 1090 Vienna, Austria

Abstract

Some 10%–15% of the population suffer from atopic diseases caused by environmental allergens, such as fecal particles from house dust mites, pollen, spores of molds, and dander from domestic animals. Pollen of the white birch (*Betula verrucosa*) is one of the main causes of IgE-mediated reactions in allergic patients. Bet v I, an allergenic protein with a molecular mass of 17 kDa, is a constituent of white birch pollen and is responsible for IgE binding in more than 95% of birch pollen allergic patients. A cDNA library was constructed from mRNA of mature birch pollen in the expression vector lambda gt11. The cDNA library was screened with IgE from a selected birch pollen allergic patient's serum for the expression of Bet v I. The nucleotide sequence of a complete cDNA clone coding for Bet v I was determined. The deduced amino acid sequence of Bet v I showed strong homologies with several pathogenesis related proteins from different plants. Furthermore, Bet v I was produced as a fusion and a nonfusion protein and the allergenicity of these proteins could be demonstrated by binding IgE from birch pollen allergic patients. The recombinant proteins may be used for better defined diagnosis and therapy and for experiments designed to investigate the regulation of the IgE response in atopic patients.

Introduction

Purified allergens are being used increasingly as well-defined tools for the diagnosis and individual therapy of allergic conditions. Studies of the molecular properties, in vitro reactions, and biological functions of these allergens will be the focus of this article.

Biochemical methods for the preparation of allergens (Table 1), with their well-known limitations (impurity of the samples; tedious preparation methods, which are time intensive and expensive; limitation in quantity of the purified allergen), are gradually losing importance compared to molecular cloning strategies. These more recent methods, which include cDNA cloning, sequence studies on the DNA and amino acid level, and expression of recombinant allergens, can provide us with much more insight and information and will help us to understand the mechanisms of allergic reactions.

Table 1. Methods for characterization and preparation of allergens.

Gel filtration
Ion exchange chromatography
CIE, CRIE
Immunoblotting
Monoclonal antibodies
cDNA cloning
Recombinant proteins
Synthetic peptides

CIE, crossed immunoelectrophoresis; CRIE, crossed radioimmunoelectrophoresis.

Table 2. Cloning of an allergen.

Selection of suitable tissues for RNA preparation
RNA isolation
Quality control of RNA
cDNA synthesis
Construction of an expression cDNA library
Screening of cDNA library with IgE from allergic patients
Sequencing of the inserts of the positive clones
Production of recombinant allergens

We have cloned and sequenced the single major allergen of white birch, *Betula verrucosa*, which has been designated Bet v I [1–3]. Therefore, this paper is based on the experience gained throughout this work. Table 2 shows one of the possible strategies that can lead to molecular cloning of an allergen. This strategy has a good chance of yielding complete clones, if the confirmation of the allergen is important for IgE binding. Genomic cloning may become more important with the advent of polymerase chain reaction (PCR) techniques. The resulting sequences may, however, contain introns and, as a consequence, the complete characterization of an allergen sequence would, on the whole, take longer with PCR than with cDNA methods.

Techniques for Allergen Cloning

RNA Isolation

One crucial point for the isolation of mRNA coding for plant allergens is the selection of tissues for mRNA preparation. In the case of Bet v I, tissue specific expression was observed. Pollen of *B. verrucosa* can be a source Bet v I mRNA, as can male inflorescences [4], although with a much smaller yield. Leaves, roots, and even callus tissue proved to be a bad choice because of the very low concentration of Bet v I mRNA. The mRNA can be of such low quantity (e.g., male inflorescences) that an in vitro translation system will yield just enough protein to be detected by immunoblotting. Therefore it was not possible to construct representative cDNA libraries from RNA of these tissues. As was first shown for *B. verrucosa*, pollen has proven to be by far the best source for allergen coding mRNA [1, 5]. For non-tree pollen it may still be necessary to devise an isolation method different from the one used for tree pollen.

It seems that non-RNA and non-protein materials, as we have found in pollen and inflorescences, form the largest obstacle in obtaining pure RNA. These compounds, which coprecipitate with the RNA, are difficult to separate from the nucleic acids. Sometimes, RNA can be purified by column chromatography. RNA from animal sources is much easier and quicker to isolate even in large quantities [6, 7]. Dog cDNA libraries are even commercially available.

It is advisable to control the quality of the isolated RNA before proceeding to the construction of the library. A Northern (RNA) blot probed with an oligodeoxynucleotide probe (constructed according to an N-terminal protein sequence of the allergen) can show whether a transcript of the gene is present in the RNA population isolated. However, if there is no sequence data, as is frequently the case, the mRNA can be translated in vitro and the synthesized proteins can be probed on a Western blot using serum IgE from patients allergic to the protein. A positive signal indicates the presence of mRNA coding for these specific allergens or parts of the proteins that contain IgE binding epitopes. If the epitopes are conformational in nature, a full length mRNA and cDNA coding for the whole protein are necessary [4, 5].

One problem associated with the wheat germ in vitro translation system is that grass pollen allergic patients may have IgE molecules that cross-react with proteins from the wheat system.

The Synthesis of cDNA

Standard methods of commercially available kits can be used to synthesize cDNAs. The mRNA should be as pure as possible because non-nucleic acid materials may inhibit reverse transcription. The cDNA synthesis can be monitored by the incorporation of ^{32}p-labeled deoxynucleotide triphosphates (dNTPs) into the nucleic acid or, simply, an aliquot of the reaction can be checked by electrophoresis on an agarose gel. Only cDNA that is visible on such gels and has sufficient length is appropriate for the construction of representative cDNA libraries.

Construction of cDNA Libraries

With the intention of immunological screening the method of choice had been the use of bacteriophage lambda gt11 [8] as a cloning vector [1, 6, 7, 9]. Now, a more recently developed lambda insertion vector, lambda ZAP II [10] (Stratagene, La Jolla, California) is being used with satisfying results. This vector allows the construction of unidirectional cDNA libraries, which are twice as likely to express fusion protein as libraries in which the cDNA is cloned in random orientation. This vector also allows convenient in vivo excision, to yield pBluescript

(Stratagene) plasmids containing the insert, without the need for subcloning of restriction fragments.

Both systems can be screened for the desired gene with sequence homologous nucleic acid probes (synthetic oligodeoxynucleotides, DNA, cDNA, RNA), but also according to antigenic properties of the expressed fusion proteins.

Screening cDNA Libraries

In standard procedures rabbit IgG raised against the desired antigen is used. However, for allergological purposes screening with IgE antibodies from allergic patients' sera is recommended. This method was successfully applied in screening for a major allergen of house dust mite, Der p II [11], and by us [1] using a single patient's serum carefully selected according to case history, RAST, skin prick test, and Western blot analyses. It is preferable to use sera from patients, whose IgE react with a single allergen on Western blots.

Lambda gt11, lambda ZAP II, or similar bacteriophage libraries can also be screened with oligonucleotides or riboprobes. These approaches will yield six times as many clones (two different orientations, three different reading frames). As a consequence the cDNA inserts obtained may not code for allergenic polypeptides of the protein. Thus, rescreening of the library with the partial clones found by the first screening of this library with oligonucleotides is a very good method for obtaining the full length clone. A problem encountered when screening with nucleic acid probes is the appearance of false positives. It is remarkable that, so far, this has never been the case when using IgEs for screening. In our experience riboprobes transcribed from the cDNA are prefered over synthetic oligodeoxynucleotides.

Sequencing

Direct sequencing is possible for lambda gt11 using lambda derived sequencing primers. However, to obtain unambiguous complete sequences, subcloning into suitable plasmids is often necessary. We subcloned the Bet v I cDNA insert from lambda gt11 into the pBluescript plasmid and sequenced both strands. The vector lambda ZAP II facilitates sequencing since subcloning is done in a single in vivo step.

Processing of Sequence Data

Computer aided predictions of epitopes on the surface of the molecule [12] are derived from the cDNA sequence and take into account such properties as hydrophilicity or hydrophobicity, charge, and flexibility of a certain part of the molecule (Fig. 1). According to the protein sequence obtained, overlapping oligopeptides can be synthesized and used to study the ability to bind IgE and monoclonal antibodies (Figs. 2 and 3). The results can then be correlated with the

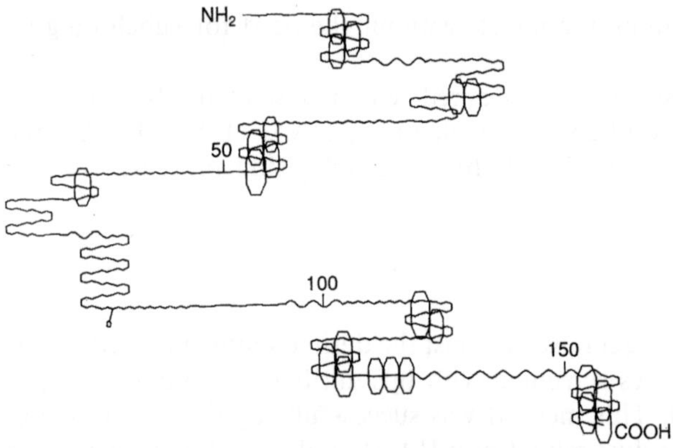

Fig. 1. Computer aided prediction of molecular characteristics of Bet v 1 following the method of Garnier, Osguthorpe, and Robson [12]. Putative epitopes have been calculated and have been marked by circles

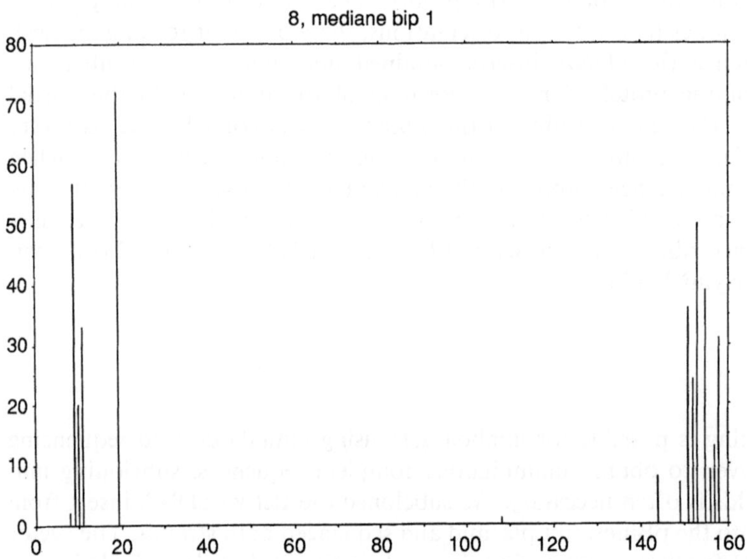

Fig. 2. Epitope mapping using overlapping octapeptides in an enzyme-linked immunoassay (ELISA) with horse radish peroxidase conjugated anti-immunoglobin antisera and 2,2′-azinobis(3-ethylbenzthiazoline sulfonic acid) as a substrate. Overlapping synthetic oligopeptides (1–160) spanning the whole Bet v I sequence were tested for their ability to bind the monoclonal antibody Bip 1 [21]. The results have been plotted as optical densities at 405 nm against the last residue in the octapeptide

computer predictions. Synthetic peptides can also be used for further studies of the antigenicity and allergenicity of certain regions of the molecule under investigation.

Computer aided sequence comparisons may also be able to provide some information about the biological functions of the protein. If the protein in question

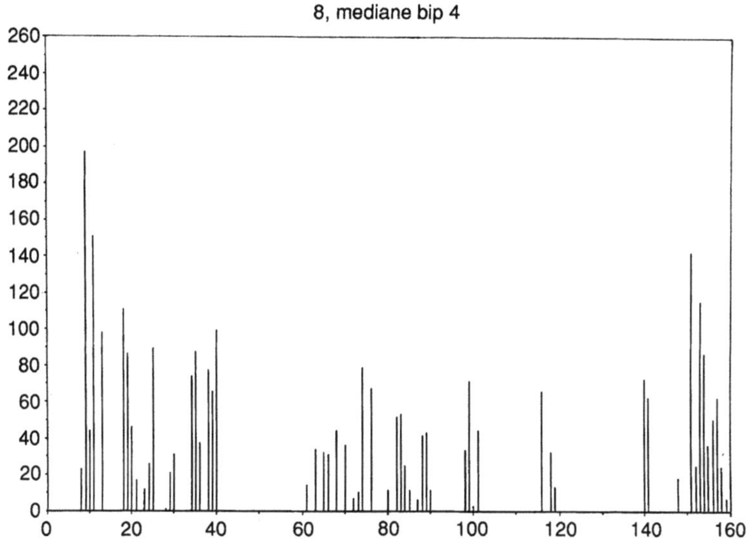

Fig. 3. Identical epitope mapping experiments were performed using the monoclonal antibody Bip 4 [22]. For details see Fig.2

shows a high homology to a protein with a known biological function, it is likely that the allergen possesses a similar function [13].

In the case of Bet v I a high homology to pathogenesis related proteins of pea [14], parsley [15], and potato [16], encoded by disease resistance response genes, was found (Fig. 4). It is tempting to speculate that Bet v I fulfills a similar function in birch and some data corroborate this view [4].

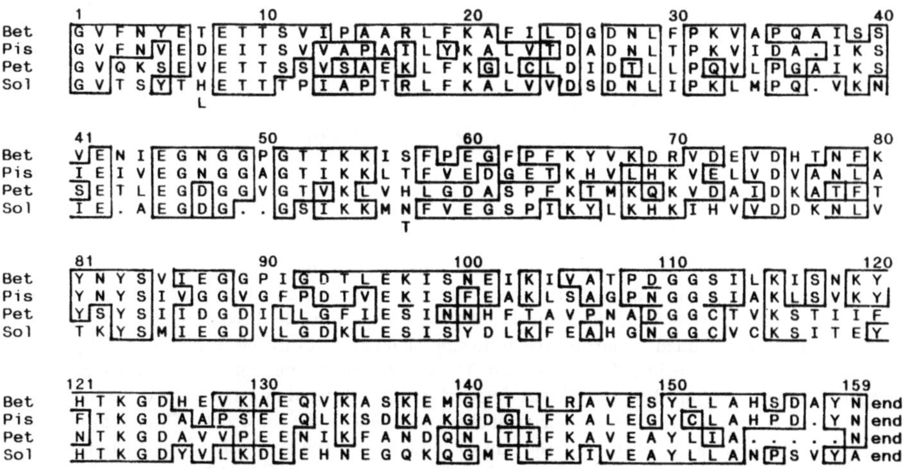

Fig. 4. Sequence comparison of Bet v I to the disease resistance response genes of pea (*Pis*), parsley (*Pet*), and potato (*Sol*). Boxes indicate identical amino acids

In Vitro Expression

To study possible applications of recombinant allergens in diagnosis and therapy and to study the mechanisms of IgE regulation in in vitro systems, large amounts of recombinant protein are needed (Table 3).

Several prokaryotic and eukaryotic systems can be used for the expression of the desired protein. It is advisable to try several approaches, since no information about the suitability of expression systems for allergological purposes is yet available. The protein under investigation can be synthesized as a fusion [17] or a non-fusion protein [18]. The fusion part of the protein will impart additional characteristics to the molecule. One problem may be the low solubility of the fusion proteins, which may lead to other problems such as a low yield. Therefore, the additional sequence should be kept as small as possible (Fig.5). If one omits the fusion part altogether, a non-fusion protein is produced which may be synthesized with less efficiency than a fusion protein.

Table 3. Use of recombinant allergens in diagnosis and therapy.

Availability of pure allergens and IgE binding proteins
Standardization of allergen extracts
Prevention of loss of unstable proteins
Production of patient-tailored allergen mixtures
Hapten inhibition therapy with synthetic peptides

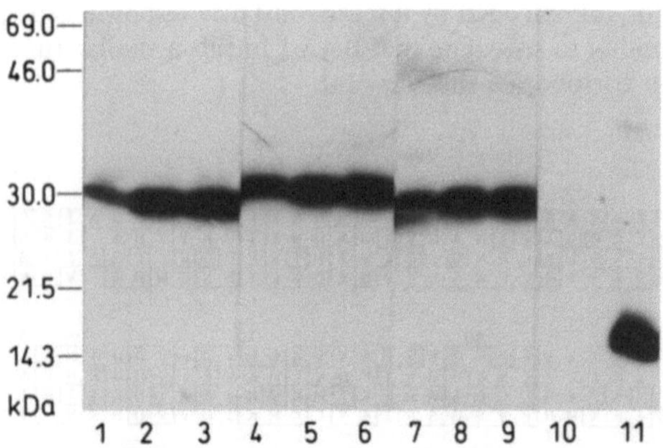

Fig. 5. Immunoblot analysis of three MS2 polymerase – Bet v I fusion protein constructs. A factor Xa cleavage site was added in frame at the 5′-end of the Bet v I coding region to facilitate the production of pure Bet v I. Upstream the sequence that codes for the Xa cleavage site; three different oligonucleotides were added imparting the following characteristics to the resulting fusion protein: *lane 1–3* basic; *lane 4–6* acidic; *lane 7–9* polar. The Western blots were probed with human IgE from an allergic patient's serum. Bound IgE was detected with ^{125}I-labeled anti-IgE. The different migratory rates may be due to the different electrical charges carried by the constructs. Three samples each were taken after 60 min, 120 min, and 180 min of induction of the synthesis of the fusion protein. *Lane 10*, the negative control, contains a protein extract from the *E. coli* host bacterium, which does not harbor the expression plasmid; *lane 11*, the positive control, contains an aqueous protein extract of birch pollen; here, the 17 kDa Bet v I band reacted strongly

Eukaryotic expression systems, such as the Chinese hamster ovarian cell system [19] and the baculovirus system [20], are much more complex and their maintenance is time consuming. Information about their use for expression of allergen molecules is very limited as their application is new in the field of allergen research.

Discussion

Standardized allergen mixtures for diagnosis and therapy have been used for several years with results which are acceptable within limits. However, it remains unsatisfying to work with extracts with undefined components, expecially when minor allergens, non-allergenic proteins, and non-protein materials are concerned. The effects of these on the immune system and on the outcome of the hyposensitization therapy are still unknown.

Well-defined and highly purified proteins seem to be the better choice. Their production by conventional biochemical methods is too expensive, time consuming, and may not be possible at all when an allergen of 100% purity is required. Recombinant DNA technologies may offer a solution to these problems and provide large quantities of the desired end product. In the near future the most important major and minor allergens will be cloned. This will allow the production of well-defined allergens for diagnostic purposes and, in the more distant future, the production of patient tailored allergen mixtures for use in hyposensitization treatments. Furthermore, the more information about allergens that is gathered, the sooner we shall be able to find out about the biological function of these allergens in plants. In the case of Der p II [13] and Bet v I [1] several interesting results have already been obtained.

More knowledge about the molecular and biological characteristics of allergens will result in a better understanding of their role in the origin and maintenance of allergies in humans. Furthermore, recombinant allergens will facilitate in vitro studies of IgE regulation.

References

1. Breiteneder H, Pettenburger K, Bito A, Valenta R, Kraft D, Rumpold H, Schreiner O, Breitenbach M (1989) The gene coding for the major birch pollen allergen Bet v I is highly homologous to a pea disease resistance response gene. EMBO J 8(7):1935–1938
2. Ipsen H, Løwenstein H (1983) Isolation and immunochemical characterization of the major allergen of birch pollen (*Betula verrucosa*). J Allergy Clin Immunol 72:150–159
3. Jarolim E, Rumpold H, Endler A, Ebner H, Breitenbach M, Scheiner O, Kraft D (1989) IgE and IgG antibodies of patients with allergy to birch pollen as tools to define the allergen profile of *Betula verrucosa*. Allergy 44:385–395
4. Pettenburger K, Breiteneder H, Valenta R, Kraft D, Rumpold H, Breitenbach N, Scheiner O (1989) Distribution of allergens and mRNAs coding for allergens isolated from various tissues of white birch. In: Sehon H, Kraft D, Kunkel G (eds) Epitopes of atopic allergens. UCB, Brussels, pp 65–68

5. Breiteneder H, Hassfeld W, Pettenburger K, Jarolim E, Breitenbach M, Rumpold H, Kraft D, Scheiner O (1988) Isolation and characterization of mRNA from male inflorescences and pollen of white birch (*Betula verrucosa*). Int Arch Allergy Appl Immunol 87:19–24
6. Thomas WR, Stewart GA, Simpson RJ, Chua KY, Plozza TM, Dilworth RJ, Nisbet A, Turner KJ (1988) Cloning and expression of DNA for the major house dust mite alleren Der p I in *Escherichia coli.* Int Arch Allergy Appl Immunol 85:127–129
7. Fang KSY, Vitale M, Fehlner P, King TP (1988) cDNA cloning and primary structure of a white-face hornet venom allergen, antigen 5. Proc Natl Acad Sci USA 85:895–899
8. Huynh TV, Young RA, Davis RW (1986) Constructing and screening cDNA libraries in lambda gt10 and lambda gt11. In: Glover DM (ed) Cloning vol 1. A practical approach. IRL, Oxford, pp 48–78
9. Walsh DJ, Matthews JA, Denmeade R, Walker MR (1989) Cloning of cDNA coding for an allergen of cocksfoot grass (*Dactylis glomerata*) pollen. Int Arch Allergy Appl Immunol 90:78–83
10. Short JM, Fernandez JM, Sorge JA, Huse WD (1988) Lambda ZAP: a bacteriophage lambda expression vector with in vivo excision properties. Nucleic Acids Res 16:7583–7600
11. Chua KY, Doyle CR, Simpson RJ, Turner KJ, Stewart GA, Thomas WR (1990) Isolation of cDNA coding for the major mite allergen Der p II by IgE plaque immunoassay. Int Arch Allergy Appl Immunol 91:118–123
12. Garnier J, Osguthorpe OJ, Robson B (1978) Analysis of the accuracy and implications of simple methods for predicting the secondary structure of globular proteins. J Mol Biol 120:97–120
13. Chua KY, Stewart GA, Thomas WR, Simpson RJ, Dilworth RJ, Plozza TM, Turner KS (1988) Sequence analysis of cDNA coding for a major house dust mite allergen Der p I. Homology with cysteine proteases. J Exp Med 167:175–182
14. Fristensky B, Horovitz D, Hadwiger LA (1988) cDNA sequence for pea disease resistance response genes. Plant Mol Biol 11:713–715
15. Somssich IE, Schmelzer E, Kawalleck P, Hahlbrock K (1988) Gene structure and in situ transcript localisation of pathogenesis-related protein 1 in parsley. Mol Gen Genet 213:93–98
16. Taylor JL, Fritzemeier KH, Häuser I, Kombrink E, Rohwer F, Schröder M, Strittmatter G, Hahlbrock K (1990) Structural analysis and activation by fungal infection of a gene encoding pathogenesis-related protein in potato. Mol Plant Microbe Interact 3 (2):72–77
17. Nagai K, Thøgersen HC (1984) Generation of β-globin by sequence-specific proteolysis of a hybrid protein produced in *Escherichia coli.* Nature 309:810–812
18. Amann E, Brosius J (1985) ATG vectors for regulated high-level expression of cloned genes in *Escherichia coli.* Gene 40:183–190
19. Uchibayashi N, Kikutani H, Barsumian EL, Hauptmann R, Schneider F-J, Schwendenwein R, Sommergruber W, Spevak W, Maurer-Fogy I, Suemura M, Kishimoto T (1989) Recombinant soluble Fcε-receptor II (FcεRII/CD23) has IgE binding activity but no B-cell growth promoting activity. J Immunol 142:3901–3908
20. Miller LK (1988) Baculoviruses as gene expression vectors. Annu Rev Microbiol 42:177–199

Molecular Structure of Allergens

X. Baur[1], G. Mazur[2], and V. Liebers[1]

[1] Berufsgenossenschaftliches Forschungsinstitut für Arbeitsmedizin (BGFA), Ruhr-Universität Bochum, Gilsingstrasse 14, W-4630 Bochum 1, Federal Republic of Germany
[2] Pneumologische Abteilung, Medizinische Klinik I, Klinikum Grosshadern, Universität München, W-8000 München 70, Federal Republic of Germany

Abstract

Inhalant allergens attack people in natural, domestic and occupational environments and consist of protein or glycoprotein mixtures, highly purified proteins (MW 5000–80000 Daltons) or low-molecular-weight chemicals. Sensitized subjects develop hypersensitivity reactions to the exposure to extremely low doses.

For Chi t I component III, an aggressive inhalant insect allergen with known primary and tertiary structures, we studied antigen-antibody interactions (IgE, IgG, mAB) as well as immunogenicity. We mapped Chi t I component III with natural and synthetic peptides and identified B and T-cell epitopes.

Using a computer display of the 3-D coordinates we localized and verified B- and T-cell epitopes in the tertiary structure.

The B-cell epitope position 1–15 is found at the N-terminal end of the molecule at the beginning of helix A. Epitope 91–101 is located between helices F and G and at the beginning of helix G. Epitope 110–135 is between helices G and H and in helix H.

A good agreement between the secondary structure elements (helices and turns) and the thermal mobility profile with the functional properties of the peptides was found.

We also applied T-cell epitope prediction methods to state T-helper sites on Chi t I component III. The capacity of tryptic and synthetic peptides to stimulate peripheral blood lymphocytes corresponds well with regions of high alpha amphipathic score (Berzofsky et al.) and/or the sequence motif according to Rothbard and Taylor.

Furthermore, we studied the immunoresponse to Chi t I allergen on a genetic basis. The HLA-DRB and -DQB genes were studied in 181 Chi t I-exposed persons of whom 58 showed IgE-mediated sensitization. We used the PCR and hybridisation with 25 sequence specific oligonucleotides to study hypervariable regions of the second exons of DRB genes and DQB genes. DQw1.1 was shown to correlate with the immunoresponse of Chi t I whereas DQw3 was negatively associated with this hyperreactivity. These associations are significant in non-atopic responders. Our results suggest a different mechanism in the immunoresponse of non-atopic and atopic subjects.

Due to new techniques in molecular genetics and protein chemistry, the primary structures of an increasing number of clinically relevant allergens have been de-

Table 1. Highly purified and (partially) characterized allergens.

Source	Allergen
Pollen	Amb a I, III, V, VI, VII, VIII; Amb t I, II; Art v I; Aln i I; Lol p I, II, III, V; Iun s I
Molds	Alt a I; Asp f I; Cla h I, II
Mites	Der p I, II; Der f I
Animal	Fel d I; Chi t I; Bla g I; Gad c I

scribed in recent years. Among them are components of pollen, molds, mites, and animal dander (Table 1). Immunogens inducing type I immune responses show particular structural properties. Their molecular weight (MW) is limited to a small range; approximately 90% of them have a MW of 10–30 kDa. Furthermore, all of them are proteins or glycoproteins. Up to now, few data exist, however, on the 3-D structures of allergens.

Primary and Tertiary Structures of the Chironomid Allergen Chi t I (component III)

An exception is the insect hemoglobin Chi t I. Its component III is the first allergen whose 3-D structure is fully known. Steigemann and Weber, from the Max Planck Institute of Biochemistry, Martinsried, FRG, performed X-ray analysis at a resolution of 1.4 angstroms [5]. Surprisingly, in spite of the enormous evolutionary distance, the tertiary structure is similar to those of vertebrate hemoglobins and myoglobins. Component III is folded into eight helical segments, with the heme group contained within a hydrophobic pocket between helices E and F. In contrast to the congruence in the tertiary structure, the amino acid sequence of Chi t I component III is quite different from that of vertebrate hemoglobins.

Analysis of B Cell Epitopes

Regarding the molecular location of *antigenic* determinants in globular proteins, it has been established that the entire surface of a protein is composed of potential antigenic epitopes [6]. Little is known, however, about the molecular location of *allergenic* determinants recognized by human IgE antibodies. Therefore, we analyzed Chi t I component III using known primary and tertiary structural probes [5] to determine the locations of allergenic epitopes in the native molecule.

By chemical and enzymatic cleavages we generated peptides of different lengths. These were isolated, identified, solid phase bound, and investigated for their IgE binding capacity. Together with Wolfgang Steigemann from the Max

Planck Institute of Biochemistry we looked at the location of the experimentally determined allergenic determinants in the 3-D structure of the molecule.

Strategy of Peptide Generation

Chemical Methods. Chemical cleavage breaks the protein next to uncommon amino acid residues so that long fragments are obtained. By cleavage of Chi t I component III with cyanogen bromide at methionine we obtained four peptides: residues 1–35, 36–108, 109–131, and 132–136. After separation by liquid chromatography and identification by Edman degradation, solid phase bound peptides were investigated with the IgE-RAST method using human anti-Chi t I sera. Three IgE binding peptides were obtained (Fig. 1). One, residues 109–131, was further cleaved at tryptophan using iodobenzoic acid. The IgE binding capacity of peptide 109–121 remained at nearly 100%, whereas it was fully lost in peptide 122–131.

Protease Treatment. In order to identify the length of the allergenic epitopes we generated shorter peptides. Therefore, with specific cleavages at arginine and lysine we obtained ten peptides with a minimal length of seven amino acid residues (Fig. 1). The peptides were separated by reverse phase high-performance liquid chromatography, identified by amino acid analysis, and solid phase bound. Three peptides were obtained, residues 1–15, 91–101, 110–135, which bound to human anti-Chi t I IgE antibodies (Fig. 1). Using this protease treatment, we are able to identify relatively short allergenic epitopes with a length of 11, 13, and 25 amino acid residues.

Application of Synthetic Peptides. Our next intention was to look for further overlapping peptides in order to find additional epitopes which may be cleaved by protease treatment. We applied synthetic peptides in the same experimental manner as described for natural peptides. To date, three synthetic peptides have been analyzed by the IgE-RAST method. Only peptide 91–101 bound to human IgE antibodies (Fig. 1). This approach enabled us to verify results obtained by the analysis of natural peptides.

Synthetic peptide 91–101 is not only recognized by human IgE but also by rabbit IgG and mouse subclass IgG1 monoclonal antibodies [3]. In inhibition

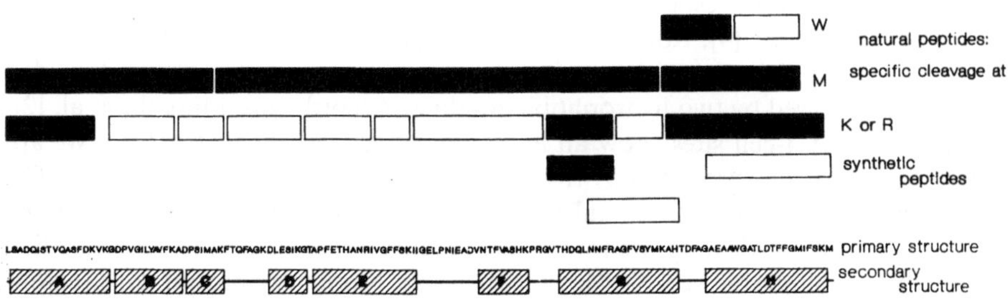

Fig. 1. B-cell analysis of Chi t I component III

studies, we found that human IgE antibodies and monoclonal antibodies show reciprocal inhibition indicating that they bind to the same epitope. Extensive studies with two monoclonal antibodies among 33 different chironomid species demonstrate the presence of this B-cell epitope in nearly all of the related species of the genera *Chironomus* and *Glyptotendipes* [1].

Comparing the identified B-cell epitopes of Chi t I component III with predictions for antigenic sites according to the UWGCG program (antigenic index) [7] agreement in several regions is seen. However, discrepancies exist, especially at the N-terminal site.

Location of B-Cell Epitopes in the 3-D Structure

We compared the location of the experimentally determined allergenic epitopes with the surface location, accessibility, and flexibility of these regions in the whole molecule [3]. Based on the computer display of the 3-D structure of component III, we found the allergenic peptides 1–15, 91–101, 109–121, and 110–135 were located on the surface and thus accessible to other molecules, with a flexible backbone for site specific adaptation and hydrophilic amino acids for contacts to other molecules such as antibodies. Regarding our results on the B-cell epitope analysis of component III we can conclude that allergenic epitopes fulfill the same criteria as postulated for antigenic determinants.

Analysis of T-Cell Epitopes

To demonstrate the immunogenicity of Chi t I component III at the T-cell level, we stimulated peripheral blood lymphocytes (PBL) in vitro. The stimulation indices (SI) of PBL were determined by [^{3}H] thymidine uptake. We examined allergen-exposed patients and non-exposed controls. The SI of patients ranged from 5 to 60, whereas nonexposed controls showed no reactivity ($SI \leq 5$).

It could be demonstrated that most of the investigated peptides contain T-cell epitopes relevant at least for some patients. One of these peptides, residues 98–111, was synthesized and studied in detail. In the 3-D structure it is located in the G helix. It exhibits regions with a relatively low flexibility of the main chain and side chain atoms, especially in residues 103–106. This epitope corresponds to a Rothbard motif [4]. Rothbard and Taylor [4] analyzed the primary structure of known T-cell epitopes and described a common sequence: A charged residue or glycine followed by two hydrophobic residues. According to Margalit et al. [2], the majority of T-cell sites show an amphipathic alpha helical structure. We applied the algorithms proposed by these two groups to Chi t I component III. The results are given in Fig. 2. By calculating the amphipathicity with overlapping blocks 11 amino acids long, we found seven regions with an alpha helix periodicity and an amphipathic score of higher than ten. Similarly, we found 12 regions in component III that agree with the Rothbard motif, including residues 103–106

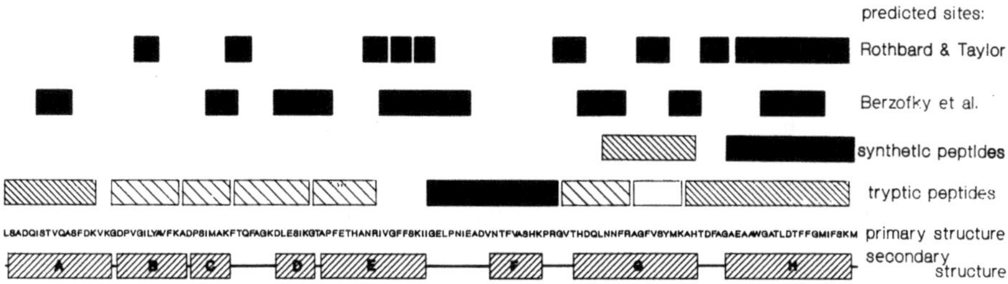

Fig. 2. Predicted T cell epitopes of Chi t I component III according to Rothbard and Berzofsky. Identified epitopes by using synthetic as well as tryptic peptides are shown in line three and four. The percentage of patients reacting to the individual peptide in the lymphocyte transformation test is indicated by the following symbols: ☐ 0%, ▧ 1–40%, ▨ 40–80%, ■ 80–100%

(Gly-Phe-Val-Ser). The latter amino acid sequence is part of a longer peptide which functions well as a T cell epitope (residues 98–111).

Genetic Basis of Immediate Type Hypersensitivity

The immune response to foreign antigens is genetically restricted due to the different structures of MHC class II molecules, which are important for the presentation of immunogenic peptides. HLA-D subtyping of 61 sensitized patients and 128 exposed healthy controls showed that the immune response to Chi t I in nonatopics is positively correlated with DR1 and DQw1.1. Furthermore, there exists a negative association in this group with DRw52a and DQw3.

Concluding Remarks

Algorithm prediction of antigenic B cell and T cell sites is helpful in identifying clinically important epitopes; however, false positive and negative predictions have to be taken into consideration. With respect to the results obtained with Chi t I component III, further investigations are necessary. It would be useful to map this allergen for B cell and T cell epitopes with a panel of overlapping peptides spanning the entire molecule. Thus far, we have analyzed several synthetic peptides and a naturally derived set of relatively small peptides. Therefore, our results may be restricted to continuous epitopes, which are composed of amino acid residues localized in the protein sequence. In contrast, assembled topographic B cell epitopes consist of amino acid residues that are brought together by the folding of the protein into its native structure.

Further, important questions include the structural relationships between individually recognized T cell epitopes, HLA-D coded polymorphic domains of surface molecules, and the hypervariable regions of T cell receptors.

References

1. Baur X, Mazur G, Becker W-M, Kagen SL, Kawai K (1990) Hemoglobin-related immunological cross-reactivity in the diptera family *Chironomidae* demonstrated with human midge- and larval-specific IgE, rabbit hyperimmune sera and monoclonal antibodies. Allergy (in press)
2. Margalit H, Spouge JL, Cornette JL, Cease KB, Delisis C, Berzofski JA (1988) Prediction of immunodominant helper T cell antigenic sites from the primary sequence. J Immunol 7:93–100
3. Mazur G, Baur X, Liebers V (1990) Hypersensitivity to hemoglobins of the diptera family *Chironomidae*: structural and functional studies of their immunogenic/allergenic sites. Monogr Allergy 28(6):121–137
4. Rothbard JB, Taylor RA (1988) A sequence pattern common to T cell epitopes. EMBO J 7:93–100
5. Steigemann W, Weber E (1979) Structure of erythrocruorin in different ligand states refined at 1.4 Å resolution. J Mol Biol 127:309–338
6. Van Regenmortel MHV (1988) Structural and functional approaches to the study of protein antigenicity. Immunol Today 10(8):266–271
7. Wolf H, Modrow S, Motz M, Jameson BA, Hermann G, Förtsch B (1989) An integrated family of amino acid sequence analysis programs. Cabios 4: 1987–1991

Characterization of Antigens and Allergens of Bird Feathers and Bird Sera

I. Tauer[1], G. Fruhmann[1], and X. Baur[2]

[1]Abteilung für Pneumologie, Medizinische Klinik I, Klinikum Grosshadern, Ludwig-Maximilians-Universität, Marchioninistrasse 15, W-8000 München 70, Federal Republic of Germany
[2]Berufsgenossenschaftliches Forschungsinstitut für Arbeitsmedizin, Abteilung für Pneumologie und Allergologie, Ruhr-Universität, Gilsingstrasse 14, W-4630 Bochum 1, Federal Republic of Germany

Introduction

Until now, it was widely believed that bird droppings and bird sera were the most responsible antigenic components causing asthma or allergic alveolitis in conjunction with contact. However, more recent information obtained from patients also implicates bloom, a component of the feathers that causes, for example, severe dyspnea in susceptible individuals after visiting bird exhibitions. In these cases there is insignificant contact with droppings or sera. The aim of our investigation was to identify and characterize allergens and antigens from sera and especially from bird feathers.

Methods and Patients

The methods used were double immunodiffusion, crossed immunoelectrophoresis (CIE), IgG RAST, IgE RAST, and immunoblot following SDS-PAGE [1]. The components from serum and feather extracts of various bird species were separated according to their molecular mass with a 10% SDS-PAGE. These fractions were transferred to a nitrocellulose sheet and incubated with bird fancier sera. The individual antigen-antibody reactions of each patient were detected by autoradiography using radiolabeled protein A.

The antigens were from extracts of feathers and sera of budgerigar, parrots, canaries, hens, and pigeons.

The sera used were from 16 patients sensitized to birds: 5 suffering from bronchial asthma and 11 with allergic alveolitis; both groups were clinically sensitized to birds. Furthermore, we used antisera raised in rabbits against the heavy chains of hen IgG, IgA, and IgM.

Results

The major antigens of sera and feather proteins were found to have molecular masses of about 21 – 31 kDa and 67 – 70 kDa. About eight antigenic components binding to human IgE and IgG, from patients with bronchial asthma, were identified in feather extracts and to a lesser extent also in bird sera.

In most cases the same antigenic components were detected by the sera of the 11 patients suffering from allergic alveolitis due to contact with birds [2]. However, allergic alveolitis patients did not demonstrate bird specific IgE. Immunological cross-reactivity was shown between allergens and antigens of all tested bird species (also in patients without contact to all species). Additional examinations with IgE and IgG RAST, double immunodiffusion, and CIE confirmed such cross-reactivity.

An accessory immunoblot study evaluated to what extent bird immunoglobulins act as antigens. The immunoblot tests were modified to use antisera raised in rabbits against the heavy chains of hen IgG, IgA, and IgM, instead of sera from patients. Cross-reacting antigens with the three sera (anti-IgG, -IgA, and -IgM) were identified in all bird sera. By contrast, the different feather extracts reacted preferably with anti-IgA and to a lesser extent with anti-IgM.

Conclusion

The immunoblot studies showed that there are a variety of antigenic components not only in bird sera, but also in bird feathers.

The molecular masses of major bird allergens and antigens are in the ranges of 21 – 30 kDa and 67 – 70 kDa. Immunological cross-reactivity existed between allergens and antigens of all tested bird species. Sera of asthmatic patients showed bird specific IgE and IgG, whereas sera of allergic alveolitis patients exclusively contained IgG.

IgE and IgG of patients with asthma or allergic alveolitis reacted more intensive with antigens of bird feathers than with those of bird sera. Bird IgA is a relevant or cross-reacting allergen and antigen for bird fanciers suffering from asthma or allergic alveolitis.

References

1. Baur X (1987) Asthma, Alveolitis, Aspergillose. Springer, Berlin Heidelberg New York
2. Tauer I, Baur X, Fruhmann G, Sennekamp J, Kösters J (1989) Ursächliche Antigene der Vogelhalterlunge. Atemwegs- und Lungenkrankheiten. Z Diagn Ther 6:226 – 227

Hop Allergy: Cross-Reactivity to Birch Pollen

C. M. Kalveram[1], C. Cronemeyer[2], and K. J. Kalveram[3]

[1] Küperweg 8, W-4400 Münster, Federal Republic of Germany
[2] Schlossstrasse 9, W-4500 Osnabrück, Federal Republic of Germany
[3] Hautklinik, Universität Münster, von-Esmarch-Strasse 56, W-4400 Münster, Federal Republic of Germany

Introduction

Allergy against many substances may be caused by multiple sensitizations against different allergens. However, a patient is often sensitized by one kind of allergen, especially pollen, and in the course of time reveals symptoms when coming into contact with material of quite another origin. For example, weed sensitized patients react to spices [1–6], bird serum allergic individuals do not tolerate eggs either as food or as part of a vaccine, birch pollen allergics have clinical symptoms when eating apples or nuts [2]. This "cross-reactivity of allergens" is well known and such patients have to be aware of possible additional allergens in their environment. Such cross-reactivities can be demonstrated in vitro by the RAST inhibition method [3, 4]

We now want to point out a new allergen for birch pollen allergics, hop, a main ingredient of beer and thus also a substance of importance for many western countries. Hop is a member of the botanic family *cannabiceae/urticales*, to which cannabis also belongs. Botanic relatives are elm, fig, nettle, and the rubber plant.

Case History

A 44 year old man with birch pollen allergy and corresponding symptoms in the early months of the year, stated that his health worsened when drinking beer. Small amounts of beer produced swelling of the nasal mucosa, wheezing, and symptoms of illness. These effects were produced by different brands of beer and thus could only be related to one of the main ingredients of beer, which according to the *German Reinheitsgebot* only be malt (barley), hop, yeast, and water (Fig. 1).

Materials and Methods

Skin tests were performed with commercially available materials, i.e., birch pollen, malt, yeast, hop, elm, and fig (Beecham-Wülfing, Bencard Allergie Dienst, Neuss,

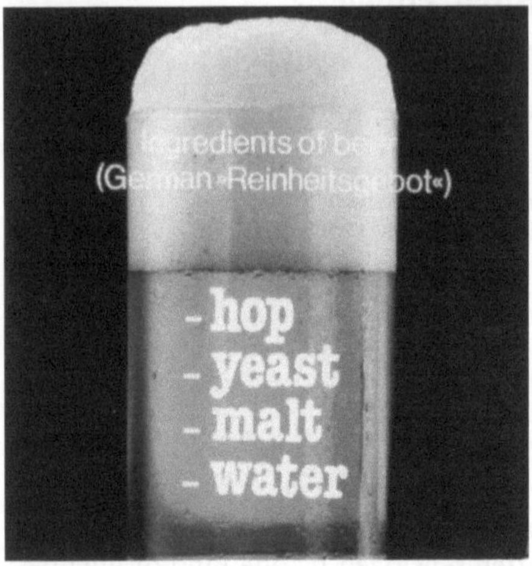

Fig. 1. Ingredients of German beer

FRG) and native substances as scratch and rub test. In vitro investigations (RAST as RIA and ELISA, RAST inhibition, and basophilic degranulation test [5] were done using identical allergens.

Results

Skin tests (Figs. 2 and 3) showed positive reactions to birch pollen and hop, not to malt and yeast. This was confirmed by RAST (Table 1) and basophilic

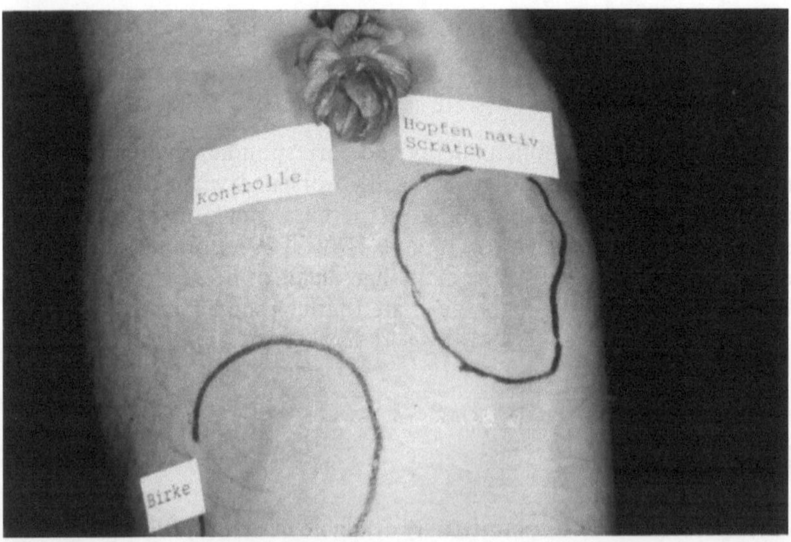

Fig. 2. Scratch test with birch pollen and hop

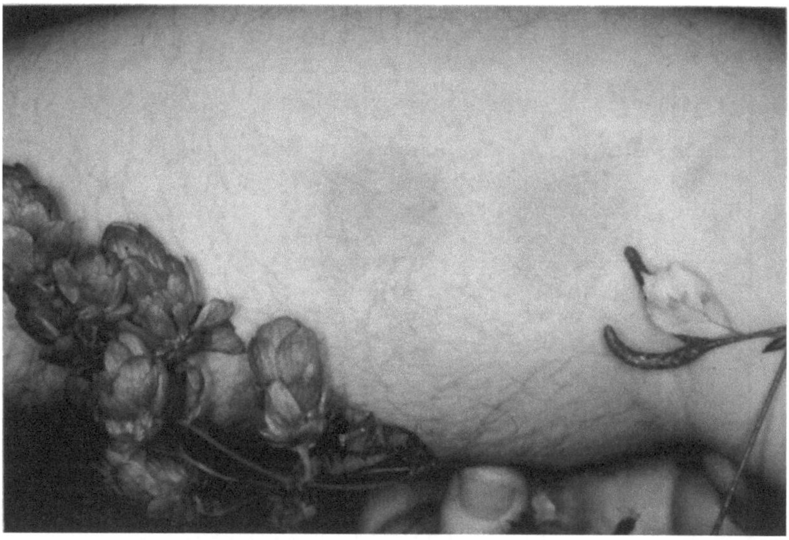

Fig. 3. Rub test with native hop pollen

Table 1. RAST (ELISA) with ingredients of beer and birch pollen.

Allergen	Score
Birch	4
Hop	3
Yeast	0
Malt	0

Table 2. Basophilic degranulation test with ingredients of beer and two brands of German beer.

Allergen	Degranulation index (%)
Malt (prick test)	18.0
Hop (native)	93.9
Veltins brand beer	92.5
DAB brand beer	95.9
Yeast	57.7

Degranulation index = $(B_0 - B_x)B_0 \times 100$.
B_0, control intact basophils; B_x, test intact basophils.

degranulation tests (Table 2), which were positive (more than 50% degranulation compared to controls) to birch, hop, and two kinds of German beer, but not to malt and yeast (borderline positive). Analogous results were achieved in a second patient. Tests with serum of control persons remained negative.

RAST inhibition methods (both, RIA and Elisa methods) with birch pollen by birch pollen (self inhibition) proved the specificity. The birch pollen RAST

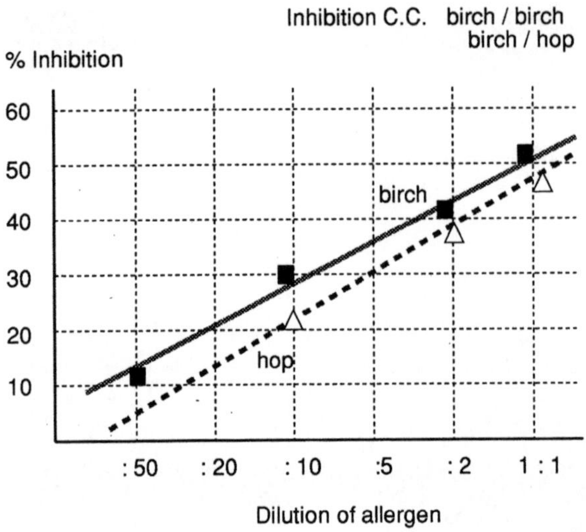

Fig. 4. Birch pollen self inhibition and RAST inhibition of birch by hop

could be inhibited by apple and hop but not by elm, fig, or other plants botanically related to yeast and malt, the other ingredients of beer (we did not test water!).

The inhibition of birch by hop (Fig. 4) was nearly as strong as the self inhibition of birch. Inhibition experiments with a serum pool of birch pollen allergic patients were negative, but we could detect three other people with sensitization and a clinical history of allergy to hop and birch.

Analogous responses could be detected by crossed immunoelectrophoresis using hop extract an anti-birch antibodies (ALK, Kopenhagen).

Discussion

Cross reactivity of birch pollen to other botanically unrelated food stuffs, such as apples and nuts, is well-known. We detected a partial cross-reactivity between birch pollen and hop.

Hop is not only a main ingredient of beer, a popular drink in Germany and many other countries, but also an important part of folk medicine and phytotherapeutics.

This sensitization could be confirmed in birch pollen allergic individuals in vivo and in vitro. Birch pollen allergic patients with hitherto unexplainable complaints outside the pollen season should be advised by their doctor of cross reactivities not only to apples or nuts, but to hop, too.

Immunoblot experiments using serum samples from such patients will reveal the common antigenic determinants. It may even be that there are more of these mutual sensitizations to birch pollen than we know of today

References

1. Dietschi R, Wüthrich B, Johansson SGO (1985) Zum sogenannten „Sellerie-Karotten-Beifuß-Gewürz-Syndrom". RAST-Untersuchungen mit neuen Gewürz-discs. Z Hautkr 62:524
2. Halmepuro L, Vuentela K, Kalimo K, Björksten F (1984) Cross-reactivity of IgE antibodies with allergens in birch pollen, fruits and vegetables. Int Arch Allergy Appl Immunol 74:235
3. Kalveram KJ, Forck G (1979) Cross-reactivity between grass and corn pollen antigens. Int Arch Allergy Appl Immunol 57:549
4. Kalveram KJ, Forck G (1979) RAST-Inhibitions-Test: Bestimmung von Antigenverwandtschaft und Antigenpotenz. Z Hautkr 54:197
5. Sennekamp HJ (1990) Allergologie
6. Thiel C (1988) Nahrungsmittelallergien bei Pollenallergikern (sogenannte pollenassoziierte Nahrungsmittelallergien. Allergologie 10:397

Immunoglobulin E Response

Possible Approaches to Controlling the IgE Antibody Response*

K. Ishizaka

La Jolla Institute for Allergy and Immunology, 11149 N. Torrey Pines RD., La Jolla, CA 92037, USA

Abstract

It is clear that IL-4 induces the switching of resting B cells to the precursors of IgE-forming cells, and that IFN_γ counteracted with IL-4 in the process. Indeed, anti-IL-4 and IFN_γ inhibited the IgE formation both in vitro and in vivo. However, the quantity of the antibody or IFN_γ required for the suppression of the in vivo IgE synthesis is too much for clinical applications. Another approach for the suppression of IgE antibody response is antigen-specific regulation. We have established an immunological maneuver for the generation of antigen-specific suppressor T cells in vitro from the antigen-primed T cell population. T cell hybridomas constructed from the suppressor T cells produced antigen-specific suppressor T cell factors upon antigenic stimulation or crosslinking of T cell receptors, and this factor suppressed the IgE antibody response in the donors of the T cells in a carrier (antigen)-specific manner.

An application of the same principle to peripheral blood lymphocytes of allergic patients provided us with allergen-specific suppressor T cells. The T cell hybridomas, which were constructed from such T cells, produced antigen-binding GIF, which would be a counter part of mouse TsF. We expect that the antigen-binding human GIF may be useful to control IgE antibody response of allergic patients who share common class II molecules with the donor of the original T cells.

Introduction

The regulation of IgE synthesis is a subject of considerable interest not only for immunologists, but also for clinicians who are interested in hypersensitivity disorders. Once the persistent antibody response is established, it is difficult to stop antibody formation. However, immunologists feel that it is, in fact, possible to regulate the formation of IgE antibodies, since only certain individuals form such antibodies against allergens. Moreover, the IgE response in the mouse can occur

* This work was supported by Al-11202 and Al-14784 from the U.S. Department of Health and Human Services.

under restricted conditions. Indeed, persistent IgE formation is obtained in mice only when genetically high responder strains are immunized with a minute dose of a potent immunogen together with an appropriate adjuvant, such as aluminum hydroxide gel or pertussis vaccine [1]. Furthermore, some immunological approaches, such as repeated injection of complete Freund's adjuvant, suppressed the IgE response without affecting the IgG response; exposure to low dose X-ray prior to immunization selectively enhanced the IgE response. These findings suggest that the IgE response is controlled by mechanisms which do not affect the IgG response. In this presentation, recent progress on the mechanisms of the IgE response will be briefly summarized, and possible approaches to controlling IgE formation will be discussed.

Role of Interleukin-4 in the IgE Response

Since the IgE response is highly T cell dependent, it is reasonable to expect that T cell derived lymphokines are involved in the differentiation of B cells to IgE-forming cells. A series of experiments carried out by Coffman et al. [2–4] indicated that interleukin-4 (IL-4) is essential for IgE production. It was known that stimulation of resting murine B cells with lipopolysaccharide (LPS) results in the differentiation of B cells that form immunoglobulins of various isotypes, except IgE. However, culture of the same B cells with LPS together with 100–500 units/ml of recombinant IL-4 resulted in the formation of IgE and selective enhancement of IgG1 formation, which was accompanied by a decrease in IgG2b and IgG3. The concentration of IL-4 required for the production of IgE by LPS stimulated B cells was about 100-fold higher than that required for the enhancement of Ia expression and was not physiological. However, Coffman et al. [4] demonstrated that the presence of IL-5 together with IL-4 diminished the minimum concentration of IL-4 needed for IgE synthesis to 5–10 units/ml.

The effect of IL-4 on IgE synthesis was also demonstrated in human peripheral blood mononuclear cells. Pene et al. [5] showed that culture of normal human peripheral blood mononuclear cells with 100 units or 10 ng/ml of human Il-4 resulted in the induction of IgE synthesis. Subsequently, Claassen et al. [6] improved the culture conditions by using Iscov's modified Dulbecco's medium. In this culture system, a much lower concentration of IL-4 was sufficient to induce IgE synthesis, and much more IgE could be synthesized by mononuclear cells from both atopic and normal individuals.

The major effect of IL-4 on IgE synthesis is probably switching of resting B cells to precursors of IgE-forming cells which bear surface IgE. Culture of pure murine B cells with LPS and IL-4 resulted in the appearance of IgE- and IgG1-bearing cells. Depletion of $SIgE^+$ B cells developed in the culture abolished IgE formation [7]. Recently, Yoshida et al. [28] studied the switching mechanisms at the DNA level using BALB/c mice infected with the nematode *Nippostrongylus brasiliensis.* If the switching is due to deletion of an immunoglobulin gene segment, one may expect the formation of circular DNA before the initiation of either IgG1 or IgE synthesis by B cells. Indeed, circular DNAs resulting from switching of IgM to IgG1 and IgG1 to IgE were detected.

An interesting finding concerning the regulation of IgE synthesis is that the effect of IL-4 on B cells is counteracted by interferon-γ (IFN-γ). This lymphokine inhibits not only the IL-4-induced increase in Ia expression of resting B cells [8], but also the formation of IgE and IgG1 by murine B cells stimulated with LPS and IL-4 [2]. As little as 1 – 10 anti-viral units/ml of IFN-γ totally inhibited IgE and IgG1 production. The IL-4 induced formation of IgE by human peripheral blood mononuclear cells was also suppressed by IFN-γ and IFN-α [4]. These findings suggest that the relative proportion of several lymphokines in the B cell environment may affect the distribution of antibodies among various isotypes and that anti-IL-4 or IFN-γ might suppress IgE synthesis in vivo.

Indeed, such attempts were made by Finkelman et al. [9] who showed that an injection of 20 mgs of monoclonal anti-IL-4 into a BALB/c mouse markedly suppressed IgE synthesis induced by *Nippostrongylus* infection. The same dose of highly purified anti-IL-4 blocked the secondary IgE response to a protein antigen, without affecting either the IgG1 or IgG2a responses [10]. These results supported the concept that IL-4 is required for IgE synthesis. However, injection of 1 – 2 mgs of the monoclonal antibody failed to affect IgE synthesis. The authors suggested that the requirement of such a large dose of anti-IL-4 may be due to the low affinity of the antibody. However, it became clear that the affinity of anti-IL-4 for IL-4 was extremely high and was comparable to the affinity of IL-4 for IL-4 receptors. These findings collectively suggest that anti-IL-4 is not useful for clinical purpose.

Finkelman et al. [11] also tried to suppress in vivo IgE synthesis induced by IFN-γ. In this experiment, IgE synthesis was enhanced by an injection of goat anti-IgD, and IFN-γ was injected intraperitoneally twice a day on days 2, 3, and 4. Their results showed that 25 000 units of IFN-γ per injection, or a total of 150 000 units, markedly suppressed both IgE and IgG1 synthesis; one-fourth of the dose did not cause a significant effect. The results of the experiments are in agreement with the in vitro effects of IL-4 and IFN-γ on IgE synthesis, although the quantities of IFN-γ required for suppression are too large for clinical application. Recently, clinical application of IFN-γ was resported by Li et al. [12] who injected up to 0.2 mg of recombinant IFN-γ three times a week into rhinitis patients allergic to ragweed. After 4 weeks of treatment, no effect was observed based on weekly symptom scores or serum IgE titers. Another course of the same treatment was given to the same patients prior to ragweed season, but no significant effect on the IgE titer was observed. The treatment failed to suppress the secondary IgE response observed after ragweed season. Considering the adverse effect of the treatment, it would be difficult to increase the dose of IFN-γ to the required level.

Why did anti-IL-4 and IFN-γ effectively suppress IgE synthesis in vitro but not antibody synthesis in vivo? As described, the persistent IgE response in the mouse is obtained with less than 1 μg of alum-absorbed antigen. It is also known that the total dose of ragweed antigen E taken into the respiratory tract during an entire ragweed season would be 1 – 2 μg. Less than 1 μg/ml of antigen is sufficient to induce cognate interaction between antigen-specific B cells and primed helper T cells but not sufficient to stimulate helper T cells to release a detectable

Table 1. Isotype distribution of polyclonal response of normal B cells to RGG-specific helper T cell clones. [From 4].

Isotype	TH_2 (ng/ml)	TH_1 (ng/ml)	TH_1 + IL-2 + anti-IFNγ (ng/ml)
IgM	98000	248	65000
IgE	187	<1	<1
IgA	487	<1	825
IgG_1	21600	<8	5280
IgG_{2a}	39	14	2760
IgG_{2b}	189	<8	135
IgG_3	354	<8	474

amount of IL-4. Thus, differentiation of B cells to IgE-forming cells in vivo appears to be triggered by cognate interaction between antigen-specific helper T cells and B cells, rather than by lymphokines released from helper T cells. In that situation, anti-IL-4 or IFN-γ has much less chance of preventing the effect of helper T cells. Nevertheless, IL-4-producing helper T cells are essential for the production of IgE by the cognate interaction. Several years ago, Mosmann et al. [13] described that mouse helper T cell clones can be classified into two subtypes, i.e., TH1 and TH2, which produce different ILs upon antigenic stimulation. TH1 cells produce IL-2, IFN-γ and lymphotoxin; TH2 produces IL-4 and IL-5. Coffman et al. [4] employed rabbit IgG-specific helper T cell clones and induced polyclonal activation of normal B cells by coculturing them with TH clones and rabbit anti-mouse antibodies. As shown in Table 1, TH2 clones were more potent inducers than TH1 clones of Ig production. The major Ig produced by B cells cocultured with TH2 clones were IgM and IgG1, but a substantial quantity of IgE was also produced. In contrast, the same B cells failed to form IgE when they were cultured with TH1 clones. Since IFN-γ suppresses Ig formation in general, these investigators added anti-IFN-γ antibody and supplemented IL-2 to the TH1system to enhance Ig production. Under this condition, substantial amounts of IgM, IgG1 and IgG2a were produced, but IgE was not detected in the supernatant. The results show that the IL-4 producing TH2 clone is essential for IgE production by cognate interaction. Accumulated evidence suggests that these two subsets do not represent distinct lineages, and a single helper T cell can develop into either TH1 or TH2. Indeed, human helper T cells cannot be classified into TH1 and TH2 subtypes. Some helper T cell clones form IL-2 and IL-4 and some others produce IL-4 and IFN-γ. Nevertheless, more IL-4 producing helper T cell clones can be obtained from lymphocytes of atopic patients than from those of normal individuals [14]. Finding the mechanisms through which IL-4-producing helper T cells preferentially develop in atopic individuals and controlling the diffentiation of helper T cells into IL-4-producing cells may allow control of the IgE response.

IgE Binding Factors

Another group of lymphokines involved in the selective regulation of IgE formation is IgE binding factors, which are derived from T cells and have an affinity for IgE [15]. The IgE-binding factors (IgE-BF) consist of two types; one selectively enhances the IgE response, while the other selectively suppresses it. These factors bind to surface IgE on the precursors of IgE-forming cells and regulate their differentiation. Since the factors do not bind to other B cells, the effect of both IgE potentiating factor and IgE suppressive factors are selective for the IgE isotype. The major differences between the IgE potentiating factors (IgE-PF) and IgE suppressive factors (IgE-SF) appear to be carbohydrate moieties in the molecules [16]. The IgE-PF bind lentil lectin and con A, while IgE-SF failed to bind these lectins. Using a T cell hybridoma clone, evidence was obtained that the same cells could produce either IgE-PF or IgE-SF depending on the conditions [17]. Furthermore, these two factors share a common structural gene, and the carbohydrate moieties in the molecules are decided during posttranslational glycosylation [18].

A series of experiments have shown that IgE-PF is formed whenever the IgE response is induced while suppression of the IgE response leads to formation of IgE-SF [15]. Analysis of the cellular mechanisms involved in the selective formation of IgE-PF or IgE-SF under various experimental conditions showed that the nature and biologic activities of IgE-BF formed by a subset of T cells are controlled by two T cell factors which either enhance or inhibit N-glycosylation of IgE-BF during their biosynthesis [19]. The glycosylation enhancing factor (GEF) appears to be a serine protease [20], while the glycosylation inhibiting factor (GIF) appears to be a derivative of phospholipase inhibitory protein [21]. This lymphokine binds to a monoclonal antibody against lipomodulin and was recovered by elution at acid pH. Recent experiments showed that the mouse GIFs are 41 kDa and 14 kDa peptides [22]. Formation of GEF is always accompanied by the formation of IgE-PF, and the formation of GIF is accompanied by the formation of IgE-SF [23]. One might speculate that the balance between GEF and GIF determines the biologic activities of IgE-BF, and these factors, in turn, regulate the IgE response.

A series of experiments on IgE-BF suggests that IgE-SF may be useful in suppressing IgE formation. However, we did not take this approach, since we were afraid that the majority of IgE-SF administered intravenously would be bound by IgE before the lymphokine reached the lymphoid tissues.

Immune Suppression by GIF

During IgE formation, T cells produce both IgE-PF and GEF. We expected that mice treated with GIF might switch the subset of T cells in vivo from those producing IgE-PF to those producing IgE-SF. Thus, BDF_1 mice were immunized with alum-absorbed ovalbumin (OVA) to stimulate persistent IgE formation and repeatedly injected with GIF. The results clearly showed that GIF suppressed not only the IgE response, but also the IgG response [24].

In order to analyze the mechanisms of immunosuppression by GIF treatment, BDF_1 mice were immunized with alum-absorbed OVA, and one group was treated with intravenous injections of GIF. Spleen cells of untreated mice formed IgE-

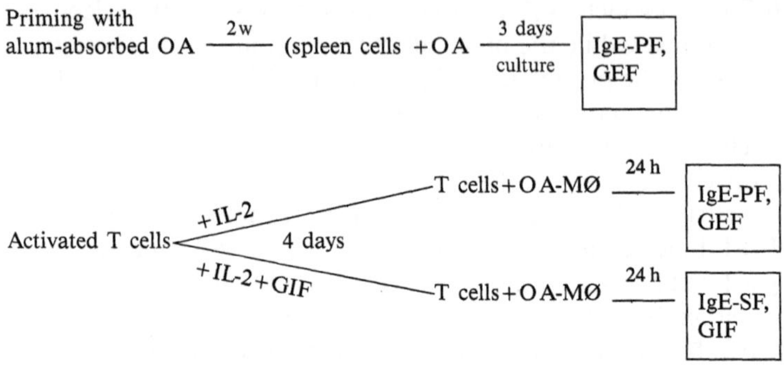

Fig. 1. Experimental design to generate GIF-producing T cells in vitro

PF and GEF upon stimulation with homologous antigen, while those of GIF treated mice formed IgE-SF and GIF. Thus, GIF treatment of the mice actually switched their splenic T cells from those producing IgE-PF to those producing IgE-SF. It was also found that spleen cells of GIF treated mice contained antigen-specific suppressor T cells [24].

In light of this latter result, attempts were made to reproduce the phenomenon in vitro. The protocols are shown in Fig. 1. BDF_1 mice were primed with alum-absorbed OVA to stimulate a persistent IgE response, and their spleen cells were stimulated with homologous antigen to activate antigen-primed T cells. These T cells were then propagated with IL-2 in the presence or absence of GIF. As expected, T cells propagated with IL-2 alone produced GEF, whereas those propagated with IL-2 in the presence of GIF produced their own GIF. Upon stimulation with antigen-pulsed syngeneic macrophages, these cells produced IgE-SF and GIF having an affinity for OVA [25].

Our separate experiments indicated that the antigen-binding GIF is composed of nonspecific GIF and antigen-binding peptide and shares several antigenic determinants with effector type, antigen-specific, suppressor T cell factor (TseF) [26]. Therefore, we constructed T cell hybridomas from the OVA-specific T cells which had been propagated in the presence of GIF and selected the hybridomas that produced antigen-binding GIF upon stimulation with OVA-pulsed syngeneic macrophages. The OVA-binding GIF from the hybridomas was purified using OVA-coupled sepharose and tested for its ability to suppress the antibody response of BDF_1 mice. The results of the experiments shown in Fig. 2 indicate that the OVA-binding GIF suppressed the anti-hapten IgE response to dinitrophenyl derivatives of OVA (DNP-OVA), but failed to suppress the anti-hapten antibody response to DNP-keyhole-limpet hemocyanin (KLH). It is clear that the OVA-binding GIF is actually an antigen- or carrier-specific suppressor factor.

Since these experiments provided us with a method of obtaining antigen-specific TsF from the lymphocytes of IgE-producing animals, we wondered whether the same method could be applied to human lymphocytes of allergic patients. We took peripheral blood mononuclear cells from allergic patients sensitive to honey-

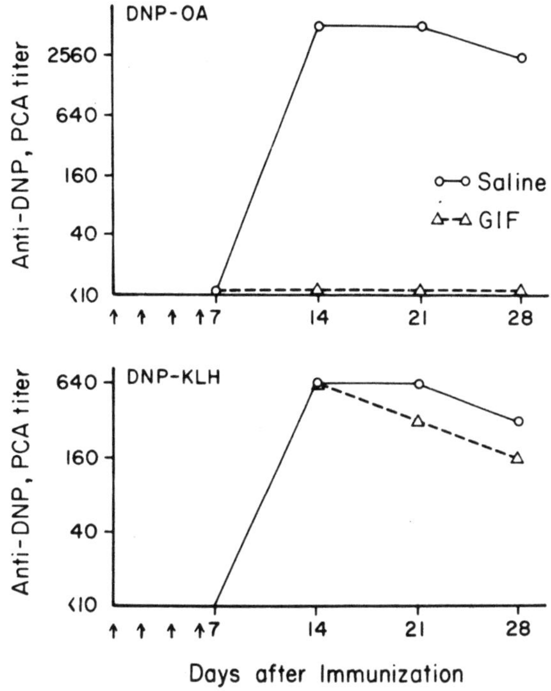

Fig. 2. Carrier-specific suppression of anti-hapten IgE antibody response by OVA-binding GIF from the T cell hybridoma. BDF_1 mice were immunized with either alum-absorbed DNP-OVA (*top*) or DNP-KLH (*bottom*). Affinity purified, OVA-binding GIF was injected intravenously on days 0, 2, 4, and 6 into both DNP-OVA-primed mice and DNP-KLH-primed mice (△ – – △). The same immunogens were used to immunize control mice (○——○) which received saline. Anti-hapten IgE antibodies were measured by PCA (passive cutaneous anaphylaxis) reactions

bee venom. Since the major allergen in the venom is phospholipase A_2, which has cytotoxic activity, we cultured the cells with a chemically modified bee venom phospholipase A_2 that had no cytotoxic effect. The cells were then propagated with human IL-2 in the presence or absence of recombinant human lipocortin, which has phospholipase A_2 inhibitory activity. T cells were then stimulated with the chemically modified bee venom antigen in the presence of autologous monocytes. As expected, T cells propagated by IL-2 alone formed IgE-PF and GEF, whereas those propagated in the presence of lipocortin formed IgE-SF and GIF [27].

We then constructed T cell hybridomas from those T cells which had been propagated in the presence of lipocortin. Since the GIF-producing hybridomas express CD3 (CD3 complex) and TcR$\alpha\beta$ (T cell receptor α, β), the hybridomas were stimulated by cross-linking of CD3 using monoclonal anti-CD3 and anti-mouse Ig. GIF produced by the cells was fractionated on bee venom phospholipase-coupled sepharose. As shown in Table 2, many of the hybridomas produced antigen-binding GIF upon cross-linking the CD3 molecules. All of the hybridomas formed nonspecific GIF when they were not stimulated. We do not have the system to evaluate the immunosuppressive effects of antigen-binding GIF from the human hybridomas. However, we believe that this lymphokine is the counterpart of antigen-binding mouse GIF which respresents antigen-specific TsF.

Immunosuppressive effects of mouse TsF is major histocompatibility class (MHC) restricted. If the same principles apply to human GIF, the lymphokines

Table 2. Formation of antigen-binding GIF by anti-CD3-treated hybridoma cells[a].

Clone	IgE-BF[b] (%)	GIF activity in PLA_2-sepharose	
		Effluent	Eluate
AC5	20	−	+
AF10	36	+	−
BA6	8	+	−
BE12	65	−	+
BF5	65	−	+
CB7	64	−	+
CE5	58	−	+

[a] Seven hybridoma clones constitutively secreted GIF. These clones were treated with OKT3 and cultured in anti-MGG (mouse IgG) coated flasks. Culture supernatants were fractionated on IgE-sepharose and proteins bound to the beads were eluted at acid pH. The effluent fraction from IgE-sepharose was fractionated on PLA_2-coupled sepharose and the effluent and eluate fractions from the immunosorbent were assessed for GIF activity using the 12H5 cells (25).
[b] Acid eluate fractions from IgE-sepharose were assessed for the presence of IgE-BF. Numbers represent percent rosette inhibition.

derived from on atopic individual may not be effective for others. Nevertheless, antigen-binding GIF from the hybridomas will regulate the IgE response of the original peripheral blood donor and that of a group of patients who share a common MHC product which restricts the function of TsF.

Acknowledgement. Experiments included in this review were carried out by Drs. Makoto Iwata, Kenji Katamura, Claudio Carini, Toru Takeuchi at the Johns Hopkins University, School of Medicine, and Drs. Peter Thomas, Akio Mori at the La Jolla Institute for Allergy and Immunology. This paper is publication No. 2 from the La Jolla Institute for Allergy and Immunology.

References

1. Ishizaka K (1976) Cellular events in the IgE antibody response. Ad Immunol 23:1
2. Coffman T, Ohara J, Bond M, Carty J, Zlotnik A, Paul WE (1986) B cell stimulatory factor – 1 enhances the IgE response of lipopolysaccharide-activated B cells. J Immunol 136:4538
3. Coffman RL Carty J (1986) A T cell activity that enhances polyclonal IgE production and its inhibition by interferon-γ. J Immunol 136:949
4. Coffman RL, Seymour BWP, Liebman DA, Hiraki DD, Christensen JA, Shrader B, Cherwinski HM, Savelkaul HF, Finkelman FD, Bond MW, Mosmann TT (1988) The role of helper T cell products in mouse B cell differentiation and isotype regulation. Immunol Rev 102:5
5. Pene J, Ronsset F, Briere F, Chretien I, Boonefoy J-Y, Spits H, Yokota T, Arai N, Arai K, Bauchereau J, DeVries JE (1988) IgE production by normal human lymphocytes is induced by interleukin-4 and suppressed by interferon-γ and α and prostaglandin E_2. Proc Natl Acad Sci USA 85:6880
6. Classen JL, Levine AD, Buckley RH (1990) A cell culture system that enhances mononuclear cell IgE synthesis induced by recombinant IL-4. J Immunol Methods 126:213
7. Snapper CM, Finkelman FP, Steany D, Conrad DH, Paul WE (1988) Interleukin-4 induces coexpression of membrane IgG1 and IgE by murine B cells stimulated by lipopolysacharide. J Immunol 141:489

8. Mond JJ, Carmen J, Sarina C, Ohara J, Finkelman FD (1986) Interferon-γ suppresses B cell stimulation factor (BSF-1) induction of class II MHC determinants on B cells. J Immunol 137:3534
9. Finkelman FD, Katona IM, Urban JF Jr, Snapper GM, Ohara J, Paul WE (1986) Suppression of in vivo polyclonal IgE responses by monoclonal antibody to the lymphokine BSF1. Proc Natl Acad Sci USA 83:9675
10. Finkelman FD, Katona IM, Urban JF, Holmes J, Ohara J, Tung AS, Sample JG, Paul WE (1988) IL-4 is required to generate and sustain in vivo IgE responses. J Immunol 141:2335
11. Finkelman FD, Katona IM, Mossmann TR, Coffman RL IFNγ regulates the isotypes of Ig secreted during in vivo humoral immune responses. J Immunol 140:1022
12. Li JTC, Yunginger JW, Reed CE, Jaffe HS, Nelson DR, Gleich GL (1990) Lack of suppression of IgE production by recombinant interferon gamma. A controlled trial in patients with allergic rhinitis. J Allergy Clin Immunol 85:934
13. Mosmann TR, Cherwinski H, Bond MW, Giedlin MA, Coffman RL (1986) Two types of murine helper T cell clone. I. Definition according to profiles of lymphokine activities and secreted proteins. J Immunol 236:2348
14. Prete GD, Maggi E, Parronchi P, Chretien I, Tiri A, Macchia D, Ricci M, Banchereau J, DeVries J, Romagniani S (1988) IL-4 is an essential factor for IgE synthesis induced in vitro by human T cell clones and their supernatants. J Immunol 140:4193
15. Ishizaka K (1984) Regulation of IgE synthesis. Ann Rev Immunol 2:159
16. Yodoi J, Hirashima M, Ishizaka K (1982) Regulatory role of IgE-binding factors from rat T lymphocytes. V. The carbohydrate moieties in IgE-potentiating factors and IgE-suppressive factors. J Immunol 128:289
17. Huff TF, Uede T, Iwata M, Ishizaka K (1983) Modulation of the biologic activities of IgE-binding factos. III. Switching of a T cell hybrid clone from the formation of IgE-suppressive factor to the formation of IgE-potentiating factor. J Immunol 131:1090
18. Martens CL, Jardieu P, Trounstein ML, Stuart SG, Ishizaka K, Moore KW (1987) Potentiating and suppressive IgE-binding factor are expressed by a single cloned gene. Proc Natl Acad Sci USA 84:809
19. Ishizaka K (1988) IgE-binding factors and regulation of the IgE antibody response. Annu Rev Immunol 6:513
20. Iwata M, Munoz JJ, Ishizaka K (1983) Modulation of the biologic activities of IgE-binding factors. IV. Identification of glycosylation enhancing factor as a kallikrein-like enzyme. J Immunol 131:1954
21. Uede T, Hirata F, Hirashima M, Ishizaka K (1983) Modulation of the biologic activities of IgE-binding factors. I. Identification of glycosylation inhibiting factor as a fragment of lipomodulin. J Immunol 130:878
22. Katamura K, Iwata M, Mori A, Ishizaka K (1990) Biochemical identification of glycosylation inhibiting factor. Proc Natl Acad Sci USA 87:1903
23. Iwata M, Huff TF, Ishizaka K (1984) Modulation of the biologic activities of IgE-binding factors. V. The role of glycosylation enhancing factor and glycosylation inhibiting factor in determining the nature of IgE-binding factors. J Immunol 132:1286
24. Akasaki M, Jardieu P, Ishizaka K (1986) Immunosuppressive effects of glycosylation inhibiting factor on the IgE and IgG antibody response. J Immunol 136:3172
25. Iwata M, Ishizaka K (1988) Construction of antigen-specific suppressor T cell hybridomas from spleen cells of mice primed for the persistent IgE formation J Immunol 141:3270
26. Jardieu P, Ishizaka K (1987) Possible relationship of an antigen-specific suppressive factor to phospholipase inhibitory protein. Immune regulation by characterized peptides. UCLA Symp 41:595
27. Carini C, Iwata M, Warner J, Ishizaka K (1990) A method to generate antigen-specific suppressor T cells in vitro from peripheral blood T cells of honeybee venom-sensitive allergic patients. J Immunol Methods 127:221
28. Yoshida K, Matsuoka M, Uenda S, Mori A, Ishizaka K, Sakano H (1990) Immunoglobulin switch circular DNA in the mouse infected with Nippostrongylus brasiliensis: evidence for successive class switching from μ to ε via γ. Proc Natl Acad Sci USA 87:7829

Human $Fc_{\varepsilon}RII$/CD23 in the Regulation of the Allergic Immune Response*

E.P. Rieber[1], U. Pirron[1], N. Endres[1], and J.C. Prinz[1,2]

[1]Institute for Immunology, University of Munich, Goethestrasse 31, W-8000 München 2, Federal Republic of Germany
[2]Department of Dermatology, University of Munich, Frauenlobstrasse 9–11, W-8000 München 2, Federal Republic of Germany

Abstract

The human low affinity receptor for IgE ($Fc_{\varepsilon}RII$), also known as the leukocyte differentiation antigen CD23 [1], is a type II integral membrane glycoprotein of 45 kDa which is constitutively expressed on resting, μ^+/δ^+ B lymphocytes and is lost after isotype switch. $Fc_{\varepsilon}RII$/CD23 is also found on follicular dendritic cells, eosinophils, platelets, alveolar macrophages and can be induced on monocytes and Langerhans cells by IL-4. Two isoforms (CD23a and CD23b) differing in the N-terminal cytoplasmic part have been identified by molecular cloning. Soluble IgE binding fragments (sCD23) are released from $CD23^+$ cells by proteolytic cleavage. Pleiotropic activities have been proposed for the $Fc_{\varepsilon}RII$/CD23 and its soluble derivatives. Although specific functions in IgE regulation have been described, the biological role of the CD23 molecule remains elusive. Two recently recognized characteristics of the $Fc_{\varepsilon}RII$/CD23 will be presented: 1) specific induction of CD23 on T-cells by allergens and 2) focusing of antigen via CD23.

1) $Fc_{\varepsilon}RII$/CD23 is not found on T-cells from healthy people. T-cells from allergic individuals, however, can be induced to express CD23 by stimulation with the specific allergen. This expression is dependent on the presence of IL-4, although IL-4 is not able to induce CD23 on T-cells. IFN-γ strongly downregulates the allergen-induced expression of CD23 on T-cells. Whether $CD23^+$ T-cells play a pivotal role in IgE regulation is presently under investigation.

2) $Fc_{\varepsilon}RII$/CD23 is also involved in antigen focusing: this was shown in experiments where B lymphocytes were incubated with tetanus toxoid (TT) complexed with IgE. The B-cells were then allowed to present the TT antigen to autologous cloned TT specific T-cells. Complexing with IgE clearly increased the antigen presenting capacity of B-cells. This finding indicates an important role of the $Fc_{\varepsilon}RII$/CD23 molecule which selectively enhances T-cell activation by IgE-bound antigens and might therefore be involved in maintaining or amplifying ongoing allergic responses.

---

* This work was supported by the Deutsche Forschungsgemeinschaft, SFB 217, and the Wilhelm Sander-Stiftung.

Structure, Tissue Distribution and Assumed Functions of the Fc_εRII/CD23

The Fc_εRII/CD23 is a type II membrane glycoprotein with a molecular mass of 45 kD, consisting of 321 (respectively 320, see below) amino acids with the carboxy terminus extracellular and the amino terminus inside the cell. The CD23 gene has been cloned and sequenced by several groups [2–5]. It consists of 11 exons which code the functional domains of the molecule. Exons 9–11 show sequence homology to a number of C type animal lectins such as the rat asialoglycoprotein receptor [6], rat mannose binding protein [7], lymphocyte homing receptor MEL-14 [8] and endothelial leukocyte adhesion molecule 1 (ELAM 1) [9]. These findings suggest that the Fc_εRII/CD23 functions as cellular adhesion molecule.

Two isoforms, CD23a and CD23b, have been identified [10]. They are generated through the use of different transcription initiation sites and alternative RNA splicing and differ only in the first seven respectively six amino acids of the intracytoplasmic aminoterminal part, the a-isoform exceeding the b-isoform by one amino acid residue. Interestingly, the a-isoform was found only in B cells, whereas the b-isoform was detected in B cells and all other cells which are able to express the low affinity Fc_ε-receptor and it is mainly the b-isoform which is induced by IL-4.

The membrane CD23 molecule is proteolytically cleaved at various positions and soluble molecules are released which retain the capacity to bind IgE. The major cleavage product has a molecular mass of 25 kDa; the cleavage site has been localized at position 149 [11].

The Fc_εRII/CD23 molecule is expressed on a variety of cell types either constitutively or after induction by different cytokines as summarized in Table 1. It is normally found on resting μ^+/δ^+ B cells and is lost after B cell activation [12]. Epstein-Barr virus transformed B cells display it at high density and the EBNA 2 protein has been shown to be responsible for its induction [13]. CD23 is not detected on resting T lymphocytes. However, as we have shown for the first time, it can clearly be induced on T cells by stimulation with the appropriate allergen [14, 15, this paper]. In addition, CD23 expression has been observed on some HTLV 1 transformed T cell lines [16]. Freshly isolated monocytes and Langerhans cells do not express CD23 but they can be induced to CD23 expression by stimulation with IL-4 [17, 18]. On the other hand, the immature monocytic cell line U 937 [19] as well as eosinophils [20] and platelets [21] display the receptor on their surface. A particularly dense expression is found on the follicular dendritic cells in germinal centers [22, own observation].

A number of different biological functions have been described for both the membrane bound and soluble form of the CD23 molecule. These have been compiled in Table 2, together with the corresponding literature references.

Table 1. Tissue distribution of $FC_{\varepsilon}RII$/CD23 and differential regulation of expression by IL-4 and IFN-γ.

Cells	Lymphokine		
	None	rIL-4	IFN-γ
$\mu^+\delta^+$ B cells	+	+ +	−
EBV transformed B cell lines	+ +	+ + +	−
Resting T cells	−	−	−
Allergen activated T cells	+	+ +	−
HTLV-1 transformed T cell lines	+	?	?
Monocytes	−	+ +	−
Monocytic cell line U937	+	+ +	+ +
Eosinophils	+	+ +	+ +
Platelets	(+)	?	+ +
Follicular dendritic cells	+ + +	?	?
Langerhans cells	−	+ +	+ +

?, data not available.

Table 2. Supposed functions of the $FC_{\varepsilon}RII$/CD23 molecule.

	Reference
Membrane bound form	
Receptor for low molecular weight B cell growth factor	[23]
Lectin: cell adhesion and binding of other factors	[3]
Low affinitiy receptor for IgE:	
IgE dependent cellular cytotoxicity against parasites	[24]
Phagocytosis of IgE coated particles	[25]
IgE mediated antigen focusing	[26]
Soluble form (sCD23)	
IgE binding factor (IgE-BF): regulation of IgE production	[27, 28]
B cell growth factor	[29, 30]
Inhibition of monocyte migration	[31]
Blockade of IgE effector functions	[32]

$Fc_{\varepsilon}RII/CD23^+$ T lymphocytes

In rodents $CD23^+$ T lymphocytes have been identified as essential components of the regulatory network of the IgE response [33], whereas in humans the expression of $Fc_{\varepsilon}RII$/CD23 on T lymphocytes is still disputed [14, 15, 34, 35]. The discordant results obtained by different groups may partially be due to technical difficulties in identifying IgE binding cells as T cells. The main reason for the discrepancies, however, is most probably the fact that $Fc_{\varepsilon}RII$/CD23 is an activation antigen on T cells and is hardly detected on resting T lymphocytes. In our investigations we used a double labeling technique which combines the identification of T cells by a fluorescein-isothiocyanate (FITC) labeled CD2 mAb with the demonstration of CD23 in a sensitive direct monoclonal antibody rosetting technique

Table 3. Induction of $Fc_{\varepsilon}RII/CD23$ on T cells by various antigens given as $Fc_{\varepsilon}RII$ expression index ($FC_{\varepsilon}R$-EI).

Blood donors	Antigen	$Fc_{\varepsilon}R$-EI [a]
Allergic to Chit I ($n = 8$)	Chit I	87.3 ± 3.5
	TT	1.3 ± 0.5
	PPD	0.6 ± 0.5
	CD3 mAb	<0.1
Allergic to phospholipase A_2 (PLA_2) from bee venom ($n = 10$)	PLA_2	99.3 ± 14.7
	TT	1.4 ± 1.6
	PPD	1.0 ± 0.8
	CD3 mAb	<0.1
Immune but not allergic to PLA_2 from bee venom ($n = 4$)	PLA_2	3.9 ± 3.0
	TT	2.2 ± 1.2
	PPD	0.6 ± 0.5
	CD3 mAb	<0.1

[a] $$Fc_{\varepsilon}R\text{-EI} = \frac{\%\ CD23^{+}\ \text{T cells} \times 100}{\text{stimulation index}}$$

[36]. As a second method two color fluorescence activated cell sorter (FACS) analysis was applied.

On resting human T cells $Fc_{\varepsilon}RII/CD23$ could not be detected. Stimulation with polyclonal mitogens or specific antigens led only to a marginal CD23 expression. Only PHA was able to induce CD23 on a subpopulation of T cells. However, when T cells from allergic individuals were stimulated with the corresponding allergen a significant proportion of the T cell blasts expressed $Fc_{\varepsilon}RII/CD23$. This expression was transient and reached its maximum on day 5. The selective induction of $Fc_{\varepsilon}RII/CD23$ on T cells by stimulation with the specific allergen becomes particularly evident when the $Fc_{\varepsilon}R$ expression index ($Fc_{\varepsilon}R$-EI) is calculated. The $Fc_{\varepsilon}R$-EI correlates the percentage of $CD23^{+}$ T cells with the stimulation index as determined by [^{3}H]thymidine uptake.

Table 3 shows the $Fc_{\varepsilon}R$-EI obtained with cells from patients allergic to fish fodder or bee venom. The cells were stimulated with purified hemoglobin from chironomid larvae (the Chit I allergen) which is the major allergen in fish fodder [37], or with phospholipase A_2, the main allergenic component of bee venom.

When the mononuclear blood cells from a patient allergic to Chit I were stimulated with Chit I, an $Fc_{\varepsilon}R$-EI of about 90 was obtained. When the same cells were stimulated with other antigens such as tetanus toxoid (TT) or purified protein derivative (PPD) only a low $Fc_{\varepsilon}R$-EI was observed. The stimulation with a monoclonal CD3 antibody was equally ineffective. Interestingly, CD3 antibodies never induced $Fc_{\varepsilon}R$-expression on T cells although they led to a marked activation and proliferation of T cells. A similar result was obtained when cells from patients allergic to bee venom were stimulated with different antigens. Only the specific allergen PLA_2 induced CD23 expression on T cell blasts. Remarkably enough, no $Fc_{\varepsilon}RII/CD23$ was expressed upon contact with PLA_2 by T cells obtained from individuals who were exposed and immunized against bee venom as

Table 4. Expression of $FC_{\varepsilon}RII$/CD23 on T cell blasts of a donor allergic to Chit I in response to different stimuli.

Stimulus	% $CD23^{+}$ T cell blasts
–	<1
CD3 mAb	<0.1
Tetanus toxoid (5 µg/ml)	4.3
PPD (5 µg/ml)	0.9
Chit I (5 µg/ml)	34.5
Chit I + rIL-4 (1 U/ml)	64
Chit I + rIFN-τ (1 U/ml)	8
Chit I + anti-IL-4 antiserum	14

Stimulated cells were stained with a PE labeled CD2 mAb and a FITC labeled CD23 mAb and analyzed by cytofluorometry on a FACScan. The gates were set for PE-CD2 mAb stained cells and cells with blast size.
PPD, purified protein derivative.

evidenced by the presence of IgG antibodies to PLA_2, but lacked specific IgE antibodies.

Mere adsorption of soluble CD23 to the T cell surface could be excluded by the demonstration of autochthonous CD23 synthesis in purified allergen stimulated T cells by northern blot analysis [15]. Very recently, we were able to prove with the help of the polymerase chain reaction (PCR) that it is exclusively the b-isoform of the $Fc_{\varepsilon}RII$ which is expressed in activated T cells [38].

The expression of $Fc_{\varepsilon}RII$/CD23 on T cells is regulated by lymphokines, particularly by IL-4 and IFN-γ.

As can be seen from Table 4 the Chit I induced $Fc_{\varepsilon}RII$/CD23 expression on T blasts was increased in the presence of recombinant IL-4 whereas it was inhibited by IFN-γ. An antiserum to IL-4 which is able to block the biological function of IL-4, reduced the allergen-induced CD23 expression on T cells. This finding indicates that IL-4 is involved in the $Fc_{\varepsilon}RII$/CD23 expression on T cells; it is, however, not capable of inducing it without the specific allergenic stimulus.

As indicated in Table 1 the influence of both lymphokines on the $Fc_{\varepsilon}RII$/CD23 expression on various cell types is quite different. rIL-4 either induces or increases the expression on almost all cells which are able to express $Fc_{\varepsilon}RII$/CD23. The effect of IFN-γ, however, varies. This cytokine inhibits $Fc_{\varepsilon}RII$/CD23 expression on B and T lymphocytes, but induces or increases the expression on the immature monocytic cell line U937, on eosinophils and on Langerhans cells. In our studies, only IL-4 was capable of inducing $Fc_{\varepsilon}R$ expression on mature blood monocytes; IFN-γ had no effect [unpublished work].

Taken together, these data clearly demonstrate that the $Fc_{\varepsilon}RII$/CD23 is selectively induced on T cells by stimulation with the specific allergen. However, the exact mechanism and the biological relevance of this phenomenon remains to be elucidated.

In a first approach to a functional characterization of the $Fc_{\varepsilon}RII$/CD23 expressing T lymphocytes we investigated their influence on the IL-4 induced differentiation of B lymphocytes into IgE secreting cells. This IL-4 mediated differ-

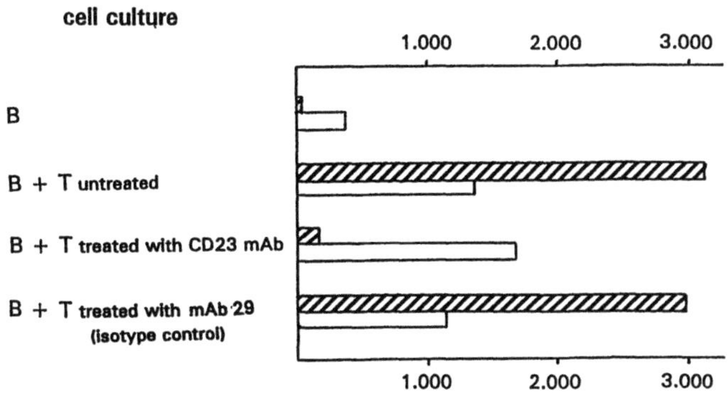

Fig. 1. Isotype specific inhibition of (anti-μ + IL-4) induced in vitro IgE synthesis by pretreatment of T cells with CD23 mAb. T and B lymphocytes were prepared from the blood of a healthy donor using the "direct monoclonal antibody rosetting technique" [36] at high purity. The T cells were treated for 1 h at 4 °C with the CD23-mAb M-L25 or with the mAB 29 as an isotype control at 10 µg/ml, washed and then added to B cells at a ratio of 1 : 1. The cells were stimulated with a combination of polyclonal anti-μ antibodies $(F(ab')_2$ fragment of rabbit antihuman μ-chain antibody (Dakopatts, Hamburg, FRG, dilution 1 : 10000) and 500 IU of rIL-4/ml. After 9 days IgE (*hatched bars*, pg/ml) and IgG (*open bars*, ng/ml) were determined in the supernatants

entiation of B cells requires an additional activation signal as well as the presence of T cells. In a first set of experiments we asked whether this collaborative role of T cells is influenced by monoclonal CD23 antibodies (CD23 mAb).

To this end peripheral blood T cells were isolated, treated with a CD23 mAb, washed and then added to purified B cells. The B cells were then stimulated with an anti-μ antibody in combination with rIL-4. After 9 days IgE and, as a control, IgG were determined in the supernatants. B cells alone were not able to produce IgE (Fig. 1). In the presence of untreated T cells, however, a marked IgE synthesis was induced. When the T cells were treated with a CD23 mAb, only background levels of IgE were observed, whereas the production of IgG was not reduced. A control mAb of the same isotype as the CD23 antibody did not inhibit the IgE response. These preliminary results suggest an important role of the $Fc_{\varepsilon}RII$ on normal T cells in the regulation of the IgE response.

Antigen Focusing Mediated by the $Fc_{\varepsilon}RII$

The capacity of the $Fc_{\varepsilon}RII/CD23$ molecule to bind IgE leads to the question of whether it can facilitate the uptake of IgE complexed antigen and is thus able to enhance the presentation of allergens to T lymphocytes. As a first approach to the involvement of $Fc_{\varepsilon}RII/CD23$ in antigen presentation we studied the uptake and presentation of IgE complexed antigen by $Fc_{\varepsilon}RII$ expressing B cells. To obviate the problem of isolating antigen specific IgE for preparing antigen IgE complexes we used a recombinant chimeric human/mouse IgE antibody (which was kindly provided by Dr. M. S. Neuberger, Cambridge, U.K.). This antibody

Table 5. Enhanced T cell activation by complexing the antigen with IgE.

Antigen	Blocking mAb	$[Ca^{2+}]_i$ (nM)
–	–	140
TT[a]	–	150
TT + IgE anti-NIP	–	160
NIP-TT[a]	–	160
NIP-TT[a] + IgE anti-NIP	–	345
NIP-TT + IgE anti-NIP	M-L25 (5 µg/ml)	155
NIP-TT + IgE anti-NIP	M-L25 (2 µg/ml)	185
NIP-TT + IgE anti-NIP	M-L25 (1 µg/ml)	245
NIP-TT + IgE anti-NIP	CD19 mAb (20 µg/ml)	335

[a] The concentration of TT or NIP-TT was 10 µg/ml.

consists of a variable part derived from a mouse monoclonal anti-NIP antibody and a constant human IgE portion [39]. The antigen NIP haptenized tetanus toxoid (NIP-TT) was complexed with the chimeric IgE antibody and then added to EBV transformed B cells which express Fc_εRII/CD23 at high density. The efficiency of antigen presentation was determined by stimulation of autologous cloned TT specific T cells. As an early parameter of T cell activation the intracellular Ca^{2+} mobilization was evaluated in Indo 1 labeled single cells by FACS analysis.

Table 5 gives the results of a representative experiment. EBV transformed B cells were incubated for 1 h at 4 °C with free or IgE complexed NIP-TT, washed and then allowed to process the antigen for 6 h at 37 °C. Subsequently they were contacted with cloned TT specific T cells and Ca^{2+} mobilization was determined by cytofluorometry. The activation of T cells at a given antigen concentration was increased about 100-fold after complexing the antigen with IgE when compared with free antigen. This increased efficiency was mediated by the low affinity Fc_εR, a fact proven by the dose dependent inhibition by the CD23 mAb M-L25 which is able to block the binding of IgE to the Fc_εR. A mAb against another B cell surface antigen such as CD19 had no effect. These data clearly show that the lymphoid Fc_εR efficiently mediates the internalization of allergens by antigen presenting cells and its subsequent processing and presentation to T cells. The amplification and maintenance of allergic immune responses may well be substantially influenced by this activity as it is schematically depicted in Fig. 2.

In its upper part Fig. 2 shows the conventional route of antigen/allergen uptake and processing by APC (monocytes, Langerhans cells) as well as by B cells, which are able to bind the antigen by their antigen specific immunoglobulin receptors. In the course of antigen processing antigenic peptides are bound to MHC class II molecules, exposed at the cell surface and presented to specific T cells. The T cells are activated and secrete a broad spectrum of lymphokines which help the B cells to differentiate into immunoglobulin secreting plasma cells. Differentiation into IgE secreting cells is propagated mainly by IL-4. Other lymphokines lead to the attraction and activation of inflammatory cells with consecutive local inflammation. This activation of T cells by allergens can be markedly enhanced by the presence of allergen specific IgE antibodies through the

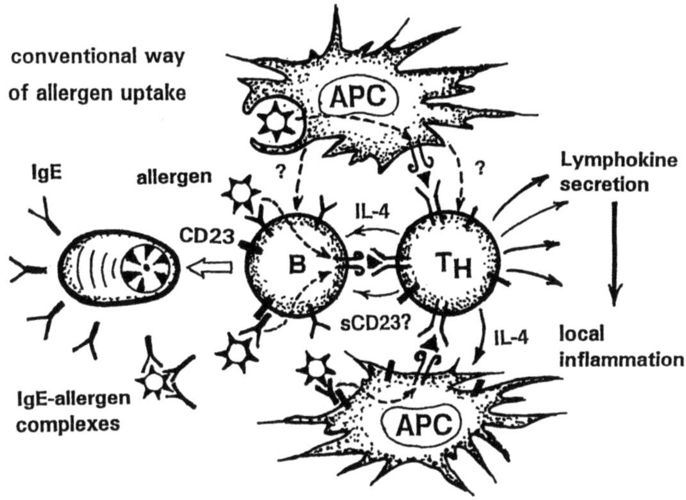

Fig. 2. IgE-CD 23 mediated enhancement of T cell activation by allergens. *APC*, antigen presenting cell; T_H, T helper cell; B, B cell

engagement of $Fc_{\varepsilon}RII$ on B lymphocytes or on other APC such as Langerhans cells where the $Fc_{\varepsilon}RII$ is also induced by the T cell lymphokine IL-4. This positive feedback loop results in maintenance or even amplification of the IgE dependent, T cell induced local inflammation such as atopic dermatitis exemplifies and can thus play an important role in the pathophysiology of allergic immune responses.

References

1. Yukawa K, Kikutani H, Owaki H, Yamasaki K, Yokota A, Nakamura H, Barsumian EL, Hardy RR, Suemura M, Kishimoto T (1987) A B cell-specific differentiation antigen CD23 is a receptor for IgE ($Fc_{\varepsilon}R$) on lymphocytes. J Immunol 138:2576
2. Kikutani H, Inui S, Sato R, Barsumian EL, Owaki H, Yamasaki K, Kaisho T, Uchibayashi N, Hardy RR, Hirano T, Tsumasawa S, Sakiyama F, Suemura M, Kishimoto T (1986) Molecular structure of human lymphocyte receptor for immunoglobulin E. Cell 47:657
3. Ikuta K, Takami M, Kim LW, Honjo T, Miyoshi T, Tagaya Y, Kawabe T, Yodoi J (1987) Human lymphocyte Fc receptor for IgE: sequence homology of its cloned cDNA with animal lectins. Proc Natl Acad Sci USA 84:819
4. Ludin C, Hofstetter H, Sarfati M, Levy CA, Suter U, Alaimo D, Kilchherr E, Frost H, Delespesse G (1987) Cloning and expression of the cDNA coding for a human lymphocyte IgE receptor. EMBO J 6:109
5. Suter U, Bastos R, Hofstetter H (1987) Molecular structure of the gene and the 5′ flanking region of the human lymphocyte immunoglobulin E receptor Nucleic Acids Res 15:7295
6. Holland EC, Leung O, Drickamer K (1984) Rat asialoglycoprotein receptor lacks a cleavable NH2-terminal sequence. Proc Natl Acad Sci USA 81:7338
7. Drickamer K, Dordal MS, Reynolds MS (1986) Mannose-binding proteins isolated from rat liver contain carbohydrate-recognition domains linked to collagen tails. J Biol Chem 261:6878

8. Lasky LA, Singer MS, Yednock TA, Dowbenko D, Fennie C, Rodriguez H, Ngueyen T, Stachel S, Rosen SD (1989) Cloning of a lymphocyte homing receptor reveals a lectin domain. Cell 56:1045
9. Bevilaqua MP, Stengelin S, Gimbrone MA, Seed B (1989) Endothelial leukocyte adhesion molecule I: an inducible receptor for neutrophils related to complement regulatory proteins and lectins. Science 243:1160
10. Yokota A, Kikutani H, Tanaka T, Sato R, Barsumian EL, Suemura M, Kishimoto T (1988) Two species of human Fcε receptor II ($Fc_εRII$/CD23): tissue-specific and IL-4-specific regulation of gene expression Cell 55:611
11. Letellier M, Sarfati M, Delespesse G (1989) Mechanisms of formation of IgE-binding factors (soluble CD23). I. $Fc_εRII$ bearing B cells generate IgE-binding factors of different molecular weights. Mol Immunol 26:1105
12. Kikutani H, Suemura M, Owaki H, Nakamura H, Sato R, Yamasaki K, Barsumian EL, Hardy RR, Kishimoto T (1986) $Fc_ε$ receptor, a specific differentiation marker transiently expressed on mature B cells prior to isotype switching. J Exp Med 164:1455
13. Wang F, Gregory CD, Rowe M, Rickinson AB, Wang D, Birkenbach M, Kikutani H, Kishimoto T, Kieff E (1987) Epstein Barr nuclear antigen 2 specifically induces expression of the B-cell activation antigen CD23. Proc Natl Acad Sci USA 84:3452
14. Prinz JC, Endres N, Rank G, Ring J, Rieber EP (1987) Expression of $Fc_ε$ receptors on activated human T lymphocytes. Eur J Immunol 17:757
15. Prinz JC, Baur X, Mazur G, Rieber EP (1990) Allergen-directed expression of Fc receptors for IgE (CD23) on human T lymphocytes is modulated by interleukin 4 and interferon-γ. Eur J Immunol 20:1259
16. Sarfati M, Nutman TB, Suter U, Hofstetter H, Delespesse G (1987) T-cell derived IgE-binding factors. II. Purification and characterization of IgE-binding factors produced by human T cell leukemia/lymphoma virus-I-transformed T lymphocytes. J Immunol 139:4055
17. Vercelli D, Jabara HH, Lee BW, Woodland N, Geha R (1988) Human recombinant interleukin-4 induces $Fc_εR2$/CD23 on normal human monocytes. J Exp Med 167:1406
18. Bieber T, Rieger A, Neuchrist C, Prinz JC, Rieber EP, Boltz-Nitulescu G, Scheiner O, Kraft D, Ring J, Stingl G (1989) Induction of $Fc_εR2$/CD23 on human epidermal Langerhans cells by human recombinant interleukin-4 and γ-interferon. J Exp Med 170:309
19. Anderson CL, Spiegelberg HL (1981) Macrophage receptors for IgE: binding of IgE to specific IgE Fc receptors on a human macrophage cell line, U937. J Immunol 126:2470
20. Capron M, Kusnierz JP, Prin L, Spiegelberg HL, Ovalque G, Gosset P, Tonnel AB, Capron A (1985) Cytophilic IgE on human blood and tissue eosinophils: detection by flow microfluorometry. J Immunol 134:3013
21. Joseph M, Capron A, Ameisen JC, Capron M, Vorng H, Pancre V, Kusnierz JP, Auriault C (1986) The receptor for IgE on blood platelets. Eur J Immunol 16:306
22. Gordon J, Flores-Romo L, Cairns JA, Millsum MJ, Lane PJ, Johnson GD, MacLennan ICM (1989) CD23: a multi-functional receptor/lymphokine? Immunol Today 10:153
23. Guy GR, Gordon J (1987) Coordinated action of IgE and a B-cell stimulatory factor on the CD23 receptor molecules upregulates B-lymphocyte growth. Proc Natl Acad Sci USA 84:6239
24. Capron A, Dessaint JP, Capron M, Joseph M, Ameisen JC, Tonnel AB (1986) From parasites to allergy: a second receptor for IgE. Immunol Today 7:13
25. Melewicz FM, Zeigger RS, Mellon MH, O'Connor RD, Spiegelberg HL (1981) Increased IgE-dependent cytotoxicity by blood mononuclear cells of allergic patients. Clin Exp Immunol 43:526
26. Pirron U, Schlunck T, Prinz JC, Rieber EP (1990) IgE-dependent antigen focusing by human B lymphocytes is mediated by the low-affinity receptor for IgE. Eur J. Immunol 20:1547
27. Pene J, Chretien I, Rousset F, Briere F, Bonnefoy JY, DeVries J (1989) Modulation of IL-4-induced human IgE production in vitro by IFN-γ and IL-5; the role of soluble CD23 (sCD23). J Cell Biochem 39:253
28. Sarfati M, Delespesse G (1988) Possible role of human lymphocyte receptor for IgE (CD23) or its soluble fragments in the in vitro synthesis of human IgE. J Immunol 141:2195
29. Gordon J, Cairns JA, Millsum MJ, Gillis S, Guy GR (1988) Interleukin 4 and soluble CD23 as progression factors for human B lymphocytes: analysis of their interaction with agonists of the phosphoinositide "dual pathway" of signalling. Eur J Immunol 18:1561

30. Thorley-Lawson DA, Swendeman SL, Edson CM (1986) Biochemical analysis suggests distinct functional roles for the Blast-1 and Blast-2 antigens. J Immunol 136:1745
31. Flores-Romo L, Cairns JA, Millsum MJ, Gordon J (1989) Soluble fragments of the low-affinity IgE receptor (CD23) inhibit the spontaneous migration of U937 monocytic cells: neutralization of MIF-activity by a CD23 antibody. Immunology 67:547
32. Suemura M, Kikutani H, Aitani M, Yamatodani A, Kuritani T, Kishimoto S, Uchibayashi N, Sugiyama K, Barusmian EL, Kishimoto T (1989) Suppression on IgE-mediated allergic reactions with recombinant soluble Fc_{ε}RII (abstract). 7th international congresson immunology. Berlin 1989, pp 19–55
33. Ishizaka K (1985) Twenty years with IgE: from the identification of IgE to regulatory factors for the IgE response. J Immunol 135:1
34. Nutman TB, Delespesse G, Sarfati M, Volkman DJ (1987) T-cell derived IgE-binding factors. I. Cloned and transformed T cells producing IgE binding factors. J Immunol 139:4049
35. Suemura M, Kikutani H, Barsumian EL, Hattori Y, Kishimoto S, Sato R, Maeda A, Nakamura H, Owaki H, Hardy RR, Kishimoto T (1986) Monoclonal anti-Fc_{ε} receptor antibodies with different specificities and studies on the expression of Fc_{ε}R on human B and T cells. J Immunol 137:1214
36. Wilhelm M, Pechumer H, Rang G, Kopp E, Riethmüller G, Rieber EP (1986) Direct monoclonal antibody rosetting: an effective method for weak antigen and large scale separation of human mononuclear cells. J Immunol Methods 90:89
37. Baur X, Aschauer H, Mazur G, Dewair M, Prelicz H, Steigemann W (1986) Structure, antigenic determinants of some clinically important insect allergens: chironomid hemoglobins. Science 233:351
38. Endres N, Prinz JC, Rieber EP (1990) T cells express the b-isoform of Fc_{ε}RII after stimulation with allergen or PHA. Immunobiology 181:152
39. Neuberger MS, Williams GT, Mitchell EB, Jouhal SS, Flanagan JG, Rabbitts TH (1985) A hapten-specific chimeric IgE antibody with human physiological effector functions. Nature 314:268

Inbred Strains of Guinea Pigs in Studies of Allergy

L.K. Poulsen[1], L. Lundberg[2], D. Sompolinsky[2], J.V. Spärck[3], M. Ploug[2], C. Bindslev-Jensen[1], and P.S. Skov[1]

[1]Laboratory of Medical Allergology, National University Hospital, Department TTA 7542, 20 Tagensvej, 2200 Copenhagen N, Denmark
[2]Institute of Medical Microbiology, University of Copenhagen, Juliane Maries Vej 22, 2100 Copenhagen Ø, Denmark
[3]Statens Serum Institut, Amager Boulevard 80, 2300 Copenhagen S, Denmark

Introduction

In investigations of basic mechanisms of allergy, animal models have frequently been employed. Several mouse and rat strains readily develop high IgE titers and have been extensively used in immunological studies. Conversely, guinea pigs are sensitive to respiratory provocation and have been used for pharmacological approaches.

The aim of the work summarized in this review has been to combine these two aspects in order to provide a sensitive and reproducible research tool for study of allergic disease and possible pharmaceutical interventions. Four inbred strains of guinea pigs have been developed and their genetic homogeneity documented. Different immunological and inflammatory parameters considered to be important in human IgE-mediated disease have been investigated. These include

- Respiratory and ocular anaphylaxis in response to an experimental antigen to which the animals had previously been sensitized
- IgE and IgG response to immunization
- Development of eosinophilia
- Development of basophilia and allergen-induced histamine release

An example of the use of this animal model is a study of the response to new forms of allergen-specific immunotherapy. Results will be shown to illustrate the suitability of guinea pigs in the study of therapeutic modalities.

Characterization of the Four Strains

More than 30 generations of guinea pigs have been bred (brother-sister mating) for production of inbred strains with different characteristics in respect to allergic disease. Using antigen-induced respiratory anaphylaxis as criterion, two high (IMM/S-209, IMM/S-740) and two low (IMM/S-201, IMM/S-203) responder strains have been developed. The animals in each of the high responder strains show a uniform ability to produce allergic asthma when sensitized with ovalbumin (OA) by inhalation or by injections of OA alone or adsorbed on alum [3]. For animals of the high responder strains the asthma is reversible and easily elicited when the animal is challenged with an aerosol containing the relevant antigen. Contrary to this, the low responder strains are refractory to the development of respiratory anaphylaxis, even after prolonged immunizations.

The homogeneity of the four strains has been demonstrated in skin transplantation experiments, in screening for erythrocyte enzyme polymorphism [16] and in examinations of the immune response to different synthetic polypeptides [4].

Immune Response

The IgE and IgG immune responses to OA were tested in the four strains (L. Lundberg et al., manuscript in preparation). IgE levels were determined by means of the passive cutaneous anaphylaxis (PCA) test according to Ovary [8]. Donor animals were challenged 14 days after passive sensitization. Heat-treated serum was regularly used as control. This test demonstrated a high reproducibility and specificity when used for testing a large number of sera [14].

In all four strains it was possible to induce an ongoing IgE response when alum or Freund's complete adjuvant (FCA) were employed as adjuvants (shown for alum in Fig. 1). This response varies between the strains, with one high responder strain (# 740) producing the highest titers. The IgE response was increased fourfold if the animals were pretreated with cyclophosphamide (150 mg/kg) 1 day prior to the immunization. As demonstrated in Table 1, the IgE and IgG_1 titers could also be increased by provocations in the eyes or in the airways.

Eosinophilia

The four strains vary in their capability to develop eosinophilia [9, 10]. One high responder strain (# 209) and one low responder (# 203) demonstrated a marked eosinophilia (up to 60%; Fig. 2). This spontaneous (age-related) eosinophilia can be accelerated by immunization with alum as adjuvant in the # 209 strain only. This is in contrast to FCA, which reduces the number of eosinophilic cells in

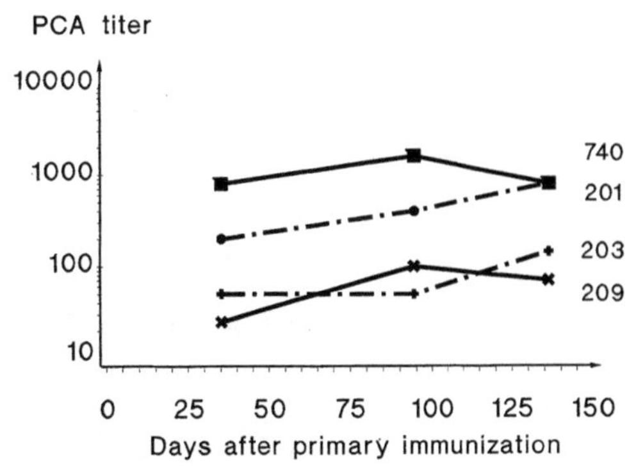

Fig. 1. Kinetics of IgE response. IgE levels as determined by the passive cutaneous anaphylaxis (*PCA*) test. Groups of animals from each of the four groups were immunized on day 0 with OA (10 µg/ml) in alum and boosted (1 µg/ml) on days 28, 56, 87, and 124). IgE titers were determined up to 134 days following the primary immunization

Table 1. Conclusions on previous and present findings.

Strain	Anaphylactic sensitivity		Eosinophilic counts			Basophilic counts		Serum IgG after OA immunizations (PCA titer)						Serum IgG_1 after OA immunizations (PCA titer)					
	Pulm	Ocul[a]	Spn	OA immunization		OA immunization		Before OA provocations			After OA provocations			Before OA provocations			After OA provocations		
				Alum	FCA	Alum	FCA	PBS	Alum	FCA	PBS	Alum	FCA	PBS	Alum	FCA	PBS	Alum	FCA
209	High	High	++	↑	↓	–	–	<13	<13	141	ND	45	130	<13	ND	400	ND	800	1600
740	High	High	–	–	↓	–	++	20	55	116	200	200	ND	25	ND	200	1600	951	ND
203	Low	High	+	–	↓	–	+	<13	<13	<13	ND	ND	ND	ND	ND	ND	ND	ND	ND
201	Low	Low	–	–	↓	–	+	ND	13	294	ND	ND	635	ND	ND	ND	ND	ND	1600

OA, ovalbumin; PCA, passive cutaneous anaphylaxis; Pulm, pulmonary; Ocul, oculary; Spn, spontaneously, without immunization; PBS, phosphate buffered saline; FCA, Freund's complete adjuvant; ND, not done; ↓, decreased compared to spontaneous; ↑, increased compared to spontaneous.
References given in text except.
[a] Lundberg et al. [5].

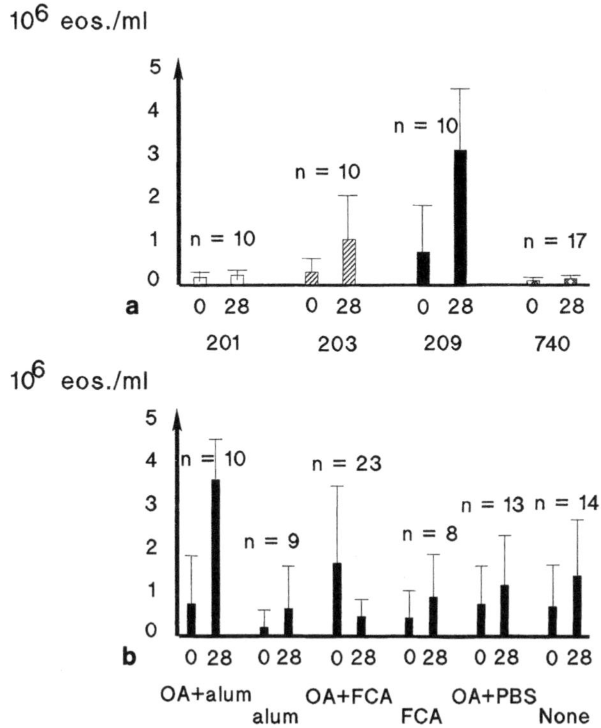

Fig. 2 a, b. Peripheral blood eosinophil count. **a**. Groups of the four strains of guinea pigs were immunized intraperitoneally with OA in alum on days 0 and 7. Eosinophils were counted in peripheral blood on days 0 and 28. **b**. Groups of guinea pigs from the 209 strain were immunized with different adjuvants (± antigen) on days 0 and 7. Eosinophils were counted in peripheral blood on days 0 and 28. *OA*, ovalbumin; *FCA*, Freund's complete adjuvant; *PBS*, phosphate-buffered saline

peripheral blood (Fig. 2). For the two remaining strains (# 740 and # 201) no abnormal cell numbers could be induced.

Basophilia and Histamine Release

When immunizations are followed by provocations in the eyes or in the airways peripheral basophilia can be induced in the guinea pigs by appropriate selection of strain and adjuvant (Fig. 3; D. Sompolinsky et al., manuscript in preparation). The two high responder strains differ in respect to the ability to form basophilia. Only #740 but not # 209 produce a marked basophilia (7%) after immunization with OA in FCA followed by nasal or ocular provocations.

To demonstrate that the basophils are actually sensitized, a histamine release assay was set up (L. Lundberg, P. Stahl Skov, D. Sompolinsky, L.K. Poulsen: Histamine release from whole blood used for evaluation of allergy in guinea pig strains (Manuscript)). A strong OA-induced histamin release was demonstrated for strain # 740, the other three strains being somewhat less responsive.

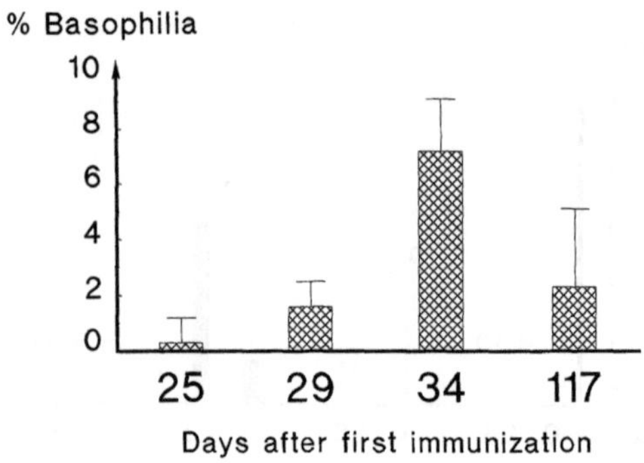

Fig. 3. Peripheral blood basophil count in strain 740 following immunization with OA in FCA (days 0 and 7) and provocation in nares (daily, days 25 to 61)

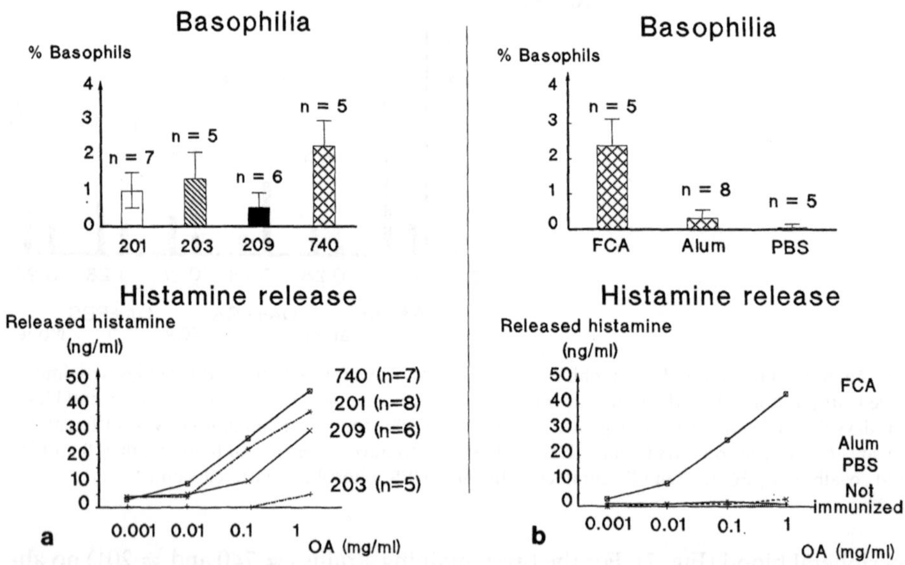

Fig. 4a, b. Peripheral blood basophil count and histamine release after immunization (OA in FCA) and repeated provocations (see legend to Fig. 3). **a** Comparison of groups of animals of the four strains. **b** Strain 740 immunized with ovalbumin (*OA*) in different adjuvants. *FCA,* Freund's complete adjuvant; *PBS,* phosphate-buffered saline

The adjuvant used for immunization strongly influenced the response in the histamine release assay (Fig. 4). A strong histamine release was obtained when the guinea pigs had previously been immunized with OA in FCA compared to alum. Neither non-immunization nor immunization with OA without adjuvant produced a response in the histamine release assay.

Therapeutic Studies: Specific Immunotherapy with Immune Complexes

Allergen-specific immunotherapy (IT) is a well-established form of treatment given to patients with a clear diagnosis of asthma or rhinitis to major inhalant allergens [6]. Almost 80 years have passed since its introduction [7], but we still do not know the mechanisms through which its effects are exerted [6, 13]. The development of "blocking antibodies" during immunotherapy was described more than 50 years ago, this "blocking" immune response being independent of the reaginic antibody titer. Later investigators demonstrated that these antibodies are of IgG type and more recently the subclass distribution of the antibodies has been elucidated [1, 13]. In our laboratory we have focused on the IgG immune response produced by patients during the first months of specific immunotherapy and have investigated the total specific reactivity against an allergen extract [1] and the IgG specifically directed against the individual allergen components [2, 15]. Based on these studies we proposed that immune complexes formed ex vivo between IgG and allergen might represent a therapeutic alternative [13].

To further test the hypothesis we carried out experiments using the guinea pig model. The strain # 209 was used for the experiments [11, 14]. An IgE-mediated allergy against OA was induced in the animals by immunization with OA in alum. Four groups of guinea pigs were treated for 36 weeks with (1) placebo, (2) passive

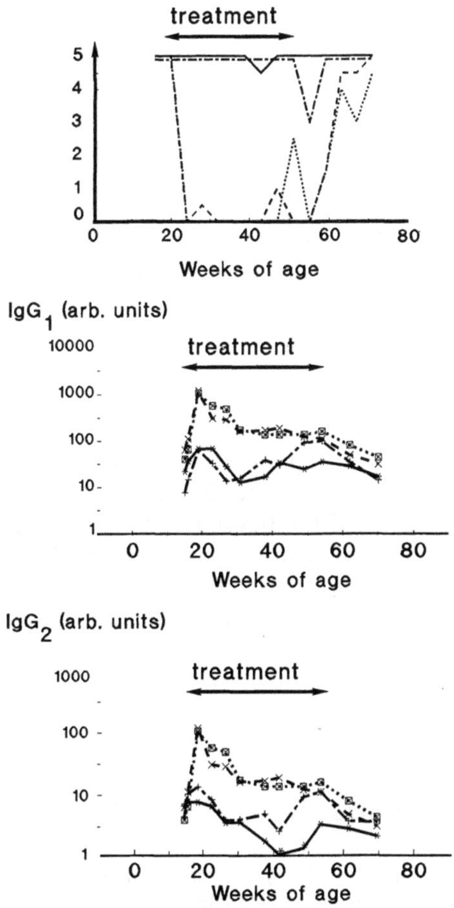

Fig. 5. Immunotherapy study. Four groups of guinea pigs (strain 209) sensitized to OA by injections with OA in alum were subsequently treated with either placebo (saline; *solid lines*; $n=5$), passive (hyperimmune IgG; *dash-dot lines*; $n=5$), active (OA; *dashed lines*; $n=6$) or combined (immune complexes between OA and IgG (*dotted lines*; $n=6$) immunotherapy. *Upper panel*, clinical response (symptom score) in bronchial provocation test in response to aerosolized OA; *Two lower panels*, serology response, i.e., OA-specific IgG_1 and IgG_2, as determined by radioimmunoassay. Antibody concentrations are given in arbitrary units

immunotherapy with anti-OA hyperimmune serum, (3) active immunotherapy with OA, and (4) immunotherapy with immune complexes between OA and hyperimmune serum.

During these experiments, it was demonstrated that antigen (OA) and immune complexes containing OA could abolish the symptoms developed during inhalation provocation test (Fig. 5, upper panel). In contrast, in guinea pigs treated with either placebo or passive immunization (hyperimmune anti-OA serum) bronchial reactivity to the antigen was not altered. The IgE-titers in the four groups were comparable, whereas the IgG_1 and IgG_2 titer increased only in the two groups given active (OA-containing) treatment. All groups were observed for additional 20 weeks after cessation of therapy and interestingly, the bronchial reactivity of the treated animals rose during this posttreatment observation period. This result suggests that duration of hyposensitization might be limited, and follow-up studies in hyposensitized patients should be performed.

The IgE and IgG immune response in the guinea pigs were evaluated by means of PCA and radioimmunoassay [14]. Animals from all four treatment groups were sensitized during the first part of the IT study and responded with a marked IgE synthesis (PCA titer 400–1600) which later stabilized on a more moderate level. In spite of noticeable reductions of symptoms in groups treated with active and combined IT, no difference in the IgE level were found between the four groups (results not shown). In contrast to IgE, mean group titers of IgG_1 and IgG_2 in the groups receiving active or combined IT rose drastically during the first part of therapy and closely paralleled the clinical response during the rest of the study period (Fig. 5, lower parts). However, as concerns the individual animals, no correlations were found between the immune response and the clinical symptoms. Thus, the strong IgG response during immunotherapy may not be causally related to the outcome of the treatment.

Conclusion

An overall summary of the features of the four strains are given in Table 1. It is tempting to ascribe the adjuvant- or strain-related differences in bronchial response and the basophilia and/or eosinophilia to different profiles of cytokine production. Thus, experiments employing inbred strains of guinea pigs could increase our understanding of some of the basic mechanisms underlying development and aggrevation of allergic diseases. Furthermore, the model provides a possibility for testing different forms of antiallergic treatments as well as possible "hypo-allergenic" products.

References

1. Djurup R (1985) The subclass nature and clinical significance of the IgG antibody response in patients undergoing allergenspecific immunotherapy. Allergy 40:469–486

2. Jarolim E, Poulsen LK, Stadler BM, Mosbech H, Østerballe O, Kraft D, Weeke B (1990) A long term follow-up study of hyposensibilization using immunoblotting. J Allergy Clin Immunol 85:996–1004
3. Lundberg L (1979) Guinea pigs inbred for studies of respiratory anaphylaxis. Acta Pathol Microbiol Immunol Scand Sect C 87:55–66
4. Lundberg L, Koch C, Magnusson M, Bertelsen C (1983) Characterization of two strains of selectively bred guinea pigs. 2. Differences in immune response to synthetic polypeptides. Acta Pathol Microbiol Immunol. Scand Sect C 91:187–195
5. Lundberg L, Bertelsen C, Zavaro A, Samrah Z, Sompolinsky D (1987) Experimental allergic conjunctivitis in inbred guinea pigs strains with high respectively low allergic reactivity. Allergy 42:262–271
6. Malling HJ (1988) Clinical efficacy of allergen immunotherapy. ISI Atlas of Science: Immunology 1:215–219
7. Noon L (1911) Prophylactic inoculation against hay fever. Lancet, June 10, i:1572–1573
8. Ovary Z, Kaplan B, Kojima S (1976) Characteristics of guinea pig IgE. Int Arch Allergy Appl Immunol 51:416–428
9. Ploug M (1989) Forskelle i udviklingen af eosinofili hos marsvin indavlede for høj eller lav respiratorisk anafylaktisk følsomhed. (Differences in development of eosinophilia by guinea pigs inbred for high or low respiratory reactivity). Thesis, University of Copenhagen
10. Ploug M, Lundberg L, Spärck JV, Katzenstein T, Sompolinsky D (1991) Genetic control of eosinophilia in guinea pig strains inbred for high or low bronchial reactivity. Allergy (in press)
11. Poulsen LK, Lundberg L, Søndergaard I, Weeke B (1988) Allergen-containing immune complexes used for immunotherapy. Preparation of complexes and evaluation of their clinical performance in guinea pigs. Allergy 44:132–142
12. Poulsen LK, Søndergaard I, Weeke B (1988) Preparation of patient-related allergens for hyposensitization. Qualitative aspects. Allergy 43:552–564
13. Poulsen LK, Søndergaard I, Weeke B (1989) Improvement of specific immunotherapy by human IgG and modified allergens (review article). Allergy 44:241–255
14. Poulsen LK, Lundberg L, Søndergaard I, Weeke B (1991) Allergen-containing immune complexes used for immunotherapy of allergic asthma. II. IgE and IgG immune response during and after hyposensitization of sensitization of sensitized guinea pigs. Allergy 46:292–303
15. Søndergaard I, Poulsen LK, Østerballe O, Weeke B (1991) A computational approach to the description of the individual immune responses. Allergen-specific IgE and IgG-subclasses formed during immunotherapy. Allergy 46:10–19
16. Sørensen M, Jørgensen PN, Lundberg L (1983) Characterization of two strains of selectively bred guinea pigs. 1. Skin transplantation experiments and screening for erythrocyte enzyme polymorphism. Acta Pathol Microbiol Immunol Scand Sect C 91:181–185

Multispecific Allergic Reactions*

J. M. Varga, G. F. Klein, and P. Fritsch

Department of Dermatology, University of Innsbruck, Anichstrasse 35, 6020 Innsbruck, Austria

Introduction

The highly prevalent allergic cross-reactions are generally explained by the presence of common allergens in different allergen preparations, shared antigenic determinants present on different allergens, and/or multiple sensitizations. It is conceivable, however, that, in addition to these mechanisms, multispecific recognition of allergens by IgE antibodies may contribute to the frequently observed lack of strict specificity in allergic reactions. We have recently initiated a project to test the role of IgE multispecificity in allergic cross-reactions by screening monoclonal IgE antibodies for multispecific ligand binding. Cross-stimulation of rat basophilic leukemia (RBL) cells, sensitized with multispecific monoclonal IgE antibodies, is then analyzed. The results show that multispecific IgEs mediate cross-stimulation of RBL cells by chemically unrelated compounds.

IgE Antibodies are Multispecific

It has been shown earlier that other classes (A, G, M) of antibodies [1] and B cell surface Igs [2] are multispecific, and that these multispecific, antigen binding receptors mediate cross-stimulation of individual B cell clones by chemically different agents to produce the same Ig species [3]. Since the same repertoire of V region genes are utilized in the various classes of immunoglobulins [4], it is anticipated, but it has not yet been shown, that IgEs are also multispecific. A recently developed solid-phase binding assay [5] was used to investigate the specificity of ligand binding to a mouse monoclonal anti-dinitrophenol (DNP) IgE [IgE (aDNP)]. In addition to DNP analogues over 2000 compounds were screened for their ability to compete with DNP for the antigen binding site of IgE(aDNP). At the concentrations used for screening (generally 1 m*M)* 59% of the compounds showed no significant inhibition, 19% inhibited the binding of IgE(aDNP) more than 50%. Several families of compounds, such as tetracyclines, polymyxins, phenothiazines, salicylates, and quinones were found to bind to the DNP binding

* These studies were supported by the Austrian Fonds zur Förderung der wissenschaftlichen Forschung and by the Mag. Mayrhofer Co.

Table 1. Affinity of DNP amino acids to IgE (aDNP).

DNP-amino acids

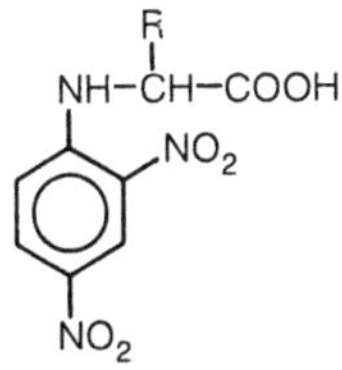

Name	Abbreviation	R	Affinity (I_{50}, μM)
DNP-Ser	S	$-CH_2-OH$	0.8
DNP-Orn	O	$-(CH_2)_3-NH_2$	1.0
DNP-Glu	D	$-CH_2-CH_2-COOH$	1.5
DNP-Gly	G	$-H$	2.0
DNP-Lys	K	$-(CH_2)_4-NH_2$	3.0
DNP-Asp	E	$-CH_2-COOH$	8.0
DNP-Arg	R	$-(CH_3)_3-NH-C(=NH)\ NH_2$	9.0
DNP-Gln	N	$-CH_2-CH_2-CONH_2$	12.0
DNP-Cys	C	$-CH_2-SH$	70.0
DNP-Trp	W	$-CH_2-$ 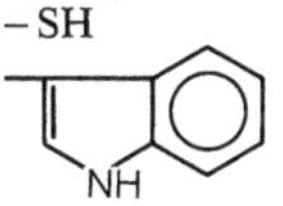	600.0
DNP-Pro	P	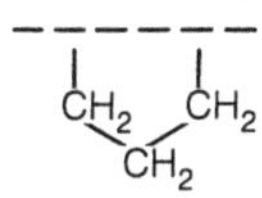	1150.0

I_{50}, Concentrations of DNP-amino acids, necessary for 50% inhibition of [^{125}I]-IgE (anti-DNP) binding to DNP-coated polystyrene microtiter plates [5].

site of IgE(aDNP). The structures of these compounds and that of DNP are shown in Tables 1, 2. Within these families of compounds, a change in the functional groups attached to the stem compound had a major influence on the affinity of binding. The IgE(aDNP) antibody did not bind indiscriminatelly to all compounds that were tested: carbohydrates, in general, and several other families of drugs, such as sulfonamides, penicillins, anesthetics, etc., had no measurable affinities. The observed frequencies of interactions of ligands with IgE(aDNP) is in good agreement with a mathematical model for multispecific ligand-antibody interactions [6]. Thus, we have demonstrated that IgE(aDNP) has multispecific ligand binding activities [7].

Ligands Chemically Unrelated to DNP Can Stimulate Release of Mediators From Sensitized RBL Cells

The functional implications of IgE multispecificity were tested by studying the stimulation of serotonin release from RBL 2H3 cells plated on polystyrene tissue culture plates coated with DNP-amino acids or with ligands that are chemically

Table 2. Binding of disparate compounds to IgE (aDNP).

No.	Name	Structure	Affinity (I_{50}, μM)
1.	Lymecycline	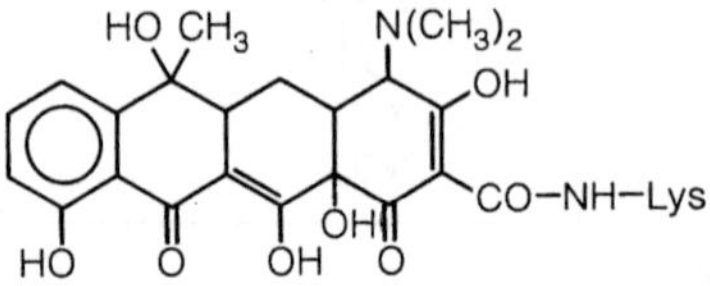	0.8
2.	Acenaphthoquinone	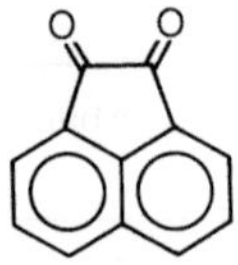	2
3.	Alizarin	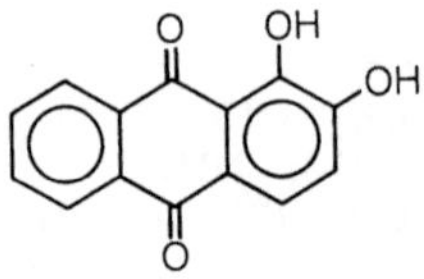	14
4.	*o-I*-Benzoic acid	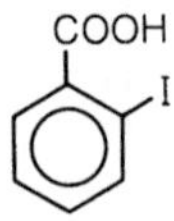	30
5.	Oxolinic acid	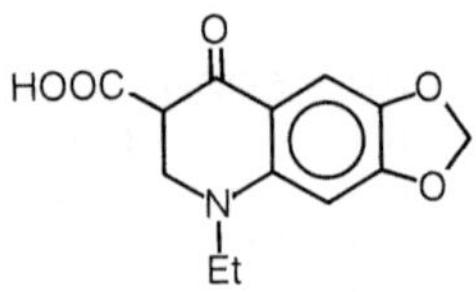	45
6.	Cyanocinnamic acid	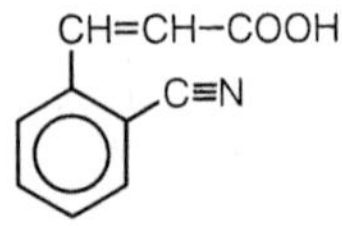	270
7.	Aspirin	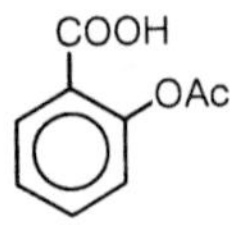	800
8.	Thiosalicylic acid	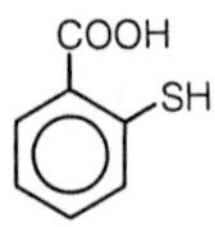	1100
9.	FMOC-Gly	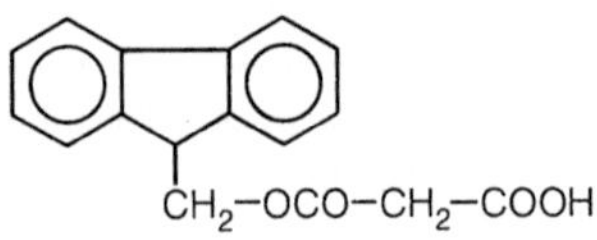	2000
10.	Dehydrocholic acid	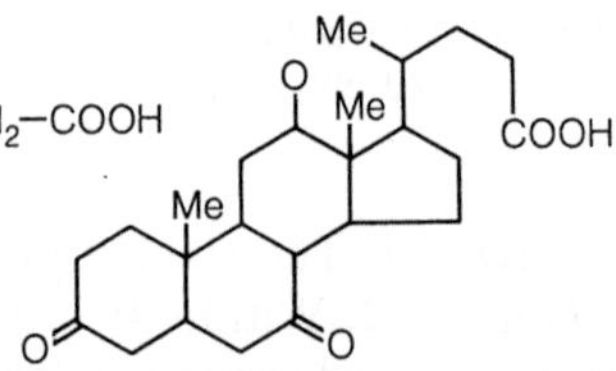	>5000

I_{50}, Concentrations of DNP-amino acids, necessary for 50% inhibition of [^{125}I]-IgE (anti-DNP) binding to DNP-coated polystyrene microtiter plates [5]
FMOC-Gly, 9-Fluorenylmethoxy-carbonyl-glycine.

unrelated to DNP [5, 8]. This new technique, presenting ligands to sensitized RBL cells in polyvalent form, allowed us to correlate ligand binding affinities with stimulation of serotonin release from RBL cells. The results are summarized in Fig. 1.

Conclusions

There is a threshold of intrinsic ligand binding affinities at a Ka of approximately 50–100 μM; ligands with lower affinities do not stimulate mediator release even if they are presented in multivalent forms. This affinity threshold for mediator

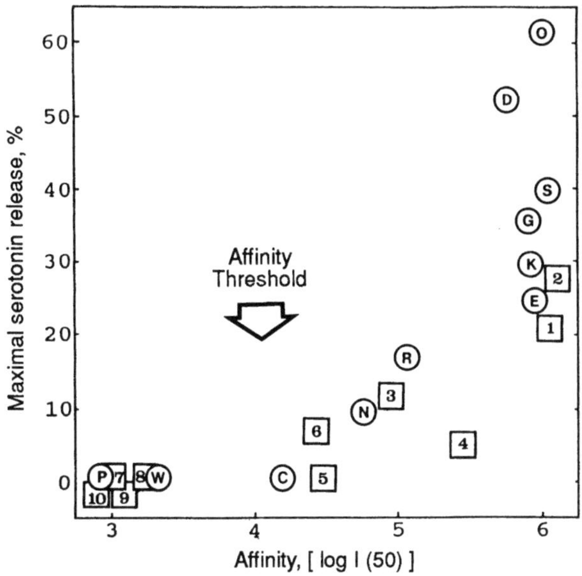

Fig. 1. Stimulation of serotonin release from RBL cells in response to DNP amino acids and a disparate set of compounds. The one letter codes for DNP amino acids are shown in Table 1; the numbers represent the compounds listed in Table 2

cell stimulation is valid for various ligands, irrespective of their chemical similarity to the immunogen. Multispecific stimulation of meditor release may contribute to the frequently observed allergic cross-reactions, false positive tests for allergies, and anaphylactic reactions to drugs upon first exposure.

Acknowledgement. We thank Ms. G. Kalchschmid for skillful technical assistance.

References

1. Varga JM, Lande S, Richards FF (1974) Immunoglobulins with multiple binding functions. II. The use of nylon-polyserine whisker disks in screening myeloma immunoglobulins for binding activity. J Immunol 112:1565–1570
2. Czaja MJ, Richards FF, Varga JM (1977) Multispecific lymphoid cell surface receptors. Proc Natl Acad Sci USA 74:1224–1228
3. Varga JM, Konigsberg WH, Richards FF (1973) Antibodies with multiple binding functions. Induction of single Ig species by structurally dissimilar haptens. Proc Natl Acad Sci USA 70:3269–3274
4. Esser C, Radbruch A (1990) Immunoglobulin class switching: molecular and cellular analysis. Ann Rev Immunol 8:717–735
5. Varga JM, Klein GF, Fritsch P (1990) Binding of a mouse monoclonal IgE (anti-DNP) antibody to radio-derivatized polystyrene-DNP complexes. FASEB J 4:2678–2684
6. Inmam JK (1978) The antibody combining region: speculations on the hypothesis of general multispecificity. In: Bell GI (ed) Theoretical immunology. Marcel Dekker, New York, pp 243–278

7. Varga JM, Kalchschmid G, Klein GF, Fritsch P (1991) Mechanism of allergic cross-reactions I. Multispecific binding of ligands to a mouse monoclonal anti DNP IgE antibody. Molecular Immunology 28:641–654
8. Varga JM, Kalchschmid G, Klein GF, Fritsch P (1991) Mechanism of allergic cross-reactions II. Cross-stimulation, by chemically unrelated ligands, of rat basophilic leukemia cells sensitized with an anti DNP IgE antibody. Molecular Immunology 28:655–659

Loss of $Fc_{\varepsilon}R2$/CD23 Expression on T and B Lymphocytes During Rush Hyposensitization

J.C. Prinz[1,2], E.P. Rieber[2], and J. Ring[3]

[1] Dermatologische Klinik und Poliklinik der Ludwig-Maximilians-Universität München, Frauenlobstrasse 9–11, W-8000 München 2, Federal Republic of Germany
[2] Institut für Immunologie der Ludwig-Maximilians-Universität München, Goetherstrasse 31, W-8000 München 2, Federal Republic of Germany
[3] Universitäts-Hautklinik Eppendorf, Martinistrasse 52, W-2000 Hamburg 20, Federal Republic of Germany

Specific hyposensitization is the only causal therapy for type I hypersensitivity reactions besides allergen avoidance. Several immunologic changes are correlated with the efficacy of this treatment. They include reduced serum levels of allergen-specific IgE and a rise of allergen specific IgG antibodies, a diminished seasonal rise of pollen specific serum-IgE, a decrease in the proliferative response to stimulation with allergen of peripheral blood mononuclear cells (PBMC), and a reduced histamine release from basophils (summarized in [1]). Despite these observations, however, the working mechanisms of hyposensitization remain ill defined.

Regulation of the IgE response is dominated by two antagonistic cytokines, interleukin 4 (IL-4) and interferon gamma (IFN-γ). Of them, IL-4 directs Ig class switching to the expression of IgE in B lymphocytes [2] and simultaneously promotes the generation of effector cells for cytophilic IgE by inducing or enhancing the expression of low affinity Fc receptors for IgE ($Fc_{\varepsilon}R2$/CD23) on monocytes [3], B cells [4], Langerhans cells of the skin [5], and on T cells [6]. Also, IL-4 in combination with IL-3 or IL-5 supports growth and maturation of mast cells and eosinophils [7]. Conversely, IL-4 induced IgE synthesis and $Fc_{\varepsilon}R2$/CD23 expression on B and T cells are strongly inhibited by IFN-γ which itself favors the production of IgG [8]. Furthermore, IL-4 and IFN-γ mutually inhibit each other's production by T cells [9]. To induce IgE secretion, however, IL-4 requires additional yet unknown regulatory signals delivered during cognate T/B interaction [2].

Recently, we have demonstrated that allergen specific T cell blasts are characterized by the selective expression of $Fc_{\varepsilon}R2$/CD23 [6, 10] and, as reported by Rieber et al. in this book ("Human $Fc_{\varepsilon}R2$/CD23 in the Regulation of the Allergic Immune Response"), that $Fc_{\varepsilon}R2/CD23^{+}$ T cells are essentially involved in the induction of in vitro IgE synthesis. A role of $Fc_{\varepsilon}R2$/CD23 in the allergic IgE response is furthermore emphasized by the observation, that the proportion of B lymphocytes bearing $Fc_{\varepsilon}R2$/CD23 is significantly enhanced in the blood of atopic patients [11]. Thus, increased $Fc_{\varepsilon}R2$/CD23 expression on B and T lymphocytes is obviously a feature of the allergic IgE response.

To better understand the working mechanisms of immunotherapy, we now have analyzed the effect of rush hyposensitization on $Fc_{\varepsilon}R2$/CD23 expression on circulating B cells and on the in vitro allergen induced proliferation and $Fc_{\varepsilon}R2$/CD23 expression of T cells. In our study we have focussed on patients allergic to bee venom. PBMC were isolated from heparinized venous blood of these patients before and after rush hyposensitization. A course of rush hyposensitization consisted of 3–4 daily subcutaneous injections of increasing doses of allergen which were continued until the maintenance dose of 100 μg bee venom/injection had been reached. For stimulation experiments, the cells were cultured in the presence of phospholipase A_2 (PLA_2, 3 μg/ml), the major allergen from bee venom, or with tetanus toxoid (TT) for control. The degree of allergen-specific proliferation was evaluated by incorporation of [^{3}H]-thymidine. Fc_εR2/CD23 expression was determined either by rosette formation or by fluorescence activated cell sorter (FACS) analysis as described. In short, the cells were stained with a phycoerythrin labeled monoclonal antibody (mAb) specific for T cells (CD2), and were subsequently rosetted with indicator erythrocytes coated with the Fc_εR2/CD23 specific mAb M-L25. Fc_εR2/CD23 expression on B cells was determined by FACS analysis of PBMC stained with a phycoerythrin labeled mAb specific for B cells (CD20) and with the fluorescein labeled Fc_εR2/CD23 specific mAb M-L25 [6, 10].

Before hyposensitization, T lymphocytes from 7 of 47 patients showed a proliferative response to stimulation with PLA_2. The maximum stimulation index (SI) ranged from 2. 4 to 4. 8, and maximum PLA_2 induced Fc_εR2/CD23 expression was observed on 2.2%–6.1% of the T lymphocytes. After rush immunotherapy, PLA_2 induced proliferation and Fc_εR2/CD23 expression were markedly reduced (Table 1). This decrease was not due to the presence of suppressor cells, since PBMC obtained after rush hyposensitization could not inhibit allergen induced proliferation and Fc_εR2/CD23 expression of T cells from before immunotherapy (data not shown). Furthermore, reduction of proliferation was allergen specific and did not affect proliferation following stimulation with TT.

In a second approach, Fc_εR2/CD23 expression on circulating B lymphocytes was determined by flow cytometry before and after rush hyposensitization. In all patients tested, the proportion of Fc_εR2/CD23$^+$ B cells was markedly reduced (Table 1). A representative example of this diminuition is shown Fig. 1.

Table 1. Change of proliferation and of Fc_εR2/CD23 expression on T and B cells after specific stimulation following rush hyposensitization with bee venom.

Patient	Phospholipase A_2 (%$Fc_\varepsilon R^+$ T cells/SI)		Tetanus toxoid (SI)		%Fc_εR2/CD23$^+$ B cells	
	Before Hy	After Hy	Before Hy	After Hy	Before Hy	After Hy
W.G.	3.9/3.1	0 /1.1	2.9	3.8	79.6	55.3
H.J.	3.8/4.0	1.2/1.2	25.7	19.5	55.4	48.9
B.L.	3.5/3.1	0 /1.3	16.3	16.3	59.0	50.0
H.P.	2.2/2.4	0 /0.9	NP	NP	85.1	72.4
A.W.	2.8/2.4	0 /0.9	77.8	53.9	61.5	53.1
E.G.	5.1/4.7	1.1/1.7	NP	NP	53.3	45.5
H.G.	6.1/4.8	0 /1.6	40.6	42.1	84.2	72.4

Hy, hyposensitization; SI, stimulation index; NP, no proliferation.

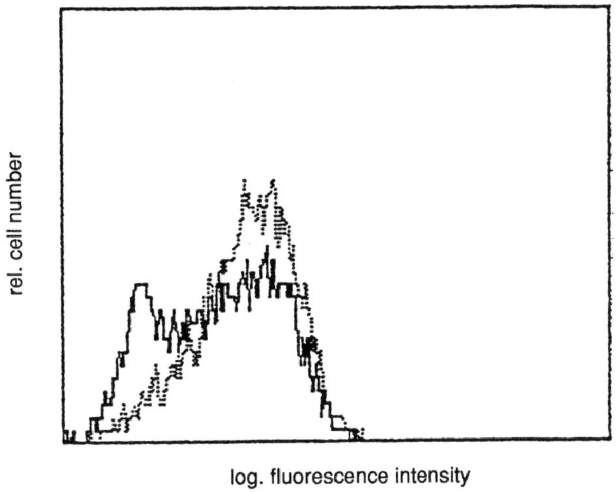

Fig. 1. Flow cytometry analysis of $Fc_{\varepsilon}R2/CD23$ expression on circulating B lymphocytes ······ before and ——— after hyposensitization

In summary, we were able to demonstrate that rush hyposensitization diminishes allergen induced proliferation and $Fc_{\varepsilon}R2/CD23$ expression of T cells and reduces the proportion of $Fc_{\varepsilon}R2/CD23^{+}$ circulating B lymphocytes. Yet, these results require further interpretation. The abated T cell proliferation could represent anergy or deletion of the allergen specific T lymphocytes. More likely, however, it results from a shift of the allergen specific T cells from the circulation to those draining lymph nodes, in which presentation of injected allergen takes places. This sight is also supported by a follow-up of pollen allergic patients during hyposensitization in whom a reconstituted or even enhanced proliferative response succeeded an initial diminuition of allergen specific proliferation (C. Jung and J. Ring, unpublished observation). The increased levels of allergen specific IgG antibodies observed in the sera of patients following immunotherapy furthermore argue against an impairment of the allergen specific T cell response. Instead, together with the decrease in IgE and the reduced $Fc_{\varepsilon}R2/CD23$ expression on B and T lymphocytes they most likely mark a change in the secretory activity of the allergen specific T cells: An augmented production of IFN-γ and a diminished secretion of IL-4, both reflected by an increased ratio of allergen specific IgG/IgE antibodies and a reduced proportion of $Fc_{\varepsilon}R2/CD23^{+}$ B and T lymphocytes, could explain many of the immunological changes induced by immunotherapy. We thus suggest that an alteration of the lymphokine pattern of the allergen specific T cells by prolonged immunization with allergen constitutes a fundamental working mechanism of immunotherapy.

References

1. Ring J (1987) Specific hyposensitization: modes of action, efficacy and safety. Allergologie 10:392–403
2. Gauchat JF, Lebman DA, Coffman RL, Gascan H, deVries JE (1990) Structure and expression of germline ε transcripts in human B cells induced by interleukin 4 to switch to IgE production. J Exp Med 172:463–473
3. Vercelli D, Jabara HH, Lee BW, Woodland N, Geha RS, Leung DYM (1989) Human recombinant interleukin 4 induces $Fc_{\varepsilon}R2$/CD23 on normal human monocytes. J Exp Med 169:1295–1307
4. Defrance T, Aubry JP, Rousset F, Vanberfliet B, Bonnefoy Y, Arai N, Takebe Y, Yokota T, Lee F, Arai K, deVries JE, Banchereau J (1986) Human recombinant interleukin 4 induces Fcε receptors (CD23) on normal human B lymphocytes. J Exp Med 165:1459–1467
5. Bieber T, Rieger A, Prinz JC, Rieber EP, Boltz-Nitulescu G, Neuchrist C, Kraft D, Ring J, Stingl G (1989) Induction of $Fc_{\varepsilon}R2$/CD23 on human epidermal Langerhans cells by human recombinant interleukin-4 and interferon-gamma. J Exp Med 170:309–314
6. Prinz JC, Baur X, Mazur G, Rieber EP (1989) Allergen-directed expression of $Fc_{\varepsilon}RII$ (CD23) on human T lymphocytes is modulated by IL-4 and IFN-g. Eur J Immunol 20:1259–1264
7. Mosmann TR, Bond MW, Coffman RL, Ohara J, Paul WE (1986) T cell and mast cell lines respond to B cell stimulatory factor 1. Proc Natl Acad Sci USA 83:5654–5658
8. Snapper CM, Paul WE (1987) Interferon gamma and B cell stimulatory factor 1 reciprocally regulate Ig isotype production. Science 236:944–947
9. Peleman R, Wu J, Fargeas H, Delespesse G (1989) Recombinant interleukin 4 suppresses the production of interferon-g by human mononuclear cells. J Exp Med 179:1751–1756
10. Prinz JC, Endres N, Rank G, Ring J, Rieber EP (1987) Expression of Fc_{ε}-receptors for IgE on activated human T lymphocytes. Eur J Immunol 17:757–761
11. Kikutani H, Suemura M, Owaki H, Nakamura, Sato R, Yamasaki K, Barsumian L, Hardy RR, Kishimoto T (1986) Fc_{ε}-receptor, a specific differentiation marker transiently expressed on mature B cells before isotype switching. J Exp Med 164:1455–1469

Construction of Human Suppressor T Cell Hybridomas That Produce Glycosylation Inhibiting Factors from Peripheral Blood Mononuclear Cells of Bee Venom Sensitive Patients

P. Thomas[1], C. Carini[2], M. Iwata[3], and K. Ishizaka[4]

[1]Dermatologische Klinik und Poliklinik der Ludwig-Maximilians-Universität, Frauenlobstrasse 9–11, W-8000 München 2, Federal Republic of Germany
[2]Cancer Biology Department, Harvard Medical School, Building 1, 9th Floor, 665 Huntington Avenue, Boston, MA 02115, USA
[3]Laboratory of Immunology, Mitsubishi Kasei Institute of Life Sciences, 11 Minamiooya, Machida-Shi, Tokyo 194, Japan
[4]La Jolla Institute for Allergy and Immunology, 11149 North Torrey Pines Road, La Jolla, CA 92037, USA

Previous experiments on the regulation of the IgE response in BDF1 mice provided a method of generating antigen specific suppressor T cells in vitro from antigen primed T cell populations [1]. Spleen cells of BDF1 mice primed with alum absorbed ovalbumin (OVA) for a persistent IgE response produced IgE potentiating factors, i.e., glycosylated IgE binding factors (IgE-BF) after antigenic stimulation but did not contain antigen-specific suppressor cells [2]. However, propagation of the antigen-activated T cells by interleukin-2 (IL-2) in the presence of glycosylation inhibiting factor (GIF) [3] or synthetic phospholipase A2 inhibitor facilitated the generation of antigen specific T cells that produced their own GIF. Stimulation of the T cells with OVA-pulsed syngeneic macrophages resulted in the formation of an IgE suppressive factor, i.e., unglycosylated IgE-BF and GIF, the latter of which had affinity for OVA. Thus, T cell hybridomas were constructed from the OVA specific T cells. Upon antigenic stimulation, some of the hybridomas formed OVA-binding GIF, which suppressed the primary IgE response of BDF1 mice to dinitrophenol (DNP)-OVA in a carrier specific manner [4] and which shared common antigenic structures with effector type, antigen specific, suppressor T cell factor (TseF) [5].

In view of the findings in the murine system and recent results with human peripheral blood mononuclear cells (PBMC) [6], attempts were made to establish GIF producing T cell hybridomas from PBMC of bee venom sensitive patients.

IgE-BF producing 12H5.7 mouse T hybridoma cells were used to detect GIF activity in test samples. This hybridoma produce glycosylated IgE-BF upon incubation with IgE. However, in the presence of GIF (enriched by affinity chromatography with 141B9 anti-lipomodulin antibody-sepharose), essentially all IgE-BF formed were unglycosylated – and thus following lentil-lectin-sepharose fractionation – IgE-BF were detected in effluent fractions by rosette inhibition assay [7]. Determination of phospholipase inhibitory activity of GIF containing samples upon dephosphorylation with porcine pancreatic phospholipase A2 (PLA2) was performed by using *E. coli* biosynthetically labeled with [^{3}H]oleic acid [8].

Since the major allergen in bee venom, PLA2, is cytotoxic, we employed PLA2 treated either with 6 M guanidine HCl in the presence of reducing agent (denatured PLA2, D-PLA2), or with cyanogen bromide (CNBr-PLA2).

To activate antigen primed T cells, PBMC of a patient allergic to bee venom were cultured for 3 days in the presence of D-PLA2. Nonadherent cells were resuspended for an additional 4 days in fresh medium containing human IL-2 and recombinant human lipocortin (PLA2 inhibitory activity similar to GIF). To construct T cell hybridomas, the activated and expanded T cells were fused at a ratio of 1:2 with BUC T lymphoma cells [9] by using polyethylene glycol. After initial culture in hypoxanthine-aminopterin-thymidine (HAT) medium, four hybrid clones were obtained, one of which (clone CL3) secreted GIF. Since CD3 expression could be detected on CL3 cells, the latter were treated with anti-CD3 antibody (OKT3) and subsequently cross-linked by culture in anti-mouse immunoglobulin-coated flasks. However, this failed to induce production of antigen specific GIF.

Thus, we constructed more T cell hybridomas from PBMC of the bee venom sensitive patient by following the same protocol, except that cells were stimulated with CNBr-PLA2. Out of the 22 hybridoma clones obtained, 10 constitutively formed GIF which bound to anti-lipomodulin (141B9) coupled sepharose. $CD3^+$ cells were enriched by cell sorting. After cross-linking of CD3 to the cells, five of the hybridomas produced GIF that bound to PLA2-sepharose (Table 1). Formation of IgE-BF could be shown by inhibition of rosette formation between $Fc\varepsilon R^+$ RPMI 8866 cells and human IgE coated ox erythrocytes.

These findings are in agreement with the observation that representative, murine GIF forming hybridomas produce antigen binding GIF upon stimulation

Table 1. Formation of antigen binding GIF by anti-CD3 treated hybridoma cells [a].

Clone	IgEBF [b] (%)	GIF activity in PLA2-sepharose [c]	
		Effluent	Eluate
AC5	20	0/21 (−)	31/0 (+)
AF10	36	19/0 (+)	0/21 (−)
BA6	8	29/0 (+)	0/24 (−)
BE12	65	0/31 (−)	25/0 (+)
BF5	65	0/27 (−)	20/0 (+)
CB7	64	0/28 (−)	17/0 (+)
CE5	58	0/28 (−)	35/0 (+)

Six out of seven clones formed IgEBF and five out of seven clones formed antigen binding GIF upon cross-linking of CD3.

GIF, glycosylation inhibiting factors; IgEBF, IgE binding factors; RFC, rosette-forming cells.

[a] T cell hybridomas were constructed by using CNBr treated bee venom PLA_2 for stimulation of PBMC. Seven hybridoma clones constitutively secreted GIF. These clones were treated with OKT3, and cultured in anti-mouse immunoglobulin coated flasks. Culture supernatants were fractionated on IgE-sepharose and proteins bound to the beads were eluted at acid pH. The effluent fraction from IgE-sepharose was fractionated on PLA_2-coupled sepharose, and the effluent and eluate fractions from the immunsorbent were assessed for GIF activity.

[b] Acid eluate fractions from IgE-sepharose were assessed for the presence of IgEBF. The proportion of IgE-RFC in the absence of IgEBF was 26.3% ± 0.6% (SD).

[c] GIF activity was determined by using the 12H5 cells. Numbers represent the percent rosette inhibition by the effluent/eluate fractions from lentil lectin sepharose. The proportion of IgE-RFC in the absence of IgEBF was 26.0% ± 0.7%; (+) indicates the presence of GIF.

with antigen-pulsed syngeneic macrophages or by cross-linking of CD3 to the cells [10] and suggest similarities between the antigen binding GIFs from the two species. In the murine system, antigen binding GIF suppressed the in vivo antibody response in a carrier (antigen) specific manner. Furthermore, both the monoclonal anti-lipomodulin antibody 141B9 and anti-I-J antibodies bound not only GIF, but also the non-antigen binding chain (I-J$^+$ chain) of effector type suppressor T cell factor (TseF) and inducer type suppressor T cell factor (TsiF) [11, 12].

Similarities between human GIF and mouse GIF suggest that the PLA2-binding GIF from human T cell hybridomas may represent molecules mediating T cell suppressor activity (TsF).

References

1. Iwata M, Ishizaka K (1988) Construction of antigen-specific suppressor T cell hybridomas from spleen cells of mice primed for the persistent IgE antibody formation. J Immunol 141:3270
2. Uede T, Hirata F, Hirashima M, Ishizaka K (1983) Modulation of the biologic activities of IgE-binding factors. I. Identification of glycosylation inhibiting factor as a fragment of lipomodulin. J Immunol 139:898
3. Ohno H, Iwata M, Nakamura T, Ishizaka K (1989) Effect of phospholipase A2 inhibitors on mouse T lymphocytes. I. Phospholipase A2 inhibitors exert similar immunological activities to glycosylation inhibiting factor. Int Immunol 1:425
4. Jardieu P, Akasaki M, Ishizaka K (1987) Carrier-specific suppression of antibody responses by antigen-specific glycosylation inhibiting factors. J Immunol 138:1494
5. Ferguson TA, Beaman KD, Iverson GM (1985) Isolation and characterization of a T suppressor factor by using a monoclonal antibody. J Immunol 134:3163
6. Carini C, Iwata M, Warner J, Ishizaka K (1990) A method to generate antigen-specific suppressor T cells in vitro from the peripheral blood T cells of honey bee venom sensitive allergic patients. J Immunol Methods 127:221
7. Iwata M, Huff TF, Ishizaka K (1984) Modulation of the biologic activities of IgE-binding factor. V. The role of glycosylation enhancing factor and glycosylation inhibiting factor in determining the nature of IgE-binding factors. J Immunol 132:1286
8. Rothut B, Russo-Marie F, Wood J, DiRosa M, Flower RJ (1983) Further characterization of the glucocorticoid induced anti-phospholipase protein "renocortin". Biochem Biophys Res Commun 117:878
9. Huff TF, Ishizaka K (1984) Formation of IgE-binding factors by human T cell hybridomas. Proc Natl Acad Sci USA 81:1514
10. Ohno H, Iwata M, Katamura K, Ishizaka K (1990) Effect of phospholipase A2 inhibitors on mouse T lymphocytes II. Phospholipase A2 inhibitor induces T cell hybridomas and a T cell clone for the formation of glycosylation inhibiting factor. Int Immunol 2:257
11. Jardieu P, Ishizaka K (1987) Possible relationship of an antigen-specific suppressor factor to phospholipase inhibitory protein. In: Goldstein G, Bach F, Wigzell H (eds) Immune regulation by characterized polypeptides. Liss, New York p 595
12. Steele JK, Kuchroo VK, Kawasaki H, Jayaraman S, Iwata M, Ishizaka K, Dorf ME (1989) A monoclonal antibody raised to lipomodulin recognizes factors in two independent hapten-specific suppressor networks. J Immunol 142:2213

Anti-IgE Autoantibodies Hide Specific IgE and Are Mistaken for Specific IgG

E. Jensen-Jarolim and B.M. Stadler

Institute of Clinical Immunology, Inselspital Bern, 3010 Bern, Switzerland

Abstract

In nonhyposensitized patients, a large proportion of specific IgE occurred in immune complexes with anti-IgE autoantibodies. These autoantibodies were mistaken for "specific IgG" in different immunoassays, such as a dot immunoassay and a RAST. Heating of immune complexes, consisting of IgE and anti-IgE autoantibodies, liberated more IgE resulting in a RAST class shift. Immune complexes of IgE and IgG anti-IgE autoantibodies contained more IgG than IgE. Radiolabeled purified anti-IgE autoantibodies specifically recognized IgE from different sources. The question whether these "hiding" autoantibodies may also represent biologically neutralizing or blocking antibodies has not yet been addressed.

Introduction

Numerous studies have assessed levels of specific IgG during hyposensitization therapy with various allergens. In a recent study using immunoblotting we showed that hyposensitization also leads to a significant increase in IgG in patients who were not successfully treated [1]. Based on the fact that a large proportion of serum IgE occurs in complexes with IgG anti-IgE autoantibodies [2], we might have mistaken IgG anti-IgE autoantibodies for specific IgG in the previous hyposensitization study. In order to test this hypothesis we investigated whether specific IgE normally occurs in immune complexes with anti-IgE autoantibodies. We would like to analyze nonhyposensitized patients for creating a basis for future studies.

Results

We fractionated serum pools of patients allergic to house dust mite using house dust mite affinity chromatography and serum pools of patients allergic to grass pollen by grass pollen affinity chromatography. Materials eluted from these columns were further passed over an anti-IgE affinity column using monoclonal antibody Le 27. Antibodies in the serum pools and eluents and effluents from the allergen and anti-IgE columns were then measured by immunodot assays for total IgE and IgG, specific IgE and IgG, and anti-IgE autoantibodies [3]. From the allergen columns specific antibodies were clearly detected. In the material further eluted from the anti-IgE column, "specific IgG" but only very low amounts of specific IgE were detected. IgG anti-IgE autoantibodies were found in the same sample. This finding questioned whether specific IgG was truly present and suggested that IgE was indeed present, but hidden within immune complexes.

In order to confirm these findings we further tested our samples using a commercial RAST (Pharmacia). Most interestingly, this assay also detected, besides specific IgE, "specific IgG" in the samples eluted from the anti-IgE column. After heating of the samples in order to disrupt immune complexes [4], more specific IgE was detected, again indicating that IgE was hidden in immune complexes by anti-IgE autoantibodies in the untreated samples.

The composition of immune complexes was examined by SDS-PAGE and immunoblotting. IgG was easily detected in effluents and eluents from the anti-IgE column, while no IgE was detected in the eluents from the anti-IgE column at the protein concentrations used, even though the immunoassays proved its presence. The ratio of IgE to IgG anti-IgE autoantibodies in immune complexes might therefore be greater than 1:1. The IgG in the effluents might represent truly specific IgG, the IgG in the eluent IgG anti-IgE autoantibodies.

Next we studied whether the IgG antibodies, which represented the majority of antibodies in the fraction eluted from the anti-IgE column, were capable of specifically reacting with IgE. Eluents and effluents from the anti-IgE column (obtained from house dust mite experiments) were therefore radiolabeled and used as revealing antibodies for immunoblotting. The labeled antibodies of the eluent fraction from the anti-IgE column reacted strongly with IgE, the labeled antibodies of the effluent fraction did not. This result indicated that the majority of antibodies eluted from the anti-IgE affinity column were anti-IgE autoantibodies.

As shown in the present study, IgG anti-IgE autoantibodies can easily be mistaken for "specific IgG" because immune complexes of IgE and autoantibody

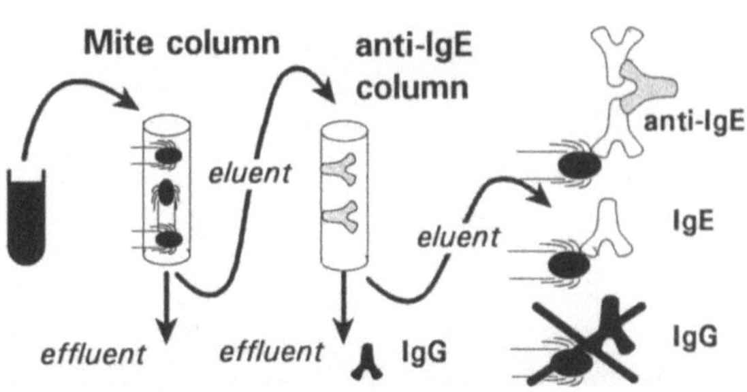

Fig. 1. Allergen specific antibody purification by affinity chromatography. If a sole immunological detection system was used to evaluate the column yield, we measured "specific" anti-allergen IgG in the subsequent eluent fractions (*crossed out immunoglobulin*). Measurements of specific IgE and anti-IgE autoantibodies revealed that most specific IgE was hidden by autoantibodies (*shaded antibody*)

bind via IgE to the allergen on the solid-phase (Fig. 1). Thus, anti-isotype autoantibodies should be considered as a major factor interfering with IgE determinations, which are based on the use of anti-IgE antibody but of the xenogeneic type. Future studies will reveal whether the increase in "specific IgG" levels during hyposensitization therapy consists of allergen specific IgG plus IgG anti-IgE autoantibody. At present we also do not know whether the masked specific IgE is also biologically neutralized. The final aim will be, of course, to evaluate whether an anti-IgE antibody, which is hiding IgE, is also a blocking antibody.

References

1. Jarolim E, Poulsen LK, Stadler BM, Mosbech H, Oesterballe O, Kraft D, Weeke B (1990) A long term follow-up study of hyposensitization with immunoblotting. J Allergy Clin Immunol 85:996–1004
2. Vassella CC, de Weck AL Stadler BM (1990) Natural anti-IgE autoantibodies interfere with diagnostic IgE determination. Clin Exp Allergy 20:295–303
3. Hong CS, Stadler BM, Wälti M, de Weck AL (1986) Dot-immunobinding assay with monoclonal anti-IgE antibodies for the detection and quantitation of human IgE. J Immunol Methods 95:195–202
4. Inganäs M, Johansson SGO, Bennich H (1981) Anti-IgE antibodies in human serum: occurrence and specificity. Int Archs Allergy Appl Immunol 65:51–61

Mast Cells and Mediator Release

In Vitro Growth of Human Mast Cells and Their Functions*

T. Ishizaka[1], T. Furitsu[1], N. Inagaki[1], and A. M. Dvorak[2]

[1]La Jolla Institute for Allergy and Immunology, 11149 N. Torrey Pins Road, La Jolla, CA 92037, USA
[2]Beth Israel Hospital, Harvard Medical School and the Charles A. Dana Research Institute, 330 Brookline Avenue, Boston, MA 02215, USA

Abstract

Long-term coculture of mononuclear cells of human umbilical cord blood with mouse skin derived 3T3 fibroblasts resulted in the development of human mast cells. These mast cells are morphologically and functionally mature, contain 1.4–2.8 μg histamine per 10^6 cells, and bear approximately 10^5 FcεR1 per cell. The mast cells sensitized with human IgE released histamine upon challenge with anti-IgE. All of the cells contained human mast cell tryptase. Electron microscopic analysis of the cells showed that they were mature human mast cells and clearly different from basophilic granulocytes. Most of the mast cells contained some granules with regular crystalline arrays and both tryptase and chymase, thus resembling human skin mast cells.

When mononuclear cells of cord blood were seeded in a millicell insert which was placed on a 3T3 fibroblast monolayer, the number of mast cells that developed in the inserts was comparable to the number that developed following coculture of the same cord blood cells with 3T3 fibroblasts, indicating that direct contact between mast cell progenitors and fibroblasts is not essential. Recent observations that mast cells developed in the presence of concentrated culture supernatants of 3T3 fibroblasts without fibroblast feeder layer confirmed that soluble factors released from 3T3 fibroblasts are essential and sufficient for the differentiation of human mast cell progenitors in vitro.

Introduction

Recent developments in recombinant DNA technology have made various recombinant cytokines available. These are powerful tools for analyzing factors involved in the differentiation and proliferation of hematopoietic cells. In the murine system, it is well established that recombinant interleukin-3 (IL-3) promotes the proliferation of mouse mast cell lines [1] and facilitates the formation of mast cell

* This work was supported by Health and Human Services grants Al 10060, Al 27517, Al 20487, and CA 28834, and a research contract with DNAX Research Institute for Molecular and Cellular Biology. This is publication no. 3 from the La Jolla Institute of Allergy and Immunology.

colonies in semisolid cultures of mouse bone marrow (BM) cells [2]. Suspension culture of murine BM cells with recombinant IL-3 results in the development of a pure mast cell population [3]. It is also known that recombinant IL-4 supports the proliferation of IL-3 dependent mouse mast cells [4], and that recombinant IL-4 is an essential factor for in vitro clonal growth of murine connective tissue type mast cells [5].

IL-3 dependent, BM derived mast cells appear to be analogous to mast cells in the gastrointestinal mucosa and different from those in connective tissues [6]. However, Levi-Schaffer et al. [7] and Dayton et al. [8] demonstrated that coculture of BM derived, IL-3 dependent mast cells with 3T3 fibroblasts, in the presence of IL-3 containing conditioned medium, resulted in a change to a phenotype resembling connective tissue mouse mast cells.

In contrast to the murine mast cell system, the growth factors and microenvironment required for the differentiation and proliferation of human mast cells and basophils are unknown. In the past 10 years, numerous attempts have been made to develop human mast cells and basophils in vitro [9–13]. Several groups, including ours, demonstrated in vitro development of human basophils from-progenitors in BM, umbilical cord blood, and fetal liver [14–17]. However, reproducible in vitro development of human mast cells has not been achieved. Recombinant human IL-3 promoted a transient selective differentiation of human basophils in suspension culture of BM and cord blood cells [18–20]. After 4 weeks of culture with IL-3, however, the majority of nonadherent cells in the culture became eosinophils, and no mast cells were detected. Furthermore, in contrast to the murine system, recombinant human IL-4 failed to promote the differentiation of either basophils or mast cells in suspension culture of cord blood cells or BM cells [18–20].

Our subsequent studies revealed that recombinant IL-1, -2, -3, -4, -5, -6, or -9 and granulocyte/macrophage colony-stimulating factor (GM-CSF), either individually or in combination, did not facilitate the differentiation of human mast cells in suspension cultures of BM or cord blood cells (unpublished data). The results suggested to us that differentiation of human mast cells may require a feeder layer or cytokine(s) from non-T cells. We explored this possibility and cocultured mononuclear cells of cord blood with various human and murine fibroblasts [21].

Coculture of Cord Blood Cells with Human and Murine Fibroblasts

Three human fibroblast cell lines, one derived from human embryo skin (Detroit 551) and two derived from human fetal lung (MRC-9 and IMR-90), were obtained from the American Type Culture Collection and tested for their ability to maintain viability and function of human lung mast cells. Since Levi-Schaffer and her co-workers demonstrated that mouse 3T3 fibroblasts were capable of maintaining viability and function of human lung mast cells [22, 23], 3T3 fibroblasts derived from Swiss albino mouse skin were also employed as a positive control. The results clearly showed that after 4 weeks of cocultures, 3T3 fibroblasts were effective in maintaining the number and viability of human lung mast cells. Fur-

Table 1. Long-term cocultures of cord blood cells with 3T3 fibroblasts.

Conditioned medium (EN)	Weeks	Viable cells per well	Differential count (%)							
			Ba	Eo	Neu	Mac	Ly	Bla	M-cells	Fib
	0	10^6	0.5	1	62.5	7.5	26	0.5	0	0
(+)	4	8.9×10^5	8	25	4.5	6.5	3	0.5	0	52.5
	8	4.8×10^5	1.4	3	2	11.8	3.2	0	3	75.6
	11	3.0×10^5	0.5	0	0	6.5	0.5	0	17.5	75
(−)	4	7.4×10^5	2.8	4.8	1.6	20.4	6	0.4	0	64
	8	2.5×10^5	1	0.2	3.8	28.2	4.6	0.4	1.6	60.2
	11	2.9×10^5	0	0	0	7.6	2.8	0	8	81.6

Ba, basophils; Eo, eosinophils; Neu, neutrophils; Mac, macrophages; Ly, lymphocytes; Bla, blasts; Fib, fibroblasts and fibroblast-like cells.

thermore, lung mast cells cocultured with 3T3 cells had the highest histamine content and gave the maximum histamine response to anti-IgE [21].

In the next series of experiments, aliquots of whole nucleated cells of cord blood were cocultured with mouse 3T3 fibroblasts or one of the three human fibroblasts cell lines in the presence or absence of conditioned medium (EN), which is a fraction of the culture supernatant of phytohemagglutinin (PHA) stimulated human T cells from which IL-2 has been eliminated [15]. Every 2 weeks, cells developed in the cultures were examined by differential counting. When the cord blood cells were cocultured with 3T3 fibroblasts, mononuclear cells containing metachromatic granules appeared after 8 weeks of culture (see Table 1). We tentatively called these mast cell-like cells M cells. The number of M cells increased by 11 weeks. In the particular cord blood cell culture containing EN, shown in Table 1, 17.5% of the total cells recovered from the well or 70% of the non-fibroblast cells were M cells. M cells also developed in the absence of EN, and subsequent studies showed that EN was not essential for the growth of M cells.

The majority of the cells that developed in the coculture of cord blood cells with human fibroblasts were basophils and eosinophils; no mast cells were detected during 11 weeks of culture [21]. When the same cord blood cells were cultured without a fibroblast feeder layer, the majority of the cells died by 11 weeks. The small number of cells remaining in the culture were macrophages [21].

Morphological and Ultrastructural Characteristics of M cells

M cells developed in 80 days of coculture of cord blood cells with 3T3 fibroblasts are shown in Fig. 1. The cells each contain a large oval or round nucleus and a cytoplasm filled with metachromatic granules. They are morphologically distinguishable from mature basophils remaining in the culture and appear to be mast cells.

Figure 2A shows an electron micrograph of an M cell developed in coculture of cord blood cells with 3T3 fibroblasts for 84 days. It has a monolobed nucleus

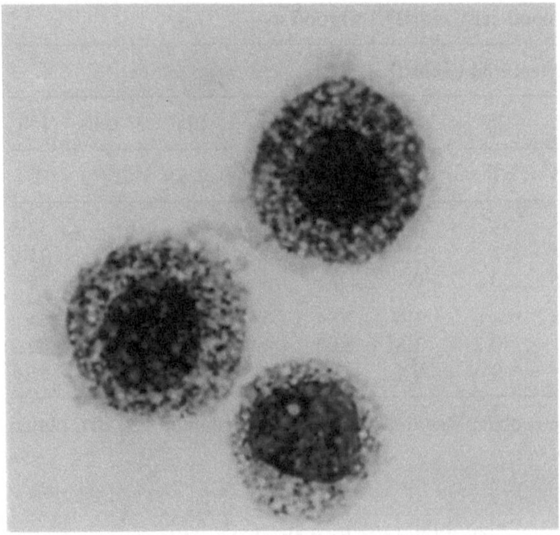

Fig. 1. Mast cells developed in a long-term coculture of cord blood nucleated cells with 3T3 cells. 80 days culture; May/Grunwald/Giemsa staining, ×3300

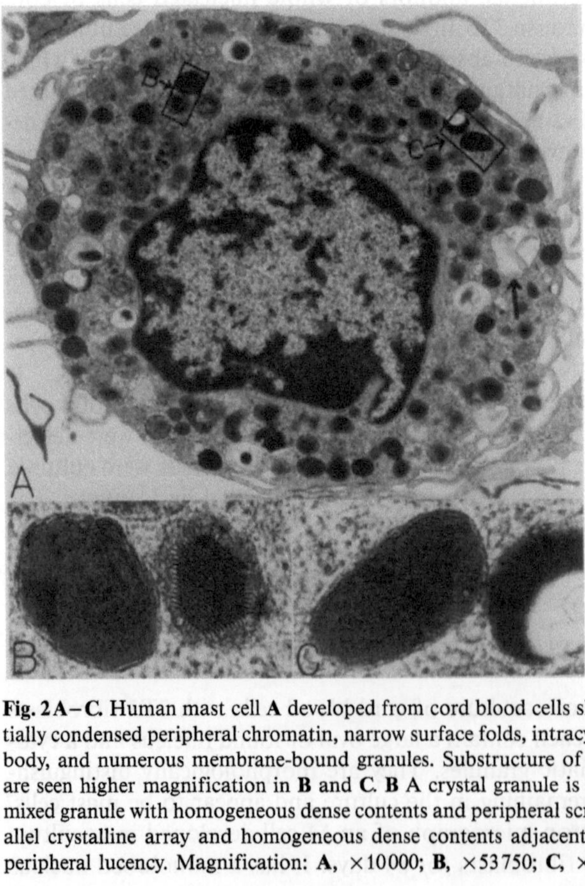

Fig. 2A–C. Human mast cell **A** developed from cord blood cells shows monolobed nucleus with partially condensed peripheral chromatin, narrow surface folds, intracytoplastic canaliculi (*arrow*), a lipid body, and numerous membrane-bound granules. Substructure of granules delineated by boxes in **A** are seen higher magnification in **B** and **C**. **B** A crystal granule is seen in cross-section adjacent to a mixed granule with homogeneous dense contents and peripheral scrolls. **C** A mixed granule shows parallel crystalline array and homogeneous dense contents adjacent to a dense lipid body, with focal peripheral lucency. Magnification: **A**, ×10000; **B**, ×53750; **C**, ×55625

with partially condensed chromatin, narrow surface folds characteristic of mast cells, a lipid body, and numerous membrane bound granules. M cells contain granules of various substructural patterns, which have been described in human mast cells studied in vivo and in isolated, purified preparations from multiple organ sources [24]. Figure 2B shows a higher magnification of two granules: a crystal granule and a mixed granule with homogeneous dense contents and peripheral lamelli. In Fig, 2C, a mixed granule with parallel crystalline arrays and homogeneous dense contents is seen adjacent to a dense lipid body. Most M cells contain some granules with regular crystalline arrays, resembling those frequently seen in mast cells from human skin [24].

Presence of Human Mast Cell Tryptase and Chymase in M Cell Granules

In order to confirm that M cells are indeed human mast cells, we examined whether granules in M cells contain human mast cell tryptase or chymase, in collaboration with Drs. Schwartz and Irani, Medical College of Virginia. In preliminary immunofluorescence experiments, it was found that granules in almost all M cells were clearly stained with monoclonal antibodies specific for human mast cell tryptase [25], while granules in cultured basophils failed to do so. Furthermore, examination of the cells by sequential double staining procedures for the detection of tryptase and chymase [26] revealed that 84% of M cells granules contained both tryptase and chymase, thus resembling human skin mast cells [21]. These findings may have some significance, since mast cells containing both tryptase and chymase predominate among the mast cells in human skin, while the majority of human lung mast cells have granules containing only tryptase [27].

Immunological Properties of M cells and Their Requirements for Growth

M cells, developed by coculture of cord blood cells witz 3T3 fibroblasts for over 10 weeks, contained 1.4 – 2.8 μg histamine per 10^6 cells. The presence of FcεRI on M cells was demonstrated by immunofluorescence and by the binding of ^{125}I-labeled human E myeloma protein (PS). The number of FcεRI was estimated to be approximately 10^5 per cell. The presence of functional FcεRI was confirmed by the fact that M cells sensitized with human IgE released histamine upon challenge with anti-IgE, whereas unsensitized cells failed to do so. It was also found that the kinetics of anti-IgE induced histamine release from M cells was similar to those of anti-IgE induced histamine release from human lung and skin mast cells [28 – 30].

The majority of mature M cells were clearly stained with monoclonal antibody YB5B8, which recognizes surface markers on human mast cells [31], while monoclonal antibody VIM12, which recognizes human basophil surface markers [32], failed to stain M cells as examined by immunofluorescence. By contrast, basophils developed in the culture were stained with VIM12; but not with YB5B8. It was also found that a monoclonal antibody against FcεRII, H107 [33] failed to stain M cells. These findings collectively indicate that M cells are indeed human mature mast cells. The results also suggest that the majority of the cells are probably of the skin mast cell type.

Although the number of mast cells developed in the cultures greatly varied from one cord blood specimen to another, the development of mast cells was quite reproducible. In 55 cultures, in which 10^6 cord blood cells were cocultured with 3T3 fibroblasts in a well, 10^3-10^5 mature mast cells per well were recovered after 8–10 weeks of culture.

Our studies also showed that neither IL-3 nor T cell derived conditioned medium was essential for the in vitro growth of human mast cells. Coculture of normal BM cells with 3T3 fibroblasts resulted in the development of mast cells, but to a lesser extent than from cord blood (0.5%–3% of the total cells after 11 weeks coculture).

Are 3T3 Fibroblasts Derived from Swiss Albino Mouse Skin the Best Feeder Layer for Human Mast Cell Growth?

Reproducible development of mature human mast cells in vitro by long term coculture of cord blood cells with 3T3 fibroblasts is the first major breakthrough in the development of human mast cells in vitro and has provided us with a valuable tool for the analysis of cytokines involved in the development of human mast cells.

To further our studies, we examined whether any other 3T3 fibroblasts could provide better support for mast cell differentiation than those derived from Swiss albino mouse skin. Thus, cord blood cells were cocultured with a derivative of NIH 3T3 fibroblasts, ψCRE [34], and the development of mast cells was followed. As shown in Table 2, mast cells were detected as early as 2–3 weeks, as determined by metachromatic and anti-tryptase staining. The number of mast cells and histamine content per well reached a maximum around 6–8 weeks. After 8 weeks, all of the metachromatic granule containing cells in the cultures were mast cells. The results clearly showed that mast cells develop earlier with ψCRE than with Swiss albino 3T3 fibroblasts.

Table 2. Development of human mast cells on ψCRE fibroblasts.

Culture (weeks)	Viable cells per well	Viability (%)	Metachromatic granule containing cells		Tryptase (+) cells (%)	Histamine content (ng/well)
			Basophils (%)	Mast cells (%)		
0	10^6	99	2.0	0	ND	0.7
2	4.2×10^5	90	2.8	1.2	1.8	14
4	3.7×10^5	94	3.8	7.4	8.1	34
6	3.0×10^5	92	0.4	24.2	27.6	72
8	3.0×10^5	93	0	28.6	30.5	123
10	2.0×10^5	95	0	26.0	29.7	118

Is Direct Contact Between 3T3 fibroblasts and Mast Cell Progenitors Essential for Their Differentiation?

The most critical question was whether direct contact with 3T3 fibroblasts was essential for differentiation of mast cell progenitors. In order to answer this question, mononuclear cells from cord blood were either seeded in a millicell insert which was placed on 3T3 monolayers, or cocultured with 3T3 cells. The development of mast cells with or without direct contact with 3T3 fibroblasts was then compared. The number of mast cells developed in the culture differed greatly from one cord blood specimen to another; however, similar numbers of mast cells developed in millicells and direct cocultures with fibroblasts, when the same cord blood were compared. The results clearly showed that differentiation of mast cell progenitor do not require direct contact with 3T3 fibroblasts and suggested that soluble factors released from 3T3 fibroblasts are sufficient for the development of human mast cells in vitro.

Since mast cells developed earlier in cocultures of cord blood cells with ψCRE fibroblasts, cord blood cells were seeded in the millicells, placed on ψCRE monolayers and the development of mast cells followed. Mast cells became detectable in the millicells within 2–3 weeks even without contact with the fibroblasts. The results suggest that ψCRE 3T3 fibroblasts may produce more growth factors for mast cells than Swiss albino 3T3 fibroblasts.

In order to confirm that soluble factors are sufficient for the differentiation of mast cell progenitors, culture supernatants of ψCRE fibroblasts were prepared under different culture conditions, and concentrated supernatants were added to cord blood cell cultures. It was found that the number of mast cells which developed during 3 weeks culture of cord blood cells in the presence of the culture supernatant was comparable to that developed in the cocultures (Table 3). The results confirmed that soluble factors released from the fibroblasts are sufficient for the differentiation of mast cell progenitors in cord blood.

Based on these findings, fractionation of the culture supernatant of 3T3 fibroblasts is underway for biochemical identification of growth factors for human mast cells

Table 3. Development of mast cells by ψCRE culture supernatant.

Culture	Mast cells developed from cord blood cells[a]	
	Cultured with 2 × culture supernatant (per well)	Coculture with ψCRE (per well)
1	1.1×10^4	6.4×10^3
2	1.1×10^4	1.7×10^4
3	7.2×10^3	1.2×10^4
4	3.1×10^4	1.5×10^4
5	1.2×10^4	1.8×10^4
Mean ± SD	$1.44\pm0.94\times10^4$	$1.37\pm0.47\times10^4$

[a] 1.5×10^6 cord blood cells were seeded per well and cultured for 3 weeks. Cord blood cells contained no mast cells.

Acknowledgements. We would like to express our sincere appreciation to: Dr. J.R. Niebyl, Dr. E. Haller, Ms. O. Wilkins, and Ms. J. Garnes of The Johns Hopkins Hospital; Ms. V. Walborn, Scripps Memorial Hospital for umbilical cord blood; Dr. D.A. Donnenberg, The Johns Hopkins Hospital for bone marrows from normal donors; Dr. M. Ogawa, University of South Carolina for his assistance in photomicroscopy; Dr. N. Arai, DNAX Research Institute for Molecular and Cellular Biology; Dr. R.L. Stevens, Harvard Medical School and Dr. K. Ishizaka, La Jolla Institute for Allergy and Immunology for their support and encouragement; Drs. L.B. Schwartz and A.M.A. Irani, Medical College of Virginia for their collaboration on analysis of proteases; Dr. L. Ashman, University of Adelaide, Dr. O. Majdic, University of Vienna, and Dr. R. Andreesen, Klinikum der Alber-Ludwigs-Universität, Freiburg for their generous supply of monoclonal antibodies, YB5B8, VIM12, and Max 1.

Our special appreciation goes to Ms. C.G.L. Ko, The Johns Hopkins University; Ms S. Kissell, Harvard Medical School; and Ms. M. Raygo, La Jolla Institute for Allergy and Immunology for their outstanding technical assistance.

References

1. Rennick DM, Lee FD, Yokota T, Arai K, Cantor H, Nabel GJ (1985) A cloned MCGF cDNA encodes a multilineage hematopoietic growth factor: multiple activities of interleukin 3. J Immunol 134:910–914
2. Rennick DM, Young G, Muller-Sieburg C, Smith C, Arai N, Tanabe Y, Gemmell L (1987) Interleukin-4 (B-cell stimulatory factor 1) can enhance or antagonize the factor-dependent growth of hemopoietic progenitor cells. Proc Natl Acad Sci USA 84:6889–6893
3. Saito H, Okajima F, Molski TFP, Shaafi RI, Ui M, Ishizaka T (1987) Effects of ADP-ribosylation of GTP-binding protein by pertussis toxin on immunoglobulin E-dependent and -independent histamine release from mast cells and basophils J Immunol 138:3927–3934
4. Smith CA, Rennick DM (1986) Characterization of a murine lymphokine distinct from interleukin-2 and interleukin-3 (IL-3) possessing a T cell growth factor activity and a mast-cell growth factor activity that synergizes with IL-3. Proc Natl Acad Sci USA 83:1857–1861
5. Hamaguohi Y, Kanakura Y, Fujita J, Takeda S, Nakano T, Tarui S, Honjo T, Kitamura Y (1987) Interleukin-4 as an essential factor for in vitro clonal growth of murine connective tissue-type mast cells. J Exp Med 165:268–273
6. Razin E, Stevens RL, Akiyama F, Schmid K, Austen KF (1982) Culture from mouse bone marrow of a subclass of mast cells possessing a distinct chondroitin sulfate proteoglycan with glycosaminoglycans rich in *N*-acetylgalactosamine-4,6-disulfate. J Biol Chem 257:7229–7236
7. Levi-Schaffer F, Austen KF, Gravallese PM, Stevens RL (1986) Coculture of interleukin-3-dependent mouse mast cells with fibroblasts results in a phenotypic change of the mast cells. Proc Natl Acad Sci USA 83:6485–6488
8. Dayton ET, Pharr P, Ogawa M, Serafin WE, Austen KF, Levi-Schaffer F, Stevens RL (1988) 3T3 fibroblasts induce cloned interleukin-3-dependent mouse mast cells to resemble connective tissue mast cells in granular constituency. Proc Natl Acad Sci USA 85:569–572
9. Horton MA, O'Brien AW (1983) Characterization of human mast cells in long-term culture. Blood 62:1251–1260
10. Czarnetzki BM, Figor CG, Kolde G, Vroom T, Aalberse R, deVries JE (1984) Development of human connective tissue mast cells from purified blood monocytes. Immunology 51:549–554
11. Yuen E, Brown RD, van der Lubbe L, Richard KA, Kronenberg H (1988) Identification and characterization of human hemopoietic mast cell colonies. Int Soc Exp Hematol 16:896–902
12. Kirshenbaum AR, Goff JP, Dreskin SC, Irani AMA, Schwartz LB, Metcalf DD (1989) IL-3 dependent growth of basophil-like cells and mast cell-like cells from human bone marrow. J Immunol 142:2424–2429
13. Ishizaka T, Saito H, Furitsu T, Dvorak AM (1989) Growth of human basophils and mast cells in vitro. In: Galli SJ, Austen KF (eds) Mast cell and basophil differentiation and function in health and disease. Raven, New York, pp 39–47
14. Razin E, Rifkind AB, Cordon-Cardo C, Good RA (1981) Selective growth of a population of human basophil cells in vitro. Proc. Natl Acad Sci USA 78:5793–5796

15. Ogawa M, Nakahata T, Leary AG, Sterk AR, Ishizaka K, Ishizaka T (1983) Suspension culture of human mast cells/basophils from umbilical cord blood mononuclear cells. Proc Natl Acad Sci USA 80:4494–4498
16. Tadokoro K, Stadler BM, de Weck AL (1983) Factor-dependent in vitro growth of human normal bone marrow-derived basophil-like cells. J Exp Med 158:857–871
17. Seldin G, Caulfield JP, Hein A, Osathanondh R, Nabel G, Schlossman S, Stevens RL, Austen KF (1986) Biochemical and phenotypic characterization of human basophilic cells derived from dispersed fetal liver with murine T cell factors. J Immunol 136:2222–2230
18. Saito H, Hatake K, Dvorak AM, Leiferman KM, Donnenberg AD, Arai N, Ishizaka K, Ishizaka T (1988) Selective differentiation and proliferation of hematopoietic cells induced by recombinant human interleukins. Proc Natl Acad Sci USA 85:2288–2292
19. Valent P, Ashman LK, Hintenberger W, Eckersberger F, Majdic O, Lechner K, Bettelheim P (1989) Mast cell typing: demonstration of a distinct hematopoietic cell type and evidence for immunophenotypic relationship to mononuclear phagocytes. Blood 73:1778–1785
20. Dvorak AM, Saito H, Estrella P, Kissel S, Arai N, Ishizaka T (1989) Ultrastructure of eosinophils and basophils stimulated to develop in human cord blood mononuclear cell cultures containing recombinant human interleukin-5 or interleukin-3. Lab Invest 61:116–132
21. Furitsu T, Saito H, Dvorak AM, Schwartz LB, Irani AMA, Burdick JF, Ishizaka K, Ishizaka T (1989) Development of human mast cells in vitro. Proc Natl Acad Sci USA 86:10039–10043
22. Levi-Schaffer F, Austen KF, Caulfield JP, Hein A, Gravellese PM, Stevens RL (1987) Co-culture of human lung-derived mast cells with mouse 3T3 fibroblasts: morphology and IgE-mediated release of histamine, prostagladin D_2, and leukotrienes. J Immunol 139:494–500
23. Levi-Schaffer F, Austen KF, Caulfield JP, Hein A, Bloes WF, Stevens RL (1985) Fibroblasts maintain the phenotype and viability of the rat heparin-containing mast cell in vitro. J Immunol 135:3454–3462
24. Dvorak AM (1989) Human mast cells. Adv Anat Embryol Cell Biol 114:1–107
25. Schwartz LB (1985) Monoclonal antibodies against human mast cell tryptase demonstrate shared antigenic sites on subunits of tryptase and selective localization of the enzyme to mast cells. J Immunol 134:526–531
26. Castells MC, Irani AMA, Schwartz LB (1987) Evaluation of human peripheral blood leukocytes for mast cell tryptase. J Immunol 138:2184–2189
27. Irani AMA, Schecter NM, Craig SS, DeBlois G, Schwarth LB (1986) Two types of human mast cells that have distinct neutral protease compositions. Proc Natl Acad Sci USA 83:4464–4468
28. Schulman ES, MacGlashan DW, Peters SP, Schleimer RP, Newball HH, Lichtenstein LM (1982) Human lung mast cells: purification and characterization. J Immunol 129:2662–2667
29. Ishizaka T, Conrad D, Schulman E, Sterk AR, Ishizaka K (1983) Biochemical analysis of initial triggering events of IgE-mediated histamine release from human lung mast cells. J Immunol 130:2357–2362
30. Benyon RC, Lowman MA, Church MK (1987) Human skin mast cells; their dispension, purification and secretory characterization. J Immunol 138:861–867
31. Mayerhofer G, Godd SJ, Spargo LDJ, Ashman LK (1987) Specificity of a mouse monoclonal antibody raised against acute myeloid leukemia cells for mast cells in human mucosal and connective tissues. Immunol Cell Biol 65:241–250
32. Knapp W, Majdic O, Stockinger H, Bettelheim P, Liszka K, Koller U, Peschel C (1984) Monoclonal antibodies to human myelomonocyte differentiation antigens in the diagnosis of acute myeloid leukemia. Med Oncol Tumor Pharmacother 1:257–262
33. Ikuta K, Takami M, Kim C-W, Honjo T, Miyoshi T, Tagaya Y, Kawabe T. Yodoi J (1987) Human lymphocyte Fc receptor for IgE: sequence homology of its cloned cDNA with animal lectins. Proc Natl Acad Sci USA 84:819–823
34. Danos O, Mulligan RC (1988) Safe and efficient generation of recombinant retroviruses with amphotropic and ecotropic host ranges. Proc Natl Acad Sci USA 85:6460–6464

Mast Cells and Fibroblasts: Partners or Neighbors?

F. Levi-Schaffer[1] and M. Shalit[2]

[1]Department of Pharmacology, School of Pharmacy, Hadassah Medical School, The Hebrew University, Jerusalem, Israel
[2]Allergy Unit, Department of Medicine A, Hadassah University Hospital, Jerusalem, Israel

Abstract

We have previously shown that 3T3 mouse Swiss Albino skin derived fibroblasts are able to maintain viability, functional activity and typical phenotype of rat peritoneal mast cells (connective tissue type MC, CTMC) for more than a month and to change the phenotype of in vitro differentiated mucosal type MC (mouse bone marrow derived BMMC).

The CTMC/3T3 coculture system serves as a model for the in vivo situation in which CTMC are in close contact with fibroblasts. We have used this model to investigate the behavior of MC up to 21 days after non-immunologic and immunologic activation. Our findings indicate that CTMC survive activation even when 95% – 98% of their histamine content is released and slowly (weeks) resynthesize their histamine content. When activated with compound 48/80 and reactivated with this segretagogue 3 – 7 – 14 days later, CTMC released the same percentages of histamine as naive (never challenged) MC. In contrast, challenge of CTMC by crosslinking surface IgE with anti-IgE antibodies or specific antigen, led to a partial loss of MC responsiveness to rechallenge with the same immunological stimulus for 7 – 14 days after the first activation. We have also shown that in addition to 3T3 fibroblasts, normal and cGVHD (chronic Graft vs-Host Disease, that serves as a model of scleroderma) mouse skin derived fibroblasts maintain CTMC properties and change BMMC phenotype.

The only other cell type, forming monolayers in culture, that can substitute for fibroblasts is the rat osteoblast-like cell line ROS 17/2.

Next we evaluated how CTMC can influence the cocultered fibroblast properties. In an in vitro model of wound (3T3 monolayer in which a linear wound is performed by cutting along the midline and scraping one half of the monolayer) immunologically activated CTMC greatly enhanced fibroblasts migration and proliferation. Coculture of MC with 3T3 or cGVHD fibroblasts in the presence of active supernatants derived from cGVHD splenocytes induced a significant release of histamine, starting on day 5 – 8 of the experiment. In this coculture system we have studied the effect of MC presence and activation on the fibroblast proliferation. We found that the presence of CTMC for 8 days on 3T3 monolayer significantly enhanced [^{3}H]-thymidine incorporation into the 3T3 fibroblasts, while this effect was less prominent on the cGVHD fibroblasts. When both monolayers were cultured with or without CTMC for 8 days in the presence of cGVHD supernatants, there was a drastic decrease in the fibroblast DNA synthesis.

In conclusion, by using our coculture system of MC and fibroblasts we have been able to demonstrate that these two cell types are actively interacting and influencing one another.

Introduction

Interactions between mast cells (MC) and fibroblasts have been postulated since the days of Paul Ehrlich (the discoverer of MC), who made the observation that MC number increases in areas of chronic inflammation, often sites of fibrous tissue production [28]. Since then a number of clinical and experimental situations have been found in which prominent numbers of MC are associated with fibrosis. These include idiopathic [14], bleomycin [8] and irradiation [33] induced pulmonary fibrosis, keloids [32], scar tissues [15], neurofibromas [27], and scleroderma [2].

Due to their anatomical proximity in connective tissues, fibroblasts and MC have been postulated to affect each other. In the past few years it has been demonstrated that IgE receptor-bearing, histamine-containing, metachromatic cells can be obtained from mouse [7] and from rat [10] by using a mixed culture system of thymus cells on a monolayer of embryonic cells that contain fibroblasts. More recently, Jarboe et al. [12] showed that a MC committed progenitor, present in mesenteric lymph node cells of mice infected with *Nippostrongylus brasiliensis*, is able to proliferate and differentiate into a MC with a connective tissue phenotype, when cultured with 3T3 or embryonic fibroblasts or with soluble growth factors present in the supernatants of these monolayers. The presence of interleukin-3 (IL-3) in these cultures committed the MC progenitor to become a MC with a mucosal phenotype. Furitsu et al. [6] found that by coculturing nucleated cells of human umbilical cord blood with mouse skin derived 3T3 fibroblasts for 11–14 weeks, MC similar to human tissue MC could be obtained.

Recently, we have developed an in vitro defined and simplified system in which rodent MC are cocultured on 3T3 fibroblast monolayers (MC/3T3). Exploiting this coculture we have been studying both MC ontogeny and physiology and MC fibroblast interactions. This review will deal with the results of these studies.

Coculture of Mouse Bone Marrow Derived Mast Cells with 3T3 Fibroblasts Induces a Change in Phenotype

Two subclasses of MC have been characterized in rodents and more recently in humans, the connective tissue type (CTMC) and the mucosal type (MMC), so designated according to their primary anatomical locations.

CTMC and MMC display a different phenotype and can be distinguished from one another by their differential histochemical staining properties, dependence or lack of dependence on IL-3 for maintenance, the type of proteoglycans and neutral serine proteases synthesized and packaged in their respective secretory granules, their histamine content, differential activation by a number of secretagogues, and by their susceptibility to inhibition by anti-allergic drugs [29, 30].

In our studies we have been using mouse bone marrow derived mast cells (BMMC) as the in vitro counterpart of MMC and rat peritoneal MC as the ex vivo representative of CTMC.

To determine the ontogenic relationship between MMC and CTMC, we have examined the effects of culturing BMMC with 3T3 fibroblasts, which provide a connective tissue microenvironment. These coculture conditions induced a change in the BMMC phenotype towards that of CTMC. Most of the BMMC adhered to the fibroblasts within 48 h and due to the presence of IL-3 in the medium, continued to divide. Although all the granules of the starting BMMC were, like MMC, alcian blue+/safranine−, in 10−14 days all the granules of all the MC became safranine+, similar to mouse and rat CTMC. The chemical basis for the increased avidity of the granules for safranine was found to be the synthesis of heparin by the cocultured BMMC. BMMC/3T3 also increased their histamine content (approximately 15-fold) and exhibited a more homogeneous and electron dense granule appearance [22, 23]. After 21 days of coculture, BMMC displayed globopentaosylceramide (Forssmann antigen), a typical CTMC surface marker [13]. In addition the percentage of histamine released in adherent BMMC/3T3, sensitized whith IgE and challenged with the specific antigen, increased about threefold compared to BMMC in suspension. Also, the release of leukotriene (LT) B_4 and of prostaglandin (PG) D_2 increased significantly (two to threefold and three to fourfold, respectively). Similar data were obtained when the cocultured BMMC were activated with calcium ionophore [23].

By showing that cloned IL-3 dependent MC change their phenotype toward that of CTMC, we established that coculture with fibroblasts induces the described changes in the entire population of starting BMMC [3].

Rat Peritoneal Mast Cells Cocultured with 3T3 Fibroblasts Maintain Their Viability, Phenotype and Functional Activity

Since CTMC exist predominantly in connective tissues, it appeared reasonable that connective tissue cells would produce the microenvironment necessary for maintaining both the survival and the phenotype of this subclass of MC. Therefore, we cocultured isolated and purified rat peritoneal MC (as a source of CTMC) on 3T3 fibroblasts (CTMC/3T3). Under these conditions MC survived for at least 30 days but died within 2 days when cultured with fibroblast matrix, collagen, gelatin, fibronectin, or fibroblast-conditioned medium [21]. Separation of the MC from the fibroblast monolayer through Millipore filters also failed to maintain MC viability. Close contact and attachment between MC and fibroblasts is therefore needed for CTMC to be kept viable. Indeed, within 10 min after seeding onto 3T3 monolayers, MC adhere so strongly to the fibroblasts that it is impossible to separate the two cell types from one another without extensive proteolytic treatment.

CTMC cocultured with 3T3 fibroblasts did not divide, continued to synthesize heparin proteoglycans, and kept their classical morphological appearance and histochemical properties. When activated immunologically 2 weeks after seeding, MC were functionally active and could release histamine and generate PGD_2 [21].

An additional effect of coculture on rat MC is the enhancement of mediator release. When these CTMC/3T3 .were activated by various secretagogues, e.g., compound 48/80, anti-IgE antibodies, substance P, bradykinin, and neurotensin, they released higher percentages of histamine compared to freshly isolated MC [20]. This may indicate that the coculture system activates biochemical processes involved in degranulation or that some granule fusion occurs in cocultered MC which makes them better "releasers". As mentioned above, a similar enhancement of histamine release and arachidonic acid metabolite production was observed in BMMC adherent to the 3T3 monolayer [23].

Regeneration of Rat CTMC/3T3 After Activation

Little is known about the events that take place in the CTMC following degranulation, mostly because of the previous lack of in vitro systems in which activated CTMC could be maintained for long periods of time. We therefore exploited our coculture system to investigate the viability, morphological appearance, histamine synthesis, and susceptibility to a second challenge of rat peritoneal MC up to 14 days after activation carried out with immunological and nonimmunological stimuli. When activated with sufficent compound 48/80 to release approximately 90% of their histamine content, MC remained fully viable throughout the duration of the experiment. Some 3–4 h after activation, MC started reacquiring their resting morphology and in 1–2 weeks they were more densely granulated, grossly resembling nonactivated control MC [19].

Reactivation of these MC, 2 and 6 h and 7 or 14 days after the first activation event resulted in a percentage histamine release that was similar to the first one and to control MC, indicating that these MC were as alive and as functionally active as control MC. The activated MC could partially resynthesize histamine during the 14 days after activation. On day 7 their histamine content was approximately 23% and on day 14 about 40% of the initial amount they had on day 0, prior to activation [19].

In contrast, challenge of CTMC/3T3 with anti-IgE antibodies (about 20% histamine release) or with specific antigen, after presensitization of the MC with the relevant anti-IgE antibodies (about 70% histamine release), led to a partial state of desensitization to the same ligand, i.e., a decrease in histamine release upon rechallenge. Stimulation of CTMC with anti-IgE antibodies resulted in a nearly complete loss of response to a second similar challenge for up to 7 days. Presensitization of the desensitized CTMC with IgE antibodies prior to the second challenge did not overcome the state of unresponsiveness. Only by day 14,

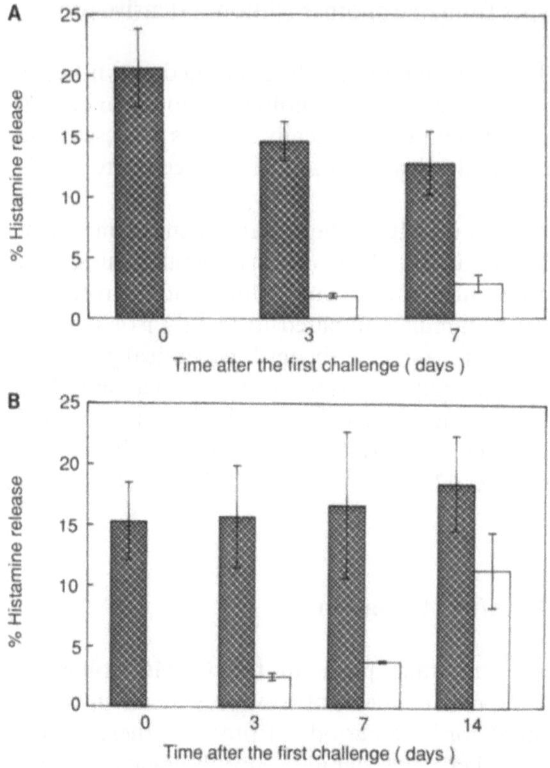

Fig. 1 A, B. Histamine release from CTMC/3T3 challenged with anti-IgE antibodies. **A** CTMC/3T3 were challenged with goat anti-rat IgE antibodies for 15 min at 37 °C on day 0 of the experiment (▩); control cultures were incubated with TG+ + buffer (Tyrode's buffer containing 0.1% gelatin, 1.8 mM $CaCl_2$ and 0.9 mM $MgCl_2$) alone. Three and 7 days later, cultures were activated with anti-IgE antibodies; experimental cultures were rechallenged (□); first challenge for control cultures (▩). **B** The same experimental protocol described in **A** was followed but CTMC/3T3 were sensitized with mouse monoclonal anti-dinitrophenol antibodies for 1 h at 37°C prior to activation with anti-IgE antibodies. Rechallenged experimental cultures (□) and control cultures challenged for the first time (▩). Results are expressed as the net percentage of histamine release, i.e., percentage of histamine released from experimental cultures minus the percentage of histamine released from cultures incubated throughout the experiment. Data are the mean ±SEM of five experiments performed in duplicate

rechallenged MC were able to release percentages of histamine comparable to those of naive, never challenged CTMC (Fig. 1). The immunologically activated MC resynthesized histamine with kinetics similar to MC challenged with compound 48/80.

Thus, following both nonimmunological and immunological activation, rat peritoneal MC remain viable and regenerate, as indicated by morphological and biochemical data. However, the kinetics of the functional regeneration are dependent upon the type of stimulus employed. Following nonimmunological activation with compound 48/80, MC can be reactivated to release high percentages of histamine as early as a few hours after the first challenge. By contrast immunological activation leads to a state of partial unresponsiveness which resolves only gradually in 14 days.

Effect of Prolonged Incubation of Mouse and Rat CTMC/3T3 with Chronic Graft-vs-host Disease Derived Splenocyte Supernatants and Cytokines

In a murine model of chronic graft-vs-host disease (cGVHD) across minor histocompatibility barriers, mice develop changes reminiscent of scleroderma, including cutaneous fibrosis and loss of fat, atrophy of dermal appendages, and a mononuclear infiltration whith T cells and macrophages [11]. Extensive MC activation and degranulation occurs coincident with the development of dermal fibrosis. An interesting feature of this model is that the CTMC reaction is slow to develop, occurring over a period of weeks and waning by 300 days [16]. We therefore investigated the long-term effects of supernatants from splenocytes of such cGVHD mice on mouse and rat CTMC/3T3 [24]. We have found that cGVHD supernatants were able to release histamine from these MC in a slow fashion starting only after 5–8 days of coculture (Table 1). This slow activation process was noncytotoxic and did not desensitize the MC to further activation with either anti-IgE antibodies or compound 48/80. Supernatants from mice in the early stages of cGVHD and with extensive fibrotic changes (days 11–28) were very active in promoting histamine release. In contrast, supernatants from mice which had cGVHD for 290 days, in whom fibrosis started to disappear and the MC had returned to full granulation, were inactive [24].

One possible explanation for the induction of histamine release by cGVHD supernatants and for the chronic activation of the MC observed in vivo in the cGVHD mice is the involvement of cytokines in the process. Indeed, it has been shown that several cytokines, including IL-1, IL-3 and granulocyte/macrophage colony-stimulating factor (GM-CSF), modulate of directly induce histamine release from human basophils [1, 25]. We therefore investigated the effects of various interleukins (IL-2, IL-3, IL-4, and a mixture of IL-3 and IL-4) on mouse and rat CTMC/3T3.

We found that the continuous presence of these cytokines for 7–9 days in the culture media was neither toxic nor growth stimulating as detected by the stability of MC numbers in culture. The lack of proliferative effects of the mixture of IL-3

Table 1. Effect of cGVHD splenocyte supernatants on histamine release from mouse CTMC/3T3 fibroblasts during long-term incubation[a].

Supernatant	Histamine in the culture medium[b] (μg)			
	Day 2	Day 4	Day 6	Day 2+4+6
cGVHD	0.083 ± 0.009	0.349 ± 0.109	0.650 ± 0.084	1.082 ± 0.190
cGVHD control	0.089 ± 0.011	0.193 ± 0.012	0.492 ± 0.135	0.711 ± 0.148
Normal BALB/c	0.034 ± 0.007	0.069 ± 0.014	0.097 ± 0.026	0.200 ± 0.024

[a] Mouse CTMC/3T3 fibroblasts were cultured in the presence of the different supernatants for up to 6 days. Every 2 days the supernatants were withdrawn, assessed for the presence of histamine, and replaced with fresh ones.
[b] Data are the mean ± SD of an experiment performed in triplicate (see [24]).

and IL-4 on the CTMC would suggest that fibroblasts provide the "final" microenvironment in which these cells cannot divide.

While short-term incubation did not cause histamine release from the MC, long-term incubation of mouse CTMC/3T3 with IL-2 (100 u/ml), IL-3 (50 u/ml), IL-4 (50 u/ml), or a mixture of IL-3 and IL-4 (25 u/ml) induced an increase in basal histamine release of 79.3% ± 19.0%, 41.0% ± 17.3%, 25.2% ± 10.4%, and 30.2% ± 3.2%, respectively, over control cells incubated with medium alone. When rat CTMC/3T3 were incubated for 7 days with the various interleukins an enhancement in histamine release similar to that observed with mouse CTMC/3T3 was found. Preincubation for 1 h of rat CTMC/3T3 with the various interleukins prior to immunologic activation with anti-IgE antibodies enhanced histamine release. The highest effect was observed with a mixture of IL-3 and IL-4 (60.4% ± 10.8% increase) followed by IL-2 (51.5% ± 4.5%), IL-4 (28.6% ± 10.4%), and IL-3 (13.2% ± 4.2%) (Fig. 2). Therefore, interleukins display a double proinflammatory effect on MC by enhancing basal and anti-IgE mediated histamine release.

In general, these two studies on MC activation upon prolonged incubation with cGVHD supernatants or with cytokines have shown that MC can undergo a novel type of stimulation. Prolonged incubation of MC with a factor(s) contained in the cGVHD splenocyte supernatants or with cytokines led to a slow and continuous release of histamine into the culture medium. Both the onset and the duration of this activation pattern are different from the anaphylactic one, which is completed within a few minutes after the addition of the secretagogue.

Interestingly, Ginsburg et al. [7] and Hammel et al. [9] also noted a similar MC "slow" activation pattern both at a biochemical (histamine release) and morphological (electron microscopy) level. They employed an in vitro system in which

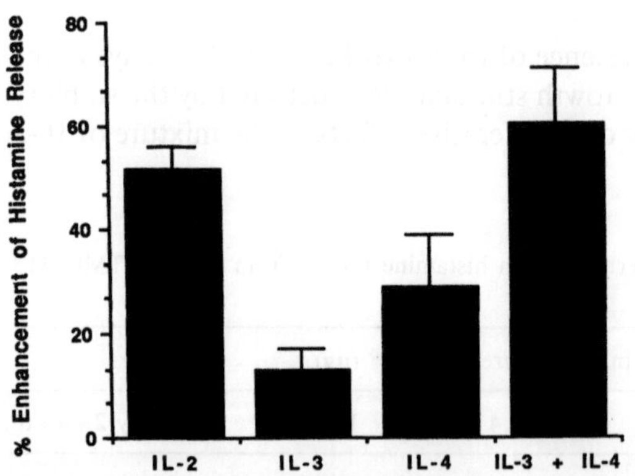

Fig. 2. Enhancement of anti-IgE induced histamine release from rat CTMC/3T3 by interleukins. Rat CTMC/3T3 were preincubated for 1 h with the various interleukins (100 u/ml) or with TG++ buffer. An optimal concentration (1:35) of goat anti-rat IgE antibodies or TG++ buffer were added for an additional 20 min. The percentages of histamine released by the cultures were calculated. Control CTMC/3T3 incubated with anti-IgE antibodies alone released 21.8% ± 4.1% histamine. Data are expressed as percentage of enhancement of histamine release of the control and are the mean ± SEM of four experiments performed in duplicate

MC were obtained from immunized mouse lymph node cells cultured on embryonic skin monolayers. When immune serum was added to this culture a gradual increase in histamine content was detected in the medium, although MC did not show any obvious characteristics of anaphylactic degranulation. More studies should be carried out to further characterize this slow nonanaphylactic type of MC activation and to assess its in vivo relevance.

Is the 3T3 Fibroblast Unique in Maintaining the CTMC and in Changing the BMMC Phenotype?

Normal mouse skin fibroblasts (from Balb/c mice) and cGVHD mouse skin fibroblasts (at day 5, before the development of fibrosis or at day 28 and 120, during fibrosis) were compared with 3T3 fibroblasts for their ability to maintain CTMC viability and functional activity and to induce a change in the BMMC phenotype. CTMC were cultured on fibroblasts monolayers for 8 days. During this time period and on all types of monolayers CTMC adhered equally well, maintained their viability, did not divide, and, when activated on the 8th day with an optimal concentration of compound 48/80, released approximately 90% of their histamine content, indicating full preserved functional activity. However, it was also found that the fibrotic cGVHD fibroblasts did not induce the cocultured CTMC to release histamine, indicating that the massive degranulation of dermal MC that occurs in cGVHD is not due to a direct activating effect of the fibroblasts on the MC.

BMMC cocultured with the different monolayers changed their phenotype toward that of CTMC, as indicated by the acquisition of safranine+ staining and by an increase in histamine content as on 3T3 monolayers. Therefore, both normal mouse fibroblasts and cGVHD derived fibroblasts, which are fibrotic and display alterations in cytokine production [26], are able, as are the 3T3 fibroblasts, to provide an adequate microenvironment to both CTMC and BMMC.

We have also investigated the specificity of the fibroblasts in maintaining CTMC viability by looking at a number of other cell types that can form monolayers in culture, such as macrophages, endothelial and epithelial cells, keratinocytes, and osteoblasts [22]. Only the rat osteoblast-like cell line ROS 17/2 was able to substitute for the 3T3 fibroblasts [17]. CTMC seeded on ROS monolayers adhered to them, remained viable for at least 2 weeks, did not divide, and were fully responsive to activation with compound 48/80. By utilizing metabolically inactive ROS cells and preventing contact between ROS and MC, we found that both release of factor(s) and cell-cell contact were required by ROS cells to exibit their MC supporting activity [17].

Thus, MC viability and functional activity are specifically maintained by fibroblastic and osteoblastic cells. The abundance of MC in bone and their participation in bone remodelling raise the possibility of physiological and pathological significance to interactions between MC and osteoblasts.

Do MC Affect Fibroblasts in the Cocultures?

From several studies it seems that MC may affect fibroblasts properties as well. For example, addition of compound 48/80 to organ cultures is followed by fibroblasts proliferation [5]. Mast cell granules are taken up by fibroblasts in vitro [31]. MC are also found in increased numbers in a series of fibrotic conditions, as earlier discussed, indicating their participation in these processes.

In our defined CTMC/3T3 coculture system we evaluated how CTMC influenced fibroblast properties in an in vitro model of wounding [18]. A linear wound was performed in confluent 3T3 or CTMC/3T3 cultures by cutting along the midline and scraping one half of the monolayer. After 42 h fibroblasts were counted in the scraped area of the wound. In the CTMC/3T3 cocultures 27.6±2.1 fibroblasts were found compared to 16.6±0.9 in the 3T3 cultures. The most significant increase in the number of fibroblasts was obtained upon activation of the MC with anti-IgE antibodies immediately after wound production (39.9±2.1). Stimulation with compound 48/80 had a weaker effect (32.7±1.5) (Fig. 3).

Incubation of 3T3 wounded monolayers with supernatants of anti-IgE, compound 48/80 activated MC, or sonicated MC induced an increase in fibroblast number similar to that found in unactivated CTMC/3T3. When [^{3}H]thymidine incorporation followed by autoradiography was performed, the highest number of fibroblasts in mitosis beyond the wound line was found in immunologically activated CTMC/3T3 followed by compound 48/80 activated CTMC/3T3 and buffer incubated CTMC/3T3 and 3T3. Upon addition of aphidicolin (antimitotic agent), MC were still effective in enhancing fibroblast migration. Thus CTMC significantly enhanced migration and proliferation of the fibroblasts showing that MC have a facilitating role in this in vitro wound model and suggesting that they may participate in the fibrotic stage of wound repair in vivo.

In another study of ours we found that, when CTMC are cocultured on intact 3T3 of cGVHD fibroblast monolayers for up to 8 days, there is an increase of

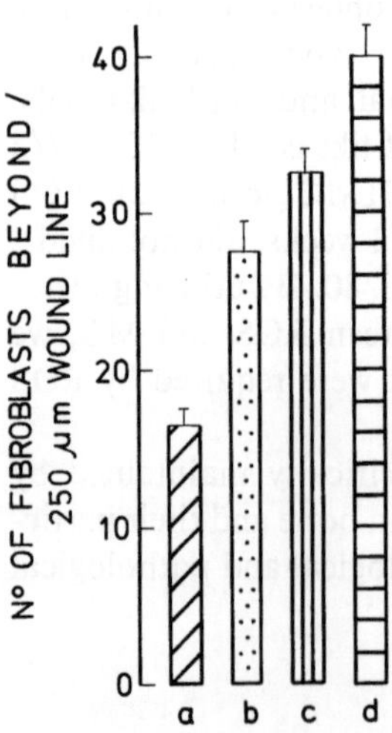

Fig. 3. Effect of unactivated and activated CTMC on fibroblasts, beyond the wound line. The number of fibroblasts found beyond the 250 µm wound line at 42 h after wounding is shown in the following cultures: 3T3 (*a*); buffer incubated CTMC/3T3 (*b*); CTMC/3T3 activated by compound 48/80 (*c*); and CTMC activated by anti-IgE (*d*). (See [18])

[^{3}H]thymidine incorporation into the fibroblast nuclei, indicating that CTMC can induce fibroblast proliferation even under conditions of contact inhibition (3T3 monolayers) or overt fibrosis (cGVHD monolayers).

BMMC also affect the biochemical properties of the cocultured fibroblasts. As mentioned earlier, after 21 days of coculture in the presence of IL-3, BMMC displayed globopentaosylceramide (Forssmann antigen), a typical CTMC surface marker. It was found that BMMC stimulated an increase in the synthesis and expression of this globopentaosylceramide on 3T3 fibroblasts. Therefore it seems that the subsequent appearance ot the marker on the surface of the BMMC is due to its secretion by fibroblasts and adsorption to the BMMC surface [13].

Moreover, during BMMC/3T3 culture, fibroblasts sloughed off the monolayer and, when examined by electron microscopy, appeared highly vacuolated in comparison to 3T3 fibroblasts cultured in the absence of BMMC. Recently, Dayton et al. [4] have demonstrated that when cocultured BMMC are maintained with IL-3 they induce the fibroblasts to multiply, resulting in an increase in collagen and proteoglycan content in the extracellular matrices of the cocultures.

Conclusions

Several observations have indicated that MC and fibroblasts can influence one another. We have demonstrated by using our defined in vitro system, in which MC are cocultured with fibroblasts, that MC and fibroblasts are indeed two actively interacting "partners". In fact, BMMC cocultured with fibroblasts change their phenotype towards that of CTMC. When cocultured with fibroblasts, CTMC are kept alive and functionally active. They become better histamine releasers and, when stimulated to degranulate, can regenerate.

Furthermore, the cocultured CTMC can be induced to slowly and chronically release histamine when incubated with cGVHD splenocyte supernantants and cytokines. Normal mouse skin and cGVHD skin fibroblasts can substitute for the 3T3 cells. Among all other cell types investigated, only the ROS osteoblastic cell line is able to maintain CTMC under in vitro conditions as fibroblasts do.

MC also influence fibroblast properties. For example, CTMC cause cocultured fibroblasts to proliferate. When CTMC are cocultured on a "wounded" fibroblast monolayer these cells are induced (by the MC presence and activation) to both proliferate and migrate. BMMC, in the presence of IL-3, induce the cocultured fibroblasts to proliferate and to synthesize more collagen and proteoglycans.

Further studies are needed to better characterize the interactions between MC and fibroblasts and to determine their role both in allergic inflammatory reactions and in other physiological and pathological conditions.

References

1. Alam R, Lett-Brown MA, Welter JB, Forsythe PA, Grany JA (1989) Comparative effect of recombinant IL-1, IL-2, IL-3, IL-4 and IL-6, IFN-γ granulocyte-macrophage-colony-stimulating factor, tumor necrosis factor-α and histamine-releasing factors on the secretion of histamine from basophils. J Immunol 142:3431–3435
2. Claman HN (1989) Mast cell changes in a case of rapidly progressing scleroderma – ultrastructural analysis. J Invest Dermatol 92:290–295
3. Dayton ET, Pharr P, Ogawa M, Serafin WE, Austen KF, Levi-Schaffer F, Stevens RL (1988) 3T3 fibroblasts induce cloned interleukin 3-dependent mouse mast cells to resemble connective tissue mast cells in granular constituency. Proc Natl Acad Sci USA 85:569–572
4. Dayton ET, Caulfield JP, Hein A, Austen KF, Stevens RL (1989) Regulation of the growth rate of mouse fibroblasts by IL-3-activated mouse bone marrow derived mast cells. J Immunol 142:4307–4313
5. Druvefors P, Norrby K (1988) Molecular aspects of mast-cell-mediated mitogenesis in fibroblasts and mesothelial cells in situ. Virchows Arch [B] 55:187–192
6. Furitsu T, Saito H, Dvorak AM, Schwartz LB, Irani AM, Burdick JF, Ishizaka K, Ishizaka T (1989) Development of human mast cells in vitro. Proc Natl Acad Sci USA 86:10039–10043
7. Ginsburg H, Nir I, Hammel I, Weisman BA, Naot Y (1978) Differentiation and activity of mast cells following immunization in cultures of lymph node cells. Immunology 35:485–502
8. Goto T, Befus D, Law R, Bienenstock J (1984) Mast cell heterogeneity and hyperplasia in bleomycin induced pulmonary fibrosis in rats. Annu Rev Respir Dis 130:797–802
9. Hammel I, Shiloh-Rabinovich H, Nir I (1988) Two populations of mast cells on fibroblast monolayers: correlation of quantitive microscopy and functional activity. J Cell Sci 91:13–19
10. Ishizaka T, Okudira H, Mauser LF, Ishizaka K (1976) Development of rat mast cells in vitro. I. Differentiation of mast cells from thymus cells. J Immunol 116:747–754
11. Jaffe BD, Claman HN (1983) Chronic graft-vs-host disease as a model for scleroderma. I. Description of model system. Cell Immunol 77:1–12
12. Jarboe DL, Marshall JS, Randolph TR, Kukolja A, Huff TF (1989) The mast cell commited progenitor. I. Description of a cell capable of IL-3-independent proliferation and differentiation without contact with fibroblasts. J Immunol 142:2405–2417
13. Katz HR, Dayton ET, Levi-Schaffer F, Benson AC, Austen KV, Stevens RL (1988) Coculture of mouse IL-3 dependent mast cells with 3T3 fibroblasts stimulates synthesis of globopentaosylceramide (Forssman glycolipid) by fibroblasts and surface expression on both populations. J Immunol 140:3090–3097
14. Kawanami O, Ferrans VJ, Fulmer JD, Crystal RG (1979) Ultrastructure of pulmonary mast cells in patients with fibrotic lung disorders. Lab Invest 40:717–734
15. Kirscher CW, Bailey JF (1972) The mast cells in hypertrophic scars. Tex Rep Biol Med 30:327–338
16. Lee Choi K, Giorno R, Claman HN (1987) Cutaneous mast cell depletion and recovery in murine graft-vs-host disease. J Immunol 138:4093–4101
17. Levi-Schaffer F, Bar-Shavit Z (1990) Osteoblast-like cell line maintains in vitro rat peritoneal mast cell viability and functional activity. Immunology 69:145–149
18. Levi-Schaffer F, Kupietzky A (1990) Mast cells enhance migration and proliferation of fibroblasts into an in vitro wound. Exp Cell Res 188:42–49
19. Levi-Schaffer F, Riesel N (1989) In vitro regneration of activated rat peritoneal mast cells cocultured with 3T3 fibroblasts. Cell Immunol 119:30–40
20. Levi-Schaffer F, Shalit M (1989) Differential release of histamine and prostaglandin D_2 in rat peritoneal mast cells activated with peptides. Int Arch Allergy Appl Immunol 90:347–357
21. Levi-Schaffer F, Austen KF, Caulfield JP, Hein A, Bloes WF, Stevens RL (1985) Fibroblasts maintain the phenotype and viability of the rat heparin-containing mast cells in vitro. J Immunol 135:3454–3465
22. Levi-Schaffer F, Austen KF, Gravallese PM, Stevens RL (1986) Coculture of interleukin 3-dependent mouse mast cells with fibroblasts results in a phenotype change of the mast cells. Proc Natl Acad Sci USA 83:6485–6488
23. Levi-Schaffer F, Dayton ET, Austen KF, Hein A, Caulfield JP, Gravallese PM, Liu FT, Stevens RL (1987) Mouse bone marrow-derived mast cells cocultured with fibroblasts. Morphology and

stimulation induced release of histamine, leukotriene B_4, leukotriene C_4, and prostaglandin D_2. J Immunol 139:3431–3441
24. Levi-Schaffer F, Mekori YA, Segal V, Claman HN (1990) Histamine release from mouse and rat mast cells cultured with supernatants from chronic murine graft-vs-host splenocytes. Cell Immunol 127:146–158
25. MacDonald SM, Schleimer RP, Kagey-Sobotka A, Gillis S, Lichtenstein LM (1989) Recombinant IL-3 induces histamine release from human basophils. J Immunol 142:3527–3532
26. Mekori YA, Huliel H, Levi-Schaffer F, Apte R (1990) Diminuished IL-1 production by dermal fibroblasts in chronic graft-vs-host disease (Abstr). J Allergy Clin Immunol 85:208
27. Riccardi VM, Eichner JE (1986) Neurofibromatosis: phenotype, natural history and pathogenesis. Johns Hopkins University Press, Baltimore
28. Riley JF (1959) The mast cells. Livingstone, Edinburgh
29. Shanahan F, Dendburg JA, Bienenstock J, Befus AD (1984) Mast cell heterogeneity. Can J Physiol Pharmacol 62:734–737
30. Stevens RL, Katz HR, Seldin DC, Austin KF (1985) Biochemical characteristics distinguish subclasses of mammalian mast cells. In: Befus AD, Bienenstock J, Denburg J (eds) Mast cell heterogeneity. Raven, New York pp 183–203
31. Subba Rao PV, Friedman MN, Atkins FM, Metcalfe DD (1983) Phagocytosis of mast cell granules by cultured fibroblasts. J Immunol 130:341–349
32. Sylven B (1945) Ester sulphuric acids on high molecular weight and mast cells in mesenchymal tumors. Acta Radiol (Stockh) 59:1–99
33. Watanabe S, Watanabe K, Ohishi T, Aiba M, Kageyama K (1974) Mast cells in the rat alveolar septa undergoing fibrosis after ionizing irradiation. Lab Invest 31:555–567

Factors Promoting Histamine and Leukotriene Release

C. A. Dahinden, M. Krieger, T. Brunner, S. Takafuji, and S. C. Bischoff

Institute of Clinical Immunology, Inselspital, 3010 Bern, Switzerland

Abstract

Basophils are known to release histamine and leukotrienes in response to IgE dependent and IgE independent agonists. Basophil degranulation and de novo synthesis of lipid mediators are clearly separately regulated. We found that the hematopoietic growth factors IL-3, IL-5, and GM-CSF profoundly modify the basophil response to diverse agonists, without inducing mediator release by themselves. The most potent, on a molar basis, is IL-3. These hematopoietic growth factors, at very low concentrations (a) enhance the releasability to all basophil agonists, (b) change the mediator profile, (c) enhance the rate of mediator release, (d) render basophils responsive to lower agonist concentrations, and (e) render basophils responsive to agonists, which by themselves are unable to activate basophils. Biologically active molecules affecting basophil function can now be divided into four groups according to their capacity to induce basophil degranulation and/or leukotriene generation: 1. complete agonists, 2. partial agonists, 3. incomplete agonists, 4. basophil response modifiers. It may be of particular relevance to the pathogenesis of allergic diseases that the same set of cytokines (IL-3, IL-5, GM-CSF) strongly modifies the function of basophils and eosinophils, the two major effector cell types found in allergic inflammatory sites.

Introduction

Basophils accumulate at inflammatory sites in allergic late phase reactions as well as in certain types of delayed type hypersensitivity reactions. An effector function of basophils in allergic late phase reactions can also be assumed based upon the mediator profile observed several hours after allergen challenge in vivo. The extent of mediator release by basophils may therefore be of particular relevance to the severity of symptoms in allergic disease. Another interesting feature of human basophils is their exceedingly high capacity to form lipid mediators in response to soluble agonists. In fact, they produce two to three orders of magnitude higher amounts of lipid mediators than any other effector leukocyte in peripheral blood. Therefore, even if the percentage of basophils present at an inflammatory site is relatively small, one must consider them a major source of inflammatory mediators [1, 2].

Results and Discussion

Human basophils are known to release preformed (e.g., histamine) as well as newly synthesized (e.g., leukotriene C4=LTC4) mediators in response to IgE dependent and IgE independent agonists. These include antigens, anti-IgE, C5a, FMLP and less defined cell derived products, so-called histamine releasing factors [3, 4]. Basophil degranulation and de novo synthesis of lipid mediators are clearly separately regulated. IgE receptor cross-linking and stimulation with the bacterial product analogue, formyl-methionyl-leucyl-phenylalanine (FMLP) promote the release of both classes of mediators. By contrast, C5a is a potent degranulating agent without inducing LTC4 formation (Fig. 1, with columns). Our recent

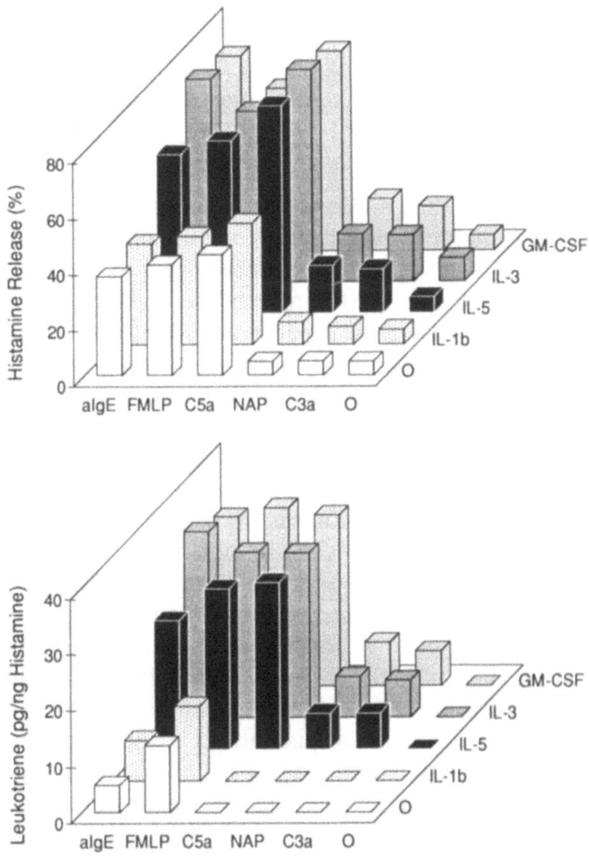

Fig. 1. Effect of cytokine preincubation upon basophil mediator release induced by various agonists. Human peripheral blood basophils were preincubated in buffer (*O*)or with cytokines (IL-5, IL-3, GM-CSF: 10 ng/ml, IL-1ß: 100 ng/ml) for 10 min and further incubated in buffer or stimulated for 20 min by C5a ($10^{-8}M$), anti-IgE (100 µg/ml), FMLP ($2.5 \times 10^{-6}M$), C3a ($10^{-6}M$), or NAP-1 ($10^{-7}M$) as second stimuli. The mean of histamine release (*upper panel*) and leukotriene generation (*lower panel*) from three separate experiments, each performed three times, with cells from representative donors is shown. The standard deviation of triplicates was less than 5% of the mean, and that of the three experiments less than 15% of the mean

Table 1. Effect of cytokines on basophil mediator release.

Cytokine	Histamine release	Leukotriene generation
IL-1	(+)	(+)
IL-2	–	–
IL-3	+ +	+ + +
IL-4	–	–
IL-5	+ +	+ + +
IL-6	–	–
GM-CSF	+ +	+ + +
γ-INF	–	–
α-INF	–	–
TNF	–	–
TGF-β	–	–

Effect of cytokines upon basophil releasability and lipid mediator synthesis in response to diverse agonists.
(+) to + + +, enhancement; –, no effect, IL, interleukin; GM-CSF, granulocyte-macrophage colony stimulating factor; INF, interferon; TNF, tumor necrosis factor; TGF, transforming growth factor.

studies have shown that hematopoietic growth factors are important regulators of lipid mediator synthesis. They are unable to induce lipid mediator synthesis by themselves but prime different cell types to produce leukotrienes and/or platelet-activating factor (PAF) in response to diverse in the respect inactive agonists [5–9]. For basophils, a particular set of cytokines, interleukins (IL-3, IL-5 and granulocyte-macrophage colony stimulating factor (GM-CSF) could be defined, which profoundly modify their response to diverse agonists (Table 1 and [9]). Interestingly, the same set of cytokines also enhances several functions of mature eosinophils [10]. Thus, IL-3, IL-5, and GM-CSF may be the most relevant cytokines involved in the pathogenesis of allergic inflammatory responses (late phase reactions). By contrast, a large number of cytokines have been examined and found to be inefficient in either inducing or modulating basophil mediator release (Table 1). The only one reported to enhance IgE dependent histamine release is IL-1 [11]. However, compared to the effects of IL-3, IL-5, and GM-CSF, this cytokine must be considered less important in influencing basophil mediator release (Fig. 1; Table 1). In basophils, IL-3, IL-5, and GM-CSF do not promote the release of relevant amounts of mediators by themselves, but modify the basophil function in a qualitatively identical manner. On a molar basis, IL-3 is the most potent priming agent within this set of cytokines. These hematopoietic growth factors (a) enhance the releasability to all agonists (Fig. 1), (b) change the mediator profile, e.g., allows LTC4 generation in response to C5a, which by itself induces histamine release only (Fig. 1), (c) enhance the rate and extent of mediator release in particular with regard to LTC4 formation [8], (d) render basophils responsive to lower agonist concentrations [8, 12], and (e) render basophils responsive to NAP-1 and C3a.

Particularly interesting is the fact that both the novel cell derived factor neutrophil activating peptide-1 (NAP-1) and the complement derived anaphylatoxin C3a are inefficient basophil agonists with regard to histamine release as well

Table 2. Classification of basophil cell agonists.

Class	Agonist	Histamine release		Leukotriene generation	
		−RM	+RM	−RM	+RM
I. "Complete" agonists	Multivalent IgE-crosslinking	++	+++	++	+++
	Divalent IgE-crosslinking	++	+++	+	+++
	FMLP	+	+++	+	+++
II. "Partial" agonists	C5a	++	+++	−	+++
III. "Incomplete" agonists	NAP-1	−	++	−	+
	NAP-2	−	+	−	−
	C3a	−	++	−	++

Classification of basophil agonists depending on their ability to induce histamine release or leukotriene generation with or without pretreatment with IL-3.
+ to +++, mediator release; −, no mediator release; FMLP, formyl-methionyl-leucyl-phenylalanine; NAP, neutrophil activating peptide; RM, "response modifiers" (IL-3, IL-5, GM-CSF) are class IV basophilic cell agonists.

as leukotriene generation, but trigger the release of both basophil mediators after preincubating the cells with IL-3, IL-5, and GM-CSF [12, 13]. The sequence of addition of these diverse factors is of crucial importance for the outcome of the release reaction. For example, if C5a is given before IL-3, no LTC4 synthesis occurs and histamine release is not, or only minimally, enhanced [5]. If the sequence of IL-3 and NAP-1 addition is reversed, no mediator release occurs at all [13]. In contrast, low concentrations of NAP-1 given before IL-3 even inhibit histamine release in response to the same factor (own unpublished result), emphasizing the importance of time and sequence of action of different agonists within the cytokine network. According to the ability of the diverse stimuli to promote the release of preformed and newly synthesized mediators either alone or when acting sequentially, we propose a classification of these agents into four categories (complete agonists, partial agonists, incomplete agonists and response modifiers) as presented in Table 2.

References

1. Denburg JA, Otsuka H, Ohnisi M, Ruhno J, Bienenstock J, Dolovich J (1987) Contribution of basophil/mastcell and eosinophil growth and differentiation to the allergic tissue inflammatory response. Int Arch Allergy Appl Immunol 82:321
2. Charlesworth EN, Iliopoulos O, MacDonald SM, Kagey-Sobotka A, Lichtenstein LM (1989) Cells and secretagogues involved in the human late-phase response. Int Arch Allergy Appl Immunol 88:50
3. Dahinden CA, Kurimoto Y, Baggiolini M, Dewald B, Walz A (1989) Histamine and sulfidoleukotriene release from human basophils: different effects of antigen, anti-IgE, C5a, f-met-leu-phe and the novel neutrophil-activating peptide NAF. Int Arch Allergy Appl Immunol 90:113

4. Alam R, Welter JB, Forsythe PA, Lett-Brown MA, Grant JA (1989) Comparative effect of recombinant IL-1, -2, -3, -4, and -6, INF-ψ, granulocyte-macrophage colony-stimulating factor, tumor necrosis factor-α, and histamine-releasing factors on the secretion of histamine from basophils. J Immunol 142:3431
5. Kurimoto Y, De Weck AL, Dahinden CA (1989) Interleukin-3 dependent mediator release in basophils triggered by C5a. J Exp Med 170:467
6. Dahinden CA, Zingg J, Maly FE, De Weck AL (1988) Leukotriene production in human neutrophils primed by recombinant human granulocyte/macrophage colony-stimulating factor and stimulated with the complement component C5a and FMLP as second signals J Exp Med 167:1281
7. Wirthmüller U, De Weck AL, Dahinden CA (1989) Platelet-activating factor production in human neutrophils by sequential stimulation with granulocyte-macrophage colony-stimulating factor and the chemotactic factors C5a or formyl-methionyl-leucyl-phenylalanine. J Immunol 142:3213
8. Kurimoto Y, De Weck AL, Dahinden CA (1991) The effect of interleukin 3 upon IgE-dependent and IgE-independent basophil degranulation and leukotriene generation. Eur J Immunol 21:361
9. Bischoff SC, Brunner T, De Weck AL, Dahinden CA (1990) Interleukin 5 modifies histamine release and leukotriene generation by human basophils in response to diverse agonists. J Exp Med 172:1577
10. Fujisawa T, Abu-Ghazaleh R, Kita H, Sanderson CJ, Gleich GJ (1990) Regulatory effect of cytokines on eosinophil degranulation. J Immunol 144:642
11. Massey WA, Randall TC, Kagey-Sobotka A, Warner JA, MacDonald SM, Gilis S, Allison AC, Lichtenstein LM (1989) Recombinant human IL-1α and IL-1β potentiate IgE-mediated histamine release from human basophils J. Immunol 143:1875
12. Bischoff SC, De Weck AL, Dahinden CA (1990) Interleukin 3 and GM-CSF render human basophils responsive to low concentrations of the complement component C3a. Proc Natl Acad Sci USA 87:6813
13. Dahinden CA, Kurimoto Y, De Weck AL, Lindley I, Dewald B, Baggiolini M (1989) The neutrophil-activating peptide NAF/NAP-1 induces histamine and leukotriene release by interleukin 3-primed basophils. J Exp Med 170:1787

Cyclosporin A Inhibits IgE Receptor Mediated Exocytosis from Rat Basophilic Leukemia Cells Without Inhibiting Phosphatidylinositol Hydrolysis, Ca^{2+} Uptake, the Rise in Cytosolic Ca^{2+} Actin Polymerization or Arachidonic Acid Release

T. Hultsch*, M. Kaliner, and R. J. Hohman

Allergic Diseases Section, Laboratory of Clinical Investigation, National Institute of Allergy and Infectious Diseases, National Institute of Health, Bethesda MD, 20892, USA

Abstract

Cyclosporin A (CSA) is produced by the fungus *Tolypocladium inflatum* and used clinically as an immunosuppressive drug. Although the mechanism of immunosuppression is unclear, CSA is generally thought to inhibit the immune response by preventing both transcription of T cell derived cytokines and cytotoxic activity in certain subpopulations of T lymphocytes. Here we report the effects of CSA in IgE receptor mediated exocytosis from rat basophilic leukemia (RBL) cells. CSA inhibited IgE receptor mediated and calcium ionophore (A23187) stimulated exocytosis from RBL cells in a dose dependent manner. Half-maximal inhibition was observed at 0.3 μ*M* CSA (≈200 ng/ml). This value falls within the range of CSA concentrations in the serum of patients undergoing immunosuppressive therapy. CSA also inhibited receptor mediated degranulation of human basophils at similar doses. Inhibition of exocytosis occurred after 2–5 min preincubation with CSA and was not reversed by washing the cells free of CSA prior to triggering. At concentrations that resulted in maximum inhibition of exocytosis, CSA did *not* inhibit IgE receptor mediated phosphatidylinositol (PI) hydrolysis, release of arachidonic acid metabolites, influx of Ca^{2+}, the rise in cytosolic free Ca^{2+}, or actin polymerization. These data demonstrate that, in addition to T lymphocytes, CSA suppresses the function of mast cells and basophils. Furthermore, these results suggest that early events in signal transduction are not affected by CSA and that its target may be an as yet unidentified late stage in exocytosis.

Introduction

Cyclosporin A (CSA) is a cyclic peptide produced by the fungus *Tolypocladium inflatum* and is used clinically as an immunosuppressive drug. The target of CSA in vivo seems to be T lymphocytes, and at least part of the immunosuppressive activity of this drug results from inhibition of transcription of cytokine mRNA

* T. H. was a recipient of a grant from the Prof. A. Schmidtmann Stiftung, Philipps Universität Marburg, Federal Republic of Germany.

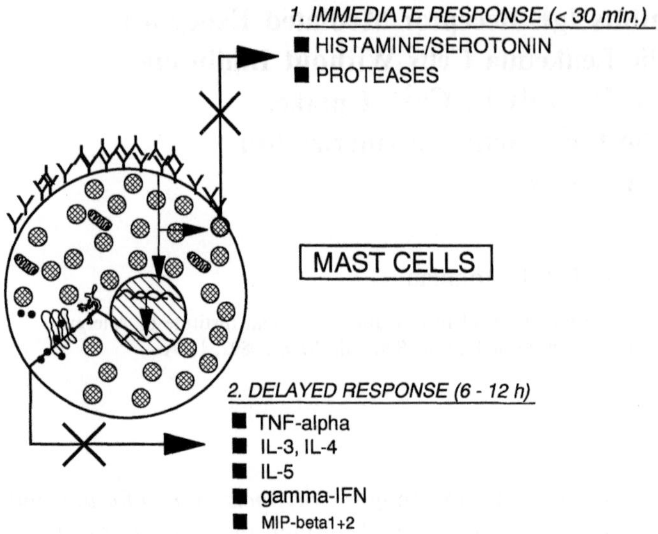

Fig. 1. CSA inhibits mast cells at multiple sites

[3, 14, 19]. However, a number of other activities of CSA have recently been reported, including inhibition of granule exocytosis in cytolytic T lymphocytes and mast cells.

A recent report by Trenn et al. [22] demonstrated that CSA inhibits various cytolytic T lymphocyte functions, including receptor mediated granule exocytosis. However, CSA did not inhibit receptor mediated PI hydrolysis, indicating that the early steps in signal transduction are not affected. These results demonstrate that CSA does than inhibit cytokine production.

In addition to the inhibition of T cell activation by CSA, mast cells and basophils seem to be a target for CSA: Inhibition of IgE receptor induced cytokine transcription has been demonstrated in several rodent mast cell lines [1, 18, 24]. Furthermore, IgE receptor mediated exocytosis is inhibited by CSA in human lung mast cells [16], skin mast cells (U. Amon, personal communication), basophils [12, 17], and RBL cells (12) (Fig. 1). Since CSA might represent a novel class of potentially useful inhibitors of mast cell activation, we examined the effects of CSA on IgE receptor mediated stimulation of RBL cells in order to further characterize the mechanism of action of CSA. Rat basophil leukemia (RBL) cells have proven to be an important model for studying the biochemical events involved in mast cell activation.

Results

CSA Inhibits Mast Cell Activation

CSA inhibits IgE receptor mediated exocytosis from RBL cells and human basophils in a dose dependent manner; 50% inhibition required $\approx$200 ng/ml

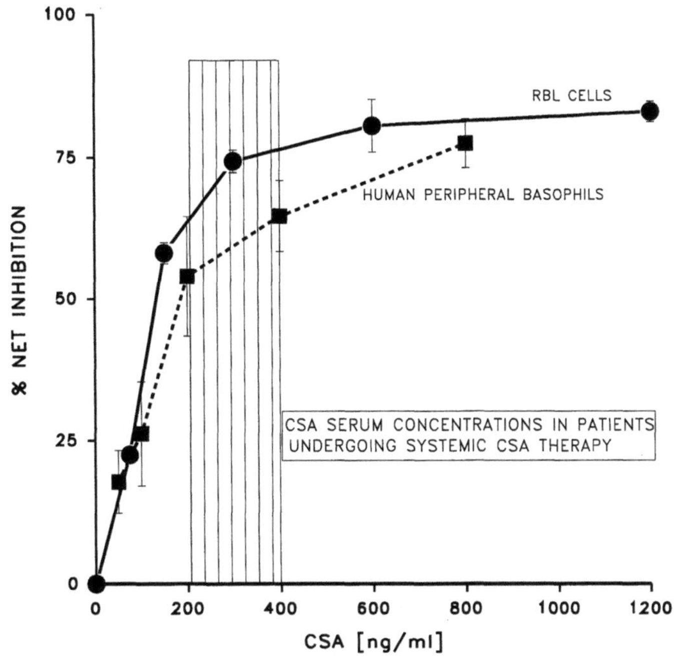

Fig. 2. CSA inhibits IgE receptor mediated exocytosis from RBL cells and human basophils in a dose dependent manner. RBL cells were preincubated for 5 min and triggered for 10 min at 37 °C; net release was 45%. Human basophils were isolated after a dextrose sedimentation, preincubated for 15 min with the indicated concentration of CSA, and then triggered for 30 min at 37 °C. Net release was approximately 30%

CSA (Fig. 2). Inhibition of IgE receptor mediated exocytosis is achieved after a short preincubation time (2–5 min) and is not reversed after removing the inhibitor from the buffer before activating the cells. In summary, CSA demonstrates all features of a potent mast cell inhibitor: effective at low concentrations, after a short preincubation time, and irreversible.

CSA Does Not Affect Signal Transduction

In contrast to the striking inhibition of exocytosis by CSA, none of the classical biochemical parameters of signal transduction are affected by CSA: Concentrations of CSA that produce 80% inhibition of IgE receptor mediated exocytosis have no effect on IgE receptor mediated PI hydrolysis, Ca^{2+} uptake (as measured by $^{45}Ca^{2+}$ uptake), or the rise in the concentration of cytosolic Ca^{2+} (as measured by quin-2). Moreover, cytoskeleton changes, assessed by measuring IgE receptor mediated actin polymerization and protein kinase C dependent myosin light chain phosphorylation (R. Adelstein, personal communication) are not inhibited by CSA.

Based on these observations, we propose that CSA specifically inhibits a late, unknown step in exocytosis. Characterization of the CSA sensitive step in the process of exocytosis should provide new insights in the mechanism of exocytosis.

Future Perspectives

Continuing studies on the inhibition of mast cell degranulation by CSA will yield important information in two separate areas: (1) the biochemistry of mast cell activation, and (2) the possible therapeutical use of CSA and CSA related drugs to treat allergic diseases.

In the mid 1980s, CSA was shown to inhibit interleukin-2 (IL-2) transcription in T lymphocytes and was therefore proposed to be a selective (T lymphocyte inhibiting) immunosuppressant [13]. During the last several years, however, additional activities of CSA have been reported. CSA inhibits receptor mediated exocytosis from cytotoxic T lymphocytes (22) and from a variety of mast cells and basophils [2, 12, 16, 17, 22, 23]. However, the molecular mechanism by which CSA mediates these effects is unknown. Binding studies performed with radioactive CSA have identified a CSA binding protein cyclophilin [8, 10, 11]. The gene for cyclophilin has now been cloned and sequenced [7, 11], and the product is identical with the enzyme peptidyl-prolyl *cis-trans* isomerase (PPIase [6, 21]). The activity of PPIase in vitro is to catalyze the folding of polypeptide chains at prolyl residues; and it has been postulated that in vivo this enzyme controls folding of proteins into their proper tertiary structure [4, 5]. Inhibition of this enzymatic activity may account for the effects of CSA in T cells and mast cells, even though ultimate proof awaits the characterization of the physiologic substrate(s) of cyclophilin(s).

Even though this *cis*→trans isomerization has been shown only in vitro, the concept of enzymatic control of protein folding in vivo [4] has drawn a great deal of interest. Enzymatic isomerization could not only accelerate protein folding, but also provide a direction for the isomerization (*cis* to *trans*, but not *trans* to *cis*). Cyclophilin(s) seem to represent a prototype of a class of enzymes, peptide bond isomerases. Two further isomerases have been demonstrated during the last year, the FK-506 binding protein [9, 20] and a new PPIase from *E. coli* [15].

The fact that isomerase inhibitors (such as CSA for cyclophilins and FK-506 for the FK-506 binding protein) do account for the inhibition of specific cellular functions (i.e., IL-2 transcription and exocytosis) in certain cell types only (T lymphocytes, mast cells, and Langerhans' cells), opens a new field of differential immunosuppressive therapy.

On the level of future therapeutical applications, CSA possibly represents a prototype of drugs that inhibit peptide bond isomerases. The selective inhibitory effect of CSA on immunocompetent cells (such as T lymphocytes, mast cells, and Langerhans' cells) makes it tempting to speculate whether this type of drug may provide an alternative to the use of corticosteroids in inflammatory skin disorders (Fig. 2). Clinical trials with topical CSA have so far been unsuccessful, mainly because CSA did not penetrate the epidermis sufficiently in order to obtain inhibitory concentrations of the drug in the dermis. The use of more potent isomerase inhibitors (such as FK-506, being ≈100 times more potent than CSA) could circumvent this problem.

References

1. Burd PR, Rogers HW, Gordon JR, Martin CA, Jayaraman KS, Wilson SD, Dvorak AM, Galli SJ, Dorf ME (1989) Interleukin 3-dependent and independent mast cells stimulated with IgE and antigen express multiple cytokines. J Exp Med 170:245–257
2. Cummins AG, Munro GH, Ferguson A (1988) Effect of cyclosporin A on rat mucosal mast cells and the associated protease RMCPII. Clin Exp Immunol 72:136–140
3. Elliott JF, Lin Y, Mizel SB, Bleackley RC, Harinsh DG, Paetkau V (1984) Induction of interleukin-2 messenger RNA inhibited by cyclosporin A. Science 226:1439–1441
4. Fischer G (1989) Slow conformational changes and their enzymology. Novo Acta Leopold 61/269:35–53
5. Fischer G, Bang H, Mech C (1984) Nachweis einer Enzymkatalyse für die cis-trans-Isomerisierung der Peptidbindung in prolinhaltigen Peptiden. Biomed Biochim Acta 43:1101–1111
6. Fischer G, Wittmann-Liebold B, Kiefhaber T, Schmid FX, Lang K (1989) Cyclophilin and peptidyl-prolyl *cis-trans* isomerase are probably identical proteins. Nature 337:476–478
7. Haendler B, Hofer-Warbinek R, Hofer E (1987) Complementary DNA for human T cell cyclophilin. EMBO J 6:947–950
8. Handschumacher RE, Harding MW, Rice J, Drugge RJ (1984) Cyclophilin: a specific cytosolic binding protein for cyclosporin A. Science 226:544–547
9. Harding MW, Galat A, Uehling DE, Schreiber SL (1989) A receptor for the immunosuppressant FK 506 is a *cis-trans* peptidyl-prolyl isomerase. Nature 341:758–760
10. Harding MW, Handschumacher RE (1988) Cyclophilin, a primary molecular target for cyclosporin. Transplantation 46:29S–35S
11. Harding MW, Handschumacher RE, Speicher DW (1986) Isolation and amino acid sequence of cyclophilin. J Biol Chem 261:8547–8555
12. Hultsch T, Rodriguez JL, Kaliner MA, Hohman RJ (1990) Cyclosporin A inhibits degranulation of rat basophilic leukemia cells and human basophils. Inhibition of mediator release without affecting PI hydrolysis or Ca++ fluxes. J Immunol 144:1000–1001
13. Kahan BD (1989) Cyclosporine. N Engl J Med 321:1725–1738
14. Kronke M, Leonard WJ, Depper JM, Arya SK, Wong-Stall F, Gallo RC, Waldmann TA, Greene WC (1984) Cyclosporin A inhibits T-cell growth factor gene expression at the level of mRNA transcription. Proc Natl Acad Sci USA 81:5214–5218
15. Liu J, Walsh CT (1990) Peptidyl-prolyl *cis-trans*-isomerase from *Escherichia coli*: a periplasmic homolog of cyclophilin that is not inhibited by cyclosporin A. Proc Natl Acad Sci USA 87:4028–4032
16. Marone G, Triggiani M, Cirillo R, Giacummo A, Siri L, Condorelli M (1988) Cyclosporin A inhibits the release of histamine and peptide leukotriene C4 from human lung mast cells. Clin Lab 18:53–57
17. Pedersen C, Permin H, Stahl Skov P, Norn S, Svenson M, Mosbech H, Bendtzen K (1985) Inhibitory effect of cyclosporin A on histamine release from human leukocytes and rat mast cells. Allergy 40:103–107
18. Plaut M, Pierce JH, Watson CJ, Hanley-Hyde J, Nordan RP, Paul WE (1989) Mast cell lines produce lymphokines in response to cross-linkage of Fc-eRI or to calcium ionophores. Nature 339:64–67
19. Shevach EM (1985) The effects of cyclosporin A on the immune system. Annu Rev Immunol 3:397–423
20. Siekierka JJ, Hung SHY, Poe M, Lin CS, Sigal NH (1989) A cytosolic binding protein for the immunosuppressant FK506 has peptidyl-prolyl isomerase activity but is distinct from cyclophilin. Nature 341:755–757
21. Takahashi N, Hayano T, Suzuki M (1989) Peptidyl-prolyl *cis-trans* isomerase is the cyclosporin A-binding protein cyclophilin. Nature 337473–475

22. Trenn G, Taffs R, Hohman RJ, Kincaid R, Shevach EM, Sitkovsky M (1989) Biochemical characterization of the inhibitory effect of CsA on cytolytic T lymphocyte effector functions. J Immunol 142:3796–3802
23. Triggiani M, Cirillo R, Lichtenstein LM, Marone G (1989) Inhibition of histamine and prostaglandin D2 release from human lung mast cells by cyclosporin A. Int Arch Allergy Appl Immunol 88:253–255
24. Wodnar-Filipowicz A, Heusser CH, Moroni C (1989) Production of the haemopoietic growth factors GM-CSF and interleukin-3 by mast cells in response to IgE receptor-mediated activation. Nature 339:150–152

Prostaglandin D Synthetase Is Localized in Antigen Presenting Cells and Mast Cells

K. Ikai[1], M. Ujihara[1], Y. Horiguchi[1], and Y. Urade[2]

[1] Department of Dermatology, Kyoto University Faculty of Medicine, Shogoin, Sakyo-ku, Kyoto 606, Japan
[2] Department of Enzymes and Metabolism, Osaka Bioscience Institute, Furuedai, Suita, Osaka 565, Japan

Introduction

Prostaglandin (PG) D_2 is a naturally occurring prostanoid that shows various kinds of pharmacological activity, such as inhibition of platelet aggregation, bronchoconstriction, sleep induction, and hypothermia, under various physiological and pathological conditions [1–3]. PGD_2 is known to be actively produced by mast cells during IgE stimulation and to modify the anaphylactic process [4].

Concerning the biosynthesis of PGD_2, at least two types of PGD synthetase (PGH_2-isomerase, EC 5.3.99.2) have been isolated from rats. One is glutathione (GSH) independent PGD synthetase purified from rat brain [5]; the other is GSH requiring PGD synthetase purified from rat spleen [6]. These enzymes are very similar, as judged by their pI value (4.7–5.2), molecular weight (26000), and self-inactivation during isomerization of PGH_2 to PGD_2, but clearly different in their amino acid compositions, catalytic properties, antigenic determinants, and mRNA structures [6, 7]. Several isozymes of GSH-*S*-transferase (EC 2.5.1.18), purified from various rat tissues, also catalyze the conversion of PGH_2 to PGD_2 to lesser but significant extents [8].

Materials and Methods

Polyclonal antibody against rat spleen PGD synthetase was prepared in rabbits as described previously [6]. Male Wistar rats were anesthetized by an i.p. injection of sodium pentobarbital (50 mg/kg) and killed by perfusion from the left ventricle of the heart with an ice-cold Krebs Ringer's solution (200 ml) followed with 4% paraformaldehyde in 0.1 *M* sodium phosphate, pH 7.5 (200 ml). Various tissues were removed, cut into slices of about 2 mm thickness, and immersed in the same fixative at 4 °C overnight. After postfixation, the tissue specimens were washed overnight with PBS containing 10%–20% sucrose and embedded in optimum cutting temperature (OCT) compound (Tissue-Tek II, Miles). Sections (thickness, 6 µm) were cut on a cryostat, mounted on albumin coated glass slides, and air-dried at 4 °C overnight [9–11]. After inactivation of endogenous peroxidase in the tissue section, the section was immunostained with anti-GSH-requiring PGD synthetase IgG (10 µg/ml PBS), followed with biotinylated anti-rabbit

IgG and the avidin-biotin peroxidase (ABC) kit. Control staining was performed in the serial section with the antibody preabsorbed with the purified enzyme or nonimmunized rabbit IgG as the first antibody. After refixation with 1% glutaraldehyde, the sections were reacted with DAB solution for 30 min and then with diaminobenzidine (DAB) hydrogen peroxide solution for 30 min, as described previously [9–11].

For immunoelectron microscopy, the immunoperoxidase stained sections were postfixed with 1% osmium tetroxide, dehydrated in an ethanol series, and embedded in polyethylene capsules of epoxy resin. The ultrathin sections were observed under a Hitachi-300 electron microscope, without electron optical counter staining, as described previously [9, 10].

Results and Discussion

The positive immunocytochemical stain was found in a number of histiocytes and/or dendritic cells in spleen, thymus, and Peyer's patch of intestine. The immunostain was also observed in such cells in lamina propria of the villus in small intestine and colon, in submuscosal layer of stomach and in Kupffer cells in liver. The immunostaining of spleen-type GSH requiring PGD synthetase was also found in the cytoplasm of tissue mast cells in connective tissue of adult rats. Such immunoreactive cells were not observed in brain, spinal cord, kidney, heart, testis, and skeletal muscle, Immunoelectron microscopy confirmed that immunoreactiv-

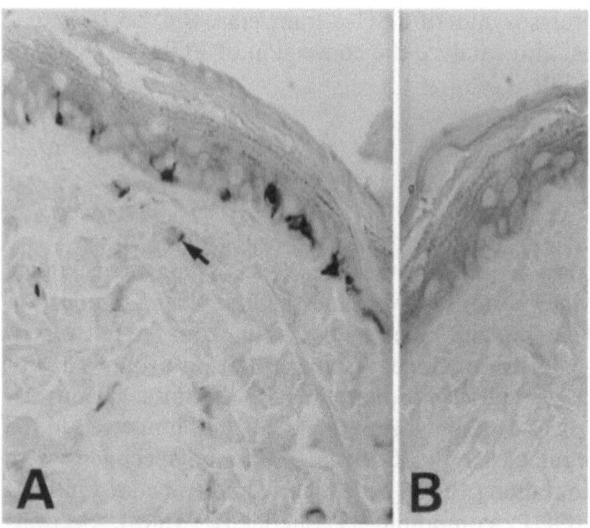

Fig. 1 A, B. Immunohistochemical distribution of PGD synthetase in rat skin by anti-rat spleen PDG synthetase antibody. **A** Cytoplasmic distribution of PGD synthetase was prominent in Langerhans' cells in the epidermis. In the dermis, infiltrating cells were stained. Immunoreactivity of mast cells (*arrow*) was positive but somewhat lower than that of the other positive cells. **B** No specific immunostaining was observed by incubation with nonimmunized rabbit IgG. (×400)

ity of this enzyme was distributed in the cytoplasm of those cells. In rat skin, cytoplasmic distribution of PGD synthetase was prominent in intraepidermal dendritic cells (Fig. 1A). In the dermis, infiltrating cells were immunohistochemically positive for PGD synthetase. The intensity of positive stain in a portion of these infiltrating cells was somewhat lower than that of the other positive cells (Fig. 1A). These weakly immunoreactive cells were identified as mast cells, since metachromasia was observed after staining with toluidine blue. Control specimens revealed no specific immunostaining (Fig. 1B).

These observations revealed that PGD_2 is produced by GSH requiring PGD synthetase localized in mast cells and antigen presenting cells, such as histiocytes, Langerhans' cells, and dendritic cells, in various tissues and contributes a dictating progression of immune responses. In the skin, PGD_2 may play an especially significant role in immunological functions, including inflammatory and immediate type immune reactions via mast cells in the dermis and delayed type immune responses via histiocytes in the dermis and Langerhans' cells in the epidermis.

References

1. Ikai K, Imamura S (1988) Prostaglandin D_2 in the skin. Int J Dermatol 27:141–149
2. Ujihara M, Urade Y, Eguchi N, Hayashi H, Ikai K, Hayaishi O (1988) Prostaglandin D_2 formation and characterization of its synthetases in various tissues of adult rat. Arch Biochem Biophys 260:521–531
3. Ito S, Narumiya S, Hayaishi O (1989) Prostaglandin D_2: a biochemical perspective. Prostaglandins Leuko Essent Fatty Acids 37:219–234
4. Lewis RA, Soter NA, Diamond PT, Austin KF, Oates JA, Roberts LJII (1982) Prostaglandin D_2 generation after activation of rat and human mast cells. J Immunol 129:1627–1631
5. Urade Y, Fumimoto N, Hayaishi O (1985) Purification and characterization of rat brain prostaglandin D synthetase. J Biol Chem 260:12410–12415
6. Urade Y, Fujimoto N, Ujihara M, Hayaishi O (1987) Biochemical and immunological characterization of rat spleen prostaglandin synthetase. J Biol Chem 262:3820–3825
7. Urade Y, Nagata A, Suzuki Y, Fujii Y, Hayaishi O (1987) Primary structure of rat brain prostaglandin D synthetase deduced from cDNA sequence. J Biol Chem 262:15132–15136
8. Ujihara M, Tsuchida S, Satoh K, Sato K, Urade Y (1988) Biochemical and immunological demonstration of prostaglandin D_2, E_2, and $F_{2\alpha}$ formation from prostaglandin H_2 by various rat glutathione S-transferase isozymes. Arch Biochem Biophys 264:428–437
9. Ujihara M, Horiguchi Y, Ikai K, Urade Y (1988) Characterization and distribution of prostaglandin D synthetase in rat skin. J Invest Dermatol 90:448–451
10. Urade Y, Ujihara M, Horiguchi Y, Ikai K, Hayaishi O (1989) The major source of endogenous prostaglandin D_2 production is likely antigen-presenting cells. J Immunol 143:2982–2989
11. Urade Y, Ujihara M, Horiguchi Y, Igarashi, Nagata A, Ikai K, Hayaishi O (1990) Mast cells contain spleen-type prostaglandin D synthetase. J Biol Chem 265:371–375

Influence of Histamine H_1, H_2, and H_3 Agonists and Antagonists on IgE Mediated Histamine Release from Human Basophils *

J. Kleine-Tebbe[1], J. Schramm[1], M. Bolz[1], H. Gagné[1], C. Josties[1], R. Lipp[2], A. Friese[2], H. Stark[2], V. Zingel[2], A. Buschauer[2], W. Schunack[2], and G. Kunkel[1]

[1]Department of Clinical Immunology and Asthma OPD, Universitätsklinikum Rudolf Virchow, Augustenburger Platz 1, W-1000 Berlin 65, Federal Republic of Germany
[2]Institut für Pharmazie, Freie Universität Berlin, Königin-Luise-Straße 2–4, W-1000 Berlin 33, Federal Republic of Germany

Introduction

Histamine has been the mediator most often ascribed to the allergic disease process since one of the central features of basophils and mast cells, besides the possession of high affinity receptors for IgE, is the possession of intracellular granules containing histamine. This primary amine evokes a variety of responses through its binding to H_1, H_2, and the recently described H_3 receptors [1, 13]. Activation of the histamine H_2 receptor has been shown to be one of the mechanisms inhibiting basophil histamine release induced by IgE cross-linking agents [2]. Receptor binding by H_2 agonists initiates an elevation of adenylate cyclase activity and a consecutive cAMP increase [3]. Stimulation of presynaptic histamine H_3 receptors will cause inhibition of histamine synthesis and release, through autofeedback in histaminergic neurons [1]. To define the role of histamine receptors on basophil leukocytes with respect to the newly developed H_3 active compounds, we studied the influence of histamine receptor stimulating (H^+) and blocking (H^-) compounds on IgE mediated release of the primary amine.

Methods and Materials

As previously described [4], peripheral leukocytes were obtained by dextran sedimentation from healthy volunteers and allergic donors with a hypersensitivity to pollen antigens. After a gentle washing procedure (three times), the basophil containing suspensions were preincubated in duplicates (37 °C, 20–120 min) with histamine receptor active compounds (Table 1) and stimulated (37 °C, 40 min) by IgE cross-linking agents (anti-IgE, Behring, FRG, and grass, birch pollen extracts, ALK SQ, Denmark), to trigger the release process (Table 1). After removal of the cells (800 x g, 4 °C, 15 min), histamine was detected by a automated fluorometric method [4].

---

* Supported by Grant No. KI 622/1-1 from the Deutsche Forschungsgemeinschaft, Bonn, FRG.

Table 1. Preincubation of histamine agonists (H^+) and antagonists (H^-) and the stimulating agents.

Preincubation (time)	Stimulation	Reference
1. H_1^+: 2-methyl-histamine, VZ 12 H_1^-: diphenhydramine (20 min) 2. H_2^+: arpromidine, BUA 75, dimaprit, FRA19, impromidine (20 min)	100 IU/ml anti-IgE	
3. H_2^+: FRA19 (20 min)	10, 30, 100 IU/ml	
4. H_2^+: FRA19 (20 min)	1, 10, 100 SQ/ml	
5./6./7. H_3^-: nos. 1–3 (N^α-acylated histamine derivatives) (120 min)		[7]
– Washed leukocytes	–	
– Cell fragments obtained by sonification	–	
– Purified eosinophils, neutrophils	–	
8. H_3^-: thioperamide, no. 4, STH7, STH19 (30 min)	100 IU/ml anti-IgE	[5]
9. H_3^+: (R)-α-methyl-histamine (30 min)	100 IU/ml anti-IgE	[7]

SQ, units of the allergen extract.

Results

1. Neither by incubation with $H_1^+ (10^{-9}-10^{-6} M)$ nor with $H_1^- (10^{-8}-10^{-4} M)$ was an influence on IgE mediated histamine release from basophils detectable. After release, histamine levels were found to reach 100% ± 7% of the controls, which had been preincubated with buffer. Conclusions on the effect of H_1^+ are limited because the compounds interfere with the assay at concentrations $\geq 10^{-7} M$.
2. Dose dependent inhibition of basophil histamine release was induced by H_2^+; differences were found in the potency of the drugs used (for IC_{30} levels see Fig. 1). Paralleled kinetics of inhibition were detectable using $10^{-5} M$ Dimaprit and $10^{-6} M$ BUA75 ($Inh_{max\,1/2}$, 5 min, Inh_{max}, 20 min, data not shown) [6].
3. The strength of the immunological stimulation by anti-IgE influenced the slope and maximum of the inhibition curves obtained by H_2 agonist FRA 19 (Fig. 2).
4. Different inhibition curves were found after activation of the H_2 receptor with FRA 19, according to the individual mediator response and the antigen dose causing the maximum of release (HR_{max}). IC_{30} levels of FRA 19 according to 1, 10, 100 SQ/ml of the allergen were 40, 150, 90 nM (HR_{max} = 10 SQ/ml) and 3, 30, 40 nM (HR_{max} = 100 SQ/ml).
5. Incubation of washed leukocytes with H_3^- no. 1–3 ($>10^{-7} M$) caused an increase in intra- and extracellular histamine levels ($2 \times 10^{-5} M$ H_3^- no. 1 induced a 6- to 10-fold elevation, $10^{-4} M$ H_3^- nos. 2 and 3 induced a 1.5- and 3-fold elevation). This increase turned out to be dose, time, and temperature dependent, but Ca^{++} and Mg^{++} independent [7].
6. Cell fragments of washed leukocytes, which were ultrasonically disrupted (2 min) before being incubated with H_3^- no. 1 ($3 \times 10^{-7} M$) produced similar elevated histamine levels (32 ± 9.5 ng/ml) compared to untreated cells (24.9 ± 8.7 ng/ml).

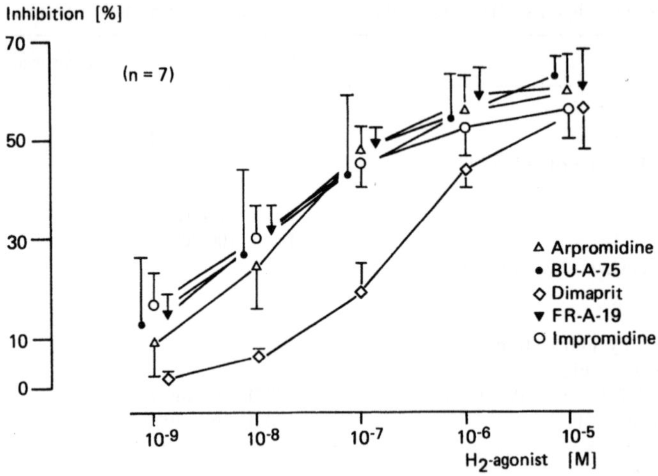

Fig. 1. H_2 agonists inhibit anti-IgE mediated histamine release in a dose dependent manner [6]. IC30-levels (n*M*): Arpromidine 20, BUA75 15, dimaprit 300, FRA19 8, impromidine 10

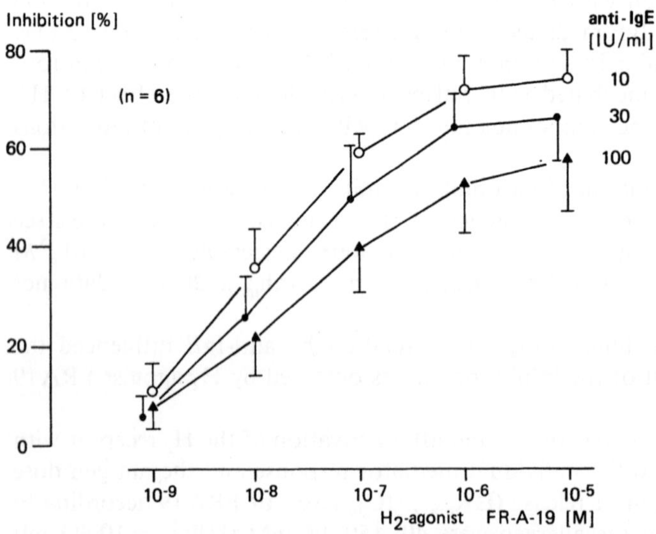

Fig. 2. H_2 receptor linked inhibition of anti-IgE induced basophil histamine release appears as a function of the strength of the immunological signal [6]

7. The histamine increase – detectable after incubation with H_3^- no.1 – appeared in the presence of highly purified eosinophils (95±3%) as well as in the presence of highly purified neutrophils (87±4%) (Fig. 3).
8. H_3^- without N^{α}-acylation (no. 4, STH7, STH19, thioperamide) neither increased histamine levels nor influenced IgE mediated histamine release from washed leukocytes (Fig. 4). Only the highest concentration of thioperamide ($10^{-4}M$) caused 25%±4.5% inhibition of leukocyte histamine release.

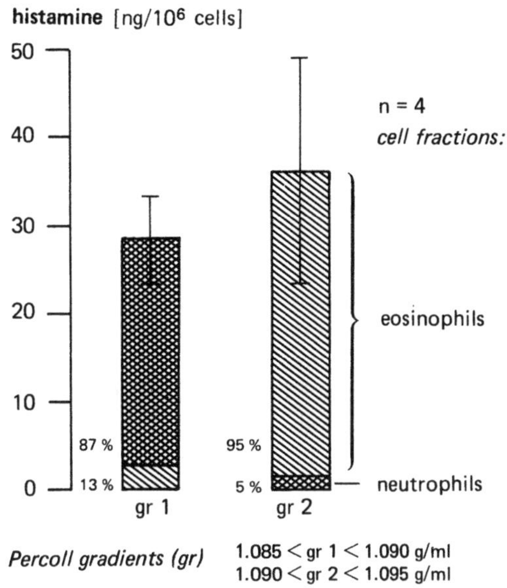

Fig. 3. In the absence of basophils N^{α}-acylated H_3 antagonist no. 1 caused elevated histamine levels after incubation with purified neutrophils and eosinophils [7]

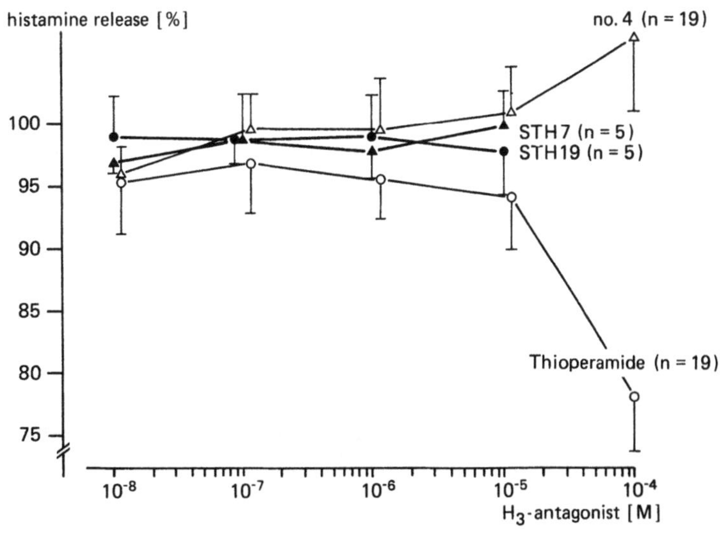

Fig. 4. Potent H_3 antagonists without a histamine moiety did not influence IgE mediated histamine release of basophil leukocytes. A decrease of approx. 25% of control release – caused by 10^{-4} *M* thioperamide – appears not to be relevant with respect to this extraordinarity high concentration of the compound

9. All investigated H_3^+ were unable to influence histamine release from human leukocytes obtained by IgE cross-linking agents (data not shown). The investigations of H_3^+ were restricted due to their histamine moiety and their subsequent fluorescence ($>10^{-7}$ *M*) in our assay.

Discussion

Comparing the potencies of H_2^+ to inhibit basophil histamine release, Dimaprit – one of the earlier H_2-agonists – is about 15- to 30-fold less potent than the newer compounds such as arpromidine, BUA 75, FRA 19 and impromidine, which are equipotent at the H_2 receptor on human basophils. Since the H_2 receptor mediated inhibition by FRA 19 and other compounds is totally blocked by potent H_2^- [2, 6], we conclude that the action of the newer agonistic compounds is only a result of their H_2 receptor specificity and not a result of other pharmacological properties. Increased in vitro potency of arpromidine and BUA 75 in other tissues [8] seems to be a result of increased H_2 receptor population or receptor subtypes with increased sensitivity in these compartments. The lipophilic character of these compounds might increase the penetration into myocardial tissues, however, no time difference was obtained in the activation of membrane bound H_2 receptors on basophils, indicating that the H_2 linked inhibition of basophil histamine release does not require lipophilic moieties. Triggering basophil histamine release with anti-IgE causes a dose response curve, which appears donor independent in a similar fashion (HR_{max} at 100 IU/ml anti-IgE) [9]. Therefore the signal for the initiation of mediator release is parallel to the absolute amount of anti-IgE: inhibition curves of anti-IgE triggered histamine release are shifted to the right in increasing signals (= increasing anti-IgE dose). The signal responsible for the maximal release probably requires a more pronounced control (i.e., cAMP-increase) and higher concentrations of the modulating compound to induce a significant inhibition of mediator release. The use of antigen as a histamine releasing agent requires a differentiated evaluation according to the individual bell-shaped dose response curve obtained by the antigen [9]. Individual varieties of mediator release might be responsible for the weak relationship between H_2 linked inhibition and the antigen dose to initiate the release process. Differences in the inhibition of mediator release by H_2^+ according to the stimulating agent (antigen or anti-IgE) have been shown using dimaprit ($Inh_{antigen} > Inh_{anti\text{-}IgE}$) [9]. Those results are in contrast to our findings ($Inh_{antigen} = Inh_{anti\text{-}IgE}$) [10]: differences in the protocol (preincubation time in [9]: 2 min) and different antigen preparations might account for this. According to earlier findings [3], classical H_1^- did not modulate basophil histamine release in concentrations below $10^{-4}M$. Nevertheless, newer histamine receptor antagonists had been shown to influence histamine release [11] by pharmacological actions, which cannot be explained by antagonist activity at the H_1 receptor on mediator containing cells.

The observation of increasing intra- and extracellular histamine levels in leukocyte preparations after incubation with N^α-acylated H_3^- [12] is not related to a receptor mediated action for several reasons: No histamine elevation was detectable using highly purified basophils [7], and specific binding to the H_3 receptor turned out to be CA^{++} dependent [1] in contrast to our observations, which appeared to be CA^{++} independent [7]. Antagonistic compounds in concentrations of several fold less are required for the binding to the H_3 receptor [13]. Elevation of histamine was not only found after cell disruption, but also in purified neutrophil and eosinophil preparations. N^α-acylated H_3^-, which has a histamine moiety and an amido group, must therefore have been cleaved into fragments by neutrophil and eosinophil enzymes and measured as histamine in our assay [7]. Because H_3^- without a histamine moiety and H_3^+ failed to modulate IgE mediated histamine release, the existence of H_3 receptors on basophils seems unlikely.

Conclusions

IgE mediated histamine release from human basophils is inhibited by activation of histamine H_2 receptor. H_2 receptor linked inhibition depends on the strength of immunological stimulation: only weak inhibition can be found in cases of maximal cell stimulation.

Activation of histamine H_1 and H_3 receptors have no effect on basophil IgE mediated histamine release. N^{α}-acylated histamine derivatives – known to be potent histamine H_3-antagonists – are not useful for the study of cell preparations containing neutrophils and eosinophils. The existence of histamine H_3 receptors on human basophils seems unlikely.

References

1. Arrang J-M, Garbarg M, Schwartz J-C (1983) Auto-inhibition of brain histamine release mediated by a novel class (H_3) of histamine receptor. Nature 302:832
2. Ring J, Sedlmeier F, von der Helm D, Mayr T, Walz U, Ibel H, Riepel H, Przybilla B, Reimann H-J, Dorsch W (1988) Histamine and allergic diseases. In: Ring J, Burg G (eds) New trends in allergy II. Springer, Berlin, Heidelberg, New York, p 44
3. Lichtenstein LM, Gillespie E (1975) The effects of the H_1- and H_2-antihistamines on "allergic" histamine release and its inhibition by histamine. J Pharmacol Exp Ther 192:441
4. Siraganian RP, Hook WA (1980) Histamine release and assay methods for the study of human allergy. In: Rose NR, Friedmann H (eds) Manual of clinical immunology. American Society for Microbiology, Washington, p 808
5. Gartner I (1980) Separation of human eosinophils in density gradients of polyvinylpyrrolidone coated silica gel (Percoll). Immunology 40:130
6. Kleine-Tebbe J, Gagné H, Josties C, Buschauer A, Friese A, Kunkel G (1990) Modulation of histamine release from human leukocytes by different histamine H_2-agonists (abstr). J Allergy Clin Immunol 85:171
7. Kleine-Tebbe J, Schramm J, Bolz M, Lipp R, Schunack W, Kunkel G (1990) Influence of histamine H_3-antagonists on human leukocytes. Agents Actions 30 (1/2):137
8. Buschauer A (1989) Synthesis and in vitro pharmacology of arpromidine and related phenyl(pyridylalkyl) guanidines, a potential new class of positive inotropic drugs. J Med Chem 32:1963
9. Marone G, Kagey-Sobotka A, Lichtenstein LM (1981) IgE-mediated histamine release from human basophils: differences between antigen E- and anti-IgE induced secretion. Int Arch Allergy Appl Immunol 65:339
10. Kleine-Tebbe J, Josties C, Gagné H, Friese A, Buschauer A, Schunack W, Kunkel G (1990) Histamine H_2-receptor-linked inhibition of IgE-mediated histamine release from human leukocytes in dependence of immunological stimulation. In: New perspectives in histamine research (Satellite Symposium of the XIth International Congress of Pharmacology/IUPHAR), The Netherlands, 1990
11. Kreutner W, Chapman, RW, Gulbenkian A, Siegel MI (1987) Antiallergic activity of loratadine, a non-sedating antihistamine. Allergy 42:57
12. Kleine-Tebbe J, Bolz M, Lipp R, Schunack W, Kunkel G (1988) Presence of histamine H_3-receptors on human basophils (abstract). N Engl Reg Allergy Proc 9:276
13. Arrang J-M, Garbarg M, Lancelot J-C, Lecomte J-M, Pollard H, Robba M, Schunack W, Schwartz JC (1987) Highly potent and selective ligands for histamine H_3-receptors. Nature 327:117

Impact of Biophysical Plasma Membrane Properties on Leukocyte/Endothelium Interaction

H.-A. Lehr[1], C. Hübner[2], J.P. Zimmer[2], A. Kohlschütter[2], and K. Messmer[1]

[1] Department of Experimental Surgery, University of Heidelberg, Im Neuenheimer Feld 347, W-6900 Heidelberg, Federal Republic of Germany
[2] Department of Pediatrics, University of Hamburg, Martinistrasse 52, W-2000 Hamburg 20, Federal Republic of Germany

Introduction

Leukocyte adhesion to the endothelium of postcapillary venules is increased in pathologic conditions such as inflammation and postischemic reperfusion injury. Enhanced adhesion results from leukocyte activation via membrane confined metabolic pathways, triggered by oxygen free radicals, complement factors, and lipid mediators [1].

The molecular structures responsible for leukocyte adhesion are molecules classified as CD 11/CD 18 glycoprotein receptors [2].

Functions of plasma membrane embedded receptors, like other integral proteins, depend on plasma membrane fluidity, affecting the degree of receptor availability for ligand interaction [3]. The idea that leukocyte adhesion receptors are likewise subject to plasma membrane fluidity is supported by several observations, in which extracellular availability of CD 11 b/CD 18 was found enhanced by substances and conditions which lead to plasma membrane rigidification

One of the pharmacological agents which reduce leukocyte/endothelium interaction, dextran sulfate (DS) [4], has been found to down-regulate Fc and CD 11 b/CD 18 receptor expression on adherent cells [5]. In order to investigate whether plasma membrane fluidization might be responsible for the down-regulation of CD 11 b/CD 18 receptors and the subsequently reduced leukocyte/endothelium interaction, we measured the effect of DS on plasma membrane fluidity of peripheral human white blood cells, using steady state fluorescence anisotropy of the classical membrane probe diphenylhexatriene [6].

Materials and Methods

Fifteen ml of whole blood was drawn from ten healthy persons (ages 23–39, 3 males and 7 females). For each probe 10 ml of blood were anticoagulated with heparin (15 I.E. ammonium heparin/ml blood) and 5 ml with the chelating agent EDTA (1.8 mg/ml blood). Peripheral blood lymphocytes (PBL) were isolated by density gradient centrifugation and washed twice in phosphate buffered saline (PBS, 21 °C). Then, 5×10^6 PBL from the heparinized blood sample and 5×10^6 PBL from the EDTA blood sample were resuspended in 5 ml of PBS each and incubated under slow rotation for 4 h and 37 °C. The 5×10^6 PBL from the heparinized blood samples were resuspended in 5 ml of PBS supplemented with 20 µg/ml (2.5 µ*M*) DS (Sigma Chemical Company, Deisenhofen, FRG) and incubated under identical conditions. After 4 h, PBL were recovered and washed twice in PBS.

Plasma membrane fluidity of intact cells was assessed by anisotropy measurements using the fluorescent marker 1,6-diphenylhexatriene (DPH) and a Shimadzu Spectrofluorophotometer RF540 [6]. PBL ($6\times10^5\pm1\times10^5$ cells/ml) were incubated for 20 min and 50 min (21 °C) in the fluorescent marker (1.0 µ*M* DPH/ml). Measurements were performed five times on each sample. In all fluorescence anisotropy measurements performed, total fluorescence intensities of each probe were monitored in order to detect differences of fluorescence lifetime of the respective probes. No differences were observed between the samples compared in this study. Statistical analysis was carried out using the Student *t*-test for paired samples.

Results

Cell viability, as assessed by trypan blue exclusion, was greater than 95% for all PBL samples after the 4 h incubation in DS supplemented and native PBS.

PBL incubated in the presence of DS showed significantly lower fluorescence anisotropy values than control PBL from the identical heparinized blood sample (0.177 ± 0.018, $n = 10$, vs 0.193 ± 0.017, $n = 10$; $p<0.01$), indicating increased plasma membrane fluidity in DS exposed cells. The increase in plasma membrane fluidity is not only based on the mean value of the pooled data, but was observed for each individual sample.

In order to rule out an effect of the anticoagulant heparin, which is structurally related to DS, we compared plasma membrane fluidity of PBL from heparin and EDTA anticoagulated blood samples. No difference in fluorescence anisotropy values was seen between control PBL isolated from heparinized blood and those isolated from EDTA blood samples (0.194 ± 0.015, $n = 10$, vs 0.193 ± 0.017, $n = 10$). The fact that under the conditions of this assay heparin exerts no plasma membrane fluidizing activity may be attributed to the low drug concentration and the short time of drug interaction with whole blood (< 30 min until PBL isolation and washing) and does not necessarily rule out a potential membrane effect of heparin under suitable in vitro conditions and in vivo.

Discussion

We found that incubation of PBL in DS supplemented medium resulted in a decrease in anisotropy of the fluorescent probe DPH, indicating increased fluidity in the hydrophobic plasma membrane interior.

Among other cellular functions, several aspects of receptor ligand interaction have been shown to be subject to alterations in membrane fluidity. Depending on the physical constraints provided by their immediate environment, embedded receptors can undergo lateral, rotational and vertical displacements within the plane of the plasma membrane, affecting their degree of exposure and availability for ligand interaction [3]. The idea that DS affects leukocyte/endothelium interaction via plasma membrane fluidization and thereby reduces availability of adherence receptors, is substantiated by the finding that DS down-regulates CD 11 b/CD 18 expression on adherent cells [5]. The fact that DS reduces CD 11 b/CD 18 mediated leukocyte adhesion to the endothelium, but at the same time does not affect binding of the receptor specific monoclonal antibody 60.3 [4], implies that DS affects ligand interaction by a nonspecific mechanism and not by direct binding to the ligand recognizing epitope on the receptors.

Conclusion

This study suggests that DS reduces leukocyte/endothelium interaction through plasma membrane fluidization and supports the concept that leukocyte adhesion receptors CD 11/CD 18 are susceptible to changes in plasma membrane fluidity. Further studies using monoclonal antibodies to CD 11/CD 18 are mandatory to establish the interrelation between plasma membrane fluidity, receptor function, and leukocyte/endothelium interaction.

References

1. Mullane KM, Salmon JA, Kraemer R (1986) Leukocyte-derived metabolites of arachidonic acid in ischemia-induced myocardial injury. Fed Proc. 46:2422–2433
2. Wallis WJ, Hickstein DD, Schwartz BR, June CH, Ochs HD, Beatty PG, Klebanoff SJ, Harlan JM (1986) Monoclonal antibody-defined function epitopes on the adhesion-promoting glycoprotein complex (CDw 18) of human neutrophils. Blood 67:1007–1013
3. Shinitzky M (1984) Membrane fluidity and cellular functions. In: Shinitzky M (ed) Physiology of membrane fluidity, vol. 1. CRC Press, Boca Raton, pp 1–51
4. Ley K, Lundgren E, Berger E, Arfors KE (1989) Shear-dependent inhibition of granulocyte adhesion to cultured endothelium by dextran sulfate. Blood 73:1324–1330
5. Hitomi M, Shimizu F (1985) Effect of mononuclear phagocyte system modulating agents on Fc and C 3 receptors of adherent cells. Br J Exp Pathol 66:371–376
6. Hübner C, Lindner SG, Albani M, Keup B, Schürmann M, Stegner H, Claussen M, Kohlschütter A (1989) Increased plasma membrane fluidity and decreased receptor availability of nonmuscle cells in myotonic dystrophy. J Neurol Sci 92:205–214

Interleukin-3 and Granulocyte/Macrophage Colony-Stimulating Factor Change the Anaphylatoxin-Induced Basophil Mediator Release Pattern

S.C. Bischoff[1], Y. Kurimoto[2], and C.A. Dahinden[1]

[1] Institute of Clinical Immunology, Inselspital, University Hospital, 3010 Bern, Switzerland
[2] Institute of Bio-Active Science, Nippon Zoki Co., Kinashi, Yashiro-cho, Hyogo, Japan

Introduction

Human basophils, albeit only a small proportion of peripheral blood leukocytes, are the only blood cells containing histamine and are by far the most prominent source of leukotrienes, as compared to other cell types [1]. Furthermore, basophils are assumed to play an important role in diverse inflammatory processes, in particular in hypersensitivity reactions [2]. Therefore, the factors and conditions necessary for inducing basophil mediator release have become a subject of increasing interest. Whereas various IgE dependent, e.g. or antigen or anti-IgE, and IgE independent, e.g. *N*-formyl-met-leu-phe (FMLP) or C5a, agonists trigger basophils for degranulation of preformed mediators, only FMLP and IgE receptor crosslinking by anti-IgE or antigen are known to induce lipid mediator synthesis [3].

The anaphylatoxins C3a and C5a are known to induce plasma exudation, smooth muscle contraction, and a wheal and flare reaction in the skin [4, 5]. In contrast to C5a, which has long been known to induce histamine release, the effects of C3a on inflammatory effector leukocytes are poorly defined and controversial, since they are weak and occur at very high concentrations. Recently, we demonstrated that C5a and C3a, both unable to induce lipid mediator synthesis by themselves, trigger the generation of large amounts of sulfidoleukotrienes (C4, D4, E4) in basophils preincubated with interleukin-3 (IL-3), a hematopoietic growth factor recently found to profoundly modify the basophil response to various cell agonists [6, 7]. Here, we examine the effect of C3a, in comparison to C5a, upon mediator release from human basophils with and without pretreatment with IL-3 or granulocyte/macrophage colony-stimulating factor (GM-CSF) another growth factor modulating anti-IgE-induced mediator release [8].

Methods

Human blood basophils from unselected volunteers were partially purified by ficoll hypaque density centrifugation (Pharmacia, Uppsala, Sweden) exactly as described previously [6] and finally suspended in HACM buffer (20 m*M* hepes, 0.5 m*M* glucose, 0.025% BSA, 125 m*M* NaCl, 5 m*M* KCl, 1 m*M* $CaCl_2$, 1 m*M*

$MgCl_2$) at a cell density of $3-5\times10^6$ cells/ml. The mediator release experiments were performed in a shaking water bath (37 °C) as described [6]. The cells were preincubated either in buffer or with cytokines for 10 min and then stimulated by the anaphylatoxins for 20 min. Recombinant human (rhu) IL-3 (bioactivity: 0.7 units/ng, determinated in a proliferation assay with leukocytes from chronic myeloid leukemia patients) and rhu GM-CSF (3.7 units/ng) were obtained from Sandoz, Basel, Switzerland and Sandoz, Vienna, Austria. C5a and C3a were purified to homogeneity from yeast-activated human serum as described [9]. The C3a preparation used contained less than 0.002% C5a.

Results and Discussion

Figure 1 shows that C5a alone (10^{-8} *M*) triggers significant histamine release in basophils, in contrast to C3a (10^{-6} *M*), which induces no or only marginal histamine release. Both anaphylatoxins are completely unable to induce the synthesis of leukotrienes. However, preincubating the cells with 10 ng/ml IL-3 for 10 min changes the basophil mediator profile dramatically: (1) the histamine release triggered by C5a is enhanced, (2) C3a becomes capable of inducing basophil degranulation, (3) IL-3 primes the basophils to produce large amounts of leukotrienes in response to C5a and, in 12 out of 21 experiments, also after stimulation with C3a. In comparison to C5a, C3a is clearly less potent in inducing either histamine or leukotriene release, but its effects are reproducible and statistically significant (*t*-test, $p<0.005$). Only two reports, from Glovsky et al., demonstrated an C3a activity in basophil degranulation [10, 11]. However, extremely high concentrations ($10^{-6}-10^{-5}$ *M*) and selected donors were used in these experiments. In addition, the moderate effect of C3a on histamine release, which we could confirm in some cases, may have been due to traces of C5a in the C3a preparation or to the cationic charge of the C3a peptide rather than to a specific

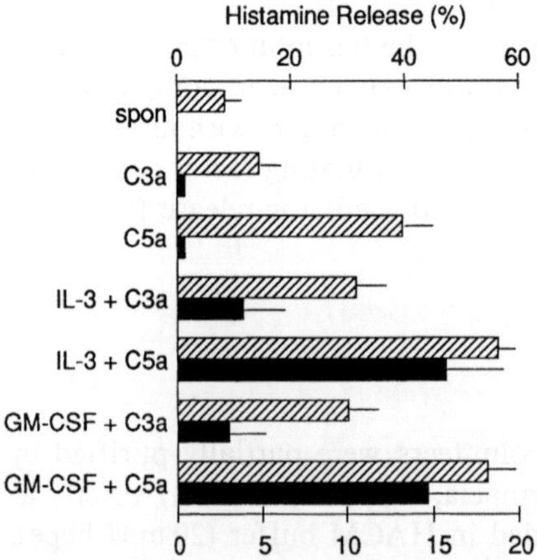

Fig. 1. Cell priming effect of IL-3 and GM-CSF on anaphylatoxin-induced basophil mediator release. Human basophils were preincubated with IL-3 (10 ng/ml) or GM-CSF (10 ng/ml) or in buffer for 10 min and then stimulated by C3a (10^{-6} *M*) or C5a (10^{-8} *M*) for 20 min. Histamine release (% of total cellular histamine, *striped columns*) and leukotriene C4 generation (pg/ng total cellular histamine, *black columns*) from 21 experiments (mean ± SD) are shown. The leukotriene production indicated for C3a or C5a alone represents the detection limit

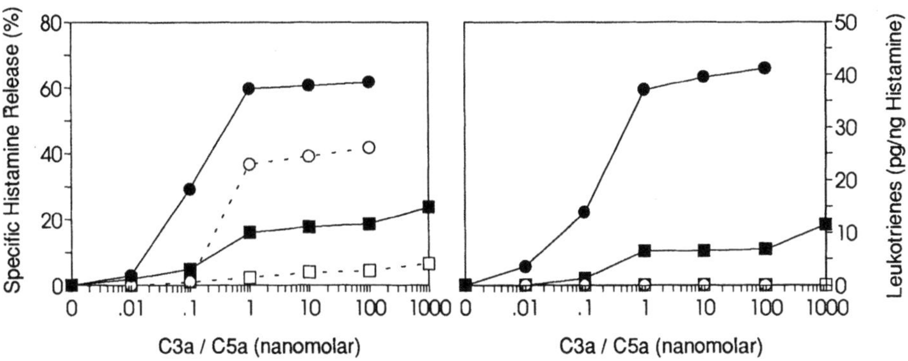

Fig. 2. Dose response of C3a and C5a with or without cytokine priming. Basophils were stimulated with C3a (*squares*) or C5a (*circles*) at the concentrations indicated, after preincubating the cells with (*closed symbols*) or without (*open symbols*) IL-3 (10 ng/ml) for 10 min. Each point represents the mean of six experiments

mechanism. GM-CSF also primes basophils for leukotriene synthesis and (enhanced) histamine release in response to the anaphylatoxins, albeit less potently than IL-3. The priming effect for leukotriene generation by anaphylatoxins occurs between 0.1–1.0 units/ml IL-3 or 0.3–33 units/ml GM-CSF for both anaphylatoxins (not shown).

The dose response curves of C3a differ from those of C5a (Fig. 2). Without cytokine priming, C3a induces marginal histamine release only at very high concentrations, whereas C5a induces basophil degranulation dose-dependently within a concentration range of $10^{-10}-10^{-7}$ *M*. Both peptides, however, are ineffective in triggering leukotriene synthesis, even at exceedingly high concentrations. By contrast, in the presence of IL-3, very low concentrations of C3a (10^{-9} *M*) induce basophil degranulation and leukotriene production. The effects of C5a occur at a concentration one order of magnitude lower than that of C3a and the maximal mediator release is about three times higher. Thus, IL-3 enhances C5a-induced histamine release, promotes a shift of the dose response curve of C5a to ten times lower concentrations, renders basophil responsive to C3a with regard to histamine release, and primes the synthesis of lipid mediators in response to the anaphylatoxins C3a or C5a.

Kinetic experiments showed that mediator release in response to anaphylatoxins occurs very rapidly, within seconds to minutes [6, 7]. The rapidity of the release reaction suggests that the anaphylatoxins act through high affinity-binding sites on IL-3-primed basophils and that cellular products from other leukocyte types are not involved in the basophil response. This is supported by our observation that an identical pattern of mediator release is obtained, with or without IL-3 preincubation [6, 7], from a cell fraction (obtained by percoll gradient centrifugation) highly enriched in basophils (40%) and contaminated exclusively with small lymphocytes, when stimulating this fraction with C3a or C5a.

Similar to C3a, another recently identified inflammatory mediator, neutrophil-activating peptide/interleukin-8 (NAP-1/IL-8), is by itself devoid of histamine-releasing activity but induces degranulation after priming with IL-3 [12].

However, relatively high concentrations of NAP-1 are needed for optimal effects on basophils. The role of the synergism of IL-3 and anaphylatoxins in vivo is not yet determined. For example, it is possible that these factors are involved in the pathogenesis of hypersensitivity reactions, particularly in the allergic late phase reaction, believed to be responsible for the major symptoms in severe asthma [1, 2]. In this context, it is interesting that tryptase, a product of mast cells which is not inhibited by classical plasma antiproteases, has the capacity to cleave C3a from complement component C3 [13]. Furthermore, granule compounds, e.g. heparin, from mast cells may associate with basic proteins. Such complexes are able to activate complement by the classical pathway. IL-3 and GM-CSF may be generated by T cells or even by mast cells after antigen exposure of an allergic individual [14]. Therefore, the combined generation of IL-3 or GM-CSF and C3a or C5a, respectively, could be, in part, responsible for the activation of basophils in allergic inflammation.

Summary

The complement cleveage products C3a and, in particular, C5a have been implicated as important effectors in inflammation, hypersensitivity reactions, and shock syndromes. Here we show the effects of C3a and C5a on human basophil mediator release with or without pretreatment with IL-3 or GM-CSF, two hematopoietic growth factors recently found to profoundly modify basophil function. C3a by itself induces no or only little histamine release, whereas C5a is a potent degranulating agent for basophils. Both anaphylatoxins fail to induce any lipid mediator synthesis by themselves. However, when the cells have been preincubated with IL-3 for 10 min, C3a, even at a nanomolar concentration, induces histamine release, both peptides, C3a and C5a, stimulate leukotriene synthesis. GM-CSF also renders basophils responsive to low concentrations of C3a and primes anaphylatoxin-induced leukotriene generation, although somewhat less efficiently than IL-3. Our results demonstrate that, in the presence of cytokines, not only C5a, but also C3a is a potent basophil activator, and furthermore show that hematopoetic growth factors are major regulators of lipid mediator synthesis. Such phenomena could be of relevance in different inflammatory processes, in particular hypersensitivity reactions.

References

1. Grant JA, Lett-Brown MA, Warner JA, Plaut M, Lichtenstein LM, Haak-Frendscho M, Kaplan AP (1986) Fed Proc 45:2653–2658
2. Naclerio RM, Proud D, Togias AG, Adkinson NF, Meyers DA, Kagey-Sobotka A, Plaut M, Norman PS, Lichtenstein LM (1985) N Engl J Med 313:65–70
3. Dahinden CA, Kurimoto Y, Baggiolini M, Dewald B, Walz A (1989) Int Arch Allergy Appl Immunol 90:113–118
4. Hugli TE, Müller-Eberhard HJ (1978) Adv Immunol 26:1–53

5. Wuepper KD, Bokisch VA, Müller-Eberhard HJ, Stoughton RB (1972) Clin Exp Immunol 11:13–20
6. Kurimoto Y, de Weck AL, Dahinden CA (1989) J Exp Med 170:467–479
7. Bischoff SC, de Weck AL, Dahinden CA (1990) Proc Natl Acad Sci USA 87:6813–6817
8. Hirai K, Morita Y, Misaki Y, Ohta K, Takaishi T, Suzuki S, Motoyoshi K, Miyamoto T (1988) J Immunol 141:3958–3964
9. Hugli TE, Gerard C, Kawahara M, Scheetz II ME, Barton R, Briggs S, Koppel G, Russell S (1981) Mol Cell Biochem 41:59–66
10. Glovsky MM, Hugli TE, Ishizaka T, Lichtenstein LM, Erickson BW (1979) J Clin Invest 64:804–811
11. Hartman CT, Glovsky MM (1981) Int Arch Allergy Appl Immunol 66:274–281
12. Dahinden CA, Kurimoto Y, de Weck AL, Lindley I, Dewald B, Baggiolini M (1989) J Exp Med 170:1787–1792
13. Schwartz LB, Kawahara MS, Hugli TE, Vik D, Fearon DT, Austen KF (1983) J Immunol 130:1891–1895
14. Plaut M, Pierce JH, Watson CJ, Hanley-Hyde J, Nordan RP, Paul WE (1989) Nature 339:64–67

Neuropeptides and Human Mast Cells*

M.K. Church and S. El-Lati

Immunopharmacology Group, Clinical Pharmacology, Centre Block, Southampton General Hospital, Southampton SO9 4XY, United Kingdom

Abstract

Unlike human mast cells associated with mucosal surfaces such as lung, adenoids, tonsils and intestine, skin mast cells may be stimulated to release histamine by the neuropeptides substance P, vasoactive intestinal polypeptide (VIP) and somatostatin or by other basic secretagogues such as morphine, poly-L-lysine and compound 48/80. Release of histamine under these conditions is rapid and accompanied by minimal generation of the eicosanoids, PGD_2 and LTC_4. Transient elevations of intracelluar calcium are associated with mediator secretion induced by both stimuli, that induced by anti-IgE being derived from extracellular sources through channels in the plasma membrane while that stimulated by neuropeptides mobilized intracellularly. Despite these biochemical and temporal differences, degranulation induced by both secretagogues proceeds by compound exocytosis which is indistinguishable under the electron microscope.

Introduction

While cross-linkage of membrane-bound immunoglobulin E (IgE) is likely to be the primary initiating stimulus for mast cell mediator release in the majority of allergic conditions, there are other conditions where there is no obvious link with a known extrinsic allergen. In the skin there is no obvious IgE-dependent or allergic basis for disorders such as a chronic idiopathic urticaria, heat-induced urticaria, cold-induced urticaria or cholinergic urticaria [1]. However, the sensitivity of these conditions to therapy with histamine H 1-receptor antagonists suggests that mast cell-derived histamine is involved in their pathogenesis [2]. In these forms of urticaria a link between nervous stimulation and inflammatory mediator release has been postulated.

The ability of peripheral nerves to induce vasodilatation by means of an axon reflex has been known for over 90 years [3–5]. These observations laid the basis for the classical paper by Lewis in 1927 [6] describing the triple response to histamine in the skin and proposing that the flare was mediated by a neurogenic mech-

* Support by Janssen Pharmaceuticals for SE-L is gratefully acknowledged.

anism probably involving axon reflexes in primary afferent neurones. More recent studies have shown these fibres to be unmyelinated C fibres [7] whose polymodal nociceptors respond to many stimuli, including pressure, heat and the local injection of histamine [8–10]. Immunocytochemical studies have shown that neuropeptides are synthesized within the cell body of sensory nerves and preferentially migrate towards the peripheral sensory endings where they concentrate [11]. The peptide first demonstrated to be released from sensory neurones following antidromic stimulation was the undecapeptide substance P [12–14]. However, substance P is not the only neuropeptide associated with sensory nerves, others including somatostatin, neurokinin A and calcitonin gene-related peptide (CGRP) have also been demonstrated in mammalian skin [15–17]. Indeed there is some evidence that substance P, neurokinin A and CGRP may co-exist within the same sensory neurones [18–20] whereas somatostatin appears to be present in different neurones [21].

Evidence that these neuropeptides may be involved in inflammatory reactions in the skin derives from their effects when injected intradermally and from the use of capsaicin to deplete the neuropeptides from primary sensory afferents [22]. Substance P, somatostatin and vasoactive intestinal polypeptide (VIP) all induce a weal and flare reaction when injected into human skin, substance P being approximately 100 times more potent than histamine [23, 24]. In contrast, CGRP causes a local persistent erythema and neurokinin A a local vasodilatation, neither of which are accompanied by flare reactions [17, 25]. The flare or vasodilatory component of the triple response is blocked by nerve section and local anaesthesia, demonstrating a neurogenic component to the response [23, 24]. Histamine H1 antagonists also markedly reduce the flare [24, 26], suggesting histamine to be involved in its development. It is clear that histamine released during the weal reaction is involved in the initiation of the flare response but whether or not it is involved directly as a vasodilator at the site of the flare is still being debated in the literature [27, 28]. Incrimination of a neuropeptide as the transmitter of the flare derives from the observation that pretreatment of the skin with capsaicin reduced flaring but not wealing on subsequent injection of histamine [23, 24].

Evidence for a direct link between neuropeptides, mast cells and some forms of urticaria has also been presented. Provocation challenge of patients with either cold- or heat-induced or cholinergic urticaria leads to an elevation in the amounts of histamine in the venous blood draining the challenged but not the control arm [29–31]. Furthermore, depletion of cutaneous neuropeptides with capsaicin attenuates both heat- and cold-induced urticaria in man [32] and heat induced oedema in rats [26].

This circumstantial evidence that neuropeptides are able to induce mediator release from skin mast cells encouraged us to examine this hypothesis and to investigate the mechansims of this interaction in vitro.

Peptide-Induced Histamine Release from Human Mast Cells

Human skin mast cells, dispersed from fresh circumcision or mastectomy specimens by incubation with a cocktail of collagenase and hyaluronidase, release histamine in response to both IgE-dependent and neuropeptide stimulation [33]. In contrast, mast cells similarly dispersed from adenoids, tonsils, intestinal muscle and the region of the intestine comprising both the mucosal surface and the immediate sub-mucosal layers responded only to the IgE-dependent stimulus, thus demonstrating functional heterogeneity between different populations of human mast cells [34, 35].

In skin mast cells, substance P, VIP and somatostatin all induce a concentration related release of histamine. The relative equipotency of these neuropeptides together with the observation that eledoisin, physalaemin, neurokinin A (NKA) and neurokinin B (NKB) induce negligible histamine release strongly suggest that the neuroreceptor on human skin mast cells does not belong to any of NK-1, NK-2 or NK-3 tachykinin receptor subtypes found on smooth muscle [36, 37]. This is supported by the observation that morphine, poly-L-lysine and the synthetic histamine releaser compound 48/80 induce a concentration related release of histamine, suggesting that the peptide sensitivity extends to other basic lipophilic substances.

Substance P is an undecapeptide in which the N-terminal amino acids Arg-Pro-Lys-Pro- constitute a positively charged area of the molecule, whereas the remaining residues and the amide-substituted C-terminal methionine provide a lipophilic area. In experiments to determine the structural requirements of substance P in releasing histamine [36] we found that the stepwise removal of N-terminal amino acids led to a progressive loss of activity, the relative potencies compared to substance P (=1) being 0.46 for SP2-11 and 0.16 for SP3-11. The fragment SP4-11 had negligible activity. This confirms the study in rat mast cells [38] which concluded that the histamine-releasing activity of substance P lay largely in the basic N-terminal region, although that SP_{1-4} was also inactive in releasing histamine from human skin mast cells demonstrates that the lipophilic C terminal is also required for the expression of activity. However, the observations that [D-Pro^2, D-$Trp^{7,9}$] substance P in human skin mast cells [36] and Arg-Pro-Lys-Pro$(CH_2)^{11}$-CH_3 in rat mast cells [39] are more effective than substance P in inducing histamine release demonstrate that the precise structure of the lipophilic groups is not critical for activity.

The ability of the neuropeptides, substance P, VIP and somatostatin, and basic substances including morphine, poly-L-lysine and compound 48/80, to cause weal and flare reactions when injected intradermally [23, 24, 40, 41] correlates with our observations of histamine release from isolated mast cells [33, 36]. In contrast, CGRP, neurotensin, bradykinin and Lys-bradykinin, none of which readily induce weal and flare reactions in the skin, caused little or no histamine release.

Evidence that neuropeptides and basic histamine releasers act through a common receptor site has been gained by the use of [D-Pro^4, D-$Trp^{7,9,10}$]SP_{4-11} (SPA), a peptide which inhibits substance P-induced histamine release from rat mast cells and substance P-induced weal and flare reactions in human skin [42].

In human skin mast cells in vitro, this peptide inhibits not only histamine release induced by substance P in a competitive manner but also that induced by VIP, somatostatin, compound 48/80, morphine and poly-L-lysine. In contrast SPA does not inhibit release induced by anti-IgE or the calcium ionophore A23187 [36]. These results suggest that human skin mast cells possess binding sites of low affinity and low specificity for neuropeptides and compounds with similar physicochemical properties and that these sites are distinct from those involved in the initiation of IgE-dependent mast cell activation.

Morphological and Temporal Aspects of Degranulation

In an electron microscopical study [43] we have observed that human dispersed skin mast cells are generally rounded with a single unilobular nucleus and a few micro paplicae extending from the cell surface. The cytoplasm is dominated by the presence of electron dense granules which occupy 47.5% of the extranuclear volume. Stimulation of these cells with anti-IgE or substance P produces identical morphological changes. The granule membranes fuse with other granule membranes and with the plasma membrane to establish communication between the granule matrices and the extracellular space. These fusions produce large labyrinths or degranulation channels through which the preformed granule-associated mediators are released from the cell. This form of degranulation, termed compound exocytosis, has been reported for both dissociated human lung and rodent mast cells [44–47] as well as in human skin biopsies [48]. Morphometric analysis of cells stimulated with anti-IgE to produce 10.2±1.7% or substance P to produce 21.4±4.0% histamine release demonstrated that degranulation channels occupied a mean of 20.9%±3.0% and 33.2%±2.8% of the cytoplasm, respectively. The reduction of granules and the formation of degranulation channels was significantly ($p<0.05$) correlated with histamine release with both stimuli [43].

Time course studies of histamine release showed that anti-IgE induces a relatively slow release of histamine which reaches a completion approximately 6 min after challenge [33, 36]. In contrast, histamine release from human skin mast cells induced by substance P is rapid, being complete within 15–20 s [33]. Similarly, mediator release by VIP, somatostatin, compound 48/80, morphine and poly-L-lysine is similarly rapid [33, 36]. Thus, although the morphological appearance of degranulation is identical, it is clear that these events proceed at widely differing rates with induction by anti-IgE and substance P.

Calcium Mobilization and Mediator Release

Calcium is a major intracellular messenger in coupling activation to a whole spectrum of cellular processes including contraction, secretion and metabolism. Indeed in mast cells facilitated introduction of calcium into the cytoplasm by use of calcium ionophores [49] or iontophoretic techniques [50] is sufficient to induce degranulation in mast cells. However, the source and mechanism of mobilization of calcium to cause elevated levels of free calcium in the cytoplasm may differ. For example in rodent mast cells, histamine release induced by IgE-dependent stimulation requires the presence of extracellular calcium, whereas histamine release induced by neuropeptides my proceed in its absence [51, 52].

To study the participation of calcium in mediator release by human skin mast cells we have performed two series of experiments. In the first series [33] we examined the requirement of extracellular calcium by measuring histamine release in the presence of 1 m*M* extracellular calcium and when extracellular calcium had been chelated with 2 m*M* EDTA for 5 min before stimulation. The results show that histamine release induced by anti-IgE had an obligatory requirement for extracellular calcium, release being negligible in the presence of EDTA. In contrast, histamine release from human skin mast cells induced by substance P, VIP, somatostatin, compound 48/80, morphine and poly-L-lysine is largely independent of the presence extracellular calcium [33, 36]. As experiments in rat mast cells have shown that depletion of intracellular calcium by long-term exposure to EDTA leads to insensitivity to neuropeptides [53], our results suggest that mobilization of intracellular calcium provides sufficient levels of this cation for substance P-induced histamine release to proceed.

In the second series of experiments, a fluorescent calcium probe, fura 2 [54], was used to confirm this hypothesis by monitoring directly the changes in intracellular calcium following cell activation. Mast cells were loaded with the probe by incubating them with 10 μ*M* fura 2 acetoxymethyl ester for 1 h at 37 °C. After thorough washing, replicates containing $3-4\times10^5$ mast cells were challenged with anti-IgE or substance P and the change in fluorescence monitored by spectrofluorimetry at 510 nm with an excitation wavelength of 340 nm. Following stimulation with anti-IgE there was a rapid elevation of intracellular calcium which reached a maximum at 20 s and which decayed exponentially to baseline by 8 min. This confirms the results obtained using rat mast cells [55, 56]. In the absence of extracellular calcium, however, there was neither a rise in intracellular calcium levels nor histamine secretion. These results suggest that with IgE-dependent provocation, the calcium necessary for activation-secretion coupling is stimulated to enter the cell by the transient opening of calcium channels in the plasma membrane. When substance P was used to activate the mast cells in the presence of extracellular calcium, similar but more rapid results were obtained to those found using anti-IgE, namely a rapid elevation of intracellular calcium which reached a maximum at 12 s and which decayed exponentially to baseline by 2 min. With neuropeptide provocation, however, a similar histamine release and intracellular calcium peak was observed in the absence of extracellular calcium clearly demonstrating that under these conditions human skin mast cells mobilize the calcium necessary for activation-secretion coupling from intracellular stores, probably the endoplasmic reticulum, rather than from extracellular sources through calcium channels in the plasma membrane. In other biological systems it has been suggested that generation of inositol 1,3,4,5-tetrakisphosphate (IP_4) is responsible for regulating calcium entry through the plasma membrane [56], whereas mobilization of intracellular calcium is regulated by inositol 1,4,5-trisphosphate [57]. How the differences in calcium mobilization in our experiments relate to differences in phosphoinositide metabolism is yet to be established.

Eicosanoid Production

In addition to differences in the time-course of mediator secretion and calcium mobilization, immunological and neuropeptide stimuli differ further in their ability to activate skin mast cells for the generation of eicosanoids. Studies using purified skin mast cells radiolabelled with [$^3H_8$]-arachidonic acid have shown that prostaglandin (PG) D_2 and leukotriene (LT) C_4 are the major cyclooxygenase and lipoxygenase products respectively generated following stimulation with either calcium ionophore A23187 or ε-chain specific anti-human IgE [58, 59]. Quantification of these eicosanoids by radioimmunoassay of supernatants from unlabelled cells stimulated for 30 min with 25 μg/ml anti-human IgE showed them to release 2897 pmol ± 368 pmol of histamine, 107 ± 15 pmol of PGD_2 and 8.0 ± 0.6 pmol of LTC_4, corresponding to molar ratios of 1000:37:3 [60]. In contrast, substance P at 30 μ*M* stimulated secretion of 4132 ± 347 pmol of histamine, 7.1 ± 1.3 pmol of PGD_2 and 0.7 ± 0.1 pmol of LTC4, giving molar ratios of 1000:1.7:2.0 [60]. Similar results occurred with VIP, somatostatin, morphine, poly-L-lysine and compound 48/80. These observations that neuropeptides and basic secretagogues caused minimal eicosanoid generation suggest a fundamental difference in the biochemical mechanisms leading to cell activation with anti-IgE and neuropeptides. There are precedents for the differential release of preformed and newly generated mediators in dog mastocytoma cells activated with compound 48/80 [61] and human basophils stimulated with the complement fragment C5a [62]. However, in basophils, priming with interleukin 3 stimulates the cells to release increased quantities of LTC_4 on activation with complement fragments [63], indicating that the biochemical processes leading to the production of newly generated mediators have the capacity to be modified in disease.

Conclusions

The ability of skin mast cells to release mediators in response to neuropeptide stimulation is evidence in favour of a neuroimmune interaction within human skin. The close association between dermal mast cells, nerves and blood vessels [64, 65] suggests that the development of skin mast cells may have been influenced by their local environment to produce a cell capable of fulfilling a homeostatic rather than a defensive role.

Knowledge of the mechanism of neuropeptide-induced mediator secretion should prove to be of great importance to our understanding of the role of skin mast cells in health and disease. An augmentation or defects in the interactions between neuropeptide-secreting neurones and skin mast cells may contribute to the aetiology of some forms of urticaria. The enhanced weal responses to various nonimmunological stimuli observed in patients with chronic idiopathic urticaria [66, 67] possibly suggests an increased mast cell sensitivity as an underlying cause of this disease.

References

1. Matthews KP (1983) Urticaria and angioedema. J Allergy Clin Immunol 72:1–14
2. Matthews KP (1985) The urticarias: current concepts in pathogenesis and treatment. Drugs 30:552–560
3. Golz F (1874) Über gefässerweiternde Nerven. Pflugers Arch 9:174–197
4. Bayliss WM (1901) On the origin from the spinal cord of the vasodilator fibres of the hind limb, and on the nature of these fibres. J Physiol (Lond) 26:173–209
5. Langley JN (1900) On axon reflexes in the preganglionic fibres of the sympathetic system. J Physiol 25:364–398
6. Lewis T (1927) The blood vessels of the human skin and their responses. Shaw, London
7. Celander O, Folkow B (1953) The nature and distribution of afferent fibres provided with the axon reflex arrangement. Acta Physiol Scand 29:359–370
8. Kenins P (1981) Identification of the unmyelinated sensory nerves which evoke plasma extravasation in response to antidromic stimulation. Neurosci Lett 25:137–141
9. Torebjork HE, Hallin RG (1974) Identification of afferent C units in intact human skin. Brain Res 67:387–403
10. Van Hees J, Gybels JM (1972) Pain related to single afferent C fibres from human skin. Brain Res 48:397–400
11. Hökfelt T, Kellerth JO, Nillson G, Pernow B (1975) Experimental immunohistochemical studies on the localization and distribution of substance P in cat primary sensory neurones. Brain Res 100:235–252
12. Keen P, Harmar AJ, Spears F, Winter E (1982) Biosynthesis, axonal transport and turnover of neuronal substance P. Substance P in the nervous system. Ciba Found Symp 91:145–164
13. Brodin E, Gazelius B, Lundberg JM, Olgart L (1983) Substance P in trigeminal nerve endings: occurrence and release. Acta Physiol Scand 111:501–503
14. White DM, Helm RP (1985) Release of substance P from peripheral nerve terminals following electrical stimulation of the sciatic nerve. Brain Res 336:27–31
15. Hartschuh W, Weihe E, Reinecke M (1983) Peptidergic (neurotensin, VIP, substance P) nerve fibres in the skin. Immunohistochemical evidence of an involvement of neuropeptides in nociception, pruritis and inflammation. Br J Dermatol 109[Suppl 25]:14–17
16. O'Shaughnessy DJ, McGregor GP, Ghatei MA, Blank MA, Springall DR, Gu J, Polak JM, Bloom SR (1983) Distribution of bombesin, somatostatin, substance P and vasoactive intestinal polypeptide in feline and porcine skin. Life Sci 32:2827–2836
17. Brain SD, Tippins JR, Morris HR, MayIntyre I, Williams TJ (1986) Potent vasodilator activity of calcitonin gene-related peptide in human skin. J Invest Dermatol 87:533–536
18. Nawa H, Hirose T, Takashima H, Inayama S, Nakanishi S (1983) Nucleotide sequences of cloned CDNA's for two types of bovine brain substance P precursor. Nature 306:32–36
19. Nawa H, Kotani H, Nakanishi S (1984) Tissue generation of two preprotachykinin mRNAs from one gene by alternative RNA spacing. Nature 312:729–734
20. Fisher J, Forssman WG, Hökfelt T et al. (1985) Immunoreactive calcitonin gene-related peptide and substance P: coexistence in sensory neurones and behavioural interaction after intrathecal administration in the rat. J Physiol (Lond) 362:29P
21. Hökfelt T, Elde R, Johansson O, Luft R, Nillson G, Arimura A (1976) Immunohistochemical evidence for separate populations of somatostatin-containing and substance P-containing primary afferent neurones in the rat. Neuroscience 1:131–136
22. Theriault E, Otsuka M, Jessel T (1979) Capsaicin-evoked release of substance P from primary sensory neurones. Brain Res 170:209–213

23. Anand P, Bloom SR, McGregor GP (1983) Topical capsaicin pretreatment inhibits axon reflex vasodilation caused by somatostatin and vasoactive polypeptide in human skin. Br J Pharmacol 78:665–669
25. Foreman JC, Jordan CC, Oehme P, Renner H (1983) Structure-activity relationships for some substance P-related peptides that cause wheal and flare reactions in human skin. J Physiol (Lond) 335:449–465
26. Foreman JC, Piotrowski W (1985) Some effects of substance P antagonists on mast cells. In: Hakanson R, Sundler F (eds) Tachykinin antagonists. Elsevier, Amsterdam, pp 405–412
26. Saria A, Lundberg JM (1983) Capsaicin pretreatment inhibits heat-induced oedema in rat skin. Naunyn Schmiedebergs Arch Pharmacol 323:341–342
27. Foreman JC (1987) Neuropeptides and the pathogenesis of allergy. Allergy 42:1–11
28. Barnes PJ, Brown MJ, Dollery CT, Fuller RW, Heavey DJ, Ind PW (1986) Histamine is released from skin by substance P but does not act as the final vasodilator in the axon reflex. Br J Pharmacol 88:741–745
29. Heavey DJ, Kobza-Black A, Barrow SE, Chappell CG, Greaves MW, Dollery CT (1986) Prostaglandin D_2 and histamine release in cold urticaria. J Allergy Clin Immunol 78:458–461
30. Koro O, Dover JS, Francis DM, Kobza-Black A, Kelly RW, Barr RM, Greaves MW (1986) Release of prostaglandin D2 and histamine in a case of localized heat urticaria and effects of treatments. Br J Dermatol 115: 721–728
31. Kaplan AP, Gray L, Shaff RE, Horakova Z, Beaven MA (1975) In vivo studies of mediator release in cold urticaria and cholinergic urticaria. J Allergy Clin Immunol 55:394–402
32. Toth-Kasa I, Jancso G, Obal F, Husz S, Simon N (1983) Involvement of sensory nerve endings in the cold and heat urticaria. J Invest Dermatol 80:34–36
33. Benyon RC, Lowman MA, Church MK (1987) Human skin mast cells: their dispersion, purification and secretory characterization. J Immunol 138:861–867
34. Lowman MA, Rees PH, Benyon RC, Church MK (1988) Human mast cell heterogeneity: histamine release from mast cells dispersed from skin, lung, adenoids, tonsils and intestinal mucosa in response to IgE-dependent and non-immunological stimuli. J Allergy Clin Immunol 81:590–597
35. Rees PH, Hillier K, Church MK (1988) The secretory characteristics of mast cells isolated from the human large intestinal mucosa and muscle. Immunology 65:437–442
36. Lowman MA, Benyon RC, Chruch MK (1988) Characterization of neuropeptide-induced histamine released from human dispersed skin mast cells. Br J Pharmacol 95:121–130
37. Lee CH, Campbell NJ, Williams BJ, Iverson LL (1986) Multiple tachykinin binding sites in peripheral tissues and in brain. Eur J Pharmacol 130:209–217
38. Fewtrell CM, Foreman JC, Jordan CC, Oehme P, Renner H, Stewart JM (1982) The effects of substance P on histamine and 5-hydroxytryptamine release in the rat. J Physiol (Lond) 330:393–411
39. Repke H, Piotrowski W, Bienert M, Foreman JC (1987) Histamine release induced by Arg-Pro-Lys-Pro$(CH_2)_{11}CH_3$ from rat peritoneal mast cells. J Pharmacol Exp Ther 243:317–321
40. Horner FA, Winkelmann RK (1968) Histamine release produced in human skin by compound 48/80. Ann Allergy 26:107–116
41. Casale TB, Bowman S, Kaliner M (1984) Induction of human cutaneous mast cell degranulation by opiates and endogenous opioid peptides: evidence for opiate and nonopiate receptor participation. J Allergy Clin Immunol 73:775–781
42. Piotrowski W, Devoy MA, Jordan CC, Foreman JC (1984) The substance P receptor on rat mast cells and in human skin. Agents Actions 14:420–424
43. Caulfield JP, El-Lati S, Thomas G, Church MK (1990) Dissociated human skin mast cells degranulate in response to anti-IgE and substance P. Lab Invest 63:502–510
44. Caulfield JP, Lewis RA, Hein A, Austen KF (1980) Secretion of dissociated human pulmonary mast cells: evidence for solubilization of granule contents before discharge. J Cell Biol 85:299–311
45. Dvorak AM, Schulman ES, Peters SP, MacGlashan DW, Newball HH, Schleimer RP, Lichtenstein LM (1984) Immunoglobulin E-mediated degranulation of human isolated lung mast cells. Lab Invest 53:45–56
46. Lagunoff D (1973) Membrane fusion during mast cell secretion. J Cell Biol 57:252–259

47. Hammel I, Lagunoff D, Bauza M, Chi EY (1983) Periodic multimodal distribution of granule volumes in mast cells. Cell Tissue Res 228:51–59
48. Kobayasi T, Asboe Hansen G (1969) Degranulation and regranulation of human mast cells: an electron microscopic analysis of whealing reaction in urticaria pigmentosa. Arch Dermatol Venereol (Stockh) 49:369–381
49. Foreman JC, Mongar JL, Gomperts BD (1973) Calcium ionophores and movements of calcium ions following the physiological stimulus to a secretory process. Nature 245:249–251
50. Kanno T, Cochrane DE, Douglas WW (1973) Exocytosis (secretory granule extrusion) induced by injection of calcium into mast cells. Can J Physiol Pharmacol 51:1001–1104
51. Foreman JC, Hallett MB, Mongar JL (1977) The relationship between histamine secretion and ^{45}calcium uptake by mast cells. J Physiol (Lond) 271:193–214
52. Tasaka K, Mio M, Okamoto M (1986) Intracellular calcium release induced by histamine releasers and its inhibition by antiallergic drugs. Ann Allergy 56:464–469
53. Shanahan F, Denburg JA, Fox J, Bienenstock J, Befus D (1985) Mast cell heterogeneity: effects of neuroenteric peptides on histamine release. J Immunol 135:1331–1337
54. Grynkiewicz G, Poenie M, Tsien RY (1985) A new generation of Ca^{2+} indicators with greatly improved fluorescence properties. J Biol Chem 260:3440–3450
55. White JR, Ishizaka T, Ishizaka K, Sha'afi RI (1984) Direct demonstration of increased intracellular concentration of free calcium as measured by quin-2 in stimulated rat peritoneal mast cell. Proc Natl Acad Sci USA 81:3978–3982
56. Irvine RF, Moor FM (1986) Microinjection of inositol-1,3,4,5-tetrakisphosphate activates sea urchin eggs by a mechanism dependent on external calcium. Biochem J 240:917–920
57. Berridge MJ, Irvine RF (1984) Inositol trisphosphate, a novel second messenger in cellular signal transduction. Nature 312:315–321
58. Benyon RC, Robinson C, Holgate ST, Church MK (1987) Prostaglandin D2 release from human skin mast cells in response to ionophore A23187. Br J Pharmacol 92:635–638
59. Robinson C, Benyon C, Agius RM, Jones DB, Wright DH, Holgate ST (1988) The immunological- and calcium-dependent release of histamine and eicosanoids from human dispersed mastocytosis spleen cells. J Invest Dermatol 90:359–365
60. Benyon CR, Robinson C, Church MK (1989) Differential release of histamine and eicosanoids from human skin mast cells activated by IgE-dependent and non-immunological stimuli. Br J Pharmacol 97:898–904
61. Goetzl EJ, Phillips MJ, Gold WM (1983) Stimulus specificity of the generation of leukotrienes by dog mastocytoma cells. J Exp Med 158:731–737
62. Schulman ES, Post TJ, Henson PM, Gicias PC (1988) Differential effects of complement peptides, C5a and C5a des arg on human basophil and lung mast cell histamine release. J Clin Invest 81:918–923
63. Kurimoto Y, DeWeck AL, Dahinden CA (1989) Interleukin 3-dependent mediator release in basophils triggered by C5a. J Exp Med 170:467–479
64. Eady RAJ, Cowen T, Marshall TF, Plummer V, Greaves MW (1979) Mast cell population density, blood vessel density and histamine content of normal human skin. Br J Dermatol 100:623–633
65. Wiesner-Menzel L, Schulz B, Vakilzadeh F, Czarnetzki BM (1981) Electron microscopical evidence for a direct contact between nerve fibres and mast cells. Acta Derm Venereol (Stockh) 61:465–469
66. Cohen RW, Rosenstreich DL (1986) Discrimination between urticaria-prone and other allergic patients by intradermal skin testing with codeine. J Allergy Clin Immunol 77:802–807
67. Bedard PM, Brunet C, Pelletier G, Hebert J (1986) Increased compound 48/80 induced local histamine release from non-lesional skin from patients with chronic urticaria. J Allergy Clin Immunol 78:1121–1125

Neuronal Interaction with Mast Cells

J. Bienenstock, M.H. Perdue, and R.H. Stead

Department of Pathology and Intestinal Diseases Research Unit, McMaster University, 2E1, 1200 Main Street West, Hamilton, Ontario L8N 3Z5, Ontario

Abstract

There is significant information available in the literature suggesting that nerves can influence mast cells. Neurotransmitters are able to cause mast cells to secrete mediators in vitro. Stimulation of nerves can result in mast cell degranulation. Stimulation of nerves ex vivo by field stimulation can result in mast cell degranulation with consequent physiological effects. In experimental situations antigen will cause IgE-dependent/mast cell-dependent/nerve-dependent effects both on intestinal and respiratory tract epithelial cell integrity and physiological changes recorded as short circuit current in Ussing chambers. In vitro co-culture of mast cells with nerves grown from superior cervical ganglia show selective association and contact with mast cells, again with physiological consequences. In Pavlovian conditioning experiments of rats, we have been able to show after suitable training, associating antigen injection in sensitized animals with an appropriate stimulus, that on exposure to the stimulus alone, intestinal mast cell degranulation occurred with physiological consequences. Many of these results suggest a bi-directional communication between mast cells and nerves and it is likely that these may have, by extrapolation, significant implications for human physiology and disease.

Introduction

There is a considerable amount of circumstantial evidence which suggests that nerves may, directly or indirectly, influence the function of mast cells [1–4]. In keeping with some of the current and developing views on communication between the nervous and immune systems [5, 6], we believe that bidirectional communication between mast cells and nerves can occur. This communication is not, we suggest, only found in unhealthy or diseased states, but also in normal healthy tissues. Most of our own work has focused on the gastrointestinal tract, but, since we have also done some work on the respiratory tract, we will focus on these two areas. In addition, there is a small amount of work which supports the contention that mast cells may communicate with nerves in other tissues such as the skin, and we will quote these data where appropriate.

At this stage of our investigations and thinking, we do not believe that all fixed tissue mast cells are in communication, directly or indirectly, with nerves. Rather, we believe that the diffusely distributed mast cell system can, where appropriately sited anatomical associations occur, contribute information to the peripheral nervous system and thereby eventually to the central nervous system for processing. Thus, it is our view that mast cells can act as relays in the sensing of information, its passage, and its transmission centrally. Similarly, mast cells may be part of the effector response system. In this manner mast cells might act as part of the diffuse neuroendocrine system which clearly communicates regularly with the peripheral and central nervous system.

Gastrointestinal Tract

Morphological Evidence

Anecdotal examples of morphological associations between nerves and mast cells abound in the literature. Perhaps the best review of this earlier information was provided by Olsson [7]. Mast cells are present in neurofibromata [8], benign nerve sheath tumours [9], and in amputation neuromas in both humans [2] and mice [10]. Mast cells are also found in association with glomus tumours where they have been observed closely apposed to unmyelinated nerve fibres [11]. In this position they often show some evidence of degranulation [12]. Some authors have found mast cells in close association with nerves in normal skin [13, 14] but the degree to which this occurs has recently been questioned [15].

Heine and Forster [13, 14] and Stach [16] observed the association of mast cells with nerves in the gastrointestinal tract. Newson et al. [17] found ultrastructural evidence for bouton formation between mast cells and enteric nerves in the rat gastrointestinal tract. Similar associations have been observed by Yonei [18] in the colonic mucosa in ulcerative colitis.

Our own studies have been in rats [19] and in humans [20]. In both the normal rat and the animal infected with *Nippostrongylus brasiliensis* we found a striking association, both by light and electron microscopy, of mast cells and enteric nerves. We showed that many of the nerves associated with mast cells were unmyelinated and peptidergic. In the light microscope most of these nerves contained both substance P and calcitonin gene-related peptide (CGRP). Many mast cells showed membrane-membrane contact with nerves. Similar confirmatory observations have recently been made by Arizono et al. [15].

In the human small bowel, appendix, and large bowel we found, by combined histoimmunocytochemical techniques, that mast cells appeared to be apposed to nerves, with an incidence ranging between 47% and 77% [20]. Confirmatory evidence was also obtained using the electron microscope.

Functional Evidence

Bani-Sacchi et al. [21] showed that field stimulation of rat ileum caused histamine release concomitant with a decrease in mast cell granule metachromasia. Furthermore, they showed that both atropine and tetrodotoxin inhibited the effect of field stimulation. This suggested that acetylcholine release was responsible, in turn, for inducing the secretion of histamine from mast cells. Ganguly et al. [22] showed that rat stomach mast cells increased their granularity following sectioning of the vagus nerve and that with pylorus ligation a decrease in tissue histamine occurred, which could be prevented by vagotomy [23]. While this study is suggestive, the cells examined could have been histamine-containing cells other than the mast cells found in the stomach. Nevertheless, this information again suggests close functional association.

There is now a growing body of information, in field stimulation experiments and in those employing antigen in sensitized animals, which suggests that mast cell products are involved in effects on epithelial cell function. Many of these experiments have been done using Ussing chambers and examining the secretion of chloride ion by the epithelium [24–28]. While rats have been used primarily, experiments in mice and guinea pigs have also produced similar results, which suggest that short circuit current (Isc) increases in response to challenge with antigen or as a result of field stimulation, indicating changes in net ion transport. Experiments using animals infected with *Nippostrongylus brasiliensis* or *Trichinella spiralis* have shown that mucosal mast cell mediators such as histamine, serotonin, and arachidonic acid metabolites are involved in these processes.

In our own studies, antigen challenge reduced both the number of stained mucosal mast cells [24] and the histamine levels in the mucosa; ion transport changes were prevented by doxantrazole, which stabilizes both mucosal and connective tissue mast cells [25], but not by cromoglycate [29], which functionally prevents degranulation of connective tissue, and not mucosal mast cells, in the rat. Several groups, including our own, have now shown that tetrodotoxin reduces the isolated jejunal ion transport abnormalities in rats sensitized and subsequently exposed to antigen [26, 28, 30]. Thus, there is a considerable amount of evidence suggesting that antigen-induced mast cell degranulation causes epithelial cell chloride ion secretion, which is dependent on intact nerves, as evidenced by nerve blocking experiments.

Recent support for these suggestions comes from the work of M. Perdue, B. Wershil, and S. Galli (submitted). The approach consists of Ussing chamber experiments using jejunal tissue from mice with the w/w^v trait or their litter-mates as controls. Galli [31] employed these animals for various studies in an attempt to see whether mast cells are involved in a variety of pathological events. The advantage of this model is that these animals are mast cell deficient, but they can be repopulated with mast cells by using normal syngeneric bone marrow or, alternatively, mast cells cultured from bone marrow to a pure population. These types of experiments have clearly shown that w/w^v animals can be induced to form sensitizing antibodies after appropriate immunization with protein antigen. They do not respond very effectively upon exposure to antigen in Ussing chambers. Nevertheless, they do have some responses which clearly cannot be mast cell-dependent. It is not known what cell is responding specifically to antigen challenge in these animals. The experiments further show that the litter-mate responses are normal and that the responses of the w/w^v animals can be restored to that of their litter-mates after reconstitution either with bone marrow or with cultured mast cells. Importantly, it was possible to show that field stimulation of the littermates caused Isc changes (as expected) and that these were blocked by tetrodotoxin, indicating that nerve stimulation could itself cause mast cell degranulation; this effect was lost in the w/w^{v} animals.

We take this type of evidence to suggest that mast cells and nerves interact in the gastrointestinal mucosa and that they do so in a functionally significant way insofar as epithelial transport activity is concerned.

Respiratory Tract

Functional Evidence

There is considerable functional evidence for mast cell association with nerves in the respiratory tract. Direct stimulation of the vidian nerve in patients with chronic hypertrophic nonallergic rhinitis causes morphological mast cell changes [32]. In such experiments, Masini et al. [32] have shown a significant decrease in tissue-based histamine and concomitant degranulation of mast cells, which normally results in vasodilatation and enhanced nasal secretion. Leff et al. [33] have shown that vagal stimulation causes an enhancement of histamine secretion from mast cells after challenge with ascaris antigen in natively allergic dog lungs.

We have performed experiments similar to those described earlier in rat intestinal mucosa with tracheal tissue in Ussing chambers [34]. After appropriate sensitization, exposure to the antigen (egg albumin) in Ussing chambers again caused an increase in Isc that was antigen specific. These changes were prevented by doxantrazole but not cromoglycate, suggesting involvement of mucosal mast cells. When we used tissues from animals that had been neonatally treated with capsaicin (which especially depletes substance P containing nerves) and subsequently sensitized the animals to ovalbumin using the same procedure, the capsaicin-treated animals had a response which was 50% lower than in the controls. Since the levels of IgE were not significantly different between the groups of animals and examination of the tracheas for numbers of mast cells showed no difference, we believe that these experiments provide evidence for the involvement of mast cells and nerves (probably substance P containing) in the regulation of tracheal epithelium homeostasis. We have performed similar studies in vivo [35]. The method used for evaluation was assessment of lung clearance of an aerosolized radiolabeled molecular probe, technetium labeled diethylenetriamine pentaacetic acid. The sensitized rats showed an approximately threefold increase in clearance 20 min after exposure to antigen. This increase remained elevated for 4 h and returned to normal after 24 h. These changes were not observed in sensitized animals exposed to the carrier or in unsensitized challenged controls. The results were antigen specific, since when we used bovine serum albumin we did not find these changes. We repeated these experiments in neonatal, capsaicin-treated, sensitized rats and again showed a major effect; capsaicin treated animals had significantly lower responses to antigen than those animals that had not received capsaicin. We believe that these data show functional consequences of nerve/mast cell associations in the lung.

Other Tissue Sites

Skofitsch et al. [36] showed close association of substance P (SP) containing nerves and mast cells in the diaphragm and mesentery. Dimlich [37] demonstrated that some mast cells appear to be closely apposed to nerves in the portal tracts of the liver. Heine and Forster [13, 14] have shown similar associations in the myocardium and some recent work from Dimitriadou et al. [38] has suggested that similar associations between type 2 cerebral mast cells and nerves may be found. Recently, Yano et al. [39] showed that in w/w^v mice, SP induced tissue swelling, vascular permeability, and granulocyte infiltration were almost entirely mast cell-dependent. Observations of a similar nature have been made by Foreman [40, 41] in the skin with regard to somatostatin and vasoactive intestinal polypeptide.

Inhibitory Effects

While many of these experiments have focused on the positive effects of nerves on mast cell function and degranulation, it is clear that the degranulation of mast cells can be accompanied by more "negative" effects. For example, Brain and Williams [42] showed, in an elegant series of experiments, that when SP was injected into rat skin at the same time as CGRP and compared to either SP or CGRP alone, the effect of CGRP on blood flow was markedly reduced as a result of degradation by mast cell proteases. This effect of mast cell and other proteases on neuropeptides such as SP have also been the focus of a considerable amount of work, particularly in the respiratory tract. Nadel's group has focused on enkephalinases, which are found under normal circumstances on the surface of the respiratory tract epithelium. Indeed, inhalation of SP by guinea pigs has been shown to have almost no bronchoconstrictive effect. The inhibition of these enzymes by proteolytic enzyme inhibitors, given at the same time or before inhalation of the same amount of SP, caused a dramatic increase in apparent activity of the SP inhaled, by up to 100-fold [43, 44]. The functional significance of these observations in relation to such conditions as asthma should need no further emphasis.

Finally, the effect of nerve stimulation is not always of a positive nature in terms of the mast cell response. Miura et al. [45] have shown that stimulation of the vagus nerve in cats natively sensitive to ascaris antigen will cause inhibition of mast cell degranulation. These experiments were performed in animals that had received atropine and propranolol prior to the experiment so as to block both cholinergic and noradrenergic nerves. The animals then received ascaris antigen by inhalation. Control animals responded by an elevation of histamine in the circulation and also by physiological evidence of bronchoconstriction. Animals that received vagal stimulation, however, showed little rise in plasma histamine, despite antigen inhalation, and almost no consequent bronchoconstriction. This information strongly suggests that there are nonadrenergic, noncholinergic nerves traveling in the vagus nerve which can give rise to efferent inhibitory regulation of mast cell degranulation.

Pavlovian Conditioning Effects

In 1886, MacKenzie [46] showed that exhibition of an artificial rose to a quiescent patient, in whom asthma had been shown to be caused by natural roses, initiated an asthmatic attack. Since then there has been much written and considerable controversy about the role of psychological factors in the regulation and induction of allergic symptoms. Considerable literature exists in regard to asthma from the point of view of psychological factor involvement. Our own experiments in animals have suggested that it is possible to psychologically condition animals in such a way as to cause mast cell degranulation [47]. Rats were sensitized to egg albumin and were trained on three successive occasions to associate the injection of antigen with an audiovisual cue. Subsequently, the animals were exposed to the audiovisual cue alone and demonstrated a significant increase in a rat mast cell protease (RMCP II) in the serum. Since the only known source of this enzyme is mucosal mast cells, we concluded that we had observed conditioned mast cell degranulation. Similar experiments have been performed by others in animals and have shown the Pavlovian conditioning of histamine release [48]. In these latter experiments, however, it was not clear whether the histamine had come from mast cells.

Discussion and Conclusions

The associations between mast cells and nerves have been described in a variety of tissues and suggest some regular and purposeful communication. In other experiments, not described or discussed in this paper, we have shown that mast cells appear to have a predilection in tissue culture for nerves [3, 4]. We believe that this is the counterpart of the experiments described here, indicating a morphological association in tissues and a functional interaction which appears to occur between mast cells and nerves when either are stimulated. Extensive literature exists suggesting that mast cells and nerves are also involved in some component of neurogenic inflammation [49, 50], although arguments against this conclusion have been recently adduced [51].

Antigen can cause a variety of cell products to be released from mast cells, which in turn can communicate with nerves and generate action potentials; for example, in ganglia removed from sensitized animals [52]. We are not sure, as described in the opening paragraphs, exactly what the role of mast cells is. They fit the general description for the amine precursor uptake and decarboxylation system (APUD) of Pearse [53]. The APUD system is diffusely located throughout the body and often thought of as being neural crest derived, whereas of course mast cells are not believed to be derived from this site of origin. APUD cells are extensively innervated and are known to be involved in the regulation of mucosal and epithelial function. It is still not clear to what extent mast cells may have the same or similar role as APUD cells. Nevertheless, we feel that sufficient circumstantial and direct evidence now suggests a role for mast cells in bidirectional communication with nerves. We further believe that these systems, which are now beginning to be described, will have important roles to play in better understanding the nature of the allergic process.

References

1. Bienenstock J, Blennerhassett MG, Marshall JS, Perdue MH, Stead RH (1989) Nerves, neuropeptides and mast cells. In: Melchers F, et al. (ed) Progress in immunology, vol 7. Springer, Berlin Heidelberg New York, pp 709–715
2. Stead RH, Perdue MH, Blennerhassett MG Kakuta Y, Sestini P, Bienenstock J (1990) The innervation of mast cells. In: Freier S (ed) The neuroendocrine-immune network. CRC, Boca Raton, pp 19–37
3. Bienenstock J, Blennerhassett MG, Kakuta Y, MacQueen G, Marshall J, Perdue M, Siegel S, Tsuda T, Denburg J, Stead R (1989) Evidence for central and peripheral nervous system interaction with mast cells. In: Galli S, Austen KF (eds) Mast cell and basophil differentiation and function in health and disease. Raven, New York, pp 275–284
4. Bienenstock J, Perdue M, Blennerhassett M, Stead R, Kakuta N, Sestini P, Vancheri C, Marshall J (1988) Inflammatory cells and the epithelium: mast cell/nerve interactions in the lung in vitro and in vivo. Am Rev Respir Dis 138:S31–S34
5. Ader R, Felten D, Cohen N (1990) Interactions between the brain and the immune system. Annu Rev Pharmacol Toxicol 30:561–602
6. Blalock JE (1989) A molecular basis for bidirectional communication between the immune and neuroendocrine systems. Physiol Rev 69:1–32
7. Olsson Y (1968) Mast cells in the nervous system. Int Rev Cytol 29:27–70
8. Pineda A (1965) Mast cells – their presence and ultrastructural characteristics in peripheral nerve tumours. Arch Neurol 13:372–382
9. Isaacson P (1976) Mast cells in benign nerve sheath tumours. J Pathol 119:193–197
10. Nennesmo I, Reinholt F (1986) Mast cells in nerve end neuromas of mice. Neurosci Lett 69:296–301
11. Kimura S (1979) Mast cells in solitary glomus tumours: a possible algogenic role. Acta Derm Venereol (Stockh) 59:415–419
12. Wiesner-Menzel L, Schulz B, Vakilzadeh F, Czarnetzki BM (1981) Electron microscopical evidence for a direct contact between nerve fibres and mast cells. Acta Derm Venereol (Stockh) 61:465–469
13. Heine H, Forster FJ (1975) Histophysiology of mast cells in skin and other organs. Arch Dermatol Res 253:225–228
14. Heine H, Forster FJ (1975) Relationships between mast cells and preterminal nerve fibres. Z Mikrosk Anat Forsch 89: S934–S937
15. Arizono N, Matsuda S, Hattori T, Kojima Y, Maeda T, Galli S (1990) Anatomical variation in mast cell nerve associations in the rat small intestine, heart, lung, and skin. Lab Invest 62:626–634
16. Stach W (1973) Über die Nervengeflechte der Duodenalzotten: Licht- und elektronenmikroskopische Untersuchungen. Acta Anat (Basel) 85:216–231
17. Newson B, Dahlstrom A, Enerback L, Ahlman H (1983) Suggestive evidence for a direct innervation of mucosal mast cells. An electron microscopic study. Neuroscience 10:565–570
18. Yonei Y (1987) Autonomic nervous alterations and mast cell degranulation in the exacerbation of ulcerative colitis. Nippon Shokakibyo Gakkai Zasshi 84:1045–1056
19. Stead RH, Tomioka M, Quinonez G, Simon GT, Felten SY, Bienenstock J (1987) Intestinal mucosal mast cells in normal and nematode-infected rat intestines are in intimate contact with peptidergic nerves. Proc Natl Acad Sci USA 84:2975–2979
20. Stead RH, Dixon MF, Bramwell NH, Riddell RH, Bienenstock J (1989) Mast cells are closely apposed to nerves in the human gastrointestinal mucosa. Gastroenterology 97:575–585
21. Bani-Sacchi T, Barattini M, Bianchi S, Blandina P, Brunelleschi S, Fantozzi R, Mannaioni PF, Masini E (1986) The release of histamine by parasympathetic stimulation in guinea pig auricle and rat ileum. J Physiol (Lond) 371:29–43

22. Ganguly AK, Sathiamoorthy SS, Bhatnagar OP (1978) Effect of subdiaphragmatic vagotomy on gastric mucosal mast cell population in pylorus ligated rats. Q J Exp Physiol 63:89–92
23. Ganguly AK, Gopinath P (1979) Vagus nerves and the gastric tissue histamine concentration in pylorus ligated albino rats. Q J Exp Physiol 64:1–6
24. Perdue MH, Chung M, Gall DG (1984) Effect of intestinal anaphylaxis on gut function in the rat. Gastroenterology 86:391–397
25. Perdue MH, Gall DG (1986) Intestinal anaphylaxis in the rat: jejunal response to in vitro antigen exposure. Am J Physiol 250:G427–G431
26. Perdue MH, Gall DG (1986) Rat jejunal mucosal response to histamine and anti-histamines in vitro. Comparison with antigen-induced changes during intestinal anaphylaxis. Agents Actions 19:5–9
27. Baird AW, Cuthbert AW, Pearce FL (1985) Immediate hypersensitivity reactions in epithelia from rats infected with *Nippostrongylus brasiliensis*. Br J Pharmacol 85:787–795
28. Castro GA, Harari Y, Russell D (1987) Mediators of anaphylaxis-induced ion transport changes in small intestine. Am J Physiol 253:G540–G548
29. Perdue MH, Gall DG (1985) Transport abnormalities during intestinal anaphylaxis in the rat: effect of antiallergic agents. J Allergy Clin Immunol 76:498–503
30. Baird AW, Cuthbert AW (1987) Neuronal involvement in type 1 hypersensitivity reaction in gut epithelia. Br J Pharmacol 92:647–655
31. Galli SJ (1990) New insights into "the riddle of mast cells": microenvironmental regulation of mast cell development and phenotypic heterogeneity. Lab Invest 62:5–33
32. Masini E, Rucci L, Cirri-Borghi MB, Giannella E, Mannaioni PF (1986) Stimulation and resection of vidian nerve in patients with chronic hypertrophic nonallergic rhinitis: effect on histamine content in nasal mucosa. Agents Actions 18:251–253
33. Leff AR, Stimler NP, Munoz NM, Shioya T, Tallet J, Dame C (1986) Augmentation of respiratory mast cell secretion of histamine caused by vagus nerve stimulation during antigen challenge. J Immunol 136:1066–1073
34. Sestini P, Bienenstock J, Crowe S, Marshall J, Stead R, Kakuta Y, Perdue M (1990) Ion transport in rat tracheal epithelium in vitro: role of capsaicin-sensitive nerves in allergic reaction. Am Rev Respir Dis 141:393–397
35. Sestini P, Dolovich M, Vancheri C, Stead RH, Marshall JS, Perdue M, Gauldie J, Bienenstock J (1989) Antigen-induced lung solute clearance in rats is dependent on capsaicin-sensitive nerves. Am Rev Respir Dis 139:401–406
36. Skofitsch G, Savitt JM, Jacobowitz DM (1985) Suggestive evidence for a functional unit between mast cells and substance P fibres in the rat diaphragm and mesentery. Histochemistry 81:5–8
37. Dimlich RVW (1984) Electron microscopic examination of mast cells and nerve processes in hepatic portal areas of the rat. In: Bailey GW (ed) Proceedings of the 42nd annual meeting of the Electron Microscopy Society of America. San Francisco Press, San Francisco, pp 230–231
38. Dimitriadou V, Aubineau P, Taxi J, Seylaz J (1987) Ultrastructural evidence for a functional unit between nerve fibres and type II celebral mast cells in the cerebral vascular wall. Neuroscience 22:621–630
39. Yano H, Wershil BK, Arizono N, Galli SJ (1989) Substance P-induced augmentation of cutaneous vascular permeability and granulocyte infiltration in mice is mast cell dependent. J Clin Invest 84:1276–1286
40. Foreman JC (1987) Substance P and calcitonin gene-related peptide: effects on mast cells and in human skin. Int Arch Allergy Appl Immunol 82:366–371
41. Piotrowski W, Foreman JC (1985) On the actions of substance P, somatostatin, and vasoactive intestinal polypeptide on rat peritoneal mast cells and in human skin. Naunyn Schmiedebergs Arch Pharmacol 331:364–368
42. Brain SD, Williams TJ (1988) Substance P regulates the vasodilator activity of calcitonin gene-related peptide. Nature 335:73–75
43. Dusser DJ, Umeno E, Graf PD, Djokic T, Borson DB, Nadel JA (1988) Airway neutral endopeptidase-like enzyme modulates tachykinin-induced bronchoconstriction in vivo. J Appl Physiol 65:2585–2591
44. Stimler-Gerard NP (1987) Neutral endopeptidase-like enzyme controls the contractile activity of substance P in guinea pig lung. J Clin Invest 79:1819–1825

45. Miura M, Inoue H, Ichinose M, Kimura K, Katsumata U, Takishima T (1990) Effect of nonadrenergic noncholinergic inhibitory nerve stimulation on the allergic reaction in cat airways. Am Rev Respir Dis 141:29–32
46. MacKenzie JN (1886) The production of the so called "rose-cold" by means of an artificial rose. Am J Med Sci 91:45–57
47. MacQueen G, Siegel S, Marshall J, Perdue M, Bienenstock J (1989) Pavlovian conditioning of rat mucosal mast cells to secrete rat mast cell protease II. Science 243:83–85
48. Russell M, Dark KA, Cummins DW, Ellman G, Callaway E, Peeke HVS (1984) Learned histamine release. Science 225:733–734
49. Kiernan JA (1975) A pharmacological and histological investigation of the involvement of mast cells in cutaneous axon reflex vasodilation. Q J Exp Physiol 60:123–130
50. Lembeck F, Holzer P (1979) Substance P as neurogenic mediator of antidromic vasodilation and neurogenic plasma extravasation. Naunyn Schmiedebergs Arch Pharmacol 310:175–183
51. Kowalski ML, Kaliner MA (1988) Neurogenic inflammation, vascular permeability, and mast cells. J Immunol 140:3905–3911
52. Weinreich D, Undem BJ (1987) Immunological regulation of synaptic transmission in isolated guinea pig autonomic ganglia. J Clin Invest 79:1529–1532
53. Pearse AGE (1966) 5-Hydroxytryptophan uptake by dog thyroid "C" cells, and its possible significance in polypeptide hormone production. Nature 211:598–600

Atopic Eczema

T Cells in Atopic Dermatitis

C. A. F. M. Bruijnzeel-Koomen, F. C. van Reijsen, and G. C. Mudde

Swiss Institute of Allergy and Asthma Research, Obere Strasse 22, 7270 Davos, Switzerland

Sofar, the role of antigen-presenting cells in atopic diseases has been underestimated. Recent observations made in the skin of patients with atopic dermatitis (AD) and in the nasal mucosa of patients with allergic rhinitis (AR) suggest that Langerhans cells (LC), being tissue-specific dendritic cells with potent antigen-presenting capacity, play an important role in the allergic inflammatory response. LC in the nasal mucosa of AR and in the skin of AD have been shown to bear IgE surface molecules. These IgE bearing LC present allergen to autologous T-cells to induce allergen-specific T-cell responses, which are responsible for the local inflammatory infiltrate. Furthermore, these IgE bearing LC may trigger the immune system directly or indirectly to guarantee ongoing IgE synthesis by B-cells.

IgE bearing LC may play a crucial role in directing the type of the allergic reaction mechanism.

Clinical evidence that atopic dermatitis (AD) is an immunologically mediated disease came from the observation that AD-like skin lesions completely disappeared after bone marrow transplantation in children with Wiskott-Aldrich syndrome [20]. Early studies concerning immunological mechanisms involved in the pathogenesis of AD were performed on T lymphocytes in peripheral blood and showed a decreased number of circulating T cells. The CD4/CD8 ratio was increased due to a decreased number of $CD8^+$ T cells [6]. This increased CD4/CD8 ratio was not present in patients with allergic asthma, allergic rhinitis, or contact dermatitis. The number of circulating T cells and the CD4/CD8 ratio were, however, correlated with both the total serum IgE level and the clinical severity of the skin lesions. The in vitro function of these T cells, e.g., their response to mitogens or recall antigens (candida, tetanus) was decreased and depended on the clinical severity of the skin lesions and the serum IgE level [5, 21].

In contrast to the in vitro response, the in vivo response to the same antigens did not normalize after clinical remission, especially in patients with serum IgE levels greater than 1000 kU/l [7]. This suggested a discrepancy between the two responses, probably due to local factors. The high incidence of viral skin infections and the depression of the mixed lymphocyte reaction, the autologous mixed lymphocyte reaction, and the autologous mixed skin lymphocyte reaction suggested a defective function of $CD8^+$ T cells, presumably due to a failure in the generation of cytotoxic T cells [11]. Furthermore, the number and function of natural killer cells (Leu 11a$^+$) was decreased up to 50% [16]. This correlated with the magnitude of the CD4/CD8 ratio. Interferon-γ production by peripheral blood mononuclear cells after phytohemagglutinin (PHA) or concanavalin A (ConA) stimulation was decreased in AD patients with highly elevated serum IgE levels. This seemed to be an intrinsically limited defect since it could not be restored by interleukin-2, calcium ionophore or phorbol ester (PMA) [17]. The decreased production of interferon-γ by T cells could explain the decreased natural killer cell function and the decreased interleukin-1 and tumor necrosis factor-alpha production observed in monocytes [9]. These decreases paralleled that of interferon-γ production by T cells and seemed not to be due to an intrinsic defect since neopterin and interleukin-6 production by monocytes was normal [18].

With respect to interleukin-2 production by T cells, Kapp et al. [9] found a decreased production after mitogenic stimulation, whereas Rousset et al. [19] measured an interleukin-2 production by T cells that was within normal limits. Even more interesting was the observation that, after mitogenic stimulation (either calcium ionophore and PMA or PHA and PMA), peripheral blood mononuclear cells produced increased levels of interleukin-4 [19]. Production of interferon-γ was decreased, and it was suggested that this was due to down-regulation by interleukin-4.

Apart from a decrease in the number and function of both CD8$^+$ T cells and natural killer cells and a defect in the function of CD4$^+$ T cells, there are signs present in AD which suggest chronic T cell stimulation. The level of soluble interleukin-2 receptor is increased, as is the number of interleukin-2 receptor positive, CD4$^+$ and CD8$^+$ T cells in the circulation, correlating with both serum IgE levels and skin involvement [23].

The presence of activated T cells in the circulation is reflected in the skin. In clinically involved AD skin, the dermis is infiltrated by activated T cells with a CD4/CD8 ratio which is even higher than that in the circulation. This suggests a selective sequestration of CD4$^+$ T cells in the skin of AD patients. Apart from T cells, many antigen presenting cells are present, e.g., CD1$^+$, RFD1$^+$ dendritic cells, and CD14$^+$ cells.

The observations made in the circulation and in the skin suggest that AD is a T cell-mediated disease in which activation of the T cell system may be of pathogenetic significance. T cell activation in the skin in AD may be due to antigens or allergens that invade the skin via the epidermis or the circulation. Another possibility is direct activation by keratinocyte-derived factors. In AD there exist in vivo and in vitro observations which suggest that allergens can activate T cells. Epicutaneous contact with allergens can induce eczematous skin lesions in AD patients with elevated serum IgE levels. The histopathology of these patch test reactions, which are specific for AD patients, is dominated by CD4$^+$ cells, CD1$^+$, cells, and eosinophils [4]. Furthermore, in the epidermis and dermis of patients with AD with elevated serum IgE levels, CD1$^+$ cells (Langerhans' cells) are present which express IgE bound to an Fc receptor [1, 3]. These IgE$^+$/CD1$^+$ epidermal cells can induce a T cell response in the presence of aeroallergens [2, 13]. In contrast CD1$^+$ cells, without cell-bound IgE from AD patients or from normal controls, cannot induce these T cell responses, although their T cells proliferate in response to aeroallergens in the presence of monocytes from peripheral blood. Furthermore, the T cell response to aeroallergens can be significantly inhibited by preincubation of the $IgE^{+}/CD1^{+}$ cells with anti-IgE and anti-light chain antibodies. This shows that the presence of cell-bound IgE on $CD1^{+}$ cells plays a key role in the antigen presenting capacity of these cells in the presence of aeroallergens.

Recently Wierenga et al. [22] have shown that house dust mite allergen-specific peripheral blood T cells from atopics, in contrast to those of nonatopics, produce increased levels of interleukin-4 and decreased levels of interferon-gamma after stimulation with house dust allergen or mitogens; these T cells provided help for IgE production by B cells. Furthermore Ramb-Lindauer et al. [15] could isolate grass pollen-specific T cells from clinically involved AD skin which also provided help for IgE synthesis by B cells.

The above mentioned observations suggest that activation of allergen-specific T cells can occur via the skin after binding to $IgE^{+}/CD1^{+}$ epidermal cells. Furthermore, activation of these T cells results in an increased production of interleukins which are involved in the regulation of IgE production.

The role of IgE antibodies in antigen presentation points to a new function for IgE [2, 14]. Kehry and Yamashita [10] demonstrated in mice that B cells presented IgE-antigen complexes 100 times more efficiently than uncomplexed antigen or antigen combined with a nonspecific IgE. In contrast binding of IgG1-antigen complexes to Fc γ receptors on B cells not only failed to promote antigen presentation, but was actually inhibitory for T cell activation. Thus, in AD, antigen-presentation by means of allergen-specific IgE, bound in Fc ε receptors on antigen presenting cells, e.g., epidermal Langerhans' cells, may induce a very effective T cell stimulation. The observation by Kehry and Yamashita [10] may explain why AD patients can be successfully treated with parenteral administration of allergen complexed to IgG, as was recently reported by Jacquemin et al. [8]. Allergen-IgG complexes may down-regulate T cell responses to the same allergen. IgE-mediated antigen presentation may play a role in the pathogenesis of atopic disorders in general, since Machiels et al. [12] could also successfully treat allergic asthma with the above mentioned allergen-IgG complexes.

References

1. Bruijnzeel-Koomen C, van Wichen D, Toonstra J, Berrens L, Bruijnzeel P (1986) The presence of IgE molecules on epidermal Langerhans cells from patients with atopic dermatitis. Arch Dermatol Res 278:199–205
2. Bruijnzeel-Koomen C, Boland G, Mudde G (1988) IgE-mediated antigen presentation by epidermal Langerhans cells from patients with atopic dermatitis. Inserm Colloq 172:335–341
3. Bruijnzeel-Koomen, van der Donk E, Bruijnzeel P, Capron M, de Gast G, Mudde G (1988) Associated expression of CD1 antigen and Fc receptor for IgE on epidermal Langerhans cells from patients with atopic dermatitis. Clin Exp Immunol 74:137–142
4. Bruijnzeel-Koomen C, van Wichen D, Spry C, Venge P, Bruijnzeel P (1988) Active participation of eosinophils in patch test reactions to inhalant allergens in patients with atopic dermatitis. Br J Dermatol 118:229–238
5. Byrom N, Timlin D (1979) Immune status in atopic eczema: a survey. Br J Dermatol 100:491

6. Cooper K, Kazmierowsky J, Wuepper K, Hanifin J (1983) Immunoregulation in atopic dermatitis: functional analysis of B-T cell interactions and the enumeration of Fc receptor bearing T cells. J Invest Dermatol 80:139–145
7. Forsbeck M, Hovmark A, Skog E (1976) Patch testing, tuberculin testing and sensitization with dinitrochlorobenzene and nitrosodiumethylaniline of patients with atopic dermatitis. Acta Derm Venereol (Stockh) 56:135–138
8. Jacquemin M, Machiels J, Lebrun P, Saint-Remy J (1990) Successful treatment of atopic dermatitis with complexes of allergen and specific antibodies. Lancet 1:1468–1469
9. Kapp A, Textor A, Krutman J, Moeller A (1990) Immunomodulating cytokines in atopic dermatitis and psoriasis: production of tumor necrosis factor and lymfotoxin by mononuclear cells in vitro. Br J Dermatol 122:587–592
10. Kehry M, Yamashita L (1990) Role of the low-affinity Fc epsilon receptor in B-lymphocyte antigen presentation. Res Immunol 141:77–81
11. Leung D, Wood N, Dubey D, Geha R (1983) Cellular basis of defective cell mediated lymphocytes in atopic dermatitis. J Immunol 130:1678–1682
12. Machiels J, Somville M, Lebrun P, Lebecque S, Jacquemin M, Saint-Remy J (1990) Allergic bronchial asthma due to Dermatophagoides pteronyssinus can be efficiently treated by inoculation of allergen-antibody complexes. J Clin Invest 85:1024–1035
13. Mudde G, van Reijsen F, Boland G, de Gast G, Bruijnzeel P, Bruijnzeel-Koomen C (1990) Allergen presentation by epidermal Langerhans cells from patients with atopic dermatitis is mediated by IgE. Immunology 69:335–341
14. Mudde G, Hansel T, van Reijsen F, Osterhof B, Bruijnzeel-Koomen C (1990) IgE: an immunoglobulin specialized in antigen capture? Immunol Today 11:440–443
15. Ramb-Lindauer C, Feldmann A, Zierz R, Neumann C (1989) Pollen reactive T cell lines from the skin of atopic dermatitis. 4th Immunodermatology Symposium, Amsterdam
16. Reinhold U, Wehrmann W, Bauer R, Kreysel H (1986) Defizit natürlicher Killerzellen im peripheren Blut bei atopischer Dermatitis. Hautarzt 37:438–443
17. Reinhold U, Pawelec G, Wehrmann W, Kukel S, Oehr P, Kreysel H (1990) Cytokine production in atopic dermatitis. Acta Derm Venereol (Stockh) 69:497–502
18. Reinhold U, Wehrmann W, Kukel S, Kreysel H (1990) Evidence that defective interferon-gamma production in atopic dermatitis patients is due to intrinsic abnormalities. Clin Exp Immunol 79:374–379
19. Rousset F, Pene J, Chretien I, Briere F, Souillet G, de Vries J (1989) The role of interleukin 4, interferon gamma and interferon alpha in the regulation of IgE synthesis by peripheral blood lymphocytes of atopic and allergic children in vitro. In: Johansson SGO (ed) IgE mediated allergy in childhood. (Pharmacia allergy research award book) AW Grafiska, Uppsala, pp 25–33
20. Saurat JH (1985) Eczema in primary immune deficiencies. Acta Derm Venereol (Stockh) 114:125–128
21. Thestrup-Pederson K, Ellegaard J, Thulin H (1977) PPD and mitogen responsiveness of lymphocytes from patients with atopic dermatitis. Clin Exp Immunol 27:118–126
22. Wierenga E, Snoek M, de Groot C, Chretien I, Bos J, Jansen H, Kapsenberg M (1990) Evidence for compartimentalization of functional subsets of CD4 positive T lymphocytes in atopic patients. J Immunol 144:4651–4656
23. Wuethrich B, Joller-Melkema H, Grob P (1990) Levels of sIL2R correlate with the severity of the atopic dermatitis. Dermatologica 181:92–97

IgE Receptor Expression on Langerhans Cells

T. Bieber

Dermatologische Klinik und Poliklinik der Ludwig-Maximilian University, Frauenlobstrasse 9, W-8000 München 2, Federal Republic of Germany

Abstract

IgE-bearing epidermal Langerhans cells (IgE+LC) have initially been described in patients with atopic eczema, suggesting that LC may be primarily involved in the pathophysiology of this disease by presenting IgE-bound aeroallergens to specific T-cells and thereby provoking an IgE mediated type IV reaction. Since normal human epidermal LC are not able to bind IgE molecules and therefore do not express any IgE receptor (FcεR), several aspects of this field were investigated recently. First of all, it is still unclear whether the high affinity FcεR1 or the low affinity FcεR2/CD23 or both or a putative third type of FcεR is expressed by LC in atopic eczema. In situ hybridization experiments will probably give the answer in the next future. In contrast, recent investigations have shown that IgE+LC are not specific for atopic eczema but found in several inflammatory skin diseases providing the patients exhibit an elevated serum IgE-level. Since it was then pointed out that cytokines locally released by infiltrating cells like T-cells may be involved in the induction/regulation of the expression of a specific receptor for IgE molecules on LC, in vitro studies on cultured LC were designed in order to induce such a Fcε on normal LC. Thereby, it became evident that T-cell derived cytokines like IL-4 and/or IFN-γ are able to induce FcεR2/CD23 on normal LC in vitro. Moreover, these cells are also able to release soluble CD23 which is probably involved in the regulation of IgE-synthesis. In vitro experiments also suggest that several epidermal cell-derived cytokines may be involved in the regulation of the FcεR2/CD23 in vivo. From these observations, it is postulated that the expression of a FcεR is not intrinsic to LC from patients with atopic eczema, but rather related to distinct signals or mediators present in inflammatory skin. Thereafter, elevated IgE levels – which are not obligatorily related to atopy – may contribute to the binding of IgE molecules on the receptor within inflammatory skin areas. However, IgE+LC are not to be considered as an epiphenomenon in atopic eczema, since in vitro studies on LC isolated from atopic eczema show that these cells are able to stimulate autologous antigen specific T-cells. Therefore, the antigen-specificity of IgE molecules bound to the receptor may be the most important feature to consider herein.

Introduction

Atopic eczema, allergic rhinoconjunctivitis, and asthma bronchiale represent the main elements of the atopic diathesis, which is classically accompanied by elevated IgE production. While the pathophysiology of IgE mediated allergic respiratory diseases is now better understood, the significance of allergic mechanisms in the pathogenesis of atopic eczema remains unclear. Due to tremendous progress in immunology during the last few years, it has become evident that distinct cytokines, such as interleukin-4 (IL-4) and interferon-γ (IFN-γ), may play a pivotal role in both the complex regulatory network of IgE production and in atopic diseases. Although it is not clear whether atopic disease can be correlated with an imbalance of the cytokine network involved in IgE synthesis and IgE mediated reactions, several aspects suggest some links between the latter and atopic eczema. However, one may only speculate about such phenomena. Nonetheless, recent findings have drawn attention to distinct, IgE-bearing, cutaneous dendritic cells, e.g., epidermal Langerhans' cells and dermal dendritic cells, which may represent the missing link.

Langerhans Cells are the Outposts of the Immune System in the Skin

Langerhans cells (LC) are dendritic, bone marrow derived cells, which presumably belong to the dendritic cell family (most aspects of LC are reviewed in [29]). They represent only 2% – 5% of the total epidermal cell population. Both the precursor cell as well as the homing mechanism of the epidermal LC are still unknown. Ultrastructurally, the LC is characterized by the presence of cytoplasmic Birbeck granules, the origin and function of which are still unclear. Recently, it has been suggested that resident LC represent immature dendritic cells, based on phenotypic and functional considerations. Resident LC strongly express CD1a but weakly CD4; they are major histocompatibility complex (MHC) class II positive, bear adhesion molecules, e.g., CD11b/CD18 and CD11c/CD18 [18], and express only the 40 kDa low affinity receptor for the Fc fragment of IgG [28] and not the receptor for IgE. Furthermore, resident LC constitutively express a 26–30 kDa variant of the early activation antigen CD69 [11]. Functionally, resident LC clearly stimulate antigen-specific autologous T cells, but are weak stimulators in the skin mixed lymphocyte reaction (SMLR). In contrast, when isolated from the skin and maintained for a few days in vitro, LC undergo a profound phenotypic and functional "maturation." Thus, they lose their Birbeck granules and most of the above mentioned surface markers, but strongly increase their MHC class I and II expression, express new surface structures common to lymphoid dendritic cells, and become potent stimulators in the SMLR [25]. From a clinical point of view, the most important and best documented function of LC is antigen presentation to T lymphocytes in contact allergic reactions. The precise location where antigen presentation to T cells occurs is still unknown. However, some observations suggest that, after antigen binding, LC move to the dermis where they may be identified as indeterminate dendritic cells or dermal dendritic cells (DDC). These cells are ultrastructurally very similar to LC but lack Birbeck granules. DDC may then leave the dermis via the lymphatics as veiled cells to present antigen by interdigitating cells to T cells in the paracortical area of the lymph node. Whereas it has been demonstrated that LC produce prostaglandin D_2 at least in vitro [26], data suggesting their ability to secrete IL-1 [27] or even IFN-γ are still a matter of discussion. Moreover, since they are difficult to isolate from the dermal compartment, nothing is known about the functional capacity of DDC. However, the above mentioned characteristics and several immunohistochemical investigations of various diseases suggest that LC and DDC play an important role in the skin immune system, in particular in antigen handling.

IgE-Bearing LC and DDC in Atopic Eczema

Quantitative studies of LC, estimated by L-Dopa staining in atopic eczema (AE), have suggested that an increased number is found in chronic skin lesions [33]. Nonetheless, using immunohistochemical techniques and enumeration of epidermal LC on cryosections by computer-assisted morphometric analysis, these results could not be confirmed and no difference in the number of LC between normal skin and skin from AE patients (acute and chronic lesions) has been detected [5].

The presence of IgE-bearing LC in AE was first described in 1986 by Bruijnzeel-Koomen et al. [12]. Since then, attention has also been drawn to IgE-bearing DDC [2, 21], which may either be LC which have left the epidermis and thereby lost their Birbeck granules or other cells which may be related to LC. One should note that, among atopic patients, IgE-bearing LC (IgE+LC) have only been found in those with AE but not in patients with asthma or rhinitis allergica, even those with a high IgE level [12]. Further studies have shown that IgE+LC are found in patients with AE and elevated IgE levels and that they can especially be observed in acute and chronic skin lesions, as well as, although to a much lesser degree, in clinically normal looking skin from these patients [6]. However, even in uninvolved skin of patients with AE, IgE+DDC are found scattered in the dermal compartment, in particular around blood vessels. In such patients, the proportion of epidermal LC able to bind IgE in lesioned skin is variable, with a maximum of 40%–70%. This suggests a limited capacity of these cells to express an adequate receptor [6], which probably depends on their maturation stage. Interestingly, epidermal anti-IgE staining progressively decreases following topical corticosteroid treatment of AE skin after 1 week and completely disappears after 2 weeks, while CD1a+LC are still present [6]. Most importantly, concerning the specificity of these findings for AE, recent investigations performed on patients with other diseases, who did not have a history of atopy or AE, have clearly shown that IgE+LC are not specific for AE. Rather, these cells can also be found in various skin diseases with dermal and/or epidermal mononuclear cell infiltrates, such as psoriasis vulgaris, cutaneous T cell lymphomas, or pseudolymphomas, provided the patients display an elevated IgE level [3]. Finally, IgE+DDC have been found in significant amounts in dermal infiltrates in skin biopsies performed in patients with actinic reticuloid with elevated serum IgE levels.

Langerhans Cells Express a Yet-To-Be-Defined Receptor for IgE in AE

Anti-IgE staining of LC or DDC in AE disappears after removal of cell-bound IgE by acid elution and can be reconstituted by incubating the skin sections with serum containing high levels of IgE, but not with serum from normal controls [7, 12]. This suggests that LC may indeed express a specific receptor for IgE molecules. Studies on LC isolated from the skin of AE patients demonstrated that IgE molecules are bound to LC via their Fc fragments [13]. These experiments further confirmed the lack of IgE binding on normal LC and showed that the FcεR expressed on LC isolated from atopic skin has relative high affinity for myeloma IgE, also binds IgG, is resistant to trypsinization, and may be spatially associated with the CD1a antigen [13]. Several of these characteristics, however, also suggest instead that LC may express a high affinity FcεR1, rather than a low affinity FcεR2. Since, as of yet, FcεR1 has been described as a constitutively expressed receptor found only on mast cells and basophils, one might expect the low affinity type receptor for IgE (FcεR2) to be present. The lack of reactivity of anti-CD23 monoclonal antibodies (mAb) on AE skin sections and the absence of inhibition in the rosette assay, using myeloma IgE coated sheep red blood cells on LC, by such mAb, however, do not support this possibility [13]. Interestingly, BB10, an mAb directed against FcεR2 on human eosinophils, platelets, and macrophages [15] has been shown to inhibit the above mentioned rosette assay [13]. Recently BB10 has been shown to react with epitopes which indeed, are common to FcεR2 [19] and adhesion molecules. Thus, it remains possible that LC express a variant of FcεR2 common to eosinophils or that the epitopes recognized by anti-CD23 mAb are hidden by other surface glycoproteins, such as CD1a, which seems to be spatially associated with FcεR on LC.

In Vitro Induction of FCεR2 on Human LC

It has been stated that normal human LC neither bind IgE molecules nor react with any anti-FcεR reagents. This indicates that in AE LC and DDC are induced to express a specific receptor for IgE. Moreover, the fact that, in uninvolved skin of patients with AE, anti-IgE staining is very weak but increases in involved areas suggests a possible role of locally released mediators in the up-regulation of the expression of this receptor. Since infiltrating cells are mostly comprised of T cells, T cell derived cytokines are presumably involved in this induction process. On the other hand, keratinocyte derived cytokines may also contribute to the regulation of this event.

The putative role of such cytokines in the induction of the FcεR2 on normal epidermal LC has been investigated [8]. While LC-enriched epidermal cells, either freshly isolated or cultured in media alone, did not react with anti-CD23 reagents, rhIL-4 as well as rhIFN-γ led to a gradual, dose-dependent emergence of CD1a/CD23 reactive cells. Furthermore, capping experiments revealed that the induced CD23 molecule is associated with CD1a (Bieber, unpublished data), as has been described for the receptor on IgE-bearing LC isolated from AE [13]. The addition of rhIL-1, rhIL-3, and rh tumor necrosis factor-α (TNF-α) decreased rhIL-4 and rhIFN-γ induced CD23 expression on LC, whereas rh granulocyte macrophage-colony stimulating factor (GM-CSF) had no effect [9]. These data show that rhIL-4 and rhIFN-γ induce FcεR2/CD23 expression on normal human LC and that epidermal cell derived cytokines may play a regulatory role in this phenomenon. It is clear that, in the epidermal compartment, LC are exposed to several cytokines which participate in a complex regulatory network. For example, in uninvolved skin of atopic patients the effect of IL-4 or IFN-γ on LC is probably counterbalanced by some epidermal cytokines, e.g. TNF-α. Thus, the presumed, locally high amount of IL-4 or IFN-γ produced by infiltrating T cells could be responsible for the increased expression of FcεR found in lesioned skin.

These in vitro results support the concept that, in atopic disease, under distinct conditions, the expression of FcεR is induced on LC which, therefore, after binding an aeroallergen, may be able to activate T cells and provoke eczematous lesions. However, the function of FcεR2 and CD23 on LC is related to the expressed receptor subtype. Recently two species of FcεR2 have been described and it has been proposed that FceR2a, which is constitutively expressed on B cells, is involved in the regulation of B cell development, whereas FcεR2b may function in effector cells involved in IgE mediated immunity [32]. Molecular biology investigations, using specific probes for each type of FcεR2, are currently in progress in order to clarify this problem. Studies on both rhIL-4 and rhIFN-γ induced CD23 expression on LC make the question why the FcεR on LC in vivo is CD23 negative even more intriguing.

Possible Role of LC in the Regulatory Network of IgE Synthesis

It remains unclear whether sensitization to aeroallergens occurs not only via the uper airways but also transepidermally. Observations based on differences in serum IgE levels, for allergens derived from house dust mite bodies and house dust mite feces in asthmatic children and children with AE, suggest that sensitization to aeroallergens may also occur via penetration of the skin [16, 31].

Recently, it was reported that, in mice, epidermal LC are capable of inducing antigen-specific T cells of the TH2 subtype which were able to produce IL-4 [20]. The pluripotent activity of IL-4 is well-documented: (1) induction of a low affinity Fc receptor for IgE not only on B cells, but also on monocytes and LC; (2) induction of normal B cells to produce soluble CD23 and IgE binding factors; (3) induction of monocytes to differentiate into dendritic cells; (4) and increasing class II MHC expression of monocytes. Hence, aeroallergens penetrating the skin bind to IgE on LC and induce a T lymphocyte response. These T cells may be involved in the induction of the eczematous response and in the regulatory network of IgE synthesis by production of IL-4. Furthermore, IL-4 may be involved in the induction of FcεRs either on monocytes, which further differentiate into dendritic cells, or directly on dendritic cells and LC in the skin, thereby amplifying the response to allergens. In vitro, IL-4 producing T cells accumulate after repeated exposure to antigen, suggesting that these cells may play a particularly important role in the immune response to antigens that persist or that are encountered repeatedly [23]. Since contact with aeroallergens occurs via direct skin contact, e.g., in upholstery, beds, and clothes [32], contact with similar environmental allergens may occur indeed frequently or even continuously.

Furthermore, recent data from our laboratory argue for a second pathway by which LC may influence IgE synthesis. It has been reported that IgE binding factors (IgE-BF) are produced by FcεR2/CD23 positive cells (reviewed in [17]). This complex consists of a 45 kDa glycoprotein which, under some conditions, is cleaved into 25–27 kDa soluble fragments referred to as IgE-BF because they are still capable of binding to IgE. They exert an inducing or suppressing activity on IgE synthesis. Both rhIL-4 and rhIFN-γ stimulated LC become FcεR2/CD23+ [8]; thus, they are, like many other FcεR2/CD23+ cells, considered to be potent producers of IgE-BF. The culture supernatants (CSN) of FceR2/CD23+LC were therefore tested for IgE-BF by radioimmunoassay using a specific noncrossreacting mAb which reacted with the cleaved moieties of CD23. These investigations have shown that: (1) CSN unstimulated LC do not contain IgE-BF; (2) CSN of rhIL-4 and rhIFN-γ stimulated LC depleted epidermal cells do not contain IgE-BF; (3) CSN of rhIL-4- and rhIFN-γ stimulated, LC enriched epidermal cells express significant amounts of IgE-BF [10]. These results indicate that rhIL-4 and rhIFN-γ not only induce the expression of FcεR2/CD23+ cells, but also the release of IgE-BF by LC in vitro. Most interestingly, IFN-γ seems to be a more potent promotor of IgE-BF release than IL-4, which rather induces surface expression of this molecule [4].

Thus, IgE+LC or DDC may play a critical role in the regulation of IgE synthesis by either stimulation of IL-4 producing T cells, production of IgE-BF, or both. However, it remains unclear where IgE-BF producing LC exert their regulatory activity. Most likely, this occurs in at least two different areas namely, in the skin and in the afferent lymph nodes. Thus, results of immunohistochemical investigations of the acutely inflamed skin of patients with atopic eczema suggest that IgE+LC may shed their IgE molecules between keratinocytes [7]. The immunological significance of this feature remains unclear, since, as far as we know, IgE synthesis has not been demonstrated in the skin. On the other hand, it has been reported that, in allergic contact dermatitis, LC may leave the epidermal compartment for the afferent lymph nodes where they probably present antigen to T cells. Therefore, we may speculate that, in AE, FcεR2/CD23+LC function the same way and participate in the regulation of IgE synthesis in lymph nodes by producing IgE-BF.

Conclusions

Pathophysiological mechanisms involved in the genesis of AE consist of a complex network resulting from the involvement of several better or lesser known factors. New hypotheses have been proposed based on the recent demonstration of IgE+LC and DDC in patients with AE. These new insights (Fig. 1) do not explain all the clinical forms of AE, especially those related to food allergy. However, sev-

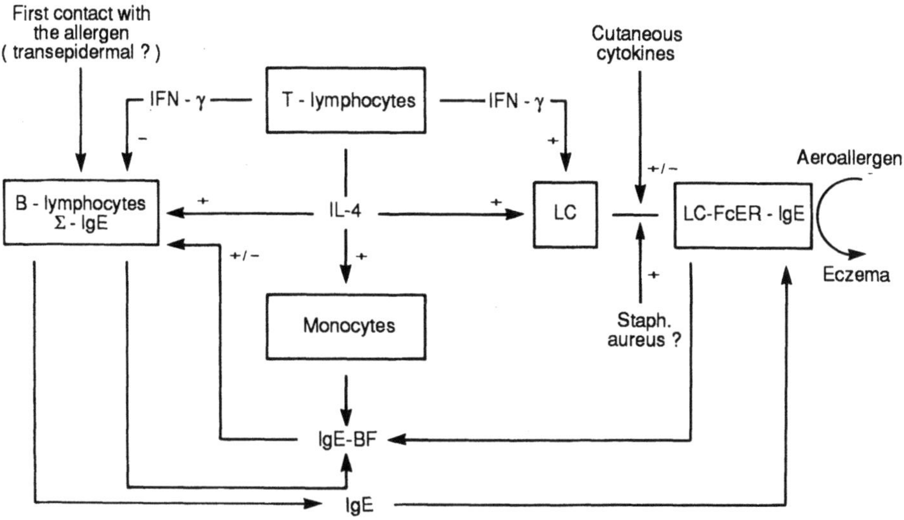

Fig. 1. Possible interrelations between IgE-bearing Langerhans cells and other cells and cytokines involved in IgE synthesis

eral arguments, resulting from clinical and laboratory studies, favor a hypothesis in which IgE+LC and DDC form an important link between type I and type IV hypersensitivity reactions in AE. Finally, further investigations will confirm the putative role of these cells in the regulatory network of IgE synthesis.

References

1. Adinoff A, Tellez P, Clark R (1988) Atopic dermatitis and aeroallergen contact sensitivity. J Allergy Clin Immunol 81:73–7426
2. Barker J, Alegre V, MacDonald DM (1988) Surface-bound immunoglobulin E on antigen presenting cells in cutaneous tissue of atopic dermatitis. J Invest Dermatol 90:117–121
3. Bieber T, Braun-Falco O (1990) IgE-bearing Langerhans are not specific for atopic exzema but are found in inflammatory skin diseases. (submitted)
4. Bieber T, Delespesse G (1991) IFN-γ preferentially promotes the release of IgE-BF (soluble CD23) by human Langerhans cells. J Invest (in press)
5. Bieber T, Ring J, Braun-Falco O (1988) Comparison of different methods for enumeration of Langerhans cells in vertical cryosections of human skin. Br J Dermatol 118:385–392
6. Bieber T, Dannenberg B, Prinz JC, Rieber EP, Stolz W, Braun-Falco O, Ring J (1989) Occurrence of IgE bearing epidermal Langerhans cells in atopic eczema: a study of the time course of the lesions and with regard to the IgE serum level. J Invest Dermatol 92:215–219
7. Bieber T, Dannenberg B, Ring J, Braun-Falco O (1989) Keratinocytes of lesional skin of atopic eczema bear HLA-DR, CD1a and IgE molecules. Clin Exp Dermatol 14:35–39
8. Bieber T, Rieger A, Neuchrist C, Prinz JC, Rieber EP, Boltz-Nitulescu G, Scheiner O, Kraft D, Ring J, Stingl G (1989) Induction of FcεR2/CD23 on human epidermal Langerhans cells by human recombinant IL-4 and IFN-γ. J Exp Med 179:309–314
9. Bieber T, Rieger A, Luger T, Stingl G (1989) Modulation of FcεR2/CD23 expression on normal human epidermal Langerhans cells by keratinocyte-derived cytokines. In: Gesellschaft für Im-

munologie (ed) 7th International Congress of Immunology, July 30–Aug 5 Berlin (West). Fischer, Stuttgart, p 589
10. Bieber T, Sarfati M, Delespesse G (1990) In vitro production of IgE-BF by human epidermal Langerhans cells. 14th Congress of the European Academy of Allergology and Clinical Immunology (in Press)
11. Bieber T, Rieger A, Wanek P, Stingl G, Strobel I (1990) Human Langerhans cells constitutively express the 26/30 kDa early activation antigen CD69. (submitted)
12. Bruijnzeel-Koomen C, van Wichen D, Toonstra J, Berrens L, Bruijnzeel P (1986) The presence of IgE molecules on epidermal Langerhans cells from patients with atopic dermatitis. Arch Dermatol Res 278:199–205
13. Bruijnzeel-Koomen C, van den Donk E, Bruijnzeel P, Capron M, de Gast G, Mudde G (1988) Associated expression of CD1 antigen and the Fc receptor for IgE on epidermal Langerhans cells from patients with atopic dermatitis. Clin Exp Immunol 74:137–142
14. Bruijnzeel-Koomen C, van Wichen D, Spry C, Venge P, Bruijnzeel P (1988) Active participation of eosinophils in patch test reactions to inhalant allergens in patients with atopic dermatitis. Br J Dermatol 118:229–238
15. Capron M, Jouault T, Prin L, Joseph M, Ameisen J, Butterworth A, Papin J, Kusnierz J, Capron A (1986) Functional study of a monoclonal antibody to IgE Fc receptor (FcεR2) on eosinophils, platelets and macrophages. J Exp Med 164:72–89
16. Carswell F, Thompson S (1986) Does natural sensitization in eczema occur through the skin? Lancet 2:13–15
17. Delespesse G, Sarfati M, Hofstetter H (1989) Human IgE-binding factors. Immunol Today 10:159–164
18. De Panfilis G, Soligo D, Manara GC, Ferrari C, Torresani C (1989) Adhesion molecules on the plasma membrane of epidermal cells. I. Resting Langerhans cells express two members of the adherence-promoting CD11/CD18 family, namely H-Mac 1 (CD11b/CD18) and gp 150,95 (CD11c/CD18). J Invest Dermatol 93:60–65
19. Grangette C, Gruart V, Ouaissi MA, Rizvi F, Delespesse G, Capron A, Capron M (1989) IgE receptor on human eosinophils (FcεR2). Comparison with B cell CD23 and association with an adhesion molecule. J Immunol 143:3580–3587
20. Hauser C, Snapper J, O'Harra W, Paul W, Katz S (1989) T helper cells grown with hapten-modified cultured Langerhans cells produce interleukin 4 and stimulate IgE production by B cells. Eur J Immunol 19:245–250
21. Leung D, Schneeberger E, Siranganian R, Geha R, Bhan AK (1987) The presence of IgE on macrophages and dendritic cells infiltrating into the skin lesions of atopic dermatitis. Clin Immunol Immunopathol 42:328–337
22. Mudde G, Bruijnzeel-Koomen C, van Reijsen F, Boland G, Bruijnzeel-Koomen P (1989) IgE dependent allergen presentation by epidermal Langerhans cells from patients with atopic dermatitis. Immunology 69:335–340
23. Powers G, Abbas A, Miller R (1988) Frequencies of IL-2 and IL-4-secreting T cells in naive and antigen-stimulated lymphocyte populations. J Immunol 140:3352–3358
24. Reitamo S, Visa K, Kahonen K, Stubb S, Salo O (1986) Eczematous reactions in atopic dermatitis patients caused by epicutaneous testing with inhalant allergens. Br J Dermatol 114:303–310
25. Romani N, Lenz A, Glassel H, Stössel H, Stanzl U, Majdic O, Fritsch P, Schuler G (1989) Cultured human Langerhans cells resemble lymphoid dendritic cells in phenotype and function. J Invest Dermatol 93:600–606
26. Ruzicka T, Auböck J (1987) Arachidonic acid metabolism in guinea pig Langerhans cells. Studies on cyclooxygenase and lipoxygenase pathways. J Immunol 138:539–543
27. Sauder D, Dinarello C, Morhenn V (1984) Langerhans cell production of interleukin-1. J Invest Dermatol 82:605–609
28. Schmitt DA, Hanau D, Bieber T, Dezutter-Dambuyant C, Schmitt D, Fabre M, Pauly G, Cazenave J-P (1990) Human epidermal Langerhans cells express only the 40 kilodalton Fcε receptor (FcRII). J Immunol 144:4284–4290
29. Stingl G, Tschachler E, Groh V, Hauser C, Wolff K (1989) The immune functions of epidermal cells. In: Norris DA (ed) Immune mechanisms in cutaneous disease. Dekker, New York, pp 4–72
30. Takigawa M, Tamamori T, Horiguchi D (1990) FcεR positive cells in atopic dermatitis. Acta Derm Venereol (Stockh) (in press)

31. Thompson S, Whitley H, Naysmith J, Carswell F (1988) IgE antibodies to *Dermatophagoides pteronyssinus* in atopic patients. Immunology 64:311–314
32. Tovey E, Chapman M, Wells C, Platts-Mills T (1981) The distribution of dust mite allergen in the houses of patients with asthma. Am Rev Respir Dis 124:630–635
33. Uno H, Hanifin J (1980) Epidermal Langerhans cells and chronic lesions of atopic dermatitis observed by L-Dopa. J Invest Dermatol 75:52–60
34. Yokota A, Kikutani H, Tanaka T, Sato R, Barsumian EL, Suemura M, Kishimoto T (1988) Two species of human Fcε receptor II (FcεR2/CD23): tissue-specific and IL-4-specific regulation of gene expression. Cell 55:611–617

Contact Sensitivity to *Pityrosporum ovale* in Patients with Atopic Dermatitis

H. Tagami, M. Rokugo, Y. Usuba, and Y. Tomita

Department of Dermatology, Tohoku University School of Medicine, 1-1 Seiryomachi, Aobaku, Sendai 980, Japan

Abstract

The cause of atopic dermatitis (AD) is unclear, but from the clinical and histopathologic resemblance to allergic contact dermatitis, as well as the nature of the cellular-infiltrate seen in the skin lesions of AD, it is suspected that inflammatory changes based on cell-mediated immunity may be involved in the pathogenesis of the skin lesions. The morphology and distribution of the skin lesions change with age. However, seborrheic area, i.e. scalp and face, are involved in most patients. Suspecting a role played by regional microorganisms in the formation of these lesions, we studied contact sensitivity and immediate hypersensitivity to extracts from *Pityrosporum ovale*. In a chamber-scarification patch test, 75 (64%) of 118 patients with AD responded positively, compared with one (3%) of 35 healthy volunteers. However, no significant statistical correlations were found between contact sensitivity to *P. ovale* in patients with AD and any of the following factors: age, sex, distribution of skin lesions, presence of pruriginous papules, history of infantile seborrheic dermatitis, or concomitance of other atopic diseases. Lymphocyte transformation test with *P. ovale* antigen confirmed that those with positive patch test reactions showed significantly high stimulation indexes.

The antigenic substances divided by gel filtration high-performance liquid chromatography were found in a fraction of components with molecular weights above 60 KD. In addition, 25 (71%) of 35 patients with AD showed a positive immediate response to *P. ovale* extract in a prick test, whereas none of 11 healthy volunteers showed any response. Although the incidence of the positive immediate responses was similar to that in contact sensitivity, there was no clear correlation between the delayed and immediate hypersensitivity reaction. Based on these results, we think that *P. ovale* may play a role in the exacerbation of the skin lesions of AD.

Introduction

Despite its high incidence among young people, the pathogenesis of atopic dermatits (AD) is still unclear. There is accumulated evidence suggesting that immunologic mechanisms contribute to its development. Due to its close association with IgE-mediated allergic diseases of the respiratory tract, such as allergic rhinitis and bronchial asthma, the role played by immediate and late-phase reactions of IgE-mediated immunity in the skin has also been emphasized [1–3]. By contrast, because of the clinical and histopathologic resemblance to allergic contact dermatitis, it has been strongly suspected that inflammatory changes based on cell-mediated immunity may be involved in the pathogenesis of AD skin lesions [4, 5].

Despite the fact that the morphology and distribution of the lesions change with age [6], the scalp and the face remain affected in most patients. Furthermore, in adult AD, pruriginous papules are frequently observed in seborrheic areas in addition to the well-known flexural eczematous lesions. According to Uehara [7] the pruriginous papules are eczematous changes that occur at the site of the follicular epithelium. Therefore, we have hypothesized a role for microorganisms colonizing the skin of seborrheic regions as well as for those colonizing the sebaceous follicles. Since *Pityrosporum ovale* and *Propionibacterium acnes* are normal microflora of such areas [8, 9], we have examined contact sensitivity reactions to these microorganisms in patients with AD [10].

Experimental Design

We tested a total of 118 patients with AD (mean age 9 years) during the remission period of their skin lesions. As controls, we also examined patients with other skin diseases in which *Pityrosporum ovale* is suspected to play a causative role [11, 12], namely, 11 patients with psoriasis vulgaris (mean age 40 years) and 11 patients with seborrheic dermatitis with excessive dandruff (mean age 52 years). There were 35 healthy volunteers (mean age 23 years) who served as normal controls.

We cultured *P. ovale* (strain IFO 0656) on Sabouraud's agar medium overlaid with a thin layer of sterile olive oil, and an antigenic extract was prepared, at a protein concentration of 20 μg/ml, in phosphate-buffered saline (PBS) from a supernatant obtained after disruption of the diethyl ether-washed organisms by sonication. Control preparations were made from uninoculated Sabouraud's agar overlaid with olive oil. *P. acnes* antigen was also prepared in the same way.

In our preliminary studies, no positive patch test responses to *P. ovale* extract were observed in patients with AD. Usually, the antigenic molecules from fungi are too large to penetrate the intact stratum corneum of normal skin and induce hypersensitivity reactions. We needed to damage, at least partially, the horny layer barrier to demonstrate contact sensitivity to fungal antigens in patients with superficial fungal infections such as dermatophytosis [13] and candidiasis [14]. Thus, in the present study we conducted chamber-scarification patch tests according to the method of Frosch and Kligman [15], to circumvent the barrier function of intact stratum corneum at the patch test site. This was done by lightly abrading the skin four times with a 27-gauge needle in a crisscross fashion. The patch test reactions were read 2, 3, and 7 days after application of the patches. In some subjects we carried out prick tests to examine immediate hypersensitivity responsiveness to *P. ovale* antigen.

To further confirm the immunologic reactivity we performed lymphocyte transformation tests by culturing lymphocytes separated from peripheral venous blood with 1 µg of *P. ovale* antigen or control preparation for 5 days and measuring [^{3}H] thymidine uptake. From the obtained data we calculated the stimulation index

Results and Discussion

In contrast to *P. acnes* antigen, to which no positive patch test response was found, 75 (64%) of 118 patients with AD showed positive eczematous patch test responses, which lasted 7 days, to *P. ovale* antigen (Table 1). Histologic studies performed in seven patients showed moderate acanthosis of the epidermis and a dense perivascular infiltrate of mononuclear cells with some intermingled eosinophils.

Although *P. ovale* is suspected to play a causative role in seborrheic dermatitis [11] and in psoriasis [12], only a few of the patients and normal healthy volunteers, including five individuals who had only allergic rhinitis but no dermatitis, showed high rates of positive patch test reactions to the *P. ovale* antigen. Even the few positive reactions in these control groups seemed to be due to primary irritation since their responses were transient and were not reproducible. Thus, the high incidence of contact sensitivity to *P. ovale* appears to be specific to patients with AD.

When we surveyed the relationships between several background factors of patients with AD and the results of the patch test with the *P. ovale* extract, we did not find any significant influence of age, sex, history of infantile seborrheic dermatitis, presence of pruriginous papules, or association with other atopic diseases, such as asthma, allergic conjunctivitis, and allergic rhinitis, on the patch test results. Thus, although children are thought to carry much fewer *P. ovale* on their skin than adults, 65% (38/61) of infant patients (less than 10 years of age, mean 2.5 years) showed positive reactions as compared with 65% (37/57) of the older age group (mean 21 years).

Recently Kieffer et al. [16] reported positive epicutaneous patch test responses to *P. ovale* in adult patients with AD, but only in a few patients. Such a low inci-

Table 1. Results of chamber-scarification patch tests in patients with atopic dermatitis and other diseases.

	Number (%) of reactors[a]	
	Pityrosporum ovale	*Propioninbacterium acnes*
Atopic dermatitis	75/118 (64)	0/20
Seborrheic dermatitis	1/11 (9)	0/7
Psoriasis vulgaris	1/11 (9)	0/8
Healthy volunteers	1/40 (2.5)	0/20

[a] Evaluated at 72 h.

dence is thought to be chiefly due to the study methods, which are totally different from ours. Instead of *P. ovale* extract they used a suspension of killed spores, which they applied on nontreated skin with an intact stratum corneum barrier, rather than on skin whose barrier function was compromised by abrasion. More than 15 years ago Imamura and Ogino [17] reported a high incidence of positive immediate and delayed hypersensitivity reactions to *P. ovale* in patients with AD, as determined by an intradermal test. However, they found a very low incidence of positive patch test reactions to *P. ovale*. This can also be explained from the poor penetration of fungal antigens through the intact stratum corneum barrier.

Patients with AD usually show decreased delayed responses to many common antigens when measured by both skin [18] and in vitro tests [19]. However, with regard to this phenomenon, Uehara and Sawai [20] recently provided evidence that actively ongoing inflammatory or immunologic processes in severe AD only reversibly block elicitation of delayed-type hypersensitivity reactions. Despite these findings, it has been shown that AD patients exhibit heightened delayed as well as immediate immune responses for several high molecular weight antigens, such as house dust mite [21], human dander [22] and other inhalant allergens [23]. In the present study we performed patch tests, with *P. ovale* antigen, commercially available house dust mite, and *Cryptomeria* pollen antigens (Torii Co, Tokyo, Japan); the latter was chosen because more than 10% of the population in our part of Japan suffer from pollinosis due to Japanese cedar pollen in the springtime. Some 51% (41/81) and 30% (12/40) of patients with AD showed a positive reaction to the mite antigen and *Cryptomeria* pollen antigen, respectively. Positive responses to mite and *P. ovale* antigen were noted in 26% and to *P. ovale* and *Cryptomeria* in 18%; triple positive responses were noted in only 10%. Thus, the demonstrability of contact sensitivity to *P. ovale* in patients with AD does not necessarily predict their sensitivity to other inhalant allergens.

In some subjects we also performed prick tests to these allergens to study immediate hypersensitivity to *P. ovale* antigen. There were 25 (54%) out of 46 patients with AD who showed a positive wheal response after 15 min, whereas 16 (64%) of 25 exhibited a positive immediate reaction to house dust mite antigen. When we divided them into two age groups, those older than 10 years of age showed a significantly higher incidence of positive immediate reactions to the *P. ovale* extract than those in the younger age group, i.e., 13 (64%) of 28 vs 7 (39%) of 18 ($p < 0.05$). This incidence in older AD patients is comparable to that reported in Europe [16, 24]. We found no relationship between the frequency of positive responses in patch tests and those in prick tests to *P. ovale* extract, i.e., 13 (65%) of 20 patients with positive prick test reactions showed positive patch test responses, while 9 (50%) of 18 negative prick test reactors had positive *P. ovale* patch test results. These finding contrasted sharply with the responses to mite antigen, which showed a correlation between the results of the prick test and the patch test [20, 22]; in the present study 7 (47%) of 15 positive prick test reactors had positive mite antigen patch tests, in contrast to only 1 (11%) of 9 negative prick test reactors ($p < 0.005$).

Our lymphocyte transformation test, which was performed to further confirm the immunologic reactivity to *P. ovale*, showed that mean stimulation indices of lymphocytes from patients with AD were much greater than those of patients with psoriasis and those of healthy volunteers. Of the patients with AD, those with positive *P. ovale* patch test results exhibited higher responses to *P. ovale* antigen than those with negative results, indicating that the positive *P. ovale* reactions noted in patients with AD are based on cellular immune reactions [10]. This was also substantiated by the finding that there was no clear relation between the lymphocyte stimulation index and the prick test responses to *P. ovale* antigen.

We further analyzed antigenic substances contained in the *P. ovale* extract by first fractioning it using gel filtration high-performance liquid chromatography and then testing the fractions on lymphocytes from AD patients with positive patch test responses. Only the fraction that contained proteins larger than 60 kD stimulated these lymphocytes.

Our results strongly suggest that *P. ovale* may play a role in AD as one of many environmental antigens. Among various environmental antigens, *P. ovale*, together with human dander, is unique in its relation to the host. Since *P. ovale* is implicated as a causative organism for dandruff and seborrheic dermatitis [12], we examined whether or not human dander antigen might share the same antigenicity with *P. ovale*. For this purpose, we immunized a rabbit to raise anti-*P. ovale* antiserum by intradermal injections of 0.6 ml *P. ovale* extracts containing 1 mg/ml protein concentration emulsified with an equal amount of Freund complete adjuvant at 12 sites on the back once a week for 6 weeks. Immune serum to *P. ovale* was obtained 1 week after the last injection. In Ouchteronly double diffusion analysis, a single broad precipitation line developed between the serum and *P. ovale* extract, but no precipitation line was formed between it and human dander antigen solution containing 70 μg/ml of protein. This finding excluded the possibility of *P. ovale* antigen sharing identical antigenic components with *P ovale*. It is interesting, however, that *P. ovale* seems to play a dual role in the pathogenesis of AD, i.e., it directly produces eczematous lesions in patients with *P. ovale* contact sensitivity. In those without such sensitivity, it induces dandruff, another important host derived antigen, which induces eczematous changes in those with contact sensitivity to human dander (Fig. 1).

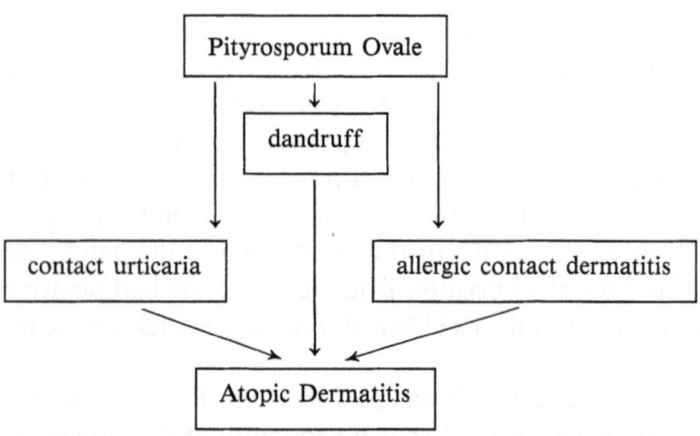

Fig. 1. Role of *Pityrosporum ovale* in atopic dermatitis

Conclusion

Based on the immediate skin reactivity to *P. ovale* Clemmensen and Hjorth [24] treated young adult AD patients showing head and neck involvement either with oral ketoconazole (200 mg) or placebo daily for 4 weeks and observed statistically significant improvement only in the ketoconazole treated group. Such a favorable clinical effect of an antifungal agent on AD also seems to support the pathogenetic importance of *P. ovale* contact sensitivity in patients with AD. The present study has demonstrated that more than half the patients with AD have contact sensitivity to the antigen derived from *P. ovale*, the incidence of which is even higher than that of house dust mite sensitivity. We do not think that *P. ovale* contact sensitivity is solely responsible for the induction of AD lesions, since most patients may have concomitant sensitivity to other environmental allergens derived from various living organisms. Thus, in the daily treatment of patients with AD we should first do our best to stop the scratching behavior of the patients, which greatly facilitates percutaneous penetration of various high molecular weight antigenic substances, including *P. ovale* antigen. At the same time, we should advise them to keep their environment as well as their skin as clean as possible.

References

1. Mitchel EB, Crow J, Williams G, Platts-Mills TAE (1986) Increase in skin mast cells following chronic house mite exposure. Br J Dermatol 114:65–73
2. Bruynzeel-Koomen C, van Wiochen DF, Spry CJF, Venge P, Bruynzeel PLB (1988) Active participation of eosinophils in patch test reactions to inhalant allergens in patients with atopic dermatitis. Br J Dermatol 118:229–238
3. Barker JNWN, Alegre VA, MacDonald DM (1988) Surface-bound immunoglobulin E on antigen-presenting cells in cutaneous tissue of atopic-determatitis. J Invest Dermatol 90:117–121
4. Leung DYM, Bhan AK, Schneeberger EE, Geha RS (1988) Characterization of the mononuclear cell infiltrate in atopic dermatitis using monoclonal antibodies. J Allergy Clin Immunol 7:47–56
5. Jonathan NW, Barker B, Donald MA (1987) Epidermal class II human lymphocyte antigen expression in atopic dermatitis: a comparison with experimental allergic contact dermatitis. J Am Acad Dermatol 16:1175–1179
6. Hanifin JM, Rajka G (1980) Diagnostic features of atopic dermatitis. Acta Derm Venereol [Suppl] (Stockh) 92:44–47
7. Uehara M (1980) Prurigo reaction in atopic dermatitis. Acta Derm Venereol [Suppl] (Stockh) 92:109–110
8. Puhvel SM, Reisner RM, Amirian DA (1975) Quantification of bacteria in isolated pilosebaceous follicles in normal skin. J Invest Dermatol 65:525–531
9. Roberts SOB (1969) Pityrosporum orbiculare: incidence and distribution on clinically normal skin. Br J Dermatol 81:264–269
10. Rokugo M, Tagami H, Usuba Y, Tomita Y (1990) Contact sensitivity to *Pityrosporum ovale* in patients with atopic dermatitis. Arch Dermatol 126:627–632
11. Rosenberg EW, Belew PW (1982) Improvement of psoriasis of the scalp with ketoconazole. Arch Dermatol 118:370–371
12. Shuster S (1984) The aetiology of dandruff and the mode of action of therapeutic angents. Br J Dermatol 111:235–242
13. Tagami H, Watanabe S, Ofuji S, Minami K (1977) Trichophytin contact sensitivity in patients with dermatophytosis. Arch Dermatol 113:1409–1414

14. Tagami H, Urano-Suehisa S, Hatchome N (1985) Contact sensitivity to *Candida albicans*: comparative studies in man and animals (guinea pigs). Br J Dermatol 113:45–53
15. Frosch PJ, Kligman AM (1976) The chamber-scarification test for irritancy. Contact Dermatitis 2:314–324
16. Kieffer A, Bergbrand I-M, Faergeman J, Jemec GBE, Ottevanger V, Skov PS, Svejgaard E (1990) Immune reactions to *Pityrosporum ovale* in adult patients with atopic and seborrheic dermatitis. J Am Acad Dermatol 22:739–742
17. Imamura S, Ogino A (1974) The response to *Pityrosporum ovale* extract in patients with atopic dermatitis: the results of intradermal skin test and patch test (in Japanese). Skin Res 16:41–43
18. Rajka G (1968) Delayed dermal and epidermal reactivity in atopic dermatitis (prurigo Besnier). III. Further studies with bacterial and viral allergens. Acta Derm Venereol (Stockh) 48:186–191
19. Jones HE, Lewis CW, Macmarlin SL (1973) Allergic contact sensitivity in atopic dermatitis. Arch Dermatol 107:217–222
20. Uehara M, Sawai T (1989) A longitudinal study of contact sensitivity in patients with atopic dermatitis. Arch Dermatol 125:366–368
21. Platts-Mills TAE, Mitchel EB, Rowntree S, Chapman MD, Wilkins SR (1983) The role of house dust mite allergens in atopic dermatitis. Clin Exp Dermatol 8:233–247
22. Uehara M, Ofuji S (1976) Patch test reactions to human dander in atopic dermatitis. Arch Dermatol 112:951–954
23. Reitamo S, Visa K, Kahonen K, Kayhko K, Stubb S, Salo OP (1986) Eczematous reactions in atopic patients caused by epicutaneous testing with inhalant allergens. Br J Dermatol 114:303–309
24. Clemmensen OJ, Hjorth N (1983) Treatment of dermatitis of the head and neck with ketoconazole in patients with type I sensitivity to *Pityrosporum orbiculare*. Semin Dermatol 2:26–29

Irritable Skin in Atopic Eczema*

R. Gollhausen

Dermatologische Klinik und Poliklinik der Ludwig-Maximilians-Universität, Frauenlobstrasse 9–11, W-8000 München 2, Federal Republic of Germany

Abstract

It is commonly accepted that the skin of patients with atopic eczema is more irritable than that of nonatopic persons. However, the definition of irritable skin lacks objectively measurable criteria. It is questionable wether irritable skin represents a single entity or whether different forms of sensitive skin have to be distinguished. The susceptibility of an individual person to skin irritation is hard to determine for a number of reasons. First, irritants can provoke different forms of skin reactions, which are influenced by numerous parameters. Second, the repeated subclinical trauma of daily stress on the skin is difficult to reproduce experimentally. Even in simple models, such as chamber tests, the intra- and interindividual variation in the skin response is very large.

Studies on skin irritability in atopic eczema patients, performed by several investigators, has led to divergent results. Frequently it was unclear if a demonstrated form of hyperirritability was specific to atopic eczema or a nonspecific sign of a "status eczematicus".

In our studies, either the cutaneous blood flow slope after UV-B irradiation or the transepidermal water loss after tenside provocation were determined. Thus, it was possible to demonstrate an increased irritability of the skin of atopic eczema patients compared to controls. However, regarding individuals, there was considerable overlap with in both groups. The clinical relevance of these test models is discussed.

Irritable Skin in Atopic Eczema

Irritable skin can be defined as skin, which is liable to eczematous reactions due to exogenous factors [30, 31, 52]. Although diagnostic criteria of atopic eczema have been established [23, 36], the diagnosis mostly depends upon the subjective clinical impression of the examining physician due to the variety of clinical forms of this disease [7, 49, 67, 96].

* This work was supported by the Bundesministerium für Forschung und Technologie, project no. 01KC8730/1.

In a person with a generalized acute flare of atopic eczema the skin is very sensitive. One of the most important therapeutic steps is therefore the diligent avoidance of irritants [14, 46, 67]. Nonetheless, it remains unclear whether the normal looking skin of an atopic eczema patient is irritable or not.

A number of clinical studies published in the last decade have convincingly shown that a personal or family history of atopy is a risk factor for the development of hand eczema [18, 20, 21, 41, 42, 48, 54, 58, 59, 69, 70, 74]. The hands are often exposed to irritants, such as chemicals, water, soil, and abrasion. The frequent involvement of the hands of adult patients with atopic eczema appears to be the result of a disposition to irritable skin and skin-irritating insults [9].

It is also possible to experimentally reproduce signs of increased irritability in sympton-free skin of patients. A number of studies, with deliberate application of irritants, such as tensides, sodium or ammonium hydroxide, or cantharidin, to the skin, have shown that normal looking skin can nonetheless be irritable in atopic eczema [4–6, 16, 32, 34, 67, 76, 78, 87, 88, 95].

Transepidermal water loss (TEWL) is used as a sign of skin barrier integrity. An elevated baseline TEWL has been measured by a number of investigators in normal looking skin of patients with atopic eczema. The average increase in relation to normals ranges from a factor of 1.12 to 4.17 (Table 1). Thus, there is ample evidence for the existense of irritability in the normal looking skin of atopic eczema patients.

Table 1. Transepidermal water loss (g/m^2 h) of uninvolved skin in patients with atopic eczema and in controls.

Reference	Method	Test area	Controls (mean ± SE)	*n*	Patients with AE (mean ± SE)	*n*	*p* value	AE/C
Abe et al. [1]	Electrohygrometry	Forearm	2.3 ± 0.3	40	3.0 ± 0.6	18	0.001	1.31
Finlay et al. [28]	Evaporimetry	Upper arm	2.9 ± 1.8	11	11.6 ± 5.0	3	0.005	4.04
Rajka [66]	Electrohygrometry	Back of hand	12.6 ± 1.3	14	16.1 ± 1.5	14	0.025	1.28
Thune [77]	Evaporimetry	Upper arm	4.8 ± 2.0	17	20.0 ± 7.8	13	Not given	4.17
Tupker [78]	Evaporimetry	Forearm	5.6 ± 1.0	18	7.6 ± 1.5	20	0.05	1.36
van der Valk et al. [87]	Evaporimetry	Forearm	6.5 ± 1.5	19	8.7 ± 2.0	10	0.004	1.34
Werner and Lindberg [91]	Evaporimetry	Back of hand	9.8 ± 2.2	16	14.6 ± 3.9	16	0.05	1.50
		Forearm	4.7 ± 1.9	16	7.6 ± 2.8	16	0.05	1.61
		Back	6.6 ± 3.0	16	7.4 ± 2.2	16	n.s.	1.12

AE, atopic eczema; C, controls.

Irritable Skin in Nonatopic Eczema

Hyperirritability, however, is not specific for atopic eczema. In many studies a lowered threshold to stimuli is also observed in the normal looking skin of patients with nonatopic eczema [4, 11, 13, 15–17, 32, 34–36, 38, 51, 56, 65, 75, 76, 87, 88, 95]. Some investigators have reported an increased hyperirritability, particularly in patients with atopic eczema, but the results are conflicting. Allison and Bettley [5] found no abnormal cantharidin response in nonatopic eczema with less than 10%–15% of the skin affected. By contrast, Sigel [75] observed a low threshold response to cantharidin in housewives' nonatopic eczema of the hands. Van der Valk et al. [87] detected an increased vulnerability of the skin to surfactants only in patients with atopic eczema, but not with irritant or allergic contact dermatitis, whereas Wahlberg et al. [88] found the irritable dose^{50} (ID_{50}) concentration of the surfactants sodium lauryl sulfate and benzalkonium chloride to be higher in patients with atopic eczema than in subjects with other dermatoses. Al-Jaberi and Marks [4] have measured a shorter minimal blistering time, i.e., a lowered resistance against the blister-causing irritant ammonium hydroxide, in patients with atopic eczema as well as in patients with contact dermatitis. They correlated an increased irritability of the skin with a reduction in the size of the corneocytes. Smaller corneocytes are the result of increased epidermal turnover.

Changes in TEWL in symptom-free skin of patients with atopic or nonatopic eczema are not unequivocal. Baker and Kligman [8] could not find an elevated baseline TEWL in patients with atopic eczema, whereas Shahidullah et al. [73] observed alterations in the TEWL in symptom-free skin of patients with nonatopic eczema. This topic is discussed below. Summarizing all the studies, there appears to be no difference between nonatopic and atopic eczematous skin with respect to irritability.

Status Eczematicus

The problem of irritability in normal looking skin of patients with eczema, even after disappearance of the dermatitis, was recognized by Jadassohn [38] and Bloch [13]. Status eczematicus [16], conditioned hyperirritability [68], and angry back or excited skin syndrome [51, 56] are terms used for the description of this puzzling phenomenon. Maibach [51] discussed this topic in the article "Excited Skin Syndrome" in the first *New Trends in Allergy 10* years ago. The term conditioned hyperirritability implies that irritable skin is the consequence rather than the cause of eczema. In his discussion of the problem of false-positive patch test reactions Mitchell [56] used the impressive title "Eczema Creates Eczema".

The extent, duration, intensity, and form of eczema necessary to agitate the entire integument are completely unknown. It can only be speculated that, in (pre) eczematous skin, mediators are released, which induce a generalized hyperirritability of the skin [40, 55, 59]. The time period required for normalization of disturbed skin after disappearance of the eczema is also unknown. The problem is that we cannot exactly determine the beginning and the end of eczema.

Dry skin can be a subclinical form of eczema [39, 82, 92]. Rystedt [69] postulates that dry and/or itchy skin, without any atopic disposition, is a high risk factor for hand eczema. According to the investigations of Diepgen et al. [23], 25% of the normal population have dry skin compared with 90% of patients with flexural eczema. Thus, there is a fluent change from irritable skin to eczema.

Irritable skin can be the cause and the consequence of eczema. The same vicious circle is found in bronchial hyperreactivity and asthma. However, pulmonologists are luckier than dermatologists since they can already measure the increased reactivity of the organ of interest, while dermatologists are still trying to do so.

Relationship Between Irritable Skin and Atopy

In the vicious circle of irritable skin and eczema (Fig. 1) we do not yet exactly know the factors which influence this concerted action either in a positive or a negative way. Persons with fair complexions and perhaps also females, Caucasians, and young people probably have more irritable skin. The phenomenon of skin hardening and the variability of responses to irritants make it even more difficult to establish a reliable clinical or experimental model for the detection of irritable skin. Atopy is certainly one factor which can facilitate the occurrence of irritable or inflamed skin [30, 31, 43, 44, 46, 47, 53, 67].

Some 75% of patients with atopic eczema have a history of mucosal atopy and 80% of these present immediate allergic skin reactions. However, a history of atopic eczema does not necessarily imply irritable skin. About 25% of persons with a history of atopic eczema, who have a job with a high risk for the development of hand eczema, e.g., cleaning, nursing, or hairdressing, never develop hand eczema [41, 58, 70]. Mucosal atopy by itself probably is not a risk factor for hand eczema since nonatopics and persons with mucosal atopy had the same risk of developing hand eczema [69].

Thus, the relationship between irritable skin and atopy remains unclear. We do not know whether there is an atopic skin unless eczema develops. In the case of eczema it is often impossible to discern whether an atopic person has an irritant dermatitis due to some atopy-unrelated factors, an atopic eczema, or a combination of both forms. In order to learn more about the pathogenesis of eczema we have to learn more about irritable skin, that is, the subclinical stages of eczema. In addition, we must compare the skin of persons without any skin problem

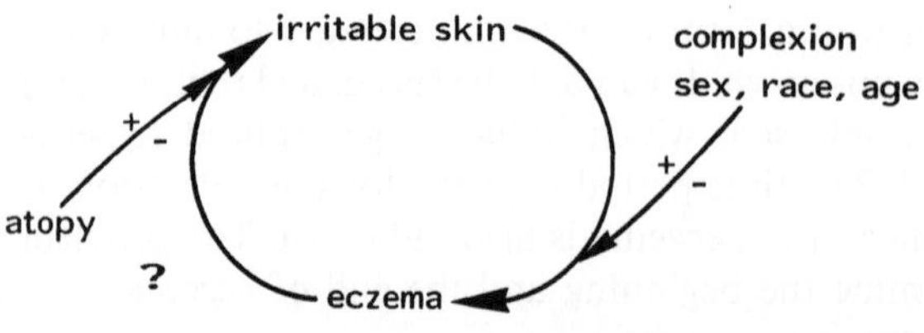

Fig. 1. Vicious circle of irritable skin and eczema with potential promoting and hampering factors

with that of patients with various forms of eczema. For this purpose, delicate instruments can be used which noninvasively measure skin properties.

Bioengineering Methods for Detection of Irritable Skin

The EP 1 evaporimeter (Servo Med, Stockholm, Sweden) is widely used for the measurement of TEWL. A number of investigators have succeeded in measuring an elevated baseline TEWL in symptom-free skin of patients with atopic eczema (Table 1). Tupker [78] was able to show that, in atopic persons with an eczema-free period of on average 15 months, the baseline TEWL was significantly higher than in persons with a history of allergic contact dermatitis or in healthy controls without any skin problems. Another author has already published exact reference ranges for TEWL: 2–6 g/m^2h for normals and 15–20 g/m^2h for patients with atopic eczema [71].

From these studies, it appears to be fairly easy to differentiate these two groups according to their TEWL. However, published mean TEWL values, obtained from the volar forearm of skin-healthy probands, range from 2.5 to 17.2 (Table 2). Our own results also do not support the possibility of clear-cut reference

Table 2. Baseline transepidermal water loss values from the volar forearm of skin-healthy probands obtained with the ServoMed EP 1 (mean ± SD).

Baseline TEWL ($g/m^2\,h$)	*n*	Reference
2.5 ± 1.0	42	van der Valk et al. [86]
2.8 ± 1.0	10	van der Valk and Maibach [84]
3.0 ± 0.6	7	Lo et al. [50]
3.2 ± 0.7	14	Lammintausta et al. [47]
3.6 ± 1.4	10	van der Valk and Maibach [83]
3.8 ± 2.0	8	Elsner et al. [27]
4.2 ± 1.3	15	Elsner et al. [25]
4.5 ± 1.7	30	Pinnegoda et al. [63]
4.7 ± ?	50	Coenraads et al. [19]
4.7 ± 0.5	9	Elsner et al. [26]
4.7 ± 1.9	16	Werner and Lindberg [91]
4.9 ± 1.9	37	Tupker et al. [79]
5.0 ± ?	33	Tupker et al. [80]
6.0 ± 1.3	35	Tupker et al. [81]
6.2 ± 1.3	27	van der Valk et al. [85]
6.5 ± 1.5	19	van der Valk et al. [87]
6.5 ± 2.1	44	Pinnegoda et al. [62]
6.6 ± ?	20	Agner and Serup [3]
7.6 ± 2.1	9	Berardesca and Maibach [10]
7.7 ± 2.9	10	Blichmann and Serup [12]
8.1 ± 2.9	21	van Neste et al. [57]
13.4 ± 1.5	15	Elsner and Maibach [24]
17.2 ± 11.6	66	Serup and Rasmussen [72]

TEWL, transepidermal water loss.

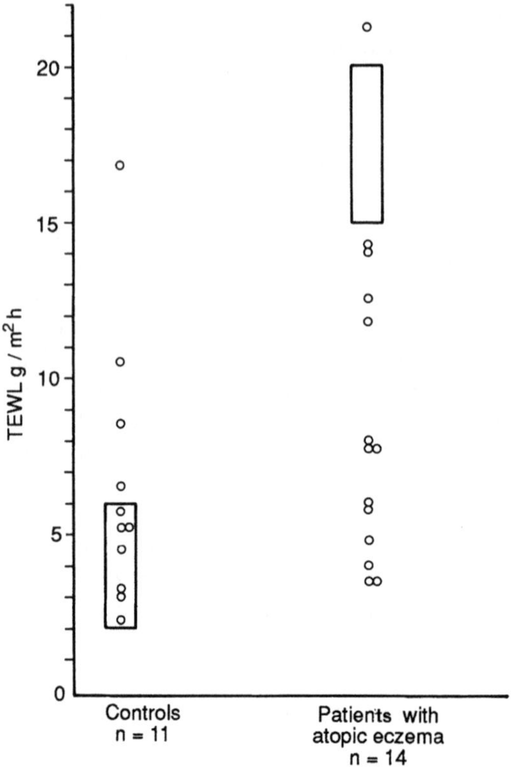

Fig. 2. Baseline transepidermal water loss measured at the volar forearm of 14 patients with atopic eczema and 11 controls. *Rectangles*, reference ranges given by Schmersahl [71]. Temperature, 20° ± 1 °C; Relative humidity 40% ± 5%

ranges: we randomly measured TEWL in in- and outpatients at our clinic, who had active dermatitis involving at least 20% of their skin and who were not receiving systemic or local treatment, for at least 1 day and compared them to nonatopic volunteers without any skin problems. A wide overlap existed between patients with atopic eczema and controls (Fig. 2); in spite of the active stage of the disease we quite often observed a low baseline TEWL in the patients. Moreover, the baseline TEWL was often higher than 6 g/m^2h in healthy volunteers without any emotional stress. In contrast to Pinnegoda et al. [62, 64], we suggest that sweating should routinely be inhibited during evaporimetry.

Patients with atopic eczema have dry skin [67, 93], which can be due to low hydration, low surface lipid level, and/or an increased roughness of the skin [39, 61]. Applying profilometry, Werner Linde et al. [93] measured an increased roughness of the skin in patients with atopic eczema. Werner Linde also detected a low water content of the stratum corneum in patients with atopic eczema using the CM 420 corneometer [90]. Gloor et al. [33], however, found an increased level of skin hydration using infrared spectroscopy. The Skicon hydrometer (I.B.S. Co., Japan) and the CM corneometer (Courage and Khazaka, Cologne, FRG) are used for measuring hydration of the stratum corneum; they use the electrophysiologic properties of the skin to measure the electrical conductance and the capacitance of the skin respectively. It is assumed that high values indicate high levels of hydration.

Table 3. CM 820 corneometer values of two duplicate rows each consisting of an untreated skin area of the volar forearm, an area irritated by 0.5% sodium lauryl sulfate (SLS) and an area irritated by 1% SLS in three volunteers.

	Subject 1 (mean ± SD)	Subject 2 (mean ± SD)	Subject 3 (mean ± SD)
Control 1	64.3 ± 2.0[a]	72.7 ± 3.6[a]	71.8 ± 2.3[a]
Control 2	73.7 ± 2.2	76.2 ± 1.8	77.7 ± 2.0
0.5% SLS 1	66.2 ± 2.8	71.5 ± 2.7	77.0 ± 4.3[a]
0.5% SLS 2	62.2 ± 2.9[b]	68.0 ± 5.2[b]	77.2 ± 1.5
1.0% SLS 1	56.2 ± 3.8[b]	65.7 ± 2.3[b]	70.2 ± 1.5
1.0% SLS 2	62.5 ± 3.5[b]	75.2 ± 1.8	74.2 ± 1.9[a]

The SLS was applied in Finn chambers for 24 h. Measurements were performed 1 h after removal of the chambers. Mean and standard deviation of six measurements are given.
[a] Significant difference between duplicate area ($p < 0.05$).
[b] Significant difference between treated and control area.

Agner and Serup [2] found the intraindividual variation of electrical conductance measurement to be so high that they questioned the use of the Skicon-100 for quantification of irritant reactions. This is in accordance with our experience using the CM 820 corneometer. In three volunteers without skin problems, two duplicate opposing rows were set on one volar forearm, each row consisting of one untreated control area and two areas irritated by 0.5% and 1% aqueous sodium lauryl sulfate (SLS), respectively. Finn chambers on Scanpor (Hermal, Reinbeck, FRG) fixted the SLS to the skin for 24 h; 1 h after removal of the chambers the SLS-irritated and two adjacent control areas were measured with the corneometer, six times each. Only half of the SLS desiccated skin areas yielded significantly lower corneometer values, but in subject 3 the value of one 0.5% SLS irritated area was, paradoxically, significantly higher than one control site. Thus, there was no reliable indication of SLS induced desiccation. Moreover, in all three subjects a significant difference was found between the two untreated control sites of the volar forearm, although they were only 8 cm apart (Table 3). Various parameters, such as skin surface structure, turgor, and thickness of the stratum corneum, probably influence the Skicon hydrometer and the CM corneometer measurements significantly.

Bioengineering Methods Combined with Provocation Tests

Sodium Lauryl Sulfate and Evaporimetry

For easier and better recognition of patients with atopic eczema by evaporimetry we propose the use of provocation tests. It is clinically known that patients with atopic eczema have a low tolerance of surfactants. Therefore, we applied a large Finn chamber filled with 1% aqueous SLS for 24 h and measured the TEWL 1 h after removal of the chamber. Although some patients did not react more to the

Table 4. Provocation test using 1% aqueous sodium lauryl sulfate applied on clinically normal skin of the volar forearm for 24 h Finn chamber.

	Baseline TEWL (g/m^2 h)	TEWL after SLS (g/m^2 h)
Patients with AE ($n = 14$)	8.9 ± 5.2	30.1 ± 15.3
Controls ($n = 11$)	6.5 ± 4.2	16.2 ± 6.1
p value	n.s.	0.01

Transepidermal water loss in irritated and nonirritated skin of 14 patients with atopic eczema and 11 controls 1 h after removal of the chamber (temperature, 20° ± 1 °C; relative humidity 40% ± 5%). TEWL, transepidermal water loss; SLS, sodium lauryl sulfate; AE, atopic eczema.

provocation test than did the controls, the test facilitates differentiation of these two groups (Table 4), in accordance with the results published by Lammintausta et al. [46].

Cutaneous Blood Flow Slope

Patients with atopic eczema often state that during acute flares of their disease they become more easily sunburned than during remission; furthermore, short periods of intensive sun exposure worsen their dermatitis. Therefore, we used UV-B radiation in another provocation test as a stimulus to more sensitively discriminate skin irritability. This method is called cutaneous blood flow slope (CBFS) because it measures the increase in blood flow after UV-B irradiation. We used the laser doppler flowmeter Periflux PF 2 (Perimed, Sweden) to determine CBFS in the following way: first the individual minimal erythema dose (MED) to polychromatic UV-B (Philips TL/12) was determined on the lower back. Then, the skin was irradiated with five fractions of the MED, increasing from 1 up to 3.0 MED in steps of 0.5. On the following day the cutaneous blood flow of each

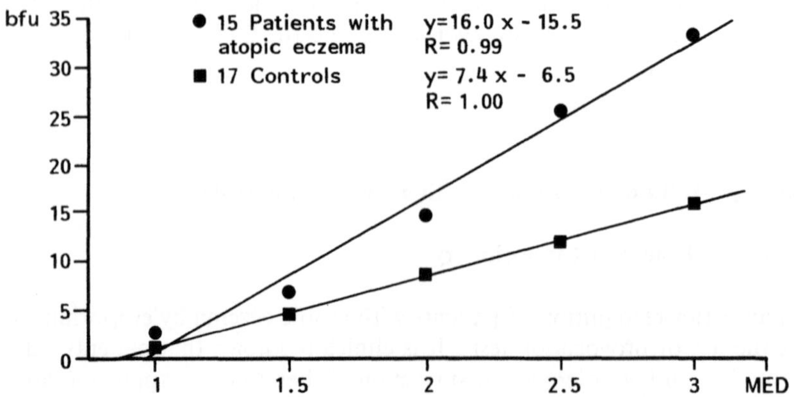

Fig. 3. Provocation test. Cutaneous blood flow slope after UV-B irradiation of 15 atopic eczema patients and 17 controls

Table 5. Cutaneous blood flow slope after UV-B irradiation and minimal erythema dose in 15 patients with atopic eczema and 17 controls.

	CBFS (bfu/MED)	MED (mJ/cm^2)
Patients with AE (n = 15)	16.5 ± 8.5	66 ± 23
Controls (n = 17)	7.6 ± 4.8	64 ± 21
p value	0.005	n.s.

CBFS, cutaneous blood flow slope; MED, minimal erythema dose; AE, atopic eczema; bfu, blood flow units.

irradiated spot was measured using the laser doppler flowmeter. The resulting dose-response curve is approximately linear in the given range. Its slope has the dimension (arbitrary) blood flow units per MED and is a sensitive parameter of skin responsiveness to UV-B light. With this method it is possible to distinguish patients with atopic eczema from controls (Fig. 3). Patients with atopic eczema have a higher CBFS, i.e., an increased vascular response to UV-B, than controls, but there is no difference in the MED (Table 5). Although it is difficult to discern whether a distinct wave length, i.e., UV-A, UV-B, or infrared, or increased sweating, exsiccation of the skin by sun and water, or other components of sunbathing induce the intolerance of strong sunlight reported by the patients, the elevated CBFS in patients with atopic eczema indicates an increased UV-B sensitivity during active states of atopic dermatitis.

Problems of Provocation Tests

Variability of Irritant Reactions

Provocation techniques have their hazards too, since the skin is very variable in its reactivity. This applies much more to irritants than to allergens [22, 47]. In our own studies ten chambers of 2.5% aqueous SLS were occlusively applied for 24 h on one volar forearm of ten healthy volunteers without any known skin problem. The following day the reactions were visually assessed using a 5 point scale (0, no visible reaction; 1, patchy erythema; 2, confluent erythema; 3, erythema and edema; 4, erythema and vesicles/erosions) 1 h after removal of the chambers. A considerable variability or response was observed (Table 6).

Compatibility of Stimulus and Instrument

It is also necessary that the stimulus used in the provocation test be compatible with the measuring device. According to van der Valk et al. [86] the EP 1 evaporimeter detects skin irritations evoked by SLS better than those evoked by phenol or benzalkonium chloride. Our own studies indicate that skin desiccation

Table 6. Variability of skin reactions to 2.5% aqueous sodium lauryl sulfate.

Subject number	Application site										Mean	SD
	a	b	c	d	e	f	g	h	i	j		
1	3	3	1	3	3	3	1	3	3	1	2.7	1.1
2	2	0	1	1	1	2	1	1	1	1	1.3	0.6
3	3	2	2	2	0	1	3	2	3	0	1.9	1.1
4	2	2	2	1	2	1	1	1	2	2	1.6	0.5
5	0	0	0	0	0	1	0	1	1	0	0.3	0.5
6	1	1	0	0	0	1	1	0	0	1	0.6	0.5
7	0	0	0	1	0	1	0	1	1	1	0.5	0.5
8	2	3	2	3	3	2	2	3	3	2	2.5	0.5
9	1	0	0	0	0	1	1	1	1	0	0.6	0.5
10	2	2	2	1	2	1	1	1	2	2	1.6	0.5

Applied in large Duhring chambers on 10 sites, labeled a to j, on the volar forearm in 10 volunteers. Visual assessment 1 h after removal of the chambers.

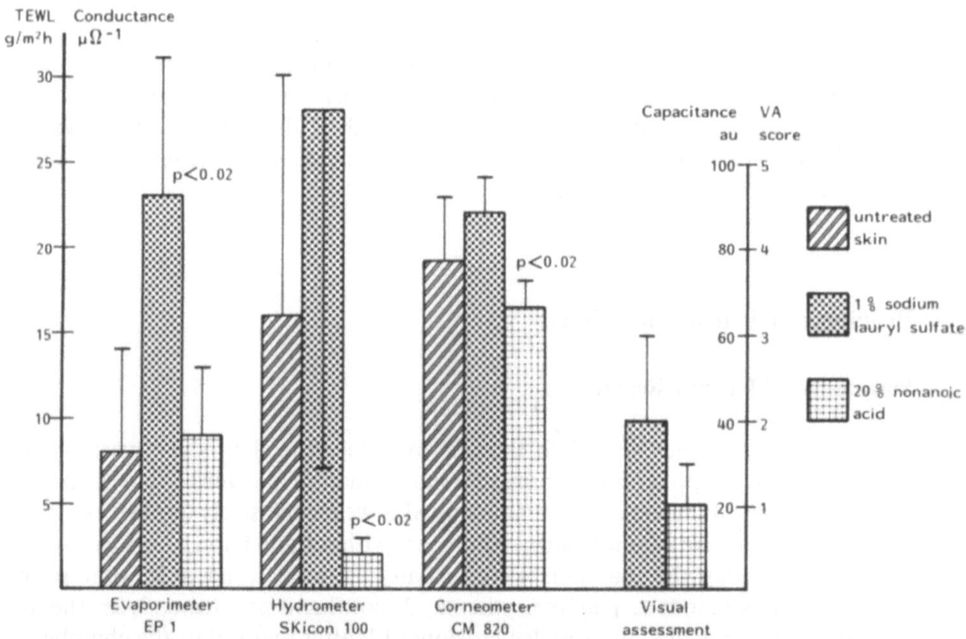

Fig. 4. Skin reactions to 1% sodium lauryl sulfate and 20% nonanoic acid, evaluated by using an EP 1 evaporimeter, a Skicon-100 hydrometer, and a CM 820 corneometer and by visual assessment. The irritants were applied in Finn chambers on the volar forearm for 24 h. Measurements were done 1 day after removal of the chambers; $n = 7$

induced by 1% SLS or by 20% nonanoic acid gives different results depending on the noninvasive technique used for evaluation. In these experiments 1% SLS and 20% nonanoic acid were occlusively applied for 24 h on the volar forearms of seven healthy volunteers without any skin problems using large Finn chambers of Scanpor. The reactions were evaluated 1 day after removal of the chambers applying four methods: visual assessment on a 6 point scale (0, no visible reaction; 1, skin surface alteration without redness, scaling, glaze, ore a "soap effect"; 2, patchy erythema; 3, distinct erythema; 4, erythema and edema; 5, erythema and vesicles/erosions) and measurement with an EP1 evaporimeter, a Skicon-100 hydrometer, and a CM820 corneometer. The results are illustrated in Fig. 4. Only a light scaling or faint erythema was visible. The evaporimeter measured a significantly elevated TEWL only at the area irritated by SLS, not at the area irritated by nonanoic acid. Conversely the Skicon-100 high frequency hydrometer or the CM820 corneometer obtained significantly lower values when measuring nonanoic acid, but not SLS. Since 20% nonanoic acid often induces a very fine scaling, whereas a low concentration of SLS makes the skin appear a little bit glazed and smooth, we believe that the Skicon-100 and the corneometer record roughness rather than dryness. Other skin properties additionally influence the results of these instruments, as discussed in a previous section. Thus, it is difficult to evaluate the water content of the skin with either of these two instruments. In addition skin irritation induced by nonanoic acid is poorly detected by an evaporimeter.

Conclusions

The problems of irritable skin and its relation to atopy are still unsolved. For a better approach to these issues noninvasive recognition of subclinical stages of eczema would be helpful. Furthermore, reliable methods for the diagnosis of irritable skin are lacking. Although promising test models for the detection of sensitive skin are being developed, their use remains experimental.

References

1. Abe T, Ohkido M, Yamamoto K (1978) Studies on skin surface barrier functions – skin surface lipids and transepidermal water loss in atopic skin during childhood. J Dermatol (Tokyo) 5:223–229
2. Agner T, Serup J (1990) Individual and instrumental variations in irritant patch-test reactions – clinical evaluation and quantification by bioengineering methods. Clin Exp Dermatol 15:29–33
3. Agner T, Serup J (1990) Transepidermal water loss and air convection. Contact Dermatitis 22:120–121
4. Al-Jaberi H, Marks R (1984) Studies of the uninvolved skin in patients with dermatitis. Br J Dermatol 111:437–443
5. Allison JH, Bettley FR (1958) Investigations into cantharidin blisters raised on apparently normal skin in normal and abnormal subjects. Br J Dermatol 70:331
6. Allison JH, Williamson DH (1960) The abnormal cantharidin blister in atopy: an explanation on its production. BR J Dermatol 72:383
7. Archer CB (1986) Atopic dermatitis – an obvious diagnosis? Clin Exp Dermatol 11:560–563
8. Baker H, Kligman AM (1967) Measurement of transepidermal water loss by electrical hygrometry. Arch Dermatol 96:441–452
9. Bandmann HJ, Agathos M (1980) Die atopische Handdermatitis. Dermatosen 28:110–113

10. Berardesca E, Maibach H (1990) Monitoring the water-holding capacity in visually nonirritated skin by plastic occlusion stress test (POST). Clin Exp Dermatol 15:107–110
11. Björnberg A (1974) Increased skin reactivity to primary irritants provoked by hand eczema. Arch Dermatol Forsch 249:389–400
12. Blichmann CW, Serup J (1987) Reproducibility and variability of transepidermal water loss measurement. Studies on the Servo med evaporimeter. Acta Derm Venereol (Stockh) 67:206–210
13. Bloch B (1924) Pathogenese des Ekzems. Arch Dermatol Syph 145:34–82
14. Braun-Falco O, Ring J (1984) Zur Therapie des atopischen Ekzems. Hautarzt 35:447–454
15. Bruynzeel DP (1983) Angry back or excited skin syndrome. Thesis, Free University, Amsterdam
16. Burckhardt W, Dorta T (1957) Die Alkaliresistenz bei Ekzemen verschiedener Genese und bei Neurodermitis. Dermatologica 114:252–257
17. Calnan CD (1964) The climate of contact dermatitis. Acta Derm Venereol (Stockh) 44:33–34
18. Coenraads PJ (1983) Prevalence of hand eczema. Association with occupational exposure especially in construction workers. Thesis, State University of Groningen
19. Coenraads PJ, Lee J, Pinnagoda J (1986) Changes in water vapor loss from the skin of metal industry workers monitored during exposure to oils. Scand J Environ Health 12:494–498
20. Cronin E (1985) Clinical patterns of hand eczema in women. Contact Dermatitis 13:153–161
21. Cronin E, Kullavanijaya P (1979) Hand dermatitis in hairdressers. Acta Derm Venereol [Suppl 59] (Stockh) 85:47–50
22. Dahl MV, Pass F, Trancik RJ (1984) Sodium lauryl sulfate irritant patch tests. II. Variations of test responses among subjects and comparison to variation of allergic responses elicited by Toxicodendron extract. J Am Acad Dermatol 11:474–477
23. Diepgen TL, Fartasch M, Hornstein OP (1989) Evaluation and relevance of atopic basic and minor features in patients with atopic dermatitis and in the general population. Acta Derm Venereol [Suppl] (Stockh) 144:50–54
24. Elsner P, Maibach HI (1990) The effect of prolonged drying on transepidermal water loss, capacitance and pH of human vulvar and forearm skin. Acta Derm Venereol (Stockh) 70:105–109
25. Elsner P, Oriba HA, Maibach HI (1989) Physiologie der Haut der Vulva: neue Aspekte. Hautarzt 40:411–417
26. Elsner P, Wilhelm D, Maibach HI (1990) Multiple parameter assessment of vulvar irritant contact dermatitis. Contact Dermatitis 23:20–26
27. Elsner P, Wilhelm D, Maibach HI (1990) Physiological skin surface water loss dynamics of human vulvar and forearm skin. Acta Derm Venereol (Stockh) 70:141–180
28. Finlay AY, Nicholls S, King CS, Marks R (1980) The "dry" non-eczematous skin associated with atopic eczema. Br J Dermatol 102:249–256
29. Forsbeck M, Skog E, Åsbrink E (1983) Atopic hand dermatitis: a comparison with atopic dermatitis without hand involvement, especially with regard to influence of work and development of contact sensitization. Acta Derm Venereol (Stockh) 63:9–13
30. Frosch PJ (1985) Hautirritation und empfindliche Haut. Grosse Berlin (Scripta 7)
31. Frosch PJ (1989) Irritant contact dermatitis. In: Frosch PJ, Dooms-Goossens A, Lachapelle JM, Rycroft RJG, Scheper RJ (eds) Current topics in contact dermatitis. Springer, Berlin Heidelberg New York, pp 385–398
32. Gehese M, Kändler-Stümer P, Gloor M (1987) Über die Bedeutung der Irritabilität der Haut für die Entstehung des berufsbedingten allergischen Kontaktekzems. Dermatol Monatsschr 173:400–404
33. Gloor M, Heymann B, Stuhlert T (1981) Infrared spectroscopic determination of the water content of the horny layer in healthy subjects and in patients suffering from atopic dermatitis. Arch Dermatol Res 271:429–436
34. Gloor M, Völlm P, Gehse M, Ringelmann R (1985) Irritationseffekt von Tensiden bei Patienten mit Gewebeekzemen im Friseur- und Krankenpflegeberuf. Vergleichsuntersuchungen mit Gesunden und Neurodermitikern. Dermatoson 33:86–89
35. Hamami I, Marks R (1988) Abnormalities in clinically normal skin – a possible explanation of the "angry back syndrome". Clin Exp Dermatol 13:328–333
36. Hamami I, Marks R (1988) Structural determinants of the response of the skin to chemical irritants. Contact Dermatitis 18:71–75
37. Hanifin JM, Rajka G (1980) Diagnostic features of atopic dermatitis. Acta Derm Venereol [Suppl] (Stockh) 92:44–47

38. Jadassohn J (1923) Bemerkungen zur Sensibilisierung und Desensibilisierung bei den Ekzemen im Anschluß an einen Fall von Odolekzem. Klin Wochenschr 36:1680–1684, 1734–1739
39. Kligman AM, Lavker RM, Grove GL, Studemayer TJ (1982) Some aspects of dry skin and its treatment. In: Kligman AM, Leyden JJ (eds) Safety and efficacy of topical drugs and cosmetics. Grune and Stratton, New York, pp 221–238
40. Kupper TS (1990) The activated keratinocyte: a model for inducible cytokine production by non-bone marrow-derived cells in cutaneous inflammatory and immune responses. J Invest Dermatol 94:146S–150S
41. Lammintausta K (1982) Risk factors for hand dermatitis in wet work. Dissertation, University of Turku
42. Lammintausta K, Kalimo K (1981) Atopy and hand dermatitis in hospital wet work. Contact Dermatitis 7:301–308
43. Lammintausta K, Maibach HI (1988) Exogenous and endogenous factors in skin irritation. Review. Int J Dermatol 27:213–222
44. Lammintausta K, Maibach HI (1990) Contact dermatitis due to irritation. General principles, etiology and histology. In: Adams RM (ed) Occupational skin disease, 2nd edn. Saunders, Philadelphia, pp 1–15
45. Lammintausta K, Maibach HI, Wilson D (1987) Irritant reactivity in males and females. Contact Dermatitis 17:276–280
46. Lammintausta K, Maibach HI, Wilson (1987) Human cutaneous irritation: induced hyporeactivity. Contact Dermatitis 17:193–198
47. Lammintausta K, Maibach HI, Wilson D (1988) Susceptibility to cumulative and acute irritant dermatitis. An experimental approach in human volunteers. Contact Dermatitis 19:84–90
48. Lantinga H, Nater JP, Coenraads PJ (1984) Prevalence, incidence and course of eczema on the hands and forearms in a sample of the general population. Contact Dermatitis 10:135–139
49. Leung DYM, Rhodes AR, Geha RS (1987) Atopic dermatitis. In: Fitzpatrick TB, Eisen AZ, Wolff K, Freedberg IM, Austen KF (eds) Dermatology in general medicine, 3rd edn. McGraw-Hill, New York, pp 1385–1408
50. Lo JS, Oriba HA, Maibach HI, Bailin PL (1990) Transepidermal potassium ion, chloride ion, and water flux across delipidized and cellophane tape-stripped skin. Dermatologica 180:66–68
51. Maibach HI (1981) The E.S.S. – excited skin syndrome (alias the "angry back"). In: Ring J, Burg G (eds) New trends in allergy. Springer, Berlin Heidelberg New York, pp 208–221
52. Maibach HI, Lammintausta K, Berardesca E, Freeman S (1989) Tendency to irritation: sensitive skin. J Am Acad Dermatol 21:833–835
53. Malten KE, den Arend JACJ (1985) Irritant contact dermatitis. Traumiterative and cumulative impairment by cosmetics, climate and other daily loads. Dermatosen 33:125–132
54. Meding B, Swanbeck G (1989) Epidemiology of different types of hand eczema in an industrial city. Acta Derm Venereol (Stockh) 69:227–233
55. Miescher G (1962) Ekzem. Histopathologie, Morphologie, Nosologie. In: Miescher G, Storck H (eds) Entzündliche Dermatosen I. Springer, Berlin Göttingen Heidelberg, pp 1–113 (Handbuch der Haut- und Geschlechtskrankheiten, vol 2/1)
56. Mitchel JC (1975) The angry back syndrome: eczema creates eczema. Contact Dermatitis 1:193–194
57. van Neste D, Mahmoud G, Masmoudi M (1987) Experimental induction of rough dermatitis skin in humans. Contact Dermatitis 16:27–33
58. Nilsson E (1986) Individual risk factors for hand eczema in hospital workers. Thesis, Uned University
59. Nilsson E, Bäck O (1986) The importance of anamnestic information of atopy, metal dermatitis and earlier hand eczema for the development of hand dermatitis in women in wet hospital work. Acta Derm Venereol (Stockh) 66:45–50
60. Nilsson E, Mikaelsson B, Andersson S (1985) Atopy, occupation and domestic work as risk factors for hand eczema in hospital workers. Contact Dermatitis 13:216–223
61. Pierard GE (1987) What does "dry skin" mean? Int J Dermatol 26:167–168
62. Pinnegoda J, Tupker RA, Coenraads PJ, Nater JP (1989) Transepidermal water loss with and without sweat gland inactivation. Contact Dermatitis 21:16–22

63. Pinnegoda J, Tupker RA, Smith JA, Coenraads PJ, Nater JP (1989) The intra- and interindividual variability and reliability of transepidermal water loss measurements. Contact Dermatitis 21:255–259
64. Pinnegoda J, Tupker RA, Agner T, Serup I (1990) Guidelines for transepidermal water loss (TEWL) measurement. Contact Dermatitis 22:164–178
65. Raffle EJ, Shahidullah M (1970) The effect of standardized 'skin insult' on transepidermal water loss. Dermatologica 141:208–214
66. Rajka G (1974) Transepidermal water loss on the hands in atopic dermatitis. Arch Dermatol Forsch 251:111–115
67. Rajka G (1989) Essential aspects of atopic dermatitis. Springer, Berlin Heidelberg New York
68. Roper SS, Jones HE (1982) A new look at conditioned hyperirritability. J Am Acad Dermatol 7:643–650
69. Rystedt I (1985) Hand eczema and long-term prognosis in atopic dermatitis. Acta Derm Venereol [Suppl] (Stockh) 117
70. Rystedt I (1990) The role of atopy in occupational skin disease. In: Adams RM (ed) Occupational skin disease, 2nd edn. Saunders, Philadelphia
71. Schmersahl P (1990) Experimentelle und klinische Untersuchungen mit einem synthetischen Gerbstoff. TW Dermatologie 20:222–227
72. Serup J, Rasmussen I (1985) Dry hands in scleroderma. Including studies of sweat gland function in healthy individuals. Acta Derm Venereol (Stockh) 65:419–423
73. Shahidullah M, Raffle EJ, Rimmer AR, Frain-Bell W (1969) Transepidermal water loss in patients with dermatitis. Br J Dermatol 81:722–730
74. Shmunes E, Keil JE (1984) The role of atopy in occupational dermatoses. Contact Dermatitis 11:174–178
75. Sigel H (1959) Threshold stimulation of the skin and house-wives eczema of the hands. Arch Dermatol 80:461–465
76. Skog E (1960) Primary irritant and allergic eczematous reactions induced in patients with different dermatoses. Acta Derm Venereol (Stockh) 40:307–316
77. Thune P (1989) Evaluation of the hydration and the water-holding capacity in atopic skin and so-called dry skin. Acta Derm Venereol [Suppl] (Stockh) 144:133–135
78. Tupker RA (1990) The influence of detergents on the human skin. A study on factors determining the individual susceptibility assessed by transepidermal water loss. Thesis, State University of Groningen
79. Tupker RA, Coenraads PJ, Pinnegoda J, Nater JP (1989) Baseline transepidermal water loss (TEWL) as a prediction of susceptibility to sodium lauryl sulfate. Contact Dermatitis 20:265–269
80. Tupker RA, Pinnegoda J, Coenraads PJ, Nater JP (1989) The influence of repeated exposure to surfactants on the human skin as determined by transepidermal water loss and visual scoring. Contact Dermatitis 20:108–114
81. Tupker RA, Pinnegoda J, Nater JP (1990) The transient and cumulative effect of sodium lauryl sulphate on the epidermal barrier assessed by transepidermal water loss: interindividual variation. Acta Derm Venereol (Stockh) 70:1–5
82. Uehara M (1986) Dry skin (sebostasis) and inflammation: heterogeneity of "dry skin" in atopic dermatitis. In: Ring J, Berg G (eds) New trends in allergy II. Springer, Berlin Heidelberg New York, pp 135–144
83. Van der Valk PGM, Maibach HI (1989) Post-application occlusion substantially increases the irritant response of the skin to repeated short-term sodium lauryl sulfate (SLS) exposure. Contact Dermatitis 21:335–338
84. Van der Valk PGM, Maibach HI (1989) Potential for irritation increases from the wrist to the cubital fossa. Br J Dermatol 121:709–712
85. Van der Valk PGM, Nater JP, Bleumink E (1984) Skin irritancy of surfactants as assessed by water vapour loss measurements. J Invest Dermatol 82:291–293
86. Van der Valk PGM, Nater JP, Bleumink E (1985) The influence of low concentrations of irritants on skin barrier function as determined by water vapour loss. Dermatosen 33:89–91
87. Van der Valk PGM, Nater JP, Bleumink E (1985) Vulnerability of the skin to surfactants in different groups of eczema patients and controls as measured by water vapour loss. Clin Exp Dermatol 10:98–103

88. Wahlberg JE, Wrangsjö K, Hietasalo A (1985) Skin irritancy from nonanoic acid. Contact Dermatitis 13:266–269
89. Wedroff NA, Dogloff AP (1935) Ein Beitrag zur Frage der Reaktionsfähigkeit der Haut bei "chemischen" Ekzemen, auf Grund von Untersuchungen bei ekzemkranken und gesunden Personen mittels der obligaten chemischen Reizmittel. Arch Dermatol Syph 171:641–646
90. Werner Y (1986) The water content of the stratum corneum in patients with atopic dermatitis. Measurement with the Corneometer CM 420. Acta Derm Venereol (Stockh) 66:281–284
91. Werner Y, Lindberg M (1985) Transepidermal water loss in dry and clinically normal skin in patients with atopic dermatitis. Acta Derm Venereol (Stockh) 65:102–105
92. Werner Linde Y (1989) "Dry" skin in atopic dermatitis. I. A clinical study. Acta Derm Venereol (Stockh) 69:311–314
93. Werner Linde Y, Bengtsson A, Lodén M (1989) "Dry" skin in atopic dermatitis. II. A surface profilometry study. Acta Derm Venereol (Stockh) 69:315–319
94. Wilkinson DS, Hambly EM (1978) Prognosis of hand eczema in hairdressing apprentices. Contact Dermatitis 4:63
95. Wilson HTH (1955) Standard patch tests in eczema and dermatitis. Br J Dermatol 67:291–298
96. Wüthrich B (1989) Neurodermatis atopica. Wien Med Wochenschr 139:156–165

Stigmata and Signs of Atopic Eczema*

T.L. Diepgen and M. Fartasch

Department of Dermatology, University of Erlangen, Hartmannstraße 14, W-8520 Erlangen, Federal Republic of Germany

Abstract

In a prospective study on atopic eczema (AE) several clinical major and minor features, including total IgE and response to Phadiatop testing, have been studied systematically and analyzed statistically with regard to diagnostic importance in patients with atopic enzema (AE) ($n = 428$) and in a sample of the normal population (NP) ($n = 628$). Total IgE was normally distributed in healthy controls, but bimodally distributed in AE. AE patients with concomitant inhalant atopy had significantly higher levels than pure AE patients. IgE and Phadiatop testing can be used to screen for inhalant atopy but not for atopic skin diathesis. Thus, the diagnosis of AE should be based on traditional anamnestic and clinical features. On the basis of chi-square values a diagnostic score system was constructed, which might help to establish a firm diagnosis of AE in patients with ambiguous cutaneous inflammatory disease. Based on this score system, patients with more than ten points should be considered as atopic, patients with more than six points are suspected of being atopic.

Introduction

For the diagnosis of atopic eczema (AE) an array of clinical major and minor features, proposed by Hanifin and Rajka [1], are in common use. However, many of them can also be found in normal individuals who never had skin problems or eczema [2, 3]. The role of IgE in the etiology of AE is still unclear [4, 5]; it may be a nonspecific feature of the disease [6]. One purpose of the present study was to determine the optimal cutoff level and to evaluate the diagnostic value of total IgE in the diagnosis of AE. The other purpose was the evaluation of atopic features in patients with clearly established (AE) compared to a normal population (NP) of young German adults.

* The study was supported by funds from the Hauptverband der gewerblichen Berufsgenossenschaften e.V., Sankt Augustin, Germany.

Material and Methods

A case control study was performed. The basis of selection was the presence or the history of chronic or relapsing flexural eczema.

Patients with AE

Patients with atopic eczema ($n = 428$; median age 22 years) were collected from the in- and outpatient divisions of our Department of Dermatology, where a special atopy service has been instituted. Patients with all degrees of severity of the disease were seen; 232 patients had pure AE (AE−) and 196 patients suffered from AE with inhalant atopy (i. e., rhinitis or asthma; AE+). All patients had clinical or anamnestical data of recurrent flexural itching and lichenified eczema. The referral area was both urban and rural.

German NP

A sample of young healthy adults (NP; $n = 628$; median age 23 years) was taken from urban and rural areas. Persons with a history or clinical picture of flexural eczema were excluded.

Clinical Examinations and Laboratory Investigations

Anamnestic and clinical atopic features were investigated in all test subjects as follows: ASTH (Asthma), CAP (cradle cap), DENNIE (Dennie-Morgan fold), DERM (white dermographism), EAR (retroauricular rhagades), ECZ (flexural eczema), FA (positive family history of atopy, first degree relatives), FACIAL (facial pallor/erythema), FOOD (food intolerance), FOOT (fissured dermatitis of the foot), HERT (Hertoghe sign), IGE150 (IgE > 150 U/ml), ITCH (itch when sweating), KERAT (keratosis pilaris), LIGHT (light phobia), METAL (history of metal sensitivity), NECK (dirty neck), NIPPL (nipple eczema), PALMS (hyperlinear palms), PERL (perlèche), PHAD (Phaditop test, a RAST for screening inhalant allergens), PITALB (pityriasis alba), RHIN (allergic rhinitis), WOOL (wool intolerance), and XERO (xerosis).

Statistics

Sensitivity and specificity were determined. The chi-square test was used to analyze cross classified data, the Kruskal-Wallis test to analyze interval and ordinal scaled data. The level of significance chosen was $p < 0.01$. A score system was constructed based on chi-square values. Odd rations and 95% confidence intervals were calculated according to Breslow and Day [7].

Results

Total IgE

Total IgE (logarithmic scale) was normally distributed in healthy controls, but bimodally distributed in AE (Fig. 1). The highest level was found in AE+ (i.e.,

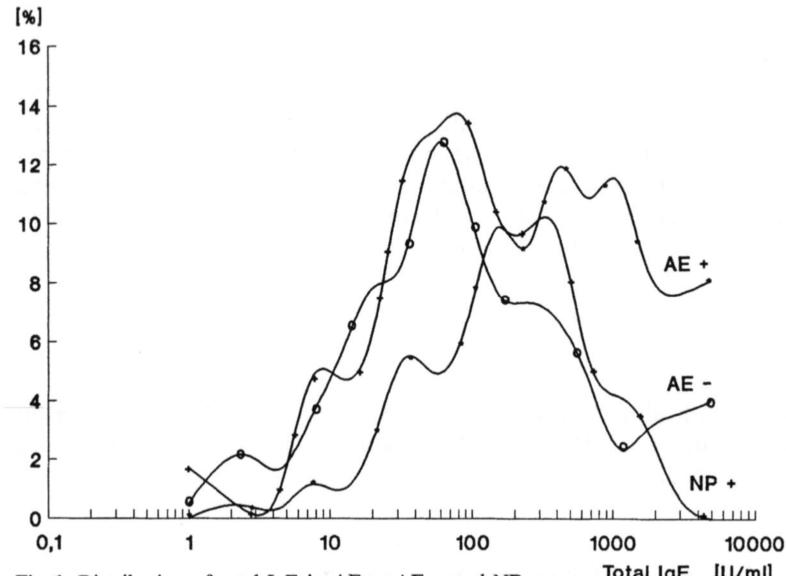

Fig. 1. Distribution of total IgE in AE+, AE−, and NP

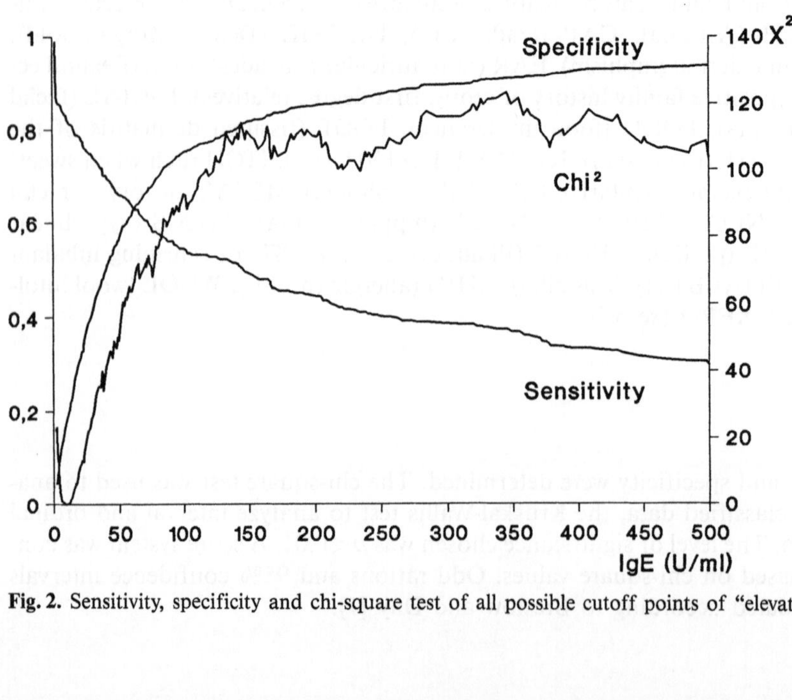

Fig. 2. Sensitivity, specificity and chi-square test of all possible cutoff points of "elevated" IgE

AE with inhalant atopy), followed by AE− (AE without inhalant atopy). The differences between all groups are statistically significant (Kruskal-Wallis test: $p < 0.001$). In Fig. 2 the sensitivity, specificity, and chi-square values are shown for all possible cutoff points to distinguish between normal and elevated total IgE. From the statistical results, the border between normal and elevated IgE should be at 150 U/ml.

Atopic Major and Minor Features

Anamnestic data as well as clinical findings of the major features of atopy in AE patients and the NP are presented in Fig. 3a, minor features (arranged according to their frequencies in AE) in Fig. 3b. Only those features which differ in a statistically significant way between both groups are shown. The chi-square values,

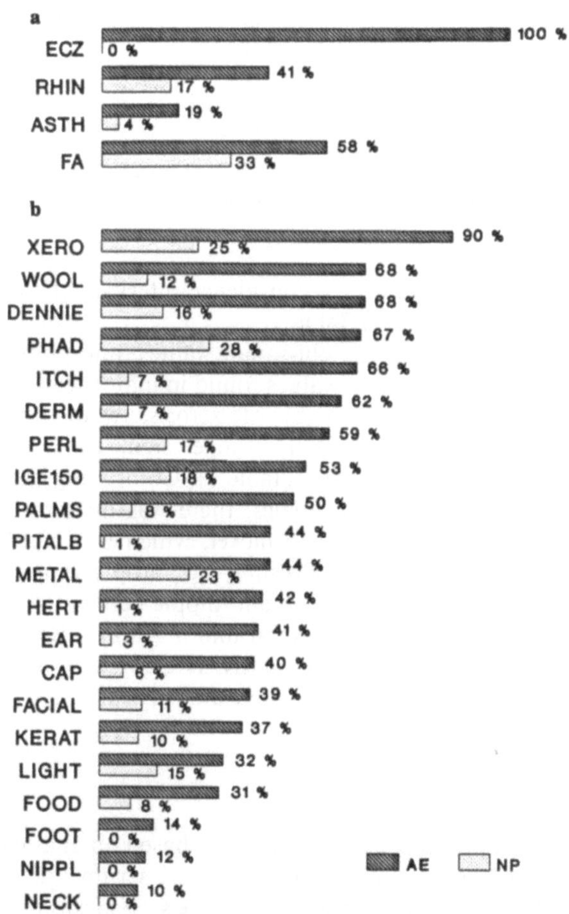

Fig. 3a, b. Frequencies of atopic major (**a**) and minor features (**b**) in AE and NP

Table 1. Chi-square test, odds ratio, and 95% confidence interval of the major and minor features of atopy.

Criteria	X^2	OR	95% CI
RHIN	65	3.1	2.7–3.6
ASTHMA	55	4.8	3.4–6.0
FA	69	2.9	2.6–3.3
XERO	429	27.9	23.2–33.8
WOOL	355	15.8	13.4–18.5
DENNIE	292	11.0	9.4–12.7
PHAD	141	5.1	4.4–5.8
ITCH	410	25.4	21.1–30.1
DERMO	357	19.3	16.2–23.2
PERL	201	7.0	6.1–8.2
IGE150	131	5.0	4.3–5.8
PALMS	242	11.7	9.8–13.9
PITALB	304	60.1	41.6–87.0
METAL	55	2.7	2.4–3.1
HERT	282	44.8	32.1–62.6
EAR	236	19.2	15.2–24.4
CAP	184	10.6	8.7–12.9
FACIAL	117	5.3	4.5–6.3
KERAT	103	4.9	4.2–5.8
LIGHT	41	2.6	2.3–3.1
FOOD	85	4.7	4.0–5.7

See text for definitions of abbreviations.

odds ratios, and 95% confidence intervals of the major and minor features of atopy are listed in Table 1.

The frequencies, chi-square values, and odds ratios of some minor features were higher than the values found in major features, especially the estimated relative risks (odds ratios) of xerosis, wool intolerance, itch when sweating (noneczematous skin), Herthoge' sign, white dermographism, pityriasis alba, retroauricular rhagades (Table 1). Comparing the frequencies of atopic features between females and males, there was no significant difference except for the anamnestic sensitivity to nickel, which was highly correlated with females and pierced ears. Specific features, e.g., atopic winter feet (AE 14%; NP 0%), dirty neck (AE 10%; NP 0%), and nipple eczema (AE 12%; NP 0%) were not often seen in AE patients. Several minor features were found to be worthless because they did not differ significantly. These were pronounced local insect reaction, herpes labialis, drug intolerance, and urticaria.

Score System

An atopic score system should be based on anamnestic and clinical features without laboratory investigations. Thus, serum IgE and Phadiatop results were not taken into consideration. The score system was based on statistical evaluation and restricted to frequently important criteria. Specific features were excluded which

Table 2. Atopy score (chi-square test).

3 Points ($X^2>300$):	XERO ITCH DERMO WOOL
2 Points ($300<X^2<200$):	PITALB DENNIE HERT PALMS EAR
1 Point ($X^2<200$):	PERL CAP FA-EKZ FACIAL KERAT FOOD RHIN ASTH METAL LIGHT

See text for definitions of abbreviations.

were less frequent than 20% in AE (atopic winter feet, nipple eczema, dirty neck). The presence of an itching flexural dermatitis was not included since this was the selection basis. On the basis of chi-square values every atopic feature received between one and three points, according to its statistical significance (Table 2). By using the proposed score system both groups were separated fairly clearly, with minimal overlapping (Fig. 4). The summarized atopic points were normally distributed in AE. There were different degrees of atopic severity based on the number of atopic points.

Discussion

The diagnostic criteria for atopic eczema proposed by Hanifin and Rajka [1] are based on traditional clinical experience. In the present prolective standardized study the occurrence of different atopic features in AE patients was compared to those in the general population, since the proposed score system is based on estimated relative risks which depend on the frequencies of atopic symptoms and signs in the general population. Some typical major features have thus been found to be of minor importance because of their high frequency in controls. A history of atopic disease in first degree relatives ranged between 58% in AE and 33% in NP (Table 1). Frequencies between 43% and 73% were obtained by other studies [8–13]. Most of the former studies did not investigate the frequencies of a positive family history in the normal population simultaneously. Kjellman [13] studied the incidence of atopic disease in a sample of children age 7 years and its relation to the family history. In our study the odds ratio of a history of atopic disease in the immediate

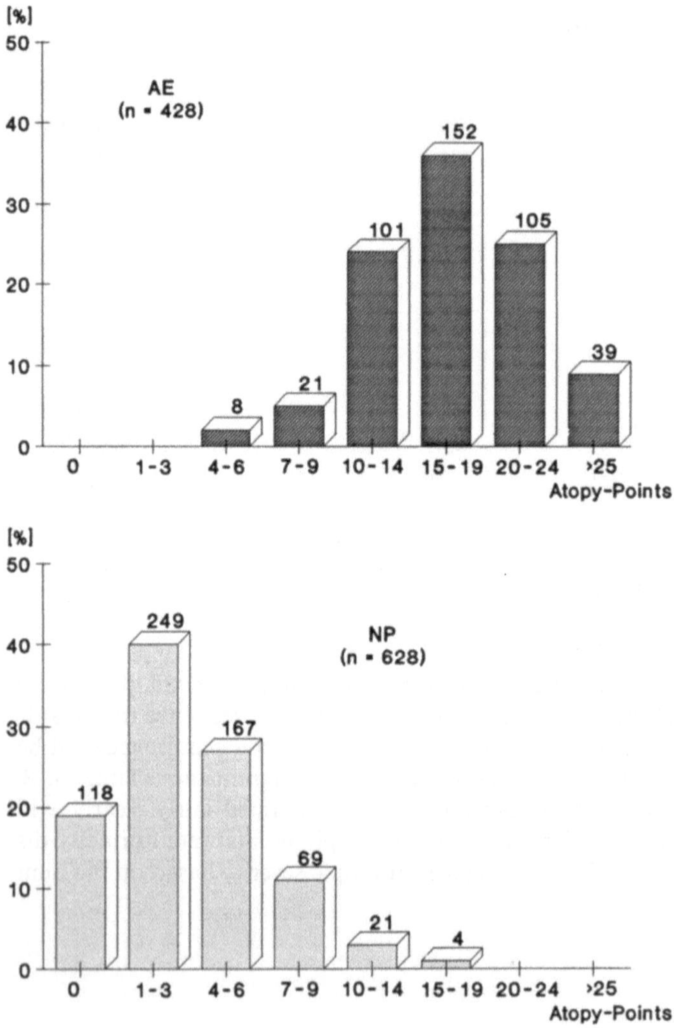

Fig. 4. Atopy score based on chi-square test

family was only 2.9 because of the high incidence in the normal population. A distant family history of atopy was found not to be of diagnostic relevance. Other minor features have emerged as important factors because of their high odds ratios. The frequency of intolerance to wool in AE (Table 1; 68%) was in good accordance with the data of Svensson et al. [8] who found irritations from textiles in 72% of AE patients and in 36% of noneczematous outpatients. In our general population of young adults, only 11% reported an intolerance to wool.

According to Hanifin and Rajka [1] an intolerance to metals is not a diagnostic feature of atopic dermatitis. Romaguera et al. [14] found an atopic history in 49% of 627 patients who complained of intolerance to metals and had a positive patch test to nickel sulfate. In our former prospective study [15], in which we investigated the occurrence of delayed-type hypersensitivity in a sample of patients with AE comparing them to control subjects similar in age and occupational distribution, atopics were found to show a significantly higher incidence of reactions to nickel. Thus, sensitivity to nickel could be regarded as another minor feature. Because on the frequency in the normal population the relative risk was only 2.7. Thus sensitivity to nickel cannot be regarded as a hard criteria for the diagnosis of AE.

According to statistical analysis, in patients with AE compared with healthy controls the cutoff between normal and elevated total IgE should be 150 U/ml or higher. IgE and Phadiatop tests can be used to screen for inhalant atopy but not for atopic skin diathesis. Thus, the diagnosis of AE should be based on traditional anamnestic and clinical features.

The purpose of the score system was to summarize atopic features in a way that best discriminated atopic risk on the basis of frequent clinical signs without laboratory investigations. Thus serum IgE and Phadiatop values or some specific signs of atopy which were less frequent than 20% were not taken into consideration. The individual atopic symptom and signs were elevated with regard to their diagnostic importance. This score system based on traditional atopic features could also be a tool to estimate the atopic risk in nonaffected individuals. A patient with more than ten points could be considered atopic, a patient with more than six points suspected of being atopic.

References

1. Hanifin JM, Rajka G (1980) Diagnostic features of atopic dermatitis. Acta Derm Venereol (Stockh) [Suppl] 92:44–47
2. Diepgen TL, Fartasch M, Bäurle G, Hornstein OP (1989) Atopiekriterien in der Normalbevölkerung – berufliche Konsequenzen. Dermatosen 37:222–223
3. Diepgen TL, Fartasch M, Hornstein OP (1989) Evaluation and relevance of atopic basic and minor features in patients with atopic dermatitis and in the general population. Acta Derm Venereol (Stockh) [Suppl] 144:50–54
4. Bruynzeel-Koomen C (1986) IgE on Langerhans cells: new insights into the pathogenesis of atopic dermatitis. Dermatologica 172:181–183
5. Hanifin J (1984) Atopic dermatitis. J Allergy Clin Immunol 73:211–222
6. Hanifin J (1983) Clinical and basic aspects of atopic dermatitis. Semin Dermatol 2:5–19
7. Breslow NE, Day NE (1980) Statistical methods in cancer research. I. The analysis of case-control studies. IARC, Lyon, p 32
8. Svensson A, Edman B, Möller H (1985) A diagnostic tool for atopic dermatitis based on clinical criteria. Acta Derm Venereol (Stockh) [Suppl] 114:33–40
9. Yates VM, Kerr REI, MacKie RM (1983) Early diagnosis of infantile seborrhoeic dermatitis and atopic dermatitis – clinical features. Br J Dermatol 108:633–638
10. Kang K, Tian R (1987) Atopic dermatitis. An evaluation of clinical and laboratory findings. Int J Dermatol 26:27–32
11. Nexmand PH (1948) Clinical studies of Besnier's Prurigo. Rosenkilde and Bagger, Copenhagen
12. Roth HL, Kierland RR (1964) The natural history of atopic dermatitis. Arch Dermatol 89:209–214
13. Kjellman NIM (1977) Atopic disease in seven-year-old children. Acta Paediatr Scand 66:465–471
14. Romaguera C, Grimalt F, Vilaplana J (1988) Contact dermatitis to nickel: an investigation of its sources. Contact Dermatitis 19:52–57
15. Huber A, Fartasch M, Diepgen TL, Bäurle G, Hornstein OP (1987) Auftreten von Kontaktallergien beim atopischen Ekzem – Zusammenhänge mit gleichzeitig gefundenen atopischen Merkmalen. Dermatosen 35:119–123

Patch Test with Immediate Type Allergens in Patients with Atopic Dermatitis

E. Vocks[1], H.-U. Seifert[2], B. Seifert[2], and M. Drosner[1]

[1] Dermatologische Klinik und Poliklinik der Technischen Universität München, Biedersteinerstrasse 29, W-8000 München 40, Federal Republic of Germany
[2] Tegernseerstrasse 35, W-8164 Hausham, Federal Republic of Germany

Abstract

The aim of this investigation was to obtain eczematous reactions in patch tests with immediate type allergens in atopic dermatitis patients. In the modified patch test (abraded skin) 65% of 100 adult patients had a positive patch test reaction with an early onset dermatitis in the test area in response to house dust mite and/or grass pollen. The correlation with the corresponding intracutaneous test was high with house dust mite and moderate with grass pollen. In the modified patch test with molds and basic foods we also obtained positive reactions, but they were fewer and weaker than those in response to mite and grass pollen.

Introduction

Same 85%–90% of atopic eczema patients show immediate type sensitizations in skin tests (prick/intracutaneous test) and/or in the RAST. Out of 100 children, 35 with atopic dermatitis develop an allergic rhinitis and 25 an allergic bronchial asthma [9]. The remaining "pure" atopic eczema patients without a clinical immediate type allergy show a 60%–70% incidence of immediate type sensitizations [9]. These are apparently without clinical manifestation, since the eczematous reaction is of the delayed type. This constellation gives rise to the question of a causal nexus between immediate type sensitizations and atopic eczema.

For years aggravation of atopic eczema after exposure to inhalant allergens, such as pollen, animal hair, and house dust mite, or after ingestion of allergenic food [1, 2, 5, 7] has been reported. Our follow-up clinical investigation was aimed at the question: Can immediate type allergens be a causal factor in atopic dermatitis?

Investigation

We performed patch tests in atopic dermatitis patients with the main (atopic) immediate type allergens: grass pollen, house dust mite, molds (*Mucores*, *Alternaria alternata*), and basic foods (egg white, cow milk, rye flour). The aim was to induce a dermatitis in the test area.

We used commercial prick solutions for the inhalant allergens and native material for the basic food. The amount was 0.1 ml per test area. The test strip was a commercial cellulose patch test strip. The test area was clinically nonaffected dorsal skin: in the first series, nontreated atopic skin; in the next series, adhesive strip abraded atopic skin. The strip was removed after 24 h; reading of the skin reaction took place after 24, 48, and 72 h and in single cases also after 6 h. Nonatopic control groups were tested also. In addition, we performed intracutaneous tests (inhalant allergens) and prick tests (food allergens) with the patch tested allergens in the same subjects. The test area was the nonaffected skin of the volar forearm; the conditions were the usual ones for these methods.

Results

The results are shown in Tables 1–4. The clinical picture was that of an early onset dermatitis exceeding the test area, with a maximum reaction occurring after

Table 1. Patch test results in response to grass pollen and house dust mite.

	Positive patch test reactions								
	Group A (untreated atopic skin)				Group B (abraded atopic skin)				Group C (control, abraded skin)
	130 adults		100 children		100 adults		30 children		30 adults
	n	%	*n*	%	*n*	%	*n*	%	*n*
House dust mite	6	5	13	13	33	33	2	6	0
Grass pollen	2	1	2	2	3	3	1	3	0
Both	1	<1	11	11	29	29	6	21	0
Total	9	7	26	26	65	65	9	30	0

Table 2. Patch test results in response to *Mucor*, *Alternaria alternata*, egg white, cow milk, and rye flour.

	Positive patch test reactions	
	Group D (abraded atopic skin) 63 adults	Group E (control, abraded skin) 10 adults
	n	*n*
Mucor	3	0
Alternaria alternata	6	0
Egg white	3	0
Cow milk	6	0
Rye flour	4	0
Total	27[a]	0

[a] 12% of 315 single tests (63 subjects, 5 tests each).

Table 3. Corresponding intracutaneous test results in response to house dust mite and grass pollen correlated with patch tests.

	Group B		
	PT+, I.C.+ (*n*)	PT+, I.C.− (*n*)	PT−, I.C.+ (*n*)
House dust mite	56	6	14
Grass pollen	24	6	30

Group C (control): No positive reactions in either test. PT, patch test; I.C., intracutaneous test.

Table 4. Corresponding intracutaneous test results in response to *Mucor*, *Alternaria alternata*, egg, milk, and rye flour correlated with patch tests.

	Group D		
	PT+, I.C.+ (*n*)	PT+, I.C.− (*n*)	PT−, I.C.− (*n*)
Mucor	2	1	14
Alternaria alternata	3	3	11
Egg white	2	1	4
Cow milk	1	5	6
Rye flour	1	3	19

Group E (control): No positive reaction in either test.

24 h. This was distinct in the patch tests using house dust mite and grass pollen, but weaker in the patch tests using allergens of the second series.

Conclusions

In response to the immediate type allergens house dust mite, grass pollen, molds and basic foods, we obtained positive patch test reactions in atopic dermatitis subjects in contrast to nonatopics. The results were significant with house dust mite and grass pollen, but not with the other allergens. The correlation with the corresponding intracutaneous test using the same allergen was also significant with house dust mite and grass pollen, but not with the other allergens. The poor results with molds and basic foods may correspond partly to the lower rate of sensitization to these allergens.

This investigation demonstrates the well known contradiction that an eczematous reaction to immediate type allergens is possible in atopic dermatitis patients. Our results correspond to those of other authors, who also observed positive patch test reactions under similar conditions [4, 6, 8]. It is unclear how much these results are applicable to natural conditions. Detection of IgE receptors on Langerhans cells in atopic dermatitis infiltrates suggests that a mixed immunological reaction contributes to the development of this disease, with features of immediate type, late phase and delayed type-hypersensitivity reactions [3].

References

1. Adinoff AD, Tellez P, Clark RAF (1988) Atopic dermatitis and aeroallergen contact sensitivity. J Allergy Clin Immunol 81:736–742
2. Atherton DJ (1983) The role of foods in atopic eczema. Clin Exp Dermatol 8:227–232
3. Bruynzeel-Koomen C (1986) IgE on Langerhans cells: New insights into the pathogenesis of atopic dermatitis. Dermatologica 172:181–183
4. Bruynzeel-Koomen C, Bruynzeel P (1988) A role for IgE in patch test reactions to inhalant allergens in patients with atopic dermatitis. Allergy 43 Suppl 5:15–21
5. Hanifin JM (1985) Atopic dermatitis. J Allergy Clin Immunol 73:211–222
6. Mitchell EB, Crow J, Rowntree S, Webster ADB, Platts-Mills TAE (1984) Cutaneous basophil hypersensitivity to inhalant allergens in atopic dermatitis patients: elicitation of delayed responses containing basophils following local transfer of immune serum but not IgE antibody. J Invest Dermatol 83:290–295
7. Rajka G (1974) Prurigo Besnier (atopic dermatitis) with special reference to the role of allergic factors II. The evaluation of the results of skin reactions. Acta Derm Venereol 54:193
8. Reitamo S, Visa K, Kähonn K, Käyhko K, Stubb S, Salo OP (1986) Eczematous reactions in atopic patients caused by epicutaneous testing with inhalant allergens. Br J Dermatol 114:303–309
9. Wüthrich B (1987) Neurodermitis atopica (atopische Dermatitis). In: Fuchs E, Schulz KH (eds) Manuale allergologicum. Dustri Dr Karl Feistle, München-Deisenhofen, V 14:1–33

Chronobiological Aspects of Atopic Disease*

E. Haen[1], T. Lederer[2], S. Bodensteiner[1], K. Woite[1], R. Hauck[4], and H. P. Emslander[3]

[1] Walther-Straub Institute of Pharmacology and Toxicology, Nussbaumstrasse 26, W-8000 München 2, Federal Republic of Germany
[2] Department of Experimental Surgery and [3] Medical Clinic I, Technical University, Ismaningerstrasse 22, W-8000 München 2, Federal Republic of Germany
[4] Medical Clinic I, Grosshadern, University of Munich, Marchioninistrasse 5, W-8000 München 70, Federal Republic of Germany

Introduction

Throughout evolution living beings have been subjected to the rhythm of light and dark. Therefore, many biological functions down to the molecular level are oscillatory in nature and follow a periodic cycle of roughly 24 h (circadian variation) [1, 2]. In humans, plasma concentrations of (neuro-)transmitter substances and hormones as well as many cardiovascular and respiratory functions, to name just a few, have been described to show such variations [3]. In clinical medicine, patients with atopic disease present with more severe skin reactions to allergens at night than during the day [4]; likewise, bronchoconstriction occurs in asthmatic patients also predominantly at night [5]. Today, only little attention is paid to these variations in the diagnosis and therapy of atopic disease or in clinical research. Chronobiological investigations are both expensive and time consuming, but we monitor patients around the clock, and in our experience it is worth the effort because

- The diagnosis of "borderline" disease is facilitated.
- Diagnostic procedures potentially dangerous to the patient may be avoided.
- Effectiveness and tolerance to drug therapy is improved through adaptation to the individual patient's needs.
- The comparison of biological variations along an appropriate time scale promotes the understanding of complex biological processes.
- The distinction between endogenous (physiological) and induced (by administration of drugs) variations can be made.

In this chapter representative examples of these approaches are presented.

Subjects and Methods

In the participating hospitals, patients suffering from atopic bronchial asthma were monitored around the clock, i.e., for 24 h and longer. At 4-h intervals respira-

* The study was supported by the German Ministry of Research and Technology (BMFT grant 01KC8806/3), by a grant from Klinge Pharma München/FRG, and by a grant from Hoechst AG Frankfurt/M., FRG.

tory function was assessed using a computer-based bedside spirometer (Spiropro 3000, Ganshorn Electronic GmbH, Münnerstadt, FRG). Just before spirometry 20 ml of venous blood was drawn. Employing a recently described procedure [6], the expression of β_2-adrenoceptors was determined on peripheral mononuclear leukocytes (pMNL). Cyclic adenosine monophosphate (cAMP) formed intracellularly in the presence of 10^{-7} mol/l isoprenaline, plasma cAMP and plasma cortisol were determined by radioimmunoassay (Amersham Buchler, Braunschweig/FRG and DRG Instruments GmbH, Marburg/FRG, respectively). A fraction of pMNL was incubated with fluorescein-isothiocyanate (FITC) labeled monoclonal antibodies (Becton Dickinson GmbH, Heidelberg/FRG) directed against specific surface epitopes termed CD 3 (T lymphocytes), CD 19 (B lymphocytes), CD 4 (T helper/inducer cells), CD 8 (T suppressor/cytotoxic cells), CD 16 (natural killer, NK cells, large granular lymphocytes) and CD 14 (monocytes, granulocytes). Cells are subsequently run on a fluorescence activated flow cytometer (FACScan, Becton Dickinson GmbH, Heidelberg/FRG) to identify the fractional distribution of pMNL subpopulations [6].

Some Illustrative Results

Diagnosis of "Borderline" Disease, Individualization of Therapy

A 19-year-old man complained of occasional shortness of breath and coughing, with these symptoms occurring predominantly at night. Routine diagnostic procedures such as spirometry performed at regular hospital staff working hours (i.e., from 8:00 a.m. to 5:00 p.m.) did not reveal any pathological findings. Only skin tests proved mildly positive for house dust mite. However, when lung function was tested at 4-h intervals on a 24-h time scale, a pronounced decrease in peak expiratory flow (PEF) could be detected between 02:00 a.m. and 06:00 a.m., whereas PEF was in the normal range between 10:00 a.m. and 10:00 p.m. (Fig. 1). The patient was then given 1050 mg/day theophylline (Bronchoretard) in an unequally divided dosage (350 mg at 08:00 a.m., 700 mg at 10:00 p.m.). After 7 days of therapy the patient felt fine, and spirometry demonstrated a successful prevention of the nocturnal decrease in respiratory function (Fig. 1).

Interaction of Physiological Variables in Complex Biological Systems

Ten male patients (19–33 year old) were admitted to the participating hospitals for diagnostic checkup. All of these patients had a history of dyspnea and/or coughing, predominantly at night. They had never been consistently treated for their complaints before, which implies that their asthma was of a mild type. Some of them had occasionally used medication, inhaled β-sympathomimetic or vagolytic drugs (one or two puffs within 3 weeks) and/or antihistamines, but usually they managed their problems without medication. The atopic nature of their asthma was verified by anamnesis, positive skin tests, demonstration of specific

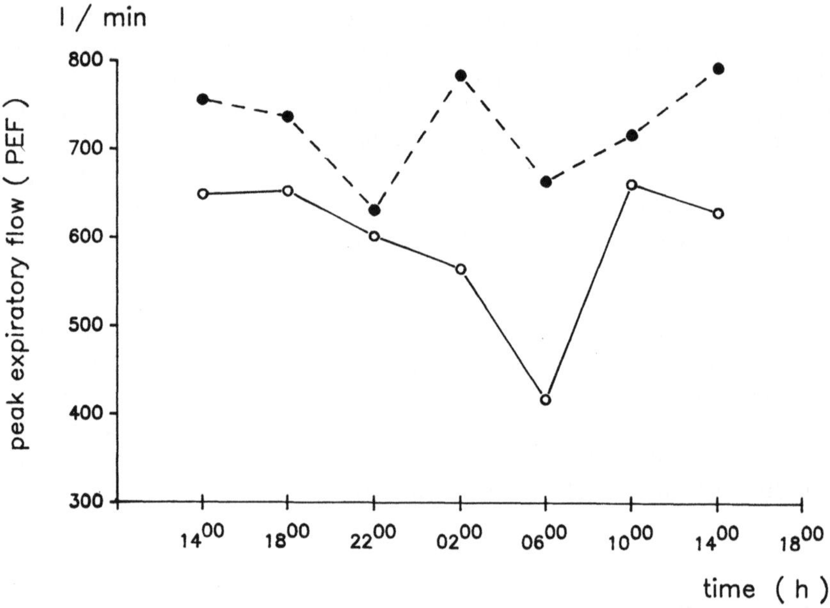

Fig. 1. Peak expiratory flow of a male asthmatic patient (19 years old) without any medication (*solid line*) and on day 7 of 1050 mg/d theophylline (Bronchoretard, 350 mg at 08:00 a.m., 700 mg at 10:00 p.m., *broken line*)

IgE antibodies and exposure to the antigen in question. Spirometry revealed considerably lower PEF rates at night than during the day. Eight male subjects (22–34 years of age; all the subjects had a negative history of asthma and were apparently healthy according to routine diagnostics) were recruited as a control group. The number of β_2-adrenoceptor expressed on pMNL did not differ between the two groups. The affinity of these receptors, however, was significantly reduced in the patients throughout the day. The decrease in affinity correlated with the cAMP content of the cells investigated, its stimulation by isoprenaline, and a reduced cAMP plasma concentration (data presented in [8] and [9]). These findings, observed in various interrelated, physiological variables of immune cells, may be taken as evidence for a reduced sympathetic tone on these cells in atopic bronchial asthma.

Distinction Between Endogenous and Induced Variations

Three asthmatic patients (68–75 years old) were investigated under therapy with inhaled and/or oral sympathomimetics. After admission, the patients were subjected to 24-h baseline monitoring (at 4-h intervals) including spirometry, differential blood counts, and lymphocyte subset evaluation. Thereafter (at 10:00 a.m. of the 2nd day), the patients received a single oral dose of 100 mg methylprednisolone (Urbasone); monitoring was continued at 1, 2, 4 and 6 h after drug administration. A decrease in the number of eosinophilic granulocytes, an increase in the number of neutrophilic granulocytes, and a reduction in the total number of lymphocytes was observed. Using flow cytometry, the latter leukocyte subpopulation was further analyzed: a decrease in the percentage of $CD3^+$ cells, $CD4^+$ cells, and $CD14^+$ cells, and an increase in the percentage of $CD8^+$ cells and $CD16^+$ cells were detected. The data following steroid administration were compared to the set of data that had been gathered during the last 24 h preceding drug administration (Fig. 2a, b). Therefore, circadian variations in the number of leukocyte subsets in peripheral blood could not be held responsible for any of the changes seen after steroid administration.

Conclusions

Diagnosis of "Borderline" Disease

Considering the patient whose respiratory function only deteriorated during the night, it might be tempting to advocate "after dark" diagnostic procedures for bronchial asthma. Patients either in an early stage of the disease and/or suffering from only a minor form of bronchial asthma might indeed benefit from such a "time switch" in diagnostics: circadian and/or nighttime testing may reveal an otherwise unapparent disease. It remains to be shown that those patients benefit from an early diagnosis by a better prognosis of their disease. In any case, drug therapy can be thus better adapted to the individual patient's needs. Administration of slow release theophylline formulations (or in the future maybe also inhalation of long-acting β-sympathomimetics) before going to bed can effectively prevent deterioration of respiratory function that has been shown to predominate in the early morning hours. Furthermore, 24-h monitoring of respiratory function may allow bronchial hyperreactivity and its reversibility to be demonstrated without affording provocation tests that may be potentially dangerous to the patient.

Interaction of Physiological Variables in Complex Biological Systems

The study of biological variations along a time scale may help to understand complex biological processes by appropriate correlating of simultaneously occurring events. Szentivanyi first suggested a reduced sympathetic tone in atopic disease [7], which has not yet been demonstrated convincingly. The aggravation of symptoms at night in bronchial asthma is caused by multifunctional processes. The data presented above suggest that one of them might actually be a reduced sympathetic tone due to a decreased affinity of β_2-adrenoceptors. This could be observed in three variables, all of them interrelated through the cells investigated: expression of β_2-adrenoceptors, stimulation of the intracellular cAMP content in these cells, as well as plasma concentrations resulting from the leakage of cAMP out of β_2-adrenoceptor bearing cells into the blood stream. This reduction in affinity of the receptors, however, does not show a circadian variation. It may rather be observed all day long, at night aggravating thereby the physiologically occur-

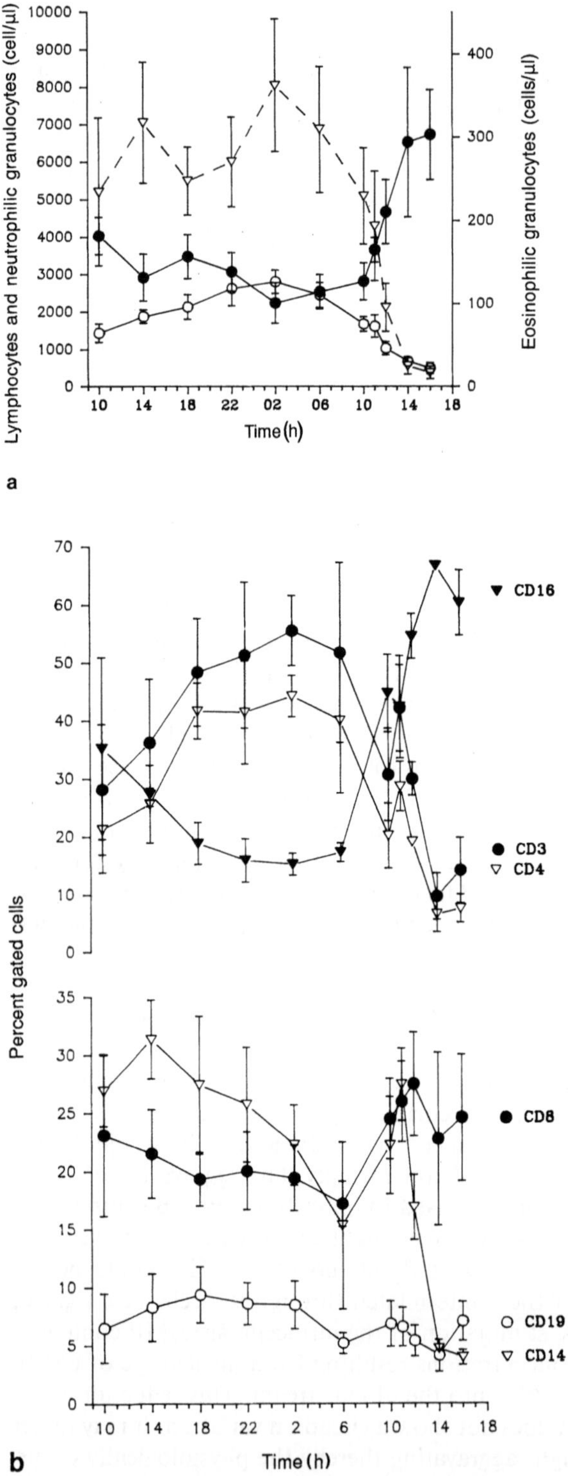

Fig. 2. a Corticosteroid effects on the circadian variation in the number of neutrophilic granulocytes (*solid circles*), eosinophilic granulocytes (*triangles*) and lymphocytes (*open circles*). **b** Corticosteroid effects on the circadian variation in lymphocyte subset distribution. Venous blood was drawn from three asthmatic patients, 68–75 years old, under therapy with β-sympathomimetic drugs. CD3, T lymphocytes; CD19, B lymphocytes; CD4, T helper/inducer cells; CD8, T suppressor/cytotoxic cells; CD16, NK cells, large granular lymphocytes; CD14, monocytes, granulocytes. Methylprednisolone (100 mg) was given orally at 10:00 a.m. on the 2nd day of the study

ring nocturnal decrease in sympathetic tone. At that time of day the parasympathetic (= bronchoconstrictive) tone increases physiologically. Under the described pathological condition this increase in bronchomotor tone cannot be sufficiently counteracted anymore by the sympathetic tone, thereby leading to bronchoconstriction [3, 8].

Distinction Between Endogenous and Induced Variations

The study of biological variations may also be used to distinguish the effects of stimuli such as drug effects from physiological variations. Since many physiological variables are subjected to endogenous oscillation, the data taken over a period of time following application of a stimulus might just reflect these physiological variations occurring during data collection. To make sure that the results of medical investigations extending over a period of time are not misinterpreted, we suggest establishing first the individual physiological oscillations of the variable under study.

References

1. Aschoff J (1954) Zeitgeber der tierischen Tagesperiodik. Naturwiss 41:49–56
2. Haen E, Halberg F (1985) Chronopharmakologie und Chronotherapie – von der experimentellen Forschung zur praktisch klinischen Anwendung. Dtsch Ärzteblatt 82:3837–3848
3. Haen E (1988) Chronopharmacology of reversible airways obstruction. Universimed, Frankfurt
4. McGovern JP, Smolensky MH, Reinberg A (1977) Circadian and circamensual rhythmicity in cutaneous reactivity to histamine and allergenic extracts. In: McGovern JP, Smolensky MH, Reinberg A (eds) Chronobiology in allergy and immunology. Thomas, Springfield, pp 79–116
5. Turner-Warwick M (1977) On observing patterns of airflow obstruction in chronic asthma. Br J Dis Chest 71:73–86
6. Haen E, Liebl B, Lederer T, Pliska V (1991) Revised radioreceptor assay for β_2-adrenoceptors expressed on peripheral mononuclear leukocytes. J Recept Res 11:129–140
7. Szentivany A (1968) The β-adrenergic theory of the atopic abnormality in bronchial asthma. J Allergy 42:203–232
8. Haen E, Emslander HP, Liebl B, Langenmayer I, Remien J (1989) Zirkadiane Variationen bei der Expression von β_2-Adrenozeptoren auf peripheren Lymphozyten von Gesunden und Asthmatikern. Atemwegs-Lungenkr 15:387–389
9. Haen E, Hauck R, Emslander HP, Langenmayer I, Liebl B, Schopohl J, Remien J, Fruhmann G (1991) Nocturnal asthma: β_2-Adrenoceptors on peripheral mononuclear leukocytes, plasma cAMP and cortisol concentrations. Chest 99 (in press)

Food Allergy

On the Diagnosis of Food Allergy in Adults – A Comparison Between DBPCFC and Intragastric Provocations*

C. Bindslev-Jensen[1], A. Norgaard[1], K. Ladefoged[2], E. Hyllander[2] and L.K. Poulsen[3]

[1] Food Allergy Unit TTA 7523, National University Hospital
[2] Medical Department P, National University Hospital
[3] Laboratory of Medical Allergology TTA 7542, National University Hospital, 20 Tagensvej, 2200 Copenhagen, Denmark

The diagnosis of immediate adverse reactions to food (food allergy) depends exclusively on the outcome of double-blind, placebo-controlled food challenges (DBPCFC) [1, 2, 4, 5 (to be published), 9]. The diagnostic value of a skin prick test (SPT), radio-allergosorbent test (RAST) and histamine release from basophils (HR) has not yet been fully elucidated and cannot replace DBPCFC [3, 6, 10]. This also applies to a new technique, the intragastric provocation under endoscopic control (IPEC), developed by Reimann and Ring [7, 8], although the authors reported a very close correlation between the results of IPEC and DBPCFC. As this new technique might prove to be more valuable than SPT, RAST, or HR in the diagnosis of food allergy, we therefore compared the outcome of IPEC with that of DBPCFC in our adult patients.

Patients

Twenty adult patients were included in the study. All had a convincing medical history of immediate objective signs within 30 min after intake of minute amounts of the offending food item. Symptoms reported were mainly rhinoconjunctivitis, asthma, urticaria, and gastrointestinal symptoms such as vomiting or diarrhea. Most patients reported adverse reactions to hen's eggs, codfish, or cow's milk, whereas some reported allergy to maize, rye, wheat, or poultry. Most of the patients had a positive result in SPT (with allergens from Allergologisk Laboratorium A/S ALK, Denmark), RAST (Pharmacia, Sweden) and/or HR (Referencelaboratoriet, Denmark). However, neither of these tests were in significant concordance with the outcome of DBPCFC [5]. The majority of the patients were also sensitized to one or more inhalant allergens.

All patients underwent a titrated DBPCFC with increasing doses of the offending food item ranging from 5 mg to 5 g (codfish), 50 g (egg) or 250 g (milk). A positive DBPCFC was defined as appearance of objective signs within 30 min after provocation with active substance and with no reaction to the appurtenant

* This study was supported by grants from Lundbeckfonden and Statens Sundhedsvidenskabelige Forskningsråd.

placebo challenge. In 12 of the 20 patients, the medical history could be verified, i.e., the patients were *clinically allergic* to the suspected food item.

Eighteen nonatopics with no history of food allergy served as controls for the IPEC histamine experiments. In none of these patients could any adverse reaction to any food item be verified.

Intragastric Provocation via Endoscope

IPEC was performed according to Reimann et al. [7]. Extracts from ALK (25 μl) were applied directly on the gastric mucosa via an Olympus GIF-Q20 gastroscope with simultaneous videorecording. Histamine hydrochloride 10 mg/ml, a suspected allergen, a negative control (saline with glycerine), and an individually tolerated allergen (nonsense allergen) were applied to all patients. The order of the provocations was blinded, and before the code was broken, the reactions in the mucosa were evaluated by two physicians. Reactions were graded from 0 (no reaction) to 3 (erythema, edema, and petechial bleedings) according to Reimann et al. [7]. In only one patient was a systemic reaction (urticaria after application of hen's egg) seen. The controls were only subjected to histamine hydrochloride and negative control applications.

Reactions of Histamine in the Gastric Mucosa

Of the 20 patients investigated, 16 exhibited a grade 2 reaction (erythema and edema) to application of histamine on the mucosa, with no reaction to the negative control. Of the remaining four, two exhibited a grade 2 reaction to all provocations, whereas the last two patients exhibited a grade 1 reaction (erythema only) to histamine. In contrast, in only 2 of the 18 nonatopic controls a grade 2 reaction was seen, whereas 7 exhibited a grade 1 reaction without reacting to the negative control. The remaining controls did not react to either histamine or the negative control. The difference in histamine reactivity between patients and control is statistically significant ($p < 0.001$, Fisher's exact test).

Reactions to Allergens in the Gastric Mucosa

The results of allergen challenge are presented in Table 1.

Table 1. Comparison of IPEC and DBPCFC results.

		DBPCFC	
		Positive	Negative
IPEC	Positive	11	14
	Negative	1	14

Of the twelve DBPCFC positive patients, one patient did not react to the offending allergen (egg) in IPEC. Six of the DBPCFC negative patients were found positive to the suspected allergen in IPEC. Furthermore, in 8 of 20 provocations with nonsense allergen a positive reaction was seen in IPEC.

Thus the overall sensitivity of IPEC was 91%, whereas the specificity only amounted to 50%.

Conclusions

From the gastric reactions to histamine it could be speculated that the gastric mucosa of atopic individuals may be "hyperreactive" as is the case with the bronchi of asthmatics, but this observation needs further elucidation before any valid conclusion can be drawn. Our data on intragastric provocation with allergen are in accordance with the high sensitivity of IPEC reporded by Reimann et al. [7, 8], but in our study we were unable to confirm its high specificity. There might be more explanations of this difference. Food extracts used for diagnostic procedures (SPT, RAST, HR, IPEC) are not standardized, thus limiting the possibility of a valid comparison. We have shown that provided the right extracts (fresh, unprocessed food items) are used, both SPT and HR are valuable tools, whereas this does not apply to the use of commercial extracts (A. Norgaard et al., manuscript in preparation). Differences in the allergen extracts used by Reimann et al. and by us might therefore explain our different outcome. On the other hand, our study included both patients with a previous food allergy, still positive in SPT, HR or RAST but without clinical allergy, as well as patients with clinical food allergy verified by a positive reaction in DBPCFC. Also we included IPEC provocation with nonsense allergens, tolerated by the patient, and this difference might account for the low specificity found in our study.

However, as stated by Reimann et al. [7] "The technique described might prove to be useful in establishing the diagnosis in doubtful cases of food allergy".

Acknowledgements. The skillful assistance of Mrs. A. Vibits, Head Nurse, and Mrs. A. Larsen, Secretary, is gratefully acknowledged.

References

1. Atkins FM, Steinberg SS, Metcalfe DD (1985) Evaluation of immediate adverse reactions to foods in adult patients. In: Correlation of demographic, laboratory, and skin prick test data with response to controlled oral food challenge. J Allergy Clin Immunol 75:348–355
2. Bernstein M, Day JH, Welsh A (1982) A double-blind food challenge in the diagnosis of food sensitivity in the adult. J Allergy Clin Immunol 70:205–211
3. Bock SA, Lee WY, Remigio L, Holst A, May CD (1978) Appraisal of skin tests with food extracts for the diagnosis of food hypersensitivity. Clin Allergy 8:559–566
4. Metcalfe DD (1987) A current practical approach to the diagnosis of suspected adverse reactions to foods. N Engl Reg Allergy Proc 8:22–26

5. Norgard A, Bindslev-Jensen C (1991) Egg and milk allergic adults – diagnosis and characterization. Insert Allergy (submitted)
6. Pastorello A, Stocchi L, Biga A, Pravettoni V, Schilke ML, Valente D, Zanussi C (1989) Value and limits of diagnostic tests in food hypersensitivity. Allergy Suppl 9:151–162
7. Reimann HJ, Ring J, Ultsch B, Wendt P (1985) Intragastric provocations under endoscopic control (IPEC) in food allergy. Mast cell and histamine changes in gastric mucosa. Clin Allergy 15:195–202
8. Reimann HJ, Lewin J (1988) Gastric mucosal reactions in patients with food allergy. Am J Gastroenterol 83:1212–1219
9. Sampson HA (1988) Immunologically mediated food allergy: the importance of food challenge procedures. Ann Allergy 60:262–269
10. Sampson HA, Albergo R (1984) Comparison of results of skin tests, RAST and double-blind placebo-controlled food challenges in children with atopic dermatitis. J Allergy Clin Immunol 74:26–34

Gastric Reactivity to Flour Extracts and *Helicobacter pylori* Associated Gastritis in Patients with Flour Allergy*

M. Kurek[1], R. Babic[1], and J. Ring[2]

[1] Department of Dermatology and Institute of Pathology, Ludwig-Maximilian University, Frauenstrasse 9–11, W-8000 München 2, Federal Republic of Germany
[2] Department of Dermatology, University Hospital Eppendorf, University of Hamburg, Martinistrasse 52, W-2000 Hamburg 20, Federal Republic of Germany

Abstract

Intragastral provocation under endoscopic control was repeated in seven bakers with occupational asthma, rhinitis and nonspecific abdominal symptoms. Flour extract which had been used for the skin test was administered to the antral mucosa. All patients had reacted positively to previous challenge of the gastric mucosa with water suspension of flour [7]. In these bakers a positive reaction was observed again after renewed administration of flour extracts, as were edema and erythema ($n = 7$), intensive gastric contractions ($n = 4$) associated with duodenal gastric reflux ($n = 2$) and abdominal pain ($n = 5$) following allergen extract administration. In addition, rhinitis ($n = 3$), asthma ($n = 2$) and conjunctivitis ($n = 2$) developed shortly after allergen administration. Biopsy specimens were taken from the antrum, corpus and duodenum before and 20 min after provocation. Microscopically, chronic active type B gastritis was diagnosed in all patients. *Helicobacter pylori* was identified in samples taken from five of the seven patients. These results suggest that (a) the stomach may be a target organ in bakers with flour allergy, (b) long-term exposure to flour in these patients may cause chronic gastritis, (c) damage to the mucosal barrier may facilitate *Helicobacter pylori* infections.

Introduction

The diagnosis of immunologically mediated adverse (allergic) reactions to food and its constituents in patients with hypersensitivity symptoms is an increasing problem in practical allergology [10, 12]. The spectrum of these symptoms ranges from gastrointestinal disturbances, urticaria, bronchial asthma, rhinitis, anaphylaxis to serum sickness type reactions with (a) arthralgia and vasculitis or (b) exacerbations of allergic contact dermatitis or (c) atopic eczema [13]. In the diagnostic procedure the exclusion of other possible causes of incompatibility and demonstration of immunologic sensitization have to be considered, and in some patients the reproducible elicitation of symptoms by the specific food is necessary.

* This work was supported in part by the Hanns-Seidel Foundation.

Different oral challenge tests may be used. In the classic oral challenge test, the patient is given the suspected agent or placebo and the general reaction is evaluated, including both objective and subjective symptoms [10]. Intragastral (i.e., intraintestinal) provocation under endoscopic control (IPEC) can be employed to confirm actual mucosal and systemic involvement in suspected food allergy [7, 11].

Investigation with this technique showed that tissue histamine content in the gastric mucosa decreased significantly after administering allergen to the mucosa, while there was no change in normal volunteers [11]. In this study, prick test extracts were used and systemic reaction in approximately one third of patients ($n = 14$) were observed. When the water suspensions of natural foods were used, these reactions appeared in approximately two thirds of patients ($n = 53$) [7]. The spectacular visible changes in the gastric mucosa, such as edema, erythema or pallor, hemorrhage with disturbances of peristalsis could not be confirmed by using nonsensitizing food suspensions in these patients [7].

Although this technique might be helpful in the diagnosis of food allergy, it has practical disadvantages: (a) it is stressful for the patient and requires specialized personel and technical effort; (b) endoscopic evaluation of mucosal and functional gastric changes is limited; and (c) histological findings such as hyperemia, edema, mucosal lesions and cell infiltrations are difficult to interpret in patients with active gastritis [8]. Interestingly, only about one fifth of our positively reacting patients ($n = 53$) suffered from chronic noncharacteristic disturbances. We found in this group 10 bakers with allergic symptoms due to long-term exposure to flour [7]. We repeated the gastric challenge in seven of these patients using intradermal flour allergen extracts and investigated the biopsy specimens taken before and after IPEC histologically and immunologically. In these patients and nonallergic controls with active gastritis the differences in the findings are doubtful [8]. We also investigated these biopsy specimens retrospectively and used the criterion of gastritis and present the findings with endoscopic and clinical evaluation of gastric reactivity in these patients.

Patients and Methods

Seven patients (five men, two women, age 21–55 years) with bronchial asthma ($n = 6$), rhinitis ($n = 5$), conjunctivitis ($n = 3$), chronic urticaria ($n = 2$) and eczema ($n = 1$) were investigated. All these patients were occupationally exposed to flour dust, and the respiratory and conjunctival symptoms appeared under professional conditions. All patients suffered from noncharacteristic gastrointestinal disturbances. Gastric and duodenal ulcers, gall bladder and bile duct diseases, parasites and gluten enteropathy were excluded. The clinical and immunological data of these patients are shown in Table 1 [8].

Intragastral Provocation. After endoscopic investigation of the stomach and high duodenum, 3–6 ml flour intradermal allergen extract was administered to the duodenal and antral mucosa. The biopsy specimens were taken from the duodenum, antrum and corpus prior to and 20 min after allergen administration [8].

Table 1. Clinical and immunological data of challenged patients.

Patient	Age (years)	Symptoms	Allergen	Intradermal skin test (+/++++)	IgE (PRIST) (KU/l)	sIgE (RAST) (class)	Leukocyte migration (max.% inhibition)
1	32	Rhinitis, asthma, atopic eczema	Maize	++++	270	2	16
2	37	Asthma, eczema	Wheat	++	47	0	59
3	21	Rhinoconjunctivitis, asthma	Wheat	++++	495	4	12
4	35	Rhinitis	Rye	++++	121	2	–
5	45	Conjunctivitis, asthma	Rye	+++	209	2	28
6	55	Rhinitis, asthma	Rye	+++	451	3	13
7	50	Rhinoconjunctivitis, asthma	Barley	++++	59	2	–

Apart from respiratory problems, all patients suffered from noncharacteristic gastrointestinal disturbances. Gastric and duodenal ulcers, gall bladder and bile duct diseases, parasites and gluten gastroenteropathy were excluded [8].
PRIST, paper radioimmunosorbent test; RAST, radioallergosorbent test.

Table 2. Endoscopic and clinical evaluation of gastric reactivity after intragstral provocation under endoscopic control (IPEC) with Score.

Score (1×5)	Symptom Score
Visible changes in the mucosa such as pallor, erythema, edema	1
Disturbances of peristalsis such as irregular contractions or duodenogastric reflux	1
Visible increase of stomach juice production	1
Abdominal pain	1
Systemic symptoms	1
Total	5

Score > 3, gastric reactivity confirmed; Score = 3, gastric reactivity probable; Score < 3, gastric reactivity doubtful.

Endoscopic and Clinical Evaluation. The visible changes in the mucosa, such as erythema, edema, remarkable disturbances of peristalsis, increase in stomach juice formation and appearance of the clinical symptoms were evaluated with Score (Table 2).

Investigation of Biopsy Specimens. Gastric biopsy specimens were stained with hematoxylin and eosin and graded for gastritis according to the criteria of the German Association of Pathologists [4]. Increased numbers of lymphocytes and plasma cells in the lamina propria were considered indicative of chronic gastritis. The features of chronic gastritis and neutrophilic infiltrate were considered to reflect the active process. Density of *Helicobacter pylori* colonization was determined semiquantitatively and Giemsa staining and Warthin-Starry silver impregnation were used. Mucosal edema and other features such as hemorrhages, erosions, atrophy and intestinal metaplasia were noted when present, but they were not considered to be of diagnostic importance.

Results

In all of the patients visible changes in the mucosa, such as erythema of varying intensity ($n = 5$), edema ($n = 4$), contractions of the stomach ($n = 4$) with duodeno-gastric reflux ($n = 2$), were observed. Remarkable abdominal pains and diverse systemic hypersensitivity symptoms appeared between 1 and 20 min after intragastral administration of allergen extract (Fig. 1, Table 3). After evaluation of these findings with Score, positive reaction was diagnosed in four patients and suspected in three. The results of IPEC with flour extracts and Score evaluation are illustrated in Table 3. The occurrence of gastric and systemic symptoms is pre-

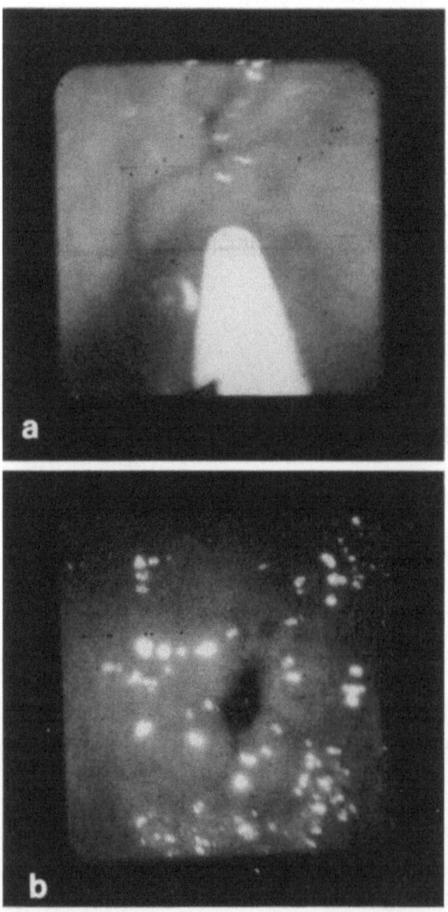

Fig. 1 a, b. Antral mucosa before (**a**) and after (**b**) intragastral provocation under endoscopic control (IPEC). After challenge the following striking findings were established: erythema of varying intensity ($n = 5$), edema ($n = 4$), contractions of stomach ($n = 4$) with duodeno-gastric reflex ($n = 2$)

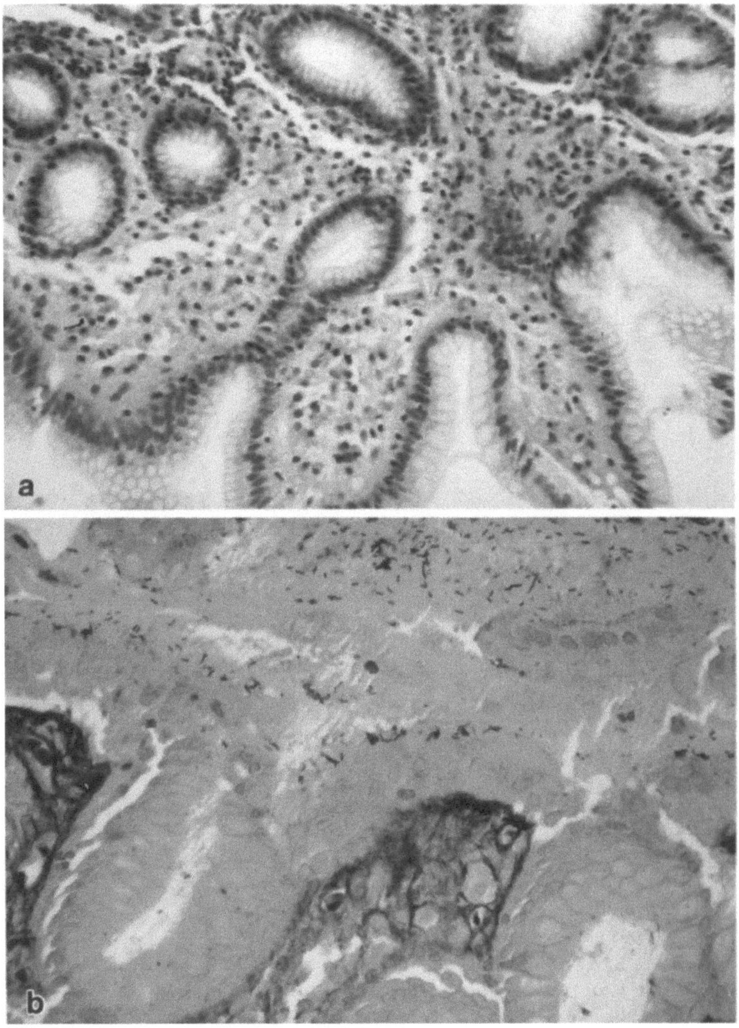

Fig. 2a, b. Active gastritis with edema **(a)**. In five patients *Helicobacter pylori* was found, in two it was suspected **(b)**

Table 3. Results of intragastral provocation under endoscopic control (IPEC) with flour extracts (Score patients).

Patient	Mucosal changes	Peristalsis disturbances	Increased fluid production	Abdominal pain	Systemic symptoms	Score
1	+	−	+	+	−	3
2	+	+	+	+	+	5
3	+	−	−	+	+	3
4	+	+	+	+	+	5
5	+	+	+	+	−	4
6	+	+	+	+	+	5
7	+	−	−	+	+	3

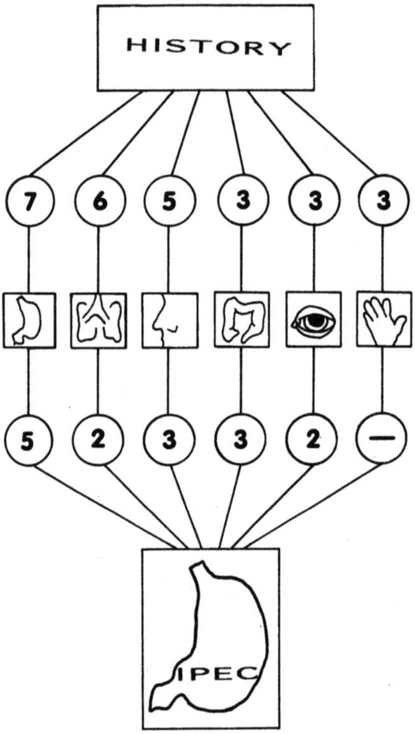

Fig. 3. Occurrence of systemic symptoms besides gastrointestinal disturbances in the history compared to intragastral provocation under endoscopic control (IPEC) with flour extracts

Table 4. Histologic findings in biopsy specimens from corpus and antrum.

Patient	Type of gastritis	Activity		Detection of *Helicobacter pylori*
		Antrum	Corpus	
1	B	Chronic, second degree	Chronic low	+ +
2	B	Chronic, second degree	Chronic low	+ +
3	B	Chronic, second degree	Chronic low	?
4	B	Chronic, first degree	Chronic minimal	+ + +
5	B	Chronic, second degree	Chronic, first degree	+
6	B	Chronic minimal	–	?
7	B	Chronic, second degree	Chronic minimal	+ + +

Microscopic edema was found in the antrum ($n = 6$) and corpus ($n = 4$).

sented in Fig. 3. Though expressed differently, active type B gastritis was diagnosed in all cases (Table 4). Microscopic edema was found in the antrum ($n = 6$) and corpus ($n = 4$). In five cases *Helicobacter pylori* was found and in two it was suspected (Table 4, Figs. 2b, 4).

Discussion

The involvement of the stomach as a "target organ" in the immediate type of allergic reaction has been confirmed by many authors [1, 5, 7, 11]. Since gastric ulceration was produced in experimental animals by a mucosal anaphylactic reaction in André's studies, it is speculated that an immediate (type I) hypersensitivity reaction might contribute to the pathogenesis of the chronic form of this disease in humans [2]. On the other hand, the immunological mechanism of ulcerprotection in the stomach has been proposed [6]. Retrospectively, we did not see gastric or duodenal ulcers in our patients who reacted positively to IPEC [7, 14]. In seven patients with flour allergy and chronic gastrointestinal disturbances, long-term exposure to inhaled and orally administered allergen might be supposed. In experimental studies 80% of radio-labeled and inhaled antigens appeared in the contents of the stomach [15]. It may also be speculated that long-term exposure to flour which has been swallowed might contribute to the pathogenesis of active chronic gastritis. Chronic active type B gastritis was microscopically diagnosed in all patients. The findings of *Helicobacter pylori* in samples taken from five of seven patients and nonidentified bacteria in two are difficult to interpret. Active chronic gastritis is characteristic of *Helicobacter pylori* colonization. There can be no doubt that *Helicobacter pylori* plays a decisive role in the etiology of type B gastritis [3]. The hypothesis that damage to the mucosal barrier may facilitate *Helicobacter pylori* colonization corresponds to our findings of gastric reactivity to flour in the allergy patients we studied [9].

References

1. André F, André C (1981) Gastric ulcer induced by mucosal anaphylaxis in ovalbumin sensitized praomys (mastomys) natalensis. Am J Pathol 102:133–135
2. André C, Moulinier B, André F et al. (1983) Evidence for anaphylactic reactions in peptic ulcer and varioliform gastritis. Ann Allergy 51:325–328
3. Dooley CP, Cohen H, Fitzgibbons PC et al. (1989) Prevalence of *Helicobacter pylori* infection and histologic gastritis in asymptomatic persons. N Engl J Med 321:1562–1566
4. Heilmann KJ, Stolte M, Borchard F et al. (1989) Gastritis – Graduierung und Klassifikation. Pathologe 10:194–196
5. Katz AJ, Twarog FJ, Zeiger RS et al. (1984) Milk-sensitive and eosinophilic gastroenteropathy: similar clinical features with contrasting mechanisms and clinical course. J Allergy Clin Immunol 74:72–78
6. Krämling HJ, Merkle T, Merkle R et al. (1988) Immunologische Reaktivität des Magens – ein neuer Mechanismus der Ulkusprotektion. Langenbecks Arch Chir 372:942–943
7. Kurek M (1985) Méthode de provocation directe de la muqueuse gastroduodénale dans le diagnostic clinique de l'allergie alimentaire. Rev Fr Allergol 25:13–17
8. Kurek M, Reimann HJ, Korenkiewicz J et al. (1986) Suivi macroscopique et histologique par endoscopies et biopsies d'une épreuve de provocation allergique gastroduodénale. Rev Fr Allergol 3:109–115
9. Malfertheiner P, Bode G (1988) Ultrastrukturelle Aspekte in der *Campylobacter-pylori*-assoziierten Pathogenese von chronischer Gastritis und peptischen Ulkus. In: Ottenjann R, Schmitt HW (eds) Aktuelle Gastroenterologie – *Campylobacter pylori*. Springer, Berlin Heidelberg New York, p 14
10. May CD, Bock SA (1980) Food sensitivity: a critical review and practical approach. Am J Dis Child 134:973–978

11. Reimann HJ, Ring J, Ultsch B et al. (1985) Intragastral provocation under endoscopic control (IPEC) in food allergy: mast cell and histamine changes in gastric mucosa. Clin Allergy 15:195–202
12. Ring J (1984) Nahrungsmittelallergie und andere Unverträglichkeiten durch Nahrungsmittel. Klin Wochenschr 62:795–802
13. Ring J (1988) Dermatologic diseases secondary to food allergy and pseudoallergy. In: Schmidt E (ed) Food allergy. Raven, New York, Nestlé nutrition workshop series, vol 17, pp 271–289
14. Romanski B (1987) The pathology of food allergy studied by gastric allergen challenge. In: Brostoff J, Challacombe SJ (eds) Food allergy and intolerance. Bailliére Tindall, London, pp 917–931
15. Van Haut C, Johnson HJ (1972) Synthesis of rat IgE by aerosol immunisation. J Immunol 108:834–836

Immediate Contact Allergy to Foods: Skin Test Based on Contact Urticaria and IgE Tests in Children with Atopic Dermatitis

A. P. Oranje[1], R. S. R. Aarsen[2], G. Liefaard[3], P. G. H. Mulder[4], and A. W. van Toorenenbergen[5]

[1] Department of Dermatology and Venereology (Division of Paediatric Dermatology), [2] Department of Paediatrics, [3] Department of Dietetics, [4] Department of Epidemiology and Biostatistics, [5] Department of Clinical Chemistry (Laboratory of Allergology), Erasmus University and University Hospital Rotterdam/Dijkzigt – Sophia Children's Hospital Rotterdam, Gordelweg 160, 3038 GE Rotterdam, The Netherlands

Introduction

The skin is often involved in the reaction pattern of food allergy (FA) [1]. Minor reactions in young children, suggesting contact urticaria (CU), consist of redness and urticaria around the mouth [2]. CU can be induced by immunological and nonimmunological mechanisms [3]. Immune-mediated CU to foods are common in children with atopic dermatitis (AD) and FA [4]. Based on this phenomenon, a test system (skin application food test) (SAFT) was applied to detect FA with the skin as the main target organ (dermal FA).

Skin Application Food Test

On symptom-free skin, 2×2 gauze, impregnated with standardized amounts of foods (0.8 ml cold pasteurized cow's milk and 1 slice, i.e., 2 g, of cold-boiled egg white) or control liquid (0.8 ml buffered saline) were fixed to the skin. After a positive reaction (often within a few minutes) the test was stopped immediately; otherwise the test was ended after 30 min. Positive tests were scored as: 2+, redness and edema (urticaria); 3+, the same but involving more than the test area; 1+, redness was scored as negative. The scores of the SAFT and IgE tests were compared by calculating the Spearman rank correlation coefficient and by Fisher's exact test.

Studies

SAFT and IgE RAST in AD

In 40 children with AD the SAFT and RAST (milk, egg) were compared (Table 1). Of the 24 children younger than 2 years, 17 were food allergic: 11 to milk and 14 to egg (8 combined). Nine children were retested after age 2. Of the 25 children 2 years and older, 16 showed food allergy: 9 to milk and 15 to egg (8 combined).

Table 1. Results of dermal food allergy testing in 40 children younger than 5 years suffering from atopic dermatitis.

Total patients	40
With FA	30 (75)
Age <2 yrs	24
≥2 yrs[a]	25
Skin symptoms	
AD	40 (100)
Related to food	19 (48)
Urticaria	21 (52)
Related to food	21 (100)

[a] Nine children were tested twice.

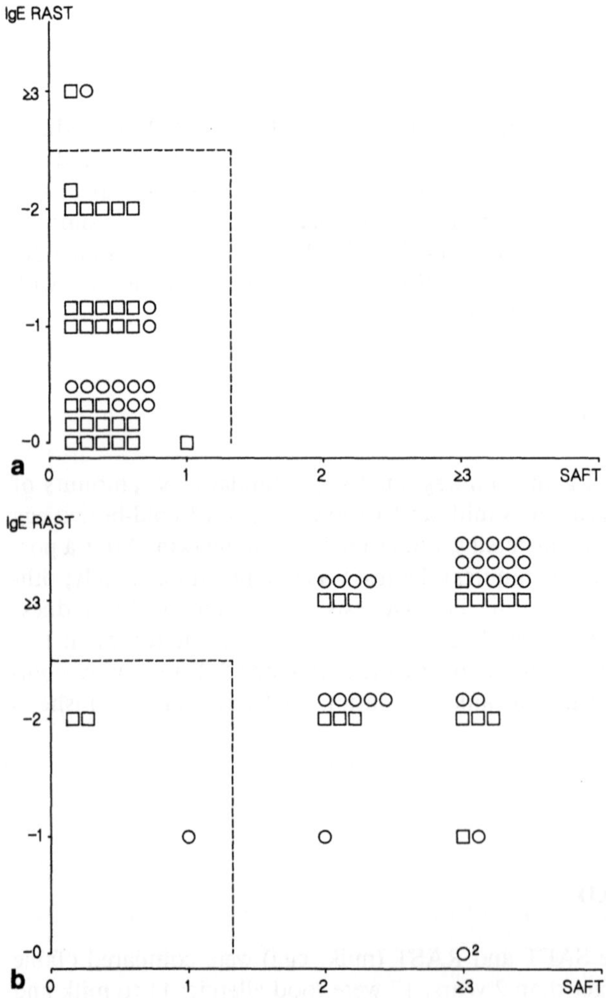

Fig. 1 a, b. IgE RAST and SAFT in children with atopic dermatitis **a** with no or lost food allergy ($n = 29$, 43 tests) or **b** with dermatitis and food allergy ($n = 30$, 47 tests). Cow's milk, ○; Egg, □

In four previously, milk allergic children, milk could be reintroduced without any problems. Milk allergy persisted in three, while egg allergy persisted in all five children retested. In four children with negative SAFT, the symptoms of eczema were not influenced by elimination diet. In 19 SAFT positive children (48%) with dermal FA, eczema improved by elimination diet. Figures 1 A and 1 B show a positive correlation between the scores of the IgE RAST and SAFT (Spearman rank correlation coefficient positive $r_s = 0.33$, $p = 0.02$).

Peanut Allergy: SAFT and IgE RAST

In 36 children, SAFT was performed with peanut butter. Of 12 children with peanut allergy SAFT was positive in 11 and IgE RAST ($\geqslant 2$) in all. The IgE RAST on peanut was, however, also positive in 12 of 22 children without symptoms.

Allergic skin reactions were observed by use of peanut oil containing bath preparations (protein ninhydrin test of bath oil preparation, weak positive) and by eating peanut butter.

SAFT, Phadiatop Pediatric, and Mixed Food RAST in AD

The Phadiatop pediatric, the mixed food RAST, and the SAFT (egg, milk, peanut) were studied in 52 children with AD, ages 0–5 years. The tests correlated well (mixed food RAST and SAFT significantly). The Phadiatop pediatric was a valuable tool for measuring atopic immune response by inhalant and food allergens.

Discussion

Specific IgE antibodies to many common foods, e.g., egg, milk, peanuts, and others, are present in at least 20%–30% of young children with AD [5, own data]. In some of them, these antibodies indicate clinically manifest food allergy (FA) [5]. AD in young children is often complicated by acute urticarial flare-ups around the mouth, i.e., CU. SAFT, as a skin provocation test, can be considered as an imitation of these symptoms. A positive SAFT may be explained by penetration of proteins through the skin. SAFT, IgE RAST, mixed food RAST, and Phadiatop pediatric correlated more or less in our different studies. CU to foods plays an important role in dermal FA. The RAST was often positive, not correlating with clinical symptoms of FA. High RAST scores corresponded more often with FA [6]. Actual IgE tests indicate atopic immune response and do not always correlate with clinical symptoms. The child-friendly SAFT seems clinically relevant for dermal FA. It supports the hypothesis of the "food-AD link" in young children.

References

1. Burks AW, Mallory SB, Williams LW et al. (1988) Atopic dermatitis: clinical relevance of food hypersensitivity reactions. J Pediatr 113:447–451
2. Oranje AP (1990) Skin provocation test (SAFT) based on contact urticaria: a marker of dermal food allergy. In: Vermeer BJ (ed) Metabolic skin disorders. Karger, Basel
3. von Krogh G, Maibach HI (1982) The contact urticaria syndrome – 1982. Sem Dermatol 1:59–66
4. Salo OP, Mäkinen-Kiljunen S, Juntunen K (1986) Milk causes a rapid urticarial reaction on the skin of children with atopic dermatitis and milk allergy. Acta Derm Venereol 66:438–442
5. Meneghini CL, Bonifazi E (1985) The role of foods in atopic dermatitis. Int J Dermatol 24:158–160
6. Renz H, Düngemann H, Rakoski J (1988) Untersuchungen über Nahrungsmittelallergien bei Kindern mit Neurodermatitis. Allergologie 11:16–21

The Prevalence of Food Allergy in Children with Atopic Dermatitis

A. Taieb, M. Debons, M.H. Cavert, M.H. Maupomé, N. Allos, D. Montaudon, and J. Maleville

Service de Dermatologie et Laboratoire de Biochimie, Hôpital des Enfants, CHU de Bordeaux, 33077 Bordeaux Cédex, France

Introduction

The relevance of food allergy (FA) in children with atopic dermatitis (AD) is still a debated matter. The practical benefit of a specialized work-up for the detection of FA is not yet established because: (1) many if not all patients in the pediatric age group greatly benefit, at very low risk, from a simple topical regimen made up of steroid ointments for eczema and water binders for dry skin [1]; thus "non-believers" in FA are numerous among dermatologists; (2) spontaneous improvement in the younger group makes any evaluation of efficacy of a diet regimen very difficult, not to mention the difficulty in obtaining reproducible scoring methods in this disease; (3) there are no simple, reliable, and standardized screening tests or diagnostic procedures for FA; (4) the relationships between type 1 hypersensitivity caused by foods and skin lesions are not clear.

However, there are important reasons not to ignore FA when managing AD children. First, parents are most concerned about this problem and diet manipulation is greatly favored among primary care physicians (general practitioners and pediatricians) especially concerning cow's milk. Second, data from the literature [2–4] clearly indicate that type 1 cutaneous, respiratory, or digestive reactions occur after double-blind challenges following an avoidance diet of suspected foods and that prolonged diet avoidance is necessary in some patients to control skin symptoms.

Our aims were to determine the prevalence of FA in AD children; examine the relevance of screening procedures, including clinical data (records to control intakes), prick testing, and chemiluminescent assay (CLA) of serum for specific IgE, food challenges being the end point of evaluation.

Patients and Methods

We report here on 105 qualified patients who completed a screening procedure between April 1989 and May 1990. The screening procedure was organized as follows: *At the first visit*, a complete history was taken, along with *clinical examination* and *scoring of disease* (taking into account pruritus, intensity, and surface involved); blood was drawn for IgE determination (Dome Hollister Stier Mast

Table 1. Skin tests for food allergy.

Patients <6 months
Negative control: glycerine
Positive control: codeine phosphate
Cow's milk, egg (white and yolk), orange, fish, pork, wheat
Patients 6–24 months
Idem plus peanut, celery, tomato, pea
Patients >24 months
Idem plus chocolate, strawberry, shrimp, artemisia vulgaris, ambrosia, apple

chemiluminescent assay system, Epernon, France) [5]. A detailed schedule for skin treatment was explained, and a short hospitalization was needed for patients with severe AD demonstrate to skin care techniques and the use of topical steroids. The parents were told to keep records in a notebook specifying meals, time of flares, and any other symptoms. The diet was continued as previously, without exclusion of any foods (also in the mother in breast-fed infants). *A second visit 1 month later* allowed checking clinical of scores and diet notebook, and performance of an *age adapted prick test battery* (Laboratoire des Stallergènes, Fresnes, France) (Table 1), chosen according to a data base provided by Dr. C. André (Lyon, France) with additions when a food not usually tested was incriminated or positive in the CLA test. In patients with at least one positive item (notebook record, prick test at least identical to codeine phosphate control, or class 1 CLA), a consultant dietitian reviewed the case and prescribed an *exclusion diet* for at least 3 weeks after a personal interview with the parents.

The challenges were performed as a single-blind, placebo controlled protocol. the patients were hospitalized, usually with their mother to minimize stress. For single blind tests, Lofarma capsules were obtained from Promedica, Levallois Perret, France. Table 2 indicates available dehydrated food allergens and doses. In most patients, only the lowest and highest doses were given because of time. For most patients in the lower age group, the capsules had to be opened and given with water sweetened with sugar. For foods not available as lyophylisates of dehy-

Table 2. Capsules for blind tests.

Capsule	Doses (mg protein/capsule)
Peanut	80, 20, 4, 0.8, 0.2
Banana	15, 6, 3
Celery	32, 16
Tomato	66, 44, 22, 11
Wheat	200, 50
Milk	85, 17, 1.7
Cod	252, 168, 84
Hazelnut	60, 15, 3, 0.6, 0.15
Soy	88, 22, 11
Ovalbumin	20, 5, 1, 0.2, 0.05
Potato	200, 50

drated proteins in capsules, open challenges were done with a quantity of food corresponding to one to two dessert spoons. All patients with negative blind challenges were rechallenged openly with a sufficient quantity of food (see above). Patients with positive blind challenges also received the food openly as a confirmation.

Results

The *characteristics of the 105 patients* (64 males) who had all screening tests completed were as follows: mean age at inclusion: 17.7 months (range 2–96); mean age at onset: 7.7 months (1–72). Severity was judged as mild in 23% (mean age at onset 10.1 months); moderate in 44% (mean age at onset 4.5 months); severe in 33% (mean age at onset 3.5 months). Nummular eczema was associated with AD in 24%. Seborrhoeic dermatitis was noted before eczema in 12%. A history of exposure to aeroallergens was present in 37% and associated asthma rhinitis in 22%. As concerns screening procedures, a total of 68/105 patients (64.7%) were suspected to react to food allergens. Table 3 shows the list of positive prick tests: egg ranks first (46/101 positive tests), then peanut (13), pork (9), and wheat and fish (7), the other positive tests being distributed among 10 different foods. Table 4 shows the list of positive specific IgE tests. Similarly, egg ranks first (22 egg white plus 7 yolk: 29/99 positive tests), then peanut (8), soy (7), fish (5), and milk, pork, potato, corn (4), the rest being distributed over 16 items.

Relevance of screening procedures was tested using food challenges (FC). In 36 patients, 86 FC were performed, some 32 patients could not be challenged because: (a) the parents rejected hospitalization, (b) the disease was too mild and already well-controlled at the second visit with a more appropriate skin care and no diet, thus introducing a bias towards more severe forms at final evaluation for FC, or (c) the diet avoidance period was not yet completed. In a total of 23 patients, 34 FC were considered as positive; 27 pure cutaneous reactions were observed: pruritus alone, pruritus plus erythema, or pruritus plus vesiculation. Six mixed reactions occurred: pruritus plus wheezing (3), pruritus or erythema plus

Table 3. Positive prick tests.

Food	(*n*)
Egg	46
Peanut	13
Pork	9
Wheat, fish	7
Milk	3
Soy, crab and shrimp, apple, strawberry, tomato, orange, pea	2
Celery, potato	1
Total	101

Table 4. Positive chemiluminescent assay tests.

Food	(*n*)
Egg white	22
Egg yolk	7
Soy	7
Fish	5
Milk, pork, potato, corn, shrimp and crab	4
Beef, wheat, pea, garlic	3
Almond, hazelnut, rice, rye, chicken, melon	2
Apple, orange, raisin, walnut, tomato, turkey	1
Total	99

Banana, bean, carrot, cabbage, chocolate, mushroom, onion, sugar, tuna, and baker's yeast were always negative.

Table 5. Clinical relevance of screening tests ($n = 68$).

Type of positive screening (*n*)	Positive FC
Clinical data only (7)	0/1
Clinical data and skin tests (9)	4/6
Clinical data, skin tests, and CLA (13)	9/12
Skin tests only (22)	3/11
Skin tests and CLA (13)	5/6
CLA only (4)	1/1

CLA, chemiluminescent assay; FC, food challenge.

Table 6. Correlations with severity of AD.

	Positive skin test	Positive CLA	Positive FC
Mild (27)	8	2	0/3
Moderate (44)	25	12	7/14
Severe (34)	23	16	15/17

CLA, chemiluminescent assay; FC, food challenge.

vomiting (2), pruritus plus diarrhea plus hyperthermia (1). The 34 positive FC included: egg (17), peanut (3), fish (3), wheat (3), soy (3), potato (2), and beef, pork, garlic (1). All reactions were observed in the first 2 h following FC. However, two patients had a delayed eczematous reaction after being challenged by egg. Table 5 shows the relevance of screening tests, indicating that most patients were screened using skin tests with or without CLA.

If we consider valid as an approximation that 23/36 patients (63.8%) are positive at FC, we would thus predict that there are $68 \times 63.8/100 = 43$ patients out of 105 who are allergic to foods (40.9%).

Table 6 shows correlations between severity, screening for FA, and results of FC. These data suggest an augmentation of prevalence of FA with severity of AD.

Discussion

The preliminary report of this ongoing study of FA in AD emphasizes a stepwise analytical approach. The population studied is very young and theoretically exposed to the highest risk concerning allergic reactions to foods [6, 7]. The main result, indicating a prevalence of 40.9% for FA in this group, is comparable to US data (33% for Burks [4]), but allergenic foods are distributed differently, probably reflecting diet differences (especially peanut). In particular, egg is prominent in our statistics. Milk, surprisingly, was rarely found at screening and has not yet been incriminated in FC. Only 9 different foods were demonstrated to cause reactions at FC from a total of 25 positive at screening tests.

At FC, some reactions appeared very specific, consisting of an intense palpable erythema with edema (fixed urticaria type), involving with predilection the large folds, the cheeks, and the ears in infants, i.e., locations not always typical for AD, but reflecting more probably areas receptive to vasoactive substances, such as histamine. Other cutaneous reactions are of good diagnostic value when associated with noncutaneous reactions (infrequent finding in our experience when compared to US data). Delayed-type reactions were detected in a minority of patients (2/34).

When screening procedures are critically evaluated, clinical records have a low sensitivity. Prick testing has been confirmed as the best screening method overall, in accordance with US data [2, 4]. The value of CLA, the novel test for specific IgE, must, however, be taken into account, since this test screens 36 food allergens with 2 ml of serum. Since not all allergens can be tested in the very young by prick testing, CLA is sometimes helpful. The sensitivity of the two methods are not the same for the same allergens and thus are complementary. CLA picked out at least three allergens not detected by pricks and subsequently found relevant at FC. The relevance of FA tests to AD was not addressed. A series of nonatopic subjects would be the best control to assess the prevalence of FA and the type of reactions in the general population. This type of study is, however, not ethically feasible in children. Indirect arguments have thus to be found. Preliminary data in some patients indicate a decrease in the use of topical steroids after prolonged selected avoidance of food allergens, as well as better clinical scores. Long-term US studies are encouraging [3]; nonetheless, it seems difficult to admit that FA remains a significant problem in older patients, in terms of prevalence, since these patients usually have aeroallergen hypersensitivity, now well-demonstrated by patch testing, which makes more sense pathogenetically.

Conclusions

Food hypersensitivity of the immediate type definitely exists in patients with AD, and probably in more than one-third of them in the age group studied. A control group, even though difficult to gather, would be necessary to check the specificity of this finding. However, FA prevalence seems to increase with severity of AD. The prevalence of food reactants is variable according to diet habits, and an analytical approach seems worthwile. How much these reactions contribute to the pathogenesis of eczema remains unclear. Late phase, IgE mediated reactions, via chronic mast cell activation and release of interleukins 4 and 5, might contribute to a vicious circle and the chronicity of lesions.

References

1. Cooper KD, Taieb A (1988) Atopic dermatitis. In:Lichtenstein LM, Fauci AS (eds) Current therapy in allergy. Immunology and Rheumatology, Dekker, Toronto, pp 177–182
2. Sampson HA (1988) The role of food allergy and mediator release in atopic dermatitis. J Allergy Clin Immunol 81:635–645
3. Sampson HA (1989) Natural history of food hypersensitivity in children with atopic dermatitis. J Pediatr 115:23–27
4. Burks AW, Mallory SB, Williams LW, Shirell MA (1988) Atopic dermatitis: clinical relevance of food hypersensitivity reactions. J Pediatr 113:447–451
5. Brown CR, Higgins KW, Frazer K, Schoelz LK, Dyminski JW, Marinkovich VA, Miller SP, Burd JF (1985) Simultaneous determination of total IgE and allergen-specific IgE in serum by the MAST chemiluminescent assay system. Clin Chem 31:1500–1505
6. André C (1980) Passage des antigènes à travers la barrière intestinale et pathologie digestive. Med Hyg 38:279–281
7. Atherton DJ (1988) Diet and atopic eczema. Clin Allergy 18:215–228

Computer System of Medical Information (KSIMPA) – Useful for an Allergological Outpatient Clinic

P. Z. Brewczyński[1,2], L. Tomica[3], and Z. Kalina[1]

[1] IInd Clinic of Internal Diseases of Silesian School of Medicine, 14, Medyków Street, 40-752 Katowice, Poland
[2] Silesian Regional Outpatient Allergic Clinic, 31, Powstańców Street, 40-038 Katowice, Poland
[3] Computer Systems Design Nexter Ltd., 1, Buczka Street, 40-955 Katowice, Poland

The medical information computer system produced by Novell NetWare, can be useful in an allergological outpatient clinic. The system covers both storage of registration data, general information useful to physicians, information regarding administrative procedures and statistical evaluation of data. The two level approach of patient history taking (level I, general data; level II, details concerning selected allergic diseases) shortens the procedure and improves the establishment of a differential diagnosis in the difficult interdisciplinary subject of allergology. The computer system's vital elements are "lexicons" containing, for example, auxiliary information (in the form of prompts) useful for the diagnosis and treatment of allergic diseases. It also provides prompts for patients with various types of allergies, including those undergoing specific immunotherapy or treated with elimination diets or steroids for a long time. The whole system was prepared for assisting in topics including bronchial asthma and allergic rhinitis, urticaria and angioedema, atopic eczema, allergic reactions to Hymenoptera, allergic reactions to foods and drugs, contact dermatitis, and occupational diseases.

The suggested configuration and spatial arrangement of equipment are also significant for quality functioning of the system.

Drug Reactions

Drug Metabolism and Drug Allergy *

H.F. Merk, D. Niederau, M. Hertl, and F. Jugert

Department of Dermatology, University of Cologne, J. Stelzmannstraße 9, W-5000 Köln 41, Federal Republic of Germany

Abstract

There are several evidences that allergic drug reactions are not due to the parent compound but to its metabolites:

a) practolol sensitive patients had an enhanced macrophage inhibition factor production in in vitro assays only after a preincubation of the drug with drug metabolizing liver microsomes;

b) patients with drug-induced hepatitis had liver-kidney-microsomal (LKM) antibodies binding specifically to cytochrome P450 isozymes capable to metabolize those drugs, which induced the hepatitis;

c) patients with the phenytoin-hypersensitivity-syndrome have an increased risk to develop allergic reactions to phenytoin, carbamazepin, sulphonamids and halothan. First results suggest that they suffer from a glutathione-transferase-deficiency;

d) in own results we improved the reactivity of the lymphocytes of patients with drug allergic reaction – indicated by positive results in the skin test or oral challenges – in the lymphocyte transformation test by a preincubation with murine liver microsomes, which are able to metabolize these drugs.

The recognition of the role of drug metabolism in type B (hypersensitivity) reactions to drugs will not only improve diagnostic in vitro tests, it will enable us to recognize individual risk factors since there is a high polymorphism of drug metabolizing enzymes especially of the cytochrome P450 isozyme system. Some of them are now detectable by restriction fraction length polymorphism (RFLP) analysis and these and other techniques may lead to the possibility to diagnose special risk factors of the patient before a special drug will be administered.

Introduction

Drug-induced toxicities can be divided into intrinsic and hypersensitivity reactions. Intrinsic reactions (type A) are related to the pharmacological properties of the drug and are based on studies using the appropriate in vitro assays and ani-

* Supported by Deutsche Forschungsgemeinschaft grant Me 939/1-1.

mal experiments [32]. Hypersensitivity (type B) is a major complication of drug therapy, since it is related both to the drug and to individual host factors. Therefore, in most patients such reactions cannot be predicted and at times may be fatal. This is especially true for immunologically mediated processes, such as allergic reactions and autoimmune diseases induced by drugs [34]. Nonetheless, much progress in clinical medicine and medical research has focused on identification of disease-associated environmental factors, especially drugs and other chemicals [6, 22]. The skin is a major target organ of drug allergic reactions and many signs and symptoms, such as urticaria, angioedema, purpura, vasculitis, or Lyell's disease, may occur [41]. Most allergic reactions to drugs are induced by small molecular weight compounds. According to the hapten hypothesis, derived from the classical studies of Landsteiner, small molecules such as drugs require covalent binding to macromolecular proteins to become immunogens [18]. The question arises whether it is the parent compound or a metabolite that is recognized by the sensitized T cells of a given patient [15, 31, 33]. Prior to metabolic transformation, such compounds usually are not very reactive and, hence, not immunogenic. Studies concerning the initiation of chemical carcinogenesis showed that a prerequisite for the binding of most xenobiotics to macromolecular compounds is their metabolism to highly reactive species [14]. Therefore, it seems reasonable to assume that similar mechanisms could play a role in some forms of drug hypersensitivity [21, 31].

The metabolic pathways of xenobiotics such as drugs are dependent on the presence of cytochrome P450 (P450) isozymes, epoxide hydrases, and transferases, especially glutathione transferases, resulting in a delicate balance between detoxification of a substrate and its toxification (Fig. 1) [14]. In most cases P450 is the first receptor for drugs and mediates the phase 1 reaction leading to the formation of highly reactive species (Fig. 1). Recent studies have shown that this enzyme system is the most complex isozyme system in biology. The amino acid

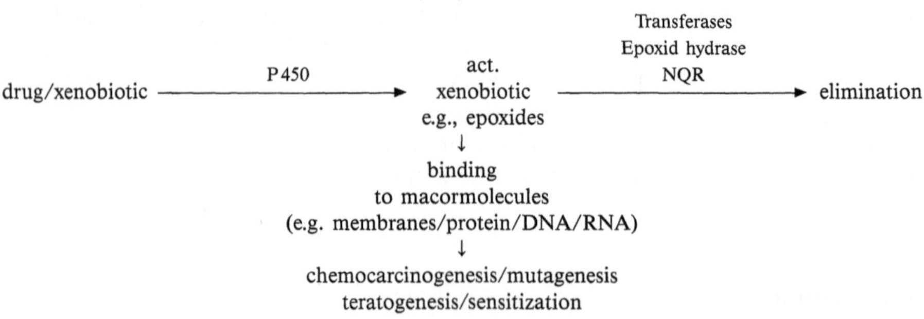

Fig. 1. Balance between cytochrome P450 (*P450*) mediated metabolism of a drug, converting the latter to a highly reactive metabolite, and its further metabolism by epoxide hydrase, transferase, or NAD(P)H-quinonereductases (*NQR*), which results in metabolites that will be eliminated. If this balance is disturbed there is a risk that the activated compound will bind to cellular macromolecules resulting in toxic effects or sensitization. The balance is dependent on multiple endogenous and exogenous factors which differ from individual to individual and which determine the activity of drug metabolizing enzymes, especially that of cytochrome P450 isozymes

sequences of at least 82 different P450 isozymes had been discovered by July 1989 – among them 26 in humans in whom the genes of nine different P450 isozymes had been located and sequenced [13]. The oldest P450 gene was formed about 3×10^9 years ago and the most recent about 1×10^6 years ago [13]. Their unit evolutionary period (UEP), that is the time in millions of years required for a 1% change in amino acid sequence, has been calculated to be 2.3–4.2. This value suggests that P450s are rapidly changing, which is typical for genes controlling proteins playing a major role in the defense of the body against xenobiotics [47]. The P450 gene superfamily consists of ten families, which are subdivided into as many as eight subfamilies. A special nomenclature for this system has recently been proposed [26, 27]. The concept that P450-dependent drug metabolism plays a role in immunologically mediated reactions to drugs is supported by several findings. These are discussed below.

Evidence for the Role of Drug Metabolites in Drug Allergic Reactions

Early experiments in the 1960s showed that known carcinogenic polycyclic hydrocarbons are able to induce contact dermatitis in guinea pigs, in contrast to noncarcinogenic polycyclic hydrocarbons [29]. This observation has been confirmed recently in mice [18]. It has also been shown that immunocompetent cells, such as lymphocytes and especially monocytes, possess P450-dependent enzyme activities [12]. Monocytes contain P450 isozymes that are different from those of lymphocytes, placenta, skin, or liver tissue, as demonstrated by studies with monoclonal antibodies to specific P450 isozymes. Moreover, monocyte P450s are very strongly induced compared to lymphocytes and even keratinocytes (Fig. 2) [12, 38].

Oculomucocutaneous Syndrome Induced by Practolol

The beta-blocking agent practolol caused a severe oculomucocutaneous syndrome characterized by inflammation of serosal tissue and psoriasis-like lesions of the skin. An antibody to a metabolite of practolol was found which was related to practolol administration, and its activity could be increased by antigenic challenge [1]. Interestingly, this metabolite was formed in microsomal preparations, known to be the main subcellular structures possessing P450 isozymes [2, 10].

Liver-Kidney-Microsomal Antibodies

Patients who developed a nonviral hepatitis after treatment with tienilic acid, a diuretic agent, had IgG autoantibodies directed against the P450 isozyme IIC8 (also called P-450meph) obtained from human liver microsomes [4]. These autoantibodies specifically inhibited the hydroxylation of tienilic acid by human liver microsomes. The authors suggested that P450, originally present in the endo-

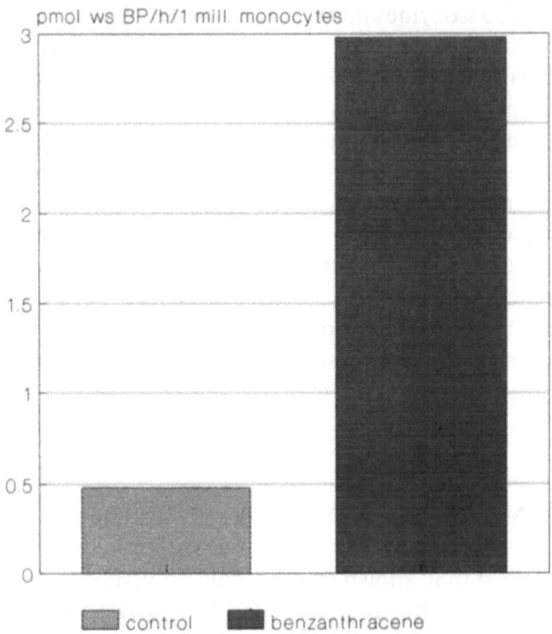

Fig. 2. Human monocytes were purified to yield a suspension of 82% anti-LeuM3 positive cells. This suspension was incubated with 2 μg benzanthracene/ml and the cytochrome P450-dependent aryl-hydrocarbon-hydroxylase (AHH) activity was determined using [^{3}H]benzo(a)pyrene as substrate. There was a sevenfold induction of the AHH activity in these antigen-presenting cells. In keratinocytes, e.g., a two- to threefold induction was observed under similar conditions (data not shown). These columns represent the mean value of three different suspensions. The variation was less than 10% [From 39]

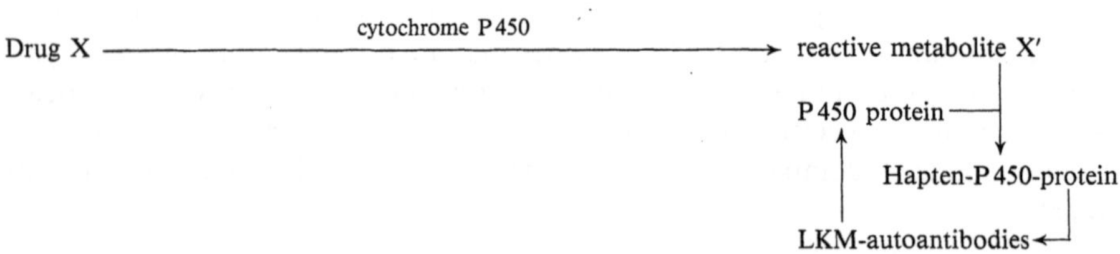

Fig. 3. Postulated initial events in autoimmune hepatitis induced by halothane, tienilic acid, or dihydralazine. Liver-kidney-microsomal antibodies (LKM), which bind to the P450 isozyme that metabolizes the involved drug (see Table 1), are formed [From 5, 7]

plasmic reticulum of the hepatocyte, could be alkylated by a reactive metabolite and migrate onto the hepatocyte membrane surface [5]. There, the modified protein could be recognized by specific T helper (Th) cells reacting to that part of the molecule derived from the reactive metabolite. These functionally active Th cells, in turn, would allow formation of IgG autoantibodies that recognize the native protein (Fig. 3). These antibodies have been termed liver-kidney-microsomal-antibodies (LKM). Besides LKM2, which reacts with P450IIC8, there is also LKM1, which is found in patients with severe hepatitis to halothane and in children with autoimmune chronic active hepatitis. LKM1 is directed against P450IID6 (Table 1) [5, 7, 20]. Recently, LKM 3 antibodies have been characterized; these were found in the sera of patients suffering from a dihydralazine-induced hepatitis. They bind with P450IA2, which metabolizes dihydralazine and is inducible up to 40-fold by smoking of charred food, suggest-

Table 1. Liver-kidney-microsomal (LKM) antibodies.

LKM antibody	Involved drug	Cytochrome P450
LKM 1	Halothane	P450IID6
LKM 2	Tienilic acid	P450IIC8/9/10
LKM 3	Dihydralazine	P450IA2

LKM are directed against different P450 isozymes in patients suffering from drug-induced hepatitis by drugs which are metabolized by these P450 isozymes [5, 7, 20].

Table 2. Drugs against which antibodies have been detected in humans and postulated or known chemically reactive metabolites formed from such drugs. [From 17, 31].

Drug	Reactive metabolite	Antibodies detected
Alcuronium		+
Amodiaquin		+
Captopril		+
Cephalosporins		+
Cyclophosphamide	Phosphoramide mustard	+
Dapsone		+
Ethynyl estradiol	*o*-Quinone	+
Ethylene oxide		+
Formaldehyde		+
Halothane	Acyl halide derivatives[a]	+
Methyldopa		+
Mianserin		+
Morphine	Morphinone (?)	+
Nomifensine		+
Paracetamol	Quinone imine	–
Penicillamine		+
Penicillin	Penicilloyl	+
Phenacetin	Hydroxylamine	–
Phenytoin	Arene oxide	–
Practolol	Epoxide derivative	+
Procainamide	Hydroxylamine	–
Quinidine		+
Quinine		+
Salicylates		+
Sulfanilamide	Hydroxylamide	–
Succinylcholine		+
Tubocurarine		+

[a] Same metabolite is formed by halothane, enflurane, and isoflurane [8, 16].

ing that the hypothesis depicted in Fig. 3 could be quite general with respect to immunoallergic drug-induced hepatitis [7].

In some patients antibodies were found against drugs known to induce hypersensitivity reactions in humans (Table 2). With some of these drugs, such as phenytoin, phenobarbital, and sulphonamides, evidence in favor of immunogenic metabolites has been presented. In most cases these metabolites are highly reactive species formed by P450 isozymes (Table 2). It is of interest that some highly reactive metabolites, such as hydroxylamine derivatives of procainamide or sulphone hydroxylamine derivatives of procainamide or sulphone derivatives, may be generated either by P450 isozymes or activated oxygen species during the oxygen burst of neutrophils [35, 37, 45, 46].

Anticonvulsant Hypersensitivity Syndrome

In the lymphocyte toxicity test the cytotoxicity of drugs to lymphocytes can be measured depending on the extent of xenobiotica metabolism. Lymphocytes are incubated with microsomes, appropriate coenzymes, and the drug. After 2 h the lymphocytes are washed and incubated for another 16h. In hypersensitivity reactions to anticonvulsive agents, such as phenytoin or carbamazepine as well as sulphonamides and halothane, increased lymphocyte toxicity was demonstrated in those patients suffering from the anticonvulsant hypersensitivity syndrome [11, 36, 43, 44].

The syndrome is characterized by eosinophilia, drug fever, skin rash, hepatitis, or Lyell's disease. Those patients who reacted to phenytoin with these symptoms had an increased risk of reacting with similar signs and symptoms to carbamazepine. However, this was not the case if the patient had an anaphylactic reaction including urticaria, angioedema, or shock (Table 3) [42]. If it is possible to reproduce this lymphocyte toxicity test in other laboratories, it might become of special interest since it permits the detection in advance of patients at high risk. Recently, Leeder et al. [19] improved the assay by using purified P450 isozymes instead of microsomes, and, in the case of sulphonamide, it was shown that the hydroxylamine metabolite elicits the hypersensitivity reaction.

Table 3. Anticonvulsant hypersensitivity syndrome symptoms.

Present[a]	Absent[b]
Eosinophilia	Urticaria
Drug fever	Angioedema
Rash	Anaphylactic shock
Hepatitis	
Lyell's disease	

Patients with the anticonvulsant hypersensitivity syndrome have an increased cytotoxicity in the lymphocyte toxicity test – described by Shear and Spielberg [42] – and have an increased risk not only to react with phenytoin but with other anticonvulsant as well beside valproic acid. Anaphylactic reactions do not belong to the anticonvulsant hypersensitivity syndrome.

[a] Alternative drug: valproic acid.

[b] Alternative drugs: carbamazepine, diazepam, and valproic acid.

Propyphenazone Allergy and the Application of the Lymphocyte Transformation Test to Drug Modified Microsomes

Allergic reactions to pyralozone derivatives are frequently observed, and patch, prick, and intracutaneous tests are not very helpful in their detection. A major problem in analyzing an allergic drug reaction by in vitro tests is the availability of reactive metabolic products [1, 21]. The costs to define and isolate all metabolites of a drug are prohibitive and thus unrealistic [1]. In consideration of these aspects we have modified the lymphocyte transformation test (LTT) by preincubating human peripheral blood mononuclear cells (PBMC) with murine liver microsomes, which are the main subcellular structures involved in xenobiotica metabolism. The preincubation generates activated metabolites which are then linked to indicator cells for use in this assay (Fig. 4) [23]. The microsomes were

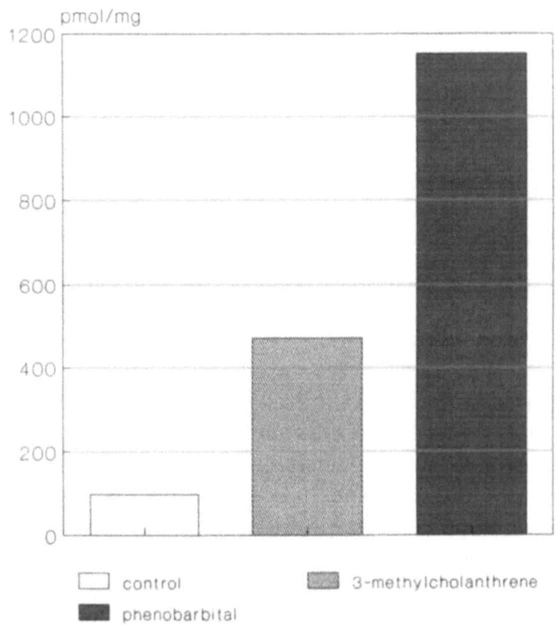

Fig. 4. Covalent binding of [^{14}C]chloramphenicol to murine liver microsomes, expressed as pmol [^{14}C]chloramphenicol/mg murine liver microsomes. Three different microsome preparations were used. *Control*, mice from which the livers were obtained were not pretreated; *3-Methylcholanthrene* or *phenobarbital*, mice were pretreated with 3-methylcholanthrene or phenobarbital, respectively. These compounds induce different cytochrome P450 isozymes [4]. The cytochrome P450-dependent aryl-hydrocarbon-hydroxylase (AHH) activities in these microsomes were 1.70 (control), 6.64 (3-methylcholanthrene), and 2.11 (phenobarbital) pmol water-soluble [^{3}H]benzo(a)pyrene metabolites/min/mg microsomal protein. Although 3-methylcholanthrene microsomes had a higher AHH activity than the phenobarbital-induced microsomes, the latter mediated more binding of chloramphenicol to the microsomes. This indicates that the P450 isozymes induced by phenobarbital (especially the P450II family) play a more important role in this reaction than P450 isozymes which are induced by 3-methylcholanthrene (P450IA family) [40]. Similar results were obtained with ethynyl estradiol, mianserin, amodiaquin, diphenylhydantoin, and practolol [From 30, 32]

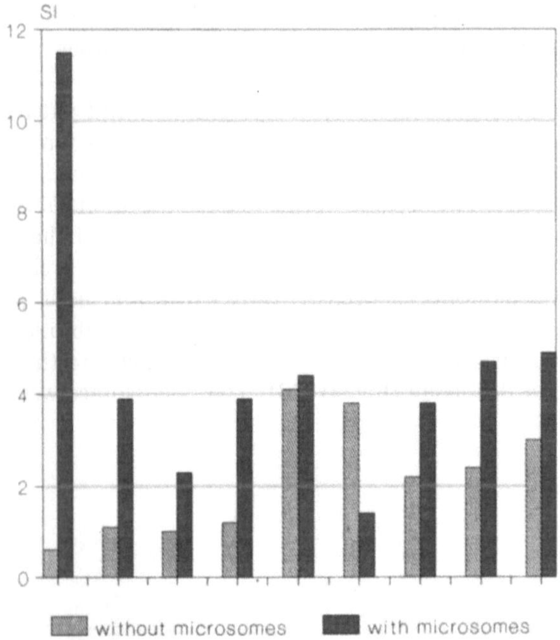

Fig. 5. Stimulation index (*SI*), which is the relation between [^{14}C]thymidine incorporation in lymphocytes with and without drug (measured in cpm), in nine lymphocyte transformation tests. The lymphocytes were obtained from propyphenazone-sensitized patients. Of 17 patients, 9 had an increased SI compared to 7 healthy controls (all SI below 1.3 not shown); 8 out of 9 patients had the highest SI after preincubation of propyphenazone with murine liver microsomes. Liver microsomes by themselves did non-influence the SI values. [From 21]

prepared from NMRI mice which were pretreated intraperitoneally for a period of 3 days with 100 μl saline solution (control) or with 80 mg/kg 3-methylcholanthrene or 50 mg/kg phenobarbital in order to induce different hepatic P450 isozymes. After preincubation with microsomes, the cells were washed and utilized in a lymphocyte proliferation assay. The proliferative response to different antigens was measured by [^{3}H]thymidine incorporation in micro- or macrocultures as previously described [23]. Murine microsomes alone had no effect on the lymphocytes. In 17 patients with a positive skin test and reaction in an oral challenge or a very suggestive history of propyphenazone allergy and no reaction in an oral challenge with acetylsalicylic acid, the modified LTT was performed. In 9 out of 17 patients we observed an increased lymphocyte proliferation. In 8 out of 9 patients the strongest proliferation was observed after preincubation with microsomes, indicating that the lymphocytes recognized propyphenazone or its metabolite as an immunogen (Fig. 5). The application of the LTT with drug-modified microsomes – at least in the case of the pyralozone derivative propyphenazone – revealed results similar to the oral challenge, which is the gold standard of diagnostic procedures in drug allergic reactions (Fig. 6). Thus, the importance of drug metabolism in drug allergy and the potential for improving in vitro tests has been demonstrated.

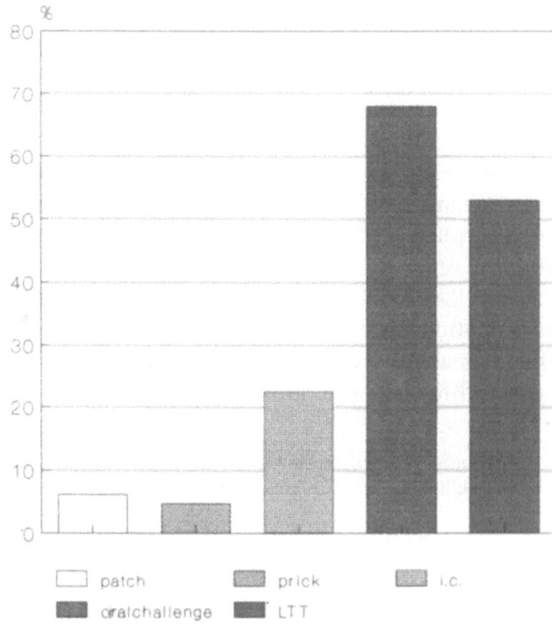

Fig. 6. Results of allergy testing in patients with a history of pyralazone-allergic reactions. In 4 out of 65 patch, 3 out of 72 prick, and 11 out of 49 intracutaneous tests, 17 out of 22 oral challenges, and 9 out of 17 lymphocyte transformation tests (LTTs) with drug-modified microsomes a propyphenazone sensitization could be shown. These data suggest that the modified LTT provides results similar to those of the oral challenge, which is the gold standard in allergy testing

Perspectives

A major problem of drug safety today is hypersensitivity reactions since unpredictable factors specific to the patient play a major role. Further research and better understanding of these individual factors will improve drug safety, especially if we become able to predict an increased risk of hypersensitivity using appropriate assay systems. At the level of preclinical drug toxicity testing, a better understanding of these individual factors is also a prerequisite for the development of new in vitro assays or animal experiments to predict potential harmful immunological effects of new drugs.

Several individual factors, such as oncogenes or the polymorphism of the major histocompatibility complex, are known to influence reactions to exogenous compounds or drugs. For example, it has been reported that in schizophrenic patients HLA-A1 is highly associated with a favorable response to chlorpromazine, whereas HLA-A2 appears to be associated with an unfavorable response [47]. In patients with affective disorders treated with lithium, HLA-A3 is associated with a high rate of relapse. In patients with rheumatoid arthritis the rate of adverse reactions to disodium aurothiomalate occurs 32 times more often in the HLA-DR3 haplotype; a similar association is found with HLA-A27 and agranulocytosis in response to levamisole and with HLA-DR4 in response to hydralazine-induced lupus erythematosis [47]. Our findings with the above mentioned modified LTT, as well as similar observations in practolol-induced disease or halothane or tienilinic acid-induced hepatitis, suggest that the metabolism of drugs by different xenobiotic-metabolizing enzymes, especially different P450 isozymes, plays an important role in drug allergic reactions [31]. The multiple P450 isozymes, belonging to at least eight gene subfamilies in mammals, are subject to complex regulation since they are dependent on endogenous and exogenous factors [13].

The dependence of drug allergic reactions on these metabolic pathways makes it possible that pharmacogenetic differences in xenobiotica-metabolizing enzymes may influence the likelihood of allergic reaction in a patient. Recently, the use of recombinant DNA techniques, such as the analysis of restriction fraction length polymorphisms of human P450 genes and genes regulating P450 levels, were proposed in order to determine the xenobiotica-metabolizing capacities of individual patients [24, 25]. If these and other methods become available for routine clinical investigations, it might become possible not only to diagnose sometimes harmful allergic reactions after their occurrence, but to predict the individual risk to a patient before such reactions occur.

Acknowledgement. The authors wish to thank Mrs. R. Schneider, H. Junginger, and B. Verwohlt for their skilled technical assistance.

References

1. Amos HE (1985) Laboratory investigation of an allergic drug reaction. Immunology 2:221–241
2. Amos HE, Lake BG, Atkinson HC (1977) Allergic drug reactions: an in vitro model using a mixed function oxidase complex to demonstrate antibodies with specificity for a practolol metabolite. Clin Allergy 7:423–428
3. Arsdel PP van, Larson EB (1989) Diagnostic tests for patients with suspected allergic disease. Utility and limitations. Ann Intern Med 110:304–312
4. Beaune PH, Guengerich FP (1988) Human drug metabolism in vitro. Pharmacol Ther 37:193–211
5. Beaune PH, Dansette PM, Mansuy D, Kiffel K, Finck M, Amar C, Leroux JP, Homberg JC (1987) Human anti-endoplasmic reticulum autoantibodies appearing in a drug-induced hepatitis are directed against a human liver P450 that hydroxylates the drug. Proc Natl Acad Sci USA 84:551–555
6. Berg PA, Daniel PT, Holzschuh J, Brattig N (1988) Medikamentöse Allergien. Diagnose und Immunpathogenese. Dtsch Med Wochenschr 113:65–73
7. Bourdi M, Larrey D, Nataf J, Bernuau J, Pessayre D, Iwasaki M, Guengerich FP, Beaune PH (1990) Anti-lever endoplasmic reticulum autoantibodies are directed against human cytochrome P-450IA2. A specific marker of dihydralazine-induced hepatitis. J Clin Invest 85:1967–1973
8. Christ DD, Satoh H, Kenna JG, Pohl LR (1987) Potential metabolic basis for enflurane hepatitis and the apparent cross-sensitization between enflurane and halothane. Drug Metab Dispos 16:135–140
9. Crabtree GR (1989) Contingent genetic regulatory events in T lymphocyte activations. Science 243:355–361
10. Davies GE (1978) Adverse reactions to practolol. In: Turk JL, Parker D (eds) Drugs and immune responsiveness. Mamcillan, London, pp 199–210
11. Farrell G, Prendergast D, Murray M (1985) Halothane hepatitis. Detection of a constitutional susceptibility factor. N Engl J Med 313:1310–1314
12. Fujino T, Park SS, Gelboin HV (1982) Phenotyping of cytochrome P-450 in human tissue with monoclonal antibodies. Proc Natl Acad Sci USA 79:3682–3686
13. Gonzalez FJ (1990) Molecular genetics of the P-450 superfamily. Pharmacol Ther 45:1–38
14. Guengerich FP, Liebler DC (1985) Enzymatic activation of chemicals to toxic metabolites. Crit Rev Toxicol 14:259–307

15. Ippen H (1964) Cutane Arzneimittelreaktionen und Arzneimittelstoffwechsel. Arch Klin Exp Dermatol 219:297–307
16. Kenna JG, Satoh H, Christ DD, Pohl LR (1988) Metabolic basis for a drug hypersensitivity: antibodies in sera from patients with halothane hepatitis recognize liver neoantigens that contain the trifluoroacetyl group derived from halothane. J Pharmacol Exp Ther 245:1103–1109
17. Kim HC, Kesarwala HH, Colvin M, Saidi P (1985) Hypersensitivity reaction to a metabolite of cyclophosphamide. J Allergy Clin Immunol 76:591–594
18. Klemme J, Craig E, Mukhtar H (1987) Induction of contact hypersensitivity to dimethylbenzanthracene and benz(a)pyrene in a tumor suspectible strain of mice. Cancer Res 47:6074–6078
19. Leeder JS, Cannon M, Nakhooda A, Spielberg SP (1988) Drug metabolite toxicity assessed in human lymphocytes with a purified, reconstituted cytochrome P-450 system. J Pharmacol Exp Ther 245:956–962
20. Manns M (1989) Autoantibodies and antigens in liver diseases – updated. J Hepatol 9:272–280
21. Merk H (1989) Arzneimittelallergie: Einfluß des Fremdstoff-Metabolismus. Allergologie 12:171–173
22. Merk H (1990) Die Haut als Signalorgan in der Entwicklung neuer Zytostatika und Antitumorstrategien. Z Hautkr 65:89–96
23. Merk H, Schneider R, Scholl P (1987) Lymphocyte stimulation by drug-modified microsomes. In: Estabrook RW, Lindenlaub E, Oesch F, de Weck AL (eds) Toxicological and immunological aspects of drug metabolism and environmental chemicals. Schattauer, Stuttgart, pp 211–219
24. Meyer UA (1990) Molecular genetics and the future of pharmacogenetics. Pharmacol Ther 46:349–355
25. Meyer UA, Skoda RC, Zanger UM (1990) The genetic polymorphism of debrisoquine/sparteine metabolism – molecular mechanisms. Pharmacol Ther 46:297–308
26. Nebert DW, Adesnik M, Coon MJ, Estabrook RW, Gonzales FJ, Guengerich FP, Gunsalus IC, Johnson EF, Kemper B, Levin W, Phillips IR, Sato R, Waterman MR (1987) The P450 gene superfamily: recommended nomenclature. DNA 6:1–11
27. Nebert DW, Nelson DR, Adesnik M, Coon MJ, Estabrook RW, Gonzales FJ, Guengerich FP, Gunsalus IC, Johnson EF, Kemper B, Levin W, Phillips IR, Sato R, Waterman MR (1989) The P450 superfamily: update on listing of all genes and recommended nomenclature of the chromosomal loci. DNA 8:1–13
28. Neuberger J, Kenna JG (1987) Halothane hepatitis: a model of immune mediated drug hepatotoxicity. Clin Sci 72:263–270
29. Old LJ, Benacerraf B, Carswell E (1963) Contact reactivity to carcinogenic polycyclic hydrocarbons. Nature 22:1215–1216
30. Orton TC, Lowery C (1981) Practolol metabolism. III. Irreversible binding of [^{14}C] practolol metabolite(s) to mammalian liver microsomes. J Pharmacol Exp Ther 219:207–212
31. Park BK, Coleman JW, Kitteringham NR (1987) Drug disposition and drug hypersensitivity. Biochem Pharmacol 36:581–590
32. Pohl LR, Satoh H, Christ DD, Kenna JG (1988) The immunologic and metabolic basis of drug hypersensitivities. Annu Rev Pharmacol 28:367–387
33. Remmer H, Schüppel R (1972) The formation of antigenic determinants. In: Samter M, Parker CW (eds) International encyclopedia of pharmacology and therapeutics, vol 1. Pergamon, Oxford, pp 67–89
34. Resch K (1988) Immunpharmakologische Grundlagen der Arzneimittelallergie. Internist (Berlin) 29:160–169
35. Rieder MJ, Uetrecht J, Shear NH, Spielberg SP (1988) Synthesis and in vitro toxicity of hydroxylamine metabolites of sulfonamides. J Pharmacol Exp Ther 244:724–728
36. Rieder MJ, Uetrecht J, Shear NH, Cannon M, Miller M, Spielberg SP (1989) Diagnosis of sulfonamide hypersensitivity reactions by in-vitro "rechallenge" with hydroxylamine metabolites. Ann Intern Med 110:286–289
37. Rubin RL, Curnutte JT (1989) Metabolism of procainamide to the cytotoxic hydroxylamine by neutrophils activated in vitro. J Clin Invest 83:1336–1343
38. Schenk V (1988) Die Aryl-Hydrocarbon-Hydroxylase und der Benz(a)pyrenmetabolismus in menschlichen Monozyten und ihre Hemmbarkeit durch Ketoconazol. Dissertation, University of Cologne

39. Schneider CH, Kasper MF, de Weck AL, Rolli H, Angst BD (1987) Diagnosis of antibody-mediated drug allergy. Allergy 42:597–603
40. Scholl P (1989) Einfluß Cytochrom P-450 abhängiger Metabolisierung an der Stimulation immunkompetenter Zellen im Lymphozytentransformationstest mit Arzneimitteln. Dissertation, University of Cologne
41. Schulz KH (1986) Allergische und pseudoallergische Reaktionen auf Arzneimittel. Internist (Berlin) 27:372–380
42. Shear NH, Spielberg SP (1988) Anticonvulsant hypersensitivity syndrome. In vitro assessment of risk. J Clin Invest 82:1826–1832
43. Shear NH, Spielberg SP, Grant DM, Tang BK, Kalow W (1986) Differences in metabolism of sulfonamides predisposing to idiosyncratic toxicity. Ann Intern Med 105:179–184
44. Spielberg SP, Gordon GB, Blake DA, Goldstein DA, Herlono HF (1981) Predisposition of phenytoin hepatoxicity assessed in vitro. N Engl J Med 305:722–727
45. Uetrecht JP, Sweetman RL, Woosley RL, Oates JA (1984) Metabolism of procainamide to hydroxylamine by rat and human hepatic microsomes. Drug Metab Dispos 12:77–81
46. Uetrecht JP, Zahid N, Shear NH, Biggar WD (1988) Metabolism of dapsone to a hydroxylamine by human neutrophils and mononuclear cells. J Pharmacol Exp Ther 245:1–6
47. Vesell ES (1984) Pharmacogenetic perspectives: genes, drugs and disease. Hepatology 4:959–965
48. Weck AL de (1988) Mechanisms of antigen formation by interaction of drugs with cell membranes. In: Estabrook RW, Linenlaub E, Oesch F, de Weck AL (eds) Toxicological and immunological aspects of drug metabolism and environmental chemicals. Symposia medica (Hoechst, vol 22) Schattauer, Stuttgart, pp 199–209

Adverse Reactions to Quinolones

D. Vieluf[1], R. Russwurm[2], B. Przybilla[3], and J. Ring[1]

[1] Hautklinik und Poliklinik des Universitäts-Krankenhauses Eppendorf, Martinistrasse 52, W-2000 Hamburg 20, Federal Republic of Germany
[2] Hoechst AG, Klinische Forschung, W-6000 Frankfurt/M 80, Federal Republic of Germany
[3] Dermatologische Klinik und Poliklinik der Ludwig-Maximilians-Universität München, Frauenlobstrasse 9–11, W-8000 München 2, Federal Republic of Germany

Abstract

The quinolones are potent bactericidal antimicrobial agents with a wide antibacterial spectrum. These antibiotics inhibit the bacterial DNA-gyrase, an enzyme related to human topoisomerase II. In the chemical structure there is no cross-reactivity to other antimicrobial substances. After oral administration quinolones are rapidly absorbed (oral bioavailability varies from 42% to 96%), reaching peak serum concentrations in 1–2 h with a half-life time below 12 h. The binding rates to plasma proteins vary from 25% to 90%. Quinolones show good penetration into the tissues as well as into human polymorphonuclear leukocytes. They are generally rapidly eliminated either unchanged or as pharmacologically still active metabolites by glomerular filtration and tubular secretion [4, 6–8, 10, 11, 15, 16, 25, 27, 28, 32].

The spectrum of adverse reactions to quinolones ranges from CNS symptoms (sleep disorders, headaches, reversible psychotic reactions such as hallucinations and agitation, convulsions), gastrointestinal complaints (nausea, abdominal pain, diarrhea) to skin symptoms (e.g., maculopapular or urticarial skin rashes, vasculitis, phototoxic/-allergic dermatitis) and anaphylactoid reactions [1–3, 5, 9, 12–14, 17, 26, 29–31, 33].

The evaluation of adverse reactions to quinolones has to follow the general principles of allergy diagnosis, namely, comprehensive case history, skin tests (prick, scratch, i.c., patch, photopatch test), in vitro methods (e.g., basophil histamine release test, BHR; lymphocyte transformation test, as possible) and provocation tests (oral administration of 10%–50%–100% of a conventional single dose in a single or double-blind, placebo-controlled manner) [20–22].

The analysis of case histories of patients with anaphylactoid reactions (AR) in connection with the oral administration of ofloxacin showed in most patients immediate onset of symptoms after first contact with the drug. Most of these patients were receiving medication with other drugs simultaneously. A personal history of atopy was found in 35% and former adverse reactions to other drugs in 25% of the patients.

Prick and intradermal tests with ofloxacin and ciprofloxacin in previously nonexposed control individuals showed a high percentage of positive test reactions.

Quinolones were found to show autofluorescence in the histamine spectrophotometric autoanalyzer, photo-induced inactivation of their antimicrobial activity as well as a photosensitizing potency in the photohemolysis test.

Although rarely, AR to quinolones may occur. The pathomechanism of these reactions is not yet established. Some facts argue for possible pseudo-allergic mechanisms (direct histamine release from skin mast cells, but not from peripheral basophiles; immediate onset of symptoms at first contact with the drug). On the other hand, the relatively rare incidence of AR together with a possible sensitization by prior exposure to quinolones in at least some patients may be regarded as hints to an allergic reaction. At present time, besides the careful history, oral provocation test (OPT) is the only reliable procedure in the diagnostic evaluation of AR to quinolones.

Introduction

Compared to the first generation of quinolones such as nalidixic acid, which was isolated from the synthesis of chloroquine, the fluorinated quinolones such as ofloxacin and ciprofloxacin are more potent bactericidal agents with a broad antibacterial spectrum (Table 1). The use of these antibiotics has significantly increased in the last few years [6–8, 10, 15, 16, 27, 28].

Pharmacology

Quinolones inhibit the activity of the bacterial DNA-gyrase, an enzyme related to human topoisomerase II. The new quinolones are fluorinated quinoline or naphthyridine carboxylic acid derivatives and show high activity against many gram-negative and gram-positive bacteria. Due to the chemical structure there is no cross-reactivity to other antimicrobial substances (Fig. 1). The fluoroquinolones are small molecules with a molecular mass of 300 to 500 daltons. Many of these compounds are so-called "zwitterions" and exhibit different solubility characteristics with changes in the pH (acid: cation, base: anion).

After oral administration the quinolones are rapidly absorbed, with a bioavailability varying from 45% to 96%, reaching peak serum concentration in 1–3 h, and with a mean terminal serum elimination half-life of between 3 and

Table 1. Quinolones.

Nonfluorinated	Fluorinated
Nalidixic acid	Norfloxacin
Oxolinic acid	Enoxacin
Cinoxacin	Ofloxacin
Flumequin	Ciprofloxacin
Rosoxacin	Pefloxacin
Pipemidic acid	Fleroxacin
	Lomefloxacin

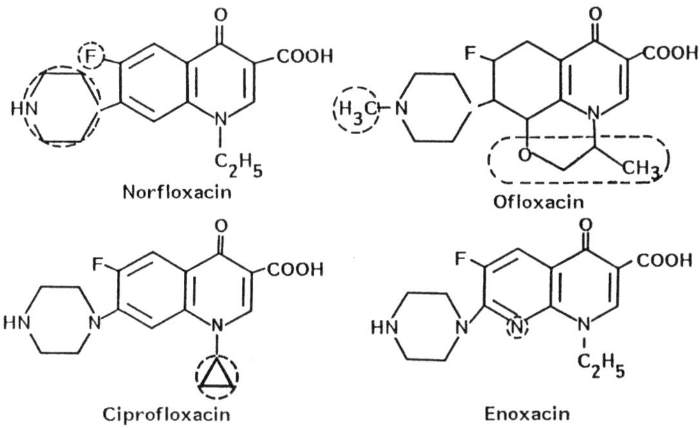

Fig. 1. Chemical structure of quinolones

12 h. The binding rates to plasma proteins vary from 20% to 50%, but the newer substances exhibit low protein binding and high penetration in body fluids and tissues (especially inflamed tissues), and they differ considerably in absorption, elimination and pharmacokinetic properties, and interaction potential. The quinolones are generally rapidly eliminated by glomerular filtration and tubular secretion, either unchanged or as pharmacologically still active metabolites, or by hepatic metabolism and gastrointestinal secretion. The quinolones may be metabolized in various quantities (ofloxacin 5%, enoxacin 14%, ciprofloxacin ~ 20%, pefloxacin > 50%) and conjugated with glucuronic acid (Fig. 2). The bile excre-

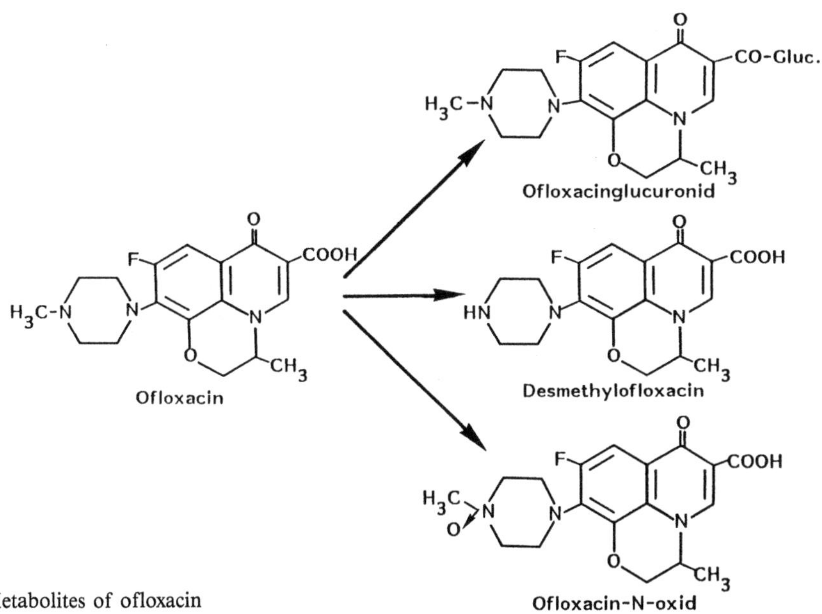

Fig. 2. Metabolites of ofloxacin

Table 2. Potential drug interactions with fluoroquinolones. [From 28].

Drug	Implications
Antacids	Decreased absorption of 4-quinolones
Theophylline, caffeine	CNS toxicity
Cyclosporine	Enhanced nephrotoxicity
Probenecid	Decreased renal clearance of 4-quinolones
Warfarin	Enhanced hypoprothrombinemic response
Cimetidine	Decreased metabolism of 4-quinolones
NSDAI	CNS toxicity

tion rate is important for the elimination of these conjugates [4, 6–8, 10, 11, 15, 16, 25, 27, 28, 32].

The absorption of quinolones is reduced by antacids by forming chelate complexes. Drug interactions of some fluoroquinolones with other drugs (Table 2) can induce toxic adverse drug reactions such as enhanced CNS toxicity in connection with theophylline or caffeine as well as a prolonged half-life of the fluoroquinolones due to probenecid or cimetidine [6–8, 10–13, 15, 16, 27, 28].

Clinical Symptoms of Adverse Drug Reactions to Quinolones

In recent years much information has accumulated concerning adverse drug reactions that may occur during treatment with quinolones. The number of spontaneously reported adverse drug reactions does not necessarily indicate the true incidence rate because the frequency of reporting is affected by various factors such as public awareness of the drug or drug group and the physician's familiarity with particular side effects. In addition, in many cases the causal relationship between the adverse reaction and the drug is questionable [12, 13].

Frequently, adverse reactions to quinolones involved the CNS with symptoms such as sleeping disorders, headaches, reversible psychotic reactions, hallucinations, and agitation. In addition, gastrointestinal complaints such as nausea, vomiting and diarrhea were noted (Table 3). Furthermore cutaneous symptoms, e.g., maculopapular rash and urticaria as well as vasculitis, were reported. A review of the literature regarding hypersensitivity reactions to quinolones also shows the possible risk of mild, and in rare cases, severe anaphylactoid reactions

Table 3. Adverse reactions to quinolones.

CNS symptoms:
Sleep disorders, insomnia, restlessness, headaches; impairment of vision, taste and smell; reversible psychotic reactions, hallucinations, agitation
Gastrointestinal complaints:
Nausea, vomiting, diarrhea, abdominal pain, gastric symptoms

Table 4. Review of the literature according to hypersensitivity reactions to quinolones.

Drug	Symptoms	Authors	Reference
Ciprofloxacin	Allergic interstitial nephritis	Rippelmeyer and Synhavsky	[23]
	Photoallergic bullous rash	Kaufmann et al.	[31]
	Vasculitis	Choe et al.	[2]
Enoxacin	Phototoxic/-allergic reaction	Schauder	[26]
	Photoallergic reaction	Kawabe	[14]
Ofloxacin	Vasculitis	Huminer	[9]

Table 5. Review of the literature according to hypersensitivity reactions to quinolones.

Drug	Symptoms (n)		Authors	Reference
Ciprofloxacin	Severe AR	(20)	Peters and Pinching	[17]
	Fatal AR	(3)		
	AR	(15)	Davis et al.	[3]
Cinoxacin	AR	(25)	Stricker et al.	[29]
Pipedemic acid	AR	(1)	Gerber	[5]
Ofloxacin	AR	(~60)	Jüngst and Mohr	[13]
Nalidixic acid	AR	(1)	Valdivieso	[30]

AR, anaphylactoid reaction.

Table 6. Anaphylactoid reaction to ofloxacin ($n = 33$).

Age	16–77 years	
Sex	15 men, 18 women	
AR after first tablet of the drug	$n = 26$	
Time interval to AR	$\leqslant 10$ min	(9)
	$\leqslant 30$ min	(10)
	$\leqslant 60$ min	(6)
	$\leqslant 4$ h	(4)
	not known	(4)
Prior oral exposition to quinolones	$n = 4$	

to different quinolones as well as phototoxic or photoallergic skin rashes [1–3, 5, 9, 12–14, 17, 26, 29–31, 33] (Tables 4, 5).

An analysis of 33 case histories of patients with anaphylactoid reactions in connection with oral administration of ofloxacin (age: 16–77 years; sex: 15 men, 18 women) showed that 26 patients had an immediate onset of symptoms after the first tablet was taken; 5 of the other 7 patients showed AR after the second or third tablet of ofloxacin while the other 2 reacted on the 5th day.

Most patients (19/29) showed an immediate onset (≤ 30 min) of symptoms after oral administration of the drug (Table 6).

Fourteen of these 33 patients reported taking other medication at the same time; only 4 patients had a history of previous oral administration of quinolones.

A personal history of atopy was found in 35% of the patients and former adverse reactions to other drugs in 25%. These data were reported spontaneously to the drug safety department of the manufacturer.

Diagnosis of Adverse Drug Reactions to Quinolones

The evaluation of adverse drug reactions to quinolones has to follow the general principles of allergy diagnosis, namely, a comprehensive case history, skin tests, in vitro methods, and oral provocation tests. The aim of these diagnostic procedures is to differentiate adverse drug reactions such as intoxication and pharmacological intolerance from pseudo-allergy or allergy (Table 7). The pharmacological intolerance is defined as a reaction with symptoms of "intoxication" after administration of a normal single dose of the drug. In contrast pseudo-allergic reactions represent a nonimmunologic hypersensitivity reaction with allergy-like symptoms [20–22].

Skin Test Results

Prick and intradermal tests with ofloxacin (brand name: Tarivid) and ciprofloxacin (brand name: Ciprobay) in previously nonexposed control individuals showed a high percentage of positive reactions. Even dilutions of Tarivid solution

Table 7. Definition of allergological terms.

Toxicity	Normal poisonousness
Allergy	Immunologic hypersensitivity
Intolerance	Hypersensitivity related to the normal pharmacologic effects
Idiosyncrasy	Nonimmunologic hypersensitivity (unrelated to pharmacologic effect)
Pseudo-allergy	Nonimmunologic hypersensitivity with "allergy-like" symptoms

Table 8. Skin tests with quinolones.

Substance	Prick	Scratch	I.D.
Tarivid tablet suspended in NaCl	6/11	3/4	n.d.
Tarivid solution undiluted	3/5	n.d.	n.d.
1:100	5/10	n.d.	8/10
1:1000	2/10	n.d.	8/10
1:10000	0/10	n.d.	0/10
Ciprobay solution undiluted	n.d.	n.d.	10/10
Ciprofloxacin suspended in NaCl	7/10	n.d.	n.d.
Ofloxacin suspended in NaCl	3/5	2/3	n.d.

I.D. = Intradermal; n.d. = not done.

(1 : 100 or 1 : 1000) evoked positive reactions in five or two controls, respectively, in the prick test and in 8 of 10 subjects in the intradermal test. Prick tests with a dilution $\geqslant$ 1 : 10000 showed no positive reactions in the control group. The other components of Tarivid tablets or solution were prick-test negative (Table 8).

The positive prick and intradermal test reactions may be due to toxic effects of the test solutions or by direct mediator release or other, yet unknown mechanisms. Because of these false-positive results skin testing with quinolones in patients with hypersensitivity reactions to quinolones have to be undertaken with high dilutions of the drug and evaluation of thresholds in comparison to controls.

In Vitro Techniques

Diagnostic test procedures in order to evaluate phototoxic or photoallergic reactions are photo patch test, photo basophil histamine release test, photohemolysis test, and systemic photoprovocation test.

We found that quinolones show autofluorescence in the ultraviolet A range, photo-induced inactivation of antimicrobial activity, as well as a possible photosensitizing potency in the photohemolysis test [1, 14, 18, 26].

Because quinolones are autofluorescent it was impossible to measure the release of histamine from basophil leukocytes using the spectrofluorometric assay in the autoanalyzer. Likewise radioimmunological measurement of released histamine was associated with methodological problems. Quinolones cross-reacted with the antibody in one radioimmunoassay KIT. In another RIA using chemical modification of histamine it was possible to measure histamine in the presence of quinolones.

Case Reports

Two patients, a 26-year-old woman (patient 1) and a 23-year-old man (patient 2) were referred to our department because of a suspected anaphylactoid reaction to Tarivid. Patient 1 had developed generalized urticaria, tachycardia and dizziness 1 – 2 min after taking the first tablet of Tarivid. She had received no other medication. She was diagnosed as atopic. She had a previous AR to the quinolone norfloxacin (brand name: Barazan) and an adverse drug reaction to doxycycline.

The second patient had suffered from generalized urticaria 30 min after oral administration of Tarivid. A prior exposure to quinolones was not known nor was there a history of adverse reactions to other drugs. The patient had noted, however, urticarial eruptions after bathing in warm water and after exercise (Table 9).

The prick tests in patient 1 showed positive reactions to aero and food allergens but no reaction to the drugs or their components. The single-blind, oral provocation test with 20 mg ofloxacin resulted in pruritus, flush, urticaria, tachycardia, dizziness, nausea, and dyspnea after 5 min while placebo elicited mild headache and chest pain after 30 min.

Table 9. Case reports: AR in relation to oral application of Tarivid.

	Patient 1 (woman, 26 years)	Patient 2 (men, 23 years)
Symptoms	Tachycardia, urticaria, dizziness	Urticaria
Time interval	1–2 min after 1st tablet	30 min after 5th tablet
Prior exposure to quinolones	AR to norfloxacin (Barazan)	?
Atopy	+	+
History of adverse reactions to other drugs	Norfloxacin (Barazan), doxycycline	–
Concomitant medication	None	None

AR, anaphylactoid reaction.

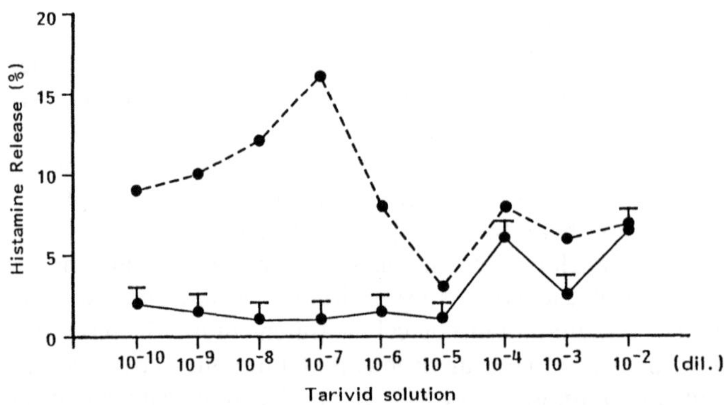

Fig. 3. Histamine release in a patient with anaphylactoid reaction to ofloxacin. *Solid line*, controls; *broken line*, patient

This patient showed an increased release of histamine from basophil leukocytes to Tarivid solution compared to the controls (Fig. 3).

In the other patient the diagnostic procedure resulted in the diagnosis of a cholinergic urticaria possibly enhanced by concomitant intake of ofloxacin in the sense of a "summation anaphylaxis".

In oral provocation tests with Tarivid in ten patients with AR to other antibiotics (single-blind, 20–100–200 mg Tarivid in gelatine capsules with a time interval of 2 h), only one patient reacted with mild subjective symptoms. This patient, however, also reacted when placebo was given.

Discussion

Quinolones are rather safe drugs with an incidence of adverse drug reactions between 2%–10% [12, 25]. AR to quinolones seem to be rare and mostly mild, but they exist [3, 5, 12, 13]. Severe or fatal AR to quinolones have been reported and

HIV patients may be at a higher risk to develop such reactions [3, 17, 25, 29, 30, 33]. The pathomechanisms of these reactions are not established [3, 5, 12, 13]. Some facts argue for possible pseudo-allergic mechanisms such as immediate onset of symptoms upon first contact with the drug and direct histamine release from skin mast cells but not from peripheral basophils. The relatively rare incidence of AR together with possible sensitization due to previous exposure to quinolones in at least some patients suggests an allergic mechanism.

Important factors influencing immune responses to antimicrobial drugs such as quinolones must be considered: the changes in activation of the immune system due to the bacterial infection at the time of exposure to the drug and due to the lysis of bacteria with a possible sudden release of endotoxins and other mediators [21, 22]. In addition, the quinolones may influence the immune system. So, ciprofloxacin has been reported to inhibit cell proliferation, immunoglobulin production and to increase the growth factor IL2 while reducing IL2 receptors on lymphocytes in vitro [4, 19, 24].

Quinolones seem to be direct mast cell activators, as measured by wheal and flare reactions after skin test procedures in healthy volunteers. In basophil leukocytes, this direct histamine release does not seem to occur. Therefore, this test might be suitable to detect actual IgE-mediated sensitization to quinolones in certain patients with anaphylactoid reactions.

A review of the literature revealed the possible risk of phototoxic or photoallergic skin eruptions as well as photoonycholysis by different quinolones. Diagnostic test procedures to evaluate such reactions are the photo patch test, photo basophil histamine release test, photohemolysis test and systemic photoprovocation test.

Presently, besides the carefully taken history, the oral provocation test is the only reliable procedure in the diagnostic evaluation of anaphylactoid reactions to quinolones. It should be considered that such a test entails a certain amount of risk and has to be undertaken in the hospital under emergency conditions.

References

1. Baran R, Brun P (1986) Photoonycholysis induced by the fluoroquinolones pefloxacine and ofloxacine. Dermatologica 173:185–188
2. Choe U, Rothschild BM, Laitman L (1989) Ciprofloxacin-induced vasculitis. N Engl J Med 257–258
3. Davis H, McGoodwin E, Reed TG (1989) Anaphylactoid reactions reported after treatment with ciprofloxacin. Ann Intern Med 111:1041–1043
4. Forsgren A, Bredberg A, Riesbeck K (1989) Effect of ciprofloxacin on human lymphocytes – laboratory findings. Scand J Infect Dis Suppl 60:39–45
5. Gerber D (1985) Anaphylaxis caused by pipemidic acid. S Afr M J 67:999
6. Gutzler F (1985) Gyrasehemmer – eine neue Klasse von Antibiotika. Inn Med 12:139–146
7. Harder S, Shah PM, Staib AH (1990) Gyrasehemmstoffe. Dtsch Med Wochenschr 115:270–273
8. Hooper DC, Wolfson JS (1985) The fluoroquinolones: pharmacological, clinical uses, and toxicities in humans. Antimicrob Agents Chemother 28:716–721
9. Huminer D, Cohen JD, Majadla R, Dux S (1989) Hypersensitivity vasculitis due to ofloxacin. Br Med J 299:303

10. Jack DB (1986) Recent advances in pharmaceutical chemistry. The 4-quinolone antibiotics. J Clin Hosp Pharm 11:75–93
11. Jaehde U, Sörgel F, Schunack W (1989) Pharmakokinetische Grundlagen der antimikrobiellen Therapie mit Gyrasehemmern. Pharm Ztg Wiss 134:171–177
12. Jüngst G, Mohr R (1987) Side effects of ofloxacin in clinical trials and in postmarketing surveillance. Drugs 34 [Suppl 1]:144–149
13. Jüngst G, Mohr R (1988) Overview of postmarketing experience with ofloxacin in Germany. J Antimicrob Chemother 22 [Suppl C]:167–175
14. Kawabe Y, Mizuno N, Sakakibara S (1989) Photoallergic reaction caused by enoxacin. Photodermatol 6:58–60
15. Lode H (1988) Chinolone. Schweiz Med Wochenschr 118:1823–1830
16. Paton JH, Reeves DS (1988) Fluoroquinolone antibiotics. Microbiology, pharmacocinetics and clinical use. Drugs 36:193–228
17. Peters B, Pinching AJ (1989) Fatal anaphylaxis associated with ciprofloxacin in a patient with AIDS related complex. Br Med J 198:605
18. Przybilla B, Georgii A, Bergner B, Ring J (1990) Demonstration of quinolone phototoxicity in vitro. Dermatologica 181:98–103
19. Riesbeck K, Andersson J, Gallberg M, Forsgren A (1989) Fluorinated 4-quinolones induce hyperproduction of interleukin 2. Proc Natl Acad Sci USA 86:2809–2813
20. Ring J (1987a) Anaphylaxis and anaphylactoid reactions. In: Baethmann A, Messmer K (eds) Surgical research: recent concepts and results. Springer, Berlin Heidelberg New York, pp 210–221
21. Ring J (1987b) Pseudo-allergische Arzneimittelreaktionen. In: Fuchs E, Schulz KH (eds) Manuale allergologicum. Dustri, München
22. Ring J (1988) Angewandte Allergologie, 2nd edn. Vieweg, München
23. Rippelmeyer DJ, Synhavsky A (1988) Ciprofloxacin and allergic interstitial nephritis. Ann Intern Med 110:866
24. Roche Y, Fay M, Gougerot-Polidalo M (1988) Enhancement of interleukin 2 production by quinolone-treated human mononuclear leukocytes. Int J Immunopharmacol 10:161–167
25. Schacht P, Arcieri G, Branotte J (1988) Worldwide clinical data on efficacy and safety of ciprofloxacin. Infection 16 [Suppl 1]:29–43
26. Schauder S (1990) Photosensitivität nach Enoxacin und Xipamid. Z Hautkr 65:253–262
27. Stahlmann R, Lode H (1987) Neuere Chinolonderivate zur Behandlung bakterieller Infektionen. Dtsch Apoth Ztg 127:541–546
28. Stein GE (1988) The 4-quinolone antibiotics: past, present, and future. Pharmacotherapy 8:301–314
29. Stricker BHC, Slagboom G, Demaeseneer R, Slootmaekers V, Thijs I, Olsson S (1988) Anaphylactic reactions to cinoxacin. Br Med J 297:1434–35
30. Valdivieso R, Pola J, Losada E, Subiza J, Armentia A, Zapata C (1988) Severe anaphylactoid reaction to nalidixic acid. Allergy 43:71–73
31. Wemmer U (1988) 46. Kölner Dermatologenabend der Universitäts-Hautklinik Köln am 25. November 1987. Kaufmann I, Hastigsputh C: Photoallergisches bullöses Lyell-artiges Arzneimittelexanthem nach Einnahme von Ciprofloxacin. Z Hautkr 63:681–690
32. Wise R, Lockley MR (1988) The pharmacocinetics of ofloxacin and a review of its tissue penetration. J Antimicrob Chemother 22 [Suppl C]:59–64
33. Wurtz RM, Abrams D, Becker S (1989) Anaphylactoid drug reactions to ciprofloxacin and rifampicin in HIV-infected patients. Lancet 1:955–956

Drug Induced Photosensitivity

E. Hölzle

Hautklinik der Heinrich-Heine-Universität Düsseldorf, Moorenstraße 5, W-4000 Düsseldorf 1, Federal Republic of Germany

Abstract

Photoreactions induced by drugs can be phototoxic, clinically characterized by erythema and whealing or an exaggerated sunburn reaction, or photoallergic showing eczematous dermatitis in a photodistribution. The term systemic chemical photosensitivity has been used for reactions which mechanisms are uncertain.

In phototoxicity cell alterations at the molecular level are induced by photoactivation of the sensitizer. Damage of DNA, cell membranes and lysosomes may occur. If oxygen is required, the reaction is designated photodynamic. In this process singlet oxygen, superoxide anion and hydroxy radical are generated as activated species. Benoxaprofen has been shown to induce such radicals. The photoaddition of a photosensitizer, e. g., psoralen, to DNA is non-photodynamic. Photoproducts of a photosensitizer, which can disrupt cell membranes, may also be generated in absence of oxygen. This may in part be the mechanism of tetracycline phototoxicity. In some instances, more than one mechanism may be involved, as has been shown for chlorpromazine.

Photoallergy requires reaction of a chemical with radiation (UVA) inducing an immune mechanism by which finally a type-IV-reaction is elicited. The method of choice to identify photoallergens is the photopatch test or, if this fails, provocative phototesting. An effort has been made to standardize substances and phototest procedures in multicenter studies in Scandinavia as well as in Germany, Switzerland and Austria. Most frequently identified photoallergic drugs are phenothiazines, nonsteroidal antiinflammatory drugs, sulfonamides and hydrochlorothiazide.

Distinction between phototoxic and photoallergic test reactions and many seemingly non-relevant reactions in the photopatch test represent as yet unsolved problems.

Introduction

Drug-induced photosensitivity is an adverse cutaneous response to the combined actions of a chemical (drug) and a physical (UV irradiation) agent. The mechanism can be either phototoxic or photoallergic. Many topical agents are known

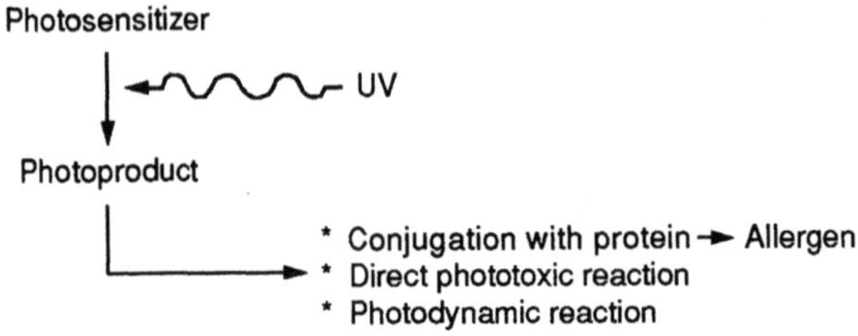

Fig. 1. Mechanisms of photosensitization

to induce photoreactions. Coal tar, acridine dyes, and furocoumarins in plants are examples of topical phototoxic compounds; disinfectants, UV absorbers, and fragrances are frequently the cause of allergic photocontact reactions. The present article emphasizes photosensitization by systemic drugs.

The concept that systemic agents induce both phototoxic and photoallergic reactions is not unequivocally accepted. Some authors [1] feel that systemic drugs react mainly as phototoxic compounds. The term systemic chemical photosensitivity has been used for reactions whose mechanisms are uncertain [2]. In the following, evidence is provided that systemic agents can indeed act by photoallergic mechanisms.

The role of the photosensitizer is to absorb UV energy, in most cases UV-A, thereby undergoing a photochemical reaction to form a photoproduct. This photoproduct can conjugate with a protein to give rise to a photoallergen, or it induces photosensitive damage to DNA, proteins, or membrane structures of the cell. Phototoxicity occurs either by direct reaction of the photosensitizer with a biological substrate or by indirect mechanisms. If oxygen is required in the process of photosensitization, the reaction is termed photodynamic (Fig. 1).

Phototoxicity

Mechanisms

In the direct photoreaction the photosensitizer acquires an excited state by absorption of UV energy and directly undergoes a photochemical reaction with the biological substrate. Examples of this mechanism are DNA damage by psoralens and chlorpromazine. In indirect photoreactions photooxidation plays an important role. Two mechanisms (type I and type II) have been described [3, 4]. In type I photooxidation the excited triplet state of the photosensitizer reacts with the substrate by either electron or hydrogen transfer. Toxic radicals are thus formed. Membrane damage by chlorpromazine and acridine dyes are examples of this mechanism. Type II photooxidation involves energy transfer from the triplet state of the sensitizer to molecular oxygen, creating active oxygen species. These comprise singlet oxygen, superoxide anion, and hydroxy radical. Membrane damage caused by protoporphyrin and chlorpromazine probably occurs by this mechanism. Chlorpromazine is an example of photosensitizers acting via different mechanisms. There is also ample evidence that, in psoralen phototoxicity, several mechanisms, in addition to direct DNA damage, are involved [5]. The most relevant phototoxic drugs are:

Psoralens
Tetracyclines
Nalidixic acid
Furosemide
Amiodarone
Benoxaprofen
Piroxicam
Carprofen
Tiaprofenic acid
Sufanilamide
Chlorpromazine

Chlorpromazine, some of the nonsteroidal anti-inflammatory drugs, and sulfanilamide may also cause photoallergic reactions.

Clinicopathologic Features

Clinical features of phototoxic reactions are immediate whealing of the skin accompanied by a burning sensation or a delayed reaction with erythema and formation of vesicles or blisters; this is followed by pigmentation. Immediate responses occur in erythropoietic protoporphyria, induced by activation of protoporphyrin in the skin, and in tar phototoxicity. The characteristic delayed phototoxic reaction mimicking exaggerated sunburn is induced by psoralens and tetracyclines. Nonsteroidal anti-inflammatory drugs may combine both immediate and delayed reactions. Examples of hyperpigmentation are berloque dermatitis and amiodarone-induced pigmentation. The active wavelengths in phototoxic reactions are mainly in the UV-A range, but sometimes also in the UV-B.

Examples of Drug-Induced Phototoxicity

Tetracyclines and amiodarone typically cause drug-induced phototoxicity.

Tetracyclines may induce phototoxic onycholysis in addition to a sunburn-like reaction (Fig. 2). The mechanism of onycholysis is not quite clear. In some cases it is the only feature of phototoxicity. The mechanisms of tetracycline phototoxicity include oxygen-dependent membrane damage, DNA damage [6, 7], and probably activation of the complement system [8]. Tetracyclines differ greatly in their phototoxic potential. Demeclocycline and doxycycline are highly phototoxic, chlortetracycline, methacycline, tetracycline, and oxytetracycline are intermediately active, and minocycline virtually lacks phototoxicity. This rank order is derived from clinical experience as well as from in vitro studies [9].

Amiodarone is the drug of choice in some patients with severe ventricular arrhythmias. Side effects of the drug involve various organ systems. Adverse cutane-

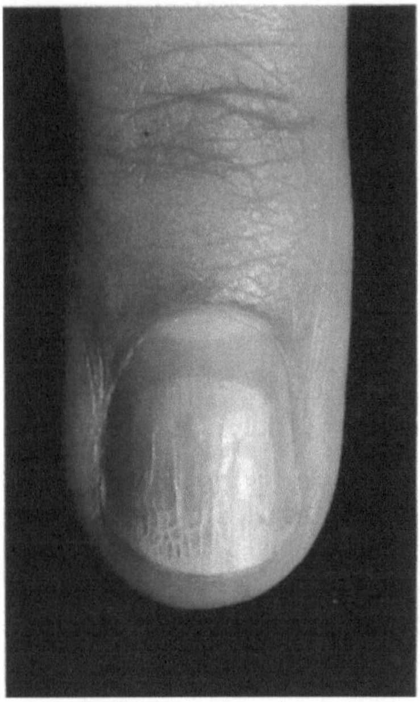

Fig. 2. Onycholysis following medication with doxycycline

ous reactions include phototoxicity and hyperpigmentation. In 30% – 50% of patients, a phototoxic reaction with immediate erythema, edema, and itching or burning has been reported [10]. The erythema might last for 1 or 2 days. This time course and the phototoxic nature of the reaction were demonstrated in one patient with suspected phototoxicity to amiodarone by phototesting her while she was still under medication (Fig. 3 A, B). Irradiation with 60 J/cm^2 UV-A (330 – 460 nm) induced brisk immediate erythema, edema, and burning. The erythema faded slowly over a period of 3 days. Histopathologic examination of a skin specimen 24 h after irradiation revealed a phototoxic reaction with dyskeratotic epidermal cells, vacuolar alteration of the basal layer, and a sparse, superficial, dermal infiltrate. The typical features of a fully developed phototoxic reaction are:

Dyskeratotic cells
Vacuolar alteration
Subepidermal edema
Sparse mononuclear infiltrate in superficial dermis, sometime neutrophils

The pathogenesis of amiodarone phototoxicity involves direct membrane damage and the formation of a phototoxic photoproduct, desethylamiodarone [11].

About 10% of patients [12] develop, in addition to phototoxicity or, rarely, independently, hyperpigmentation in light-exposed areas (Fig. 4). A greyish blue slate color is characteristic. Intracellular deposits of amiodarone, lipofuscin, and melanin are probably responsible for the discoloration [13]. Recently, intracellular phospholipid membranes were also observed by ultrastructural investigations [14].

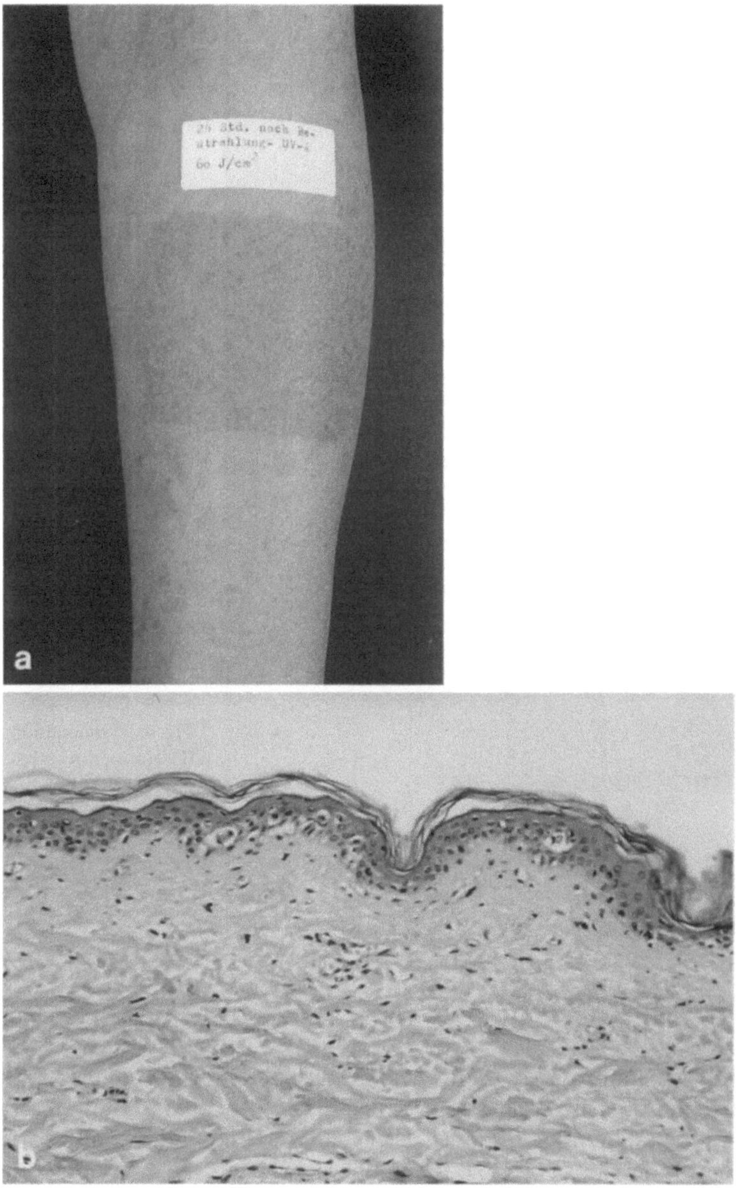

Fig. 3a, b. Provocative phototesting in a patient under medication with amiodarone. **a** Delayed erythema 24 h after 60 J/cm^2 UV-A. **b** Histopathology revealed a phototoxic reaction with dyskeratoses, vacuolar alteration, and a sparse dermal infiltrate

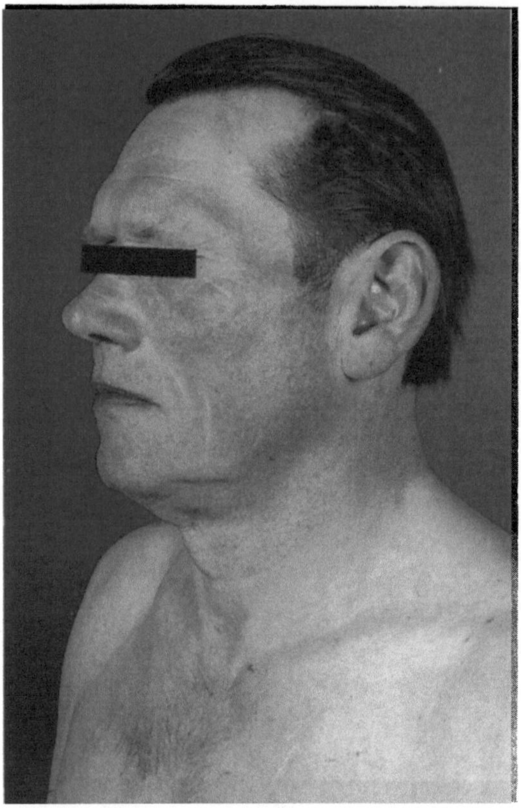

Fig. 4. Pigmentation in a photodistribution in a patient taking amiodarone

Photoallergy

Mechanism

It is generally agreed upon that, by absorption of UV energy, a photoproduct of the photosensitizer is formed which binds to a protein, thus creating the allergen. A type IV immune response is elicited and, upon reexposure, an eczematous dermatitis develops [15–17]. In animal experiments the active wavelengths for induction of systemic photosensitivity were shown to be in the UV-A and UV-B ranges for sulfanilamide and chlorpromazine [18] and in the UV-A range only for quinidine [19]. Elicitation is virtually always induced by UV-A. The most relevant systemic drugs capable of inducing photoallergic reactions are:

Chlorpromazine
Promethazine
Piroxicam
Carprofen
Tiaprofenic acid
Quinidine
Hydrochlorothiazide
Sulfanilamide

Clinicopathologic Features

The characteristic clinical picture in systemic photoallergy is eczematous dermatitis in a photodistribution. The dermatitis comprises erythema, dermal infiltrate, scaling, and eventually papulovesicles (Fig. 5). In a chronic course lichenification predominates. Itching is always present and may be incapacitating in chronic lichenified photodermatitis. Histopathology reveals spongiotic dermatitis with a superficial and sometimes deep dermal perivascular infiltrate of mononuclear cells and some eosinophils. The main histopathologic criteria are:

Parakeratosis
Akanthosis, spongiosis, exocytosis
Superficial and deep perivascular infiltrate of mononuclear cells, sometimes eosinophils

Diagnostic Procedures

To investigate a patient with suspected systemic photosensitivity, phototesting, a photopatch test, and systemic photochallenge are employed.

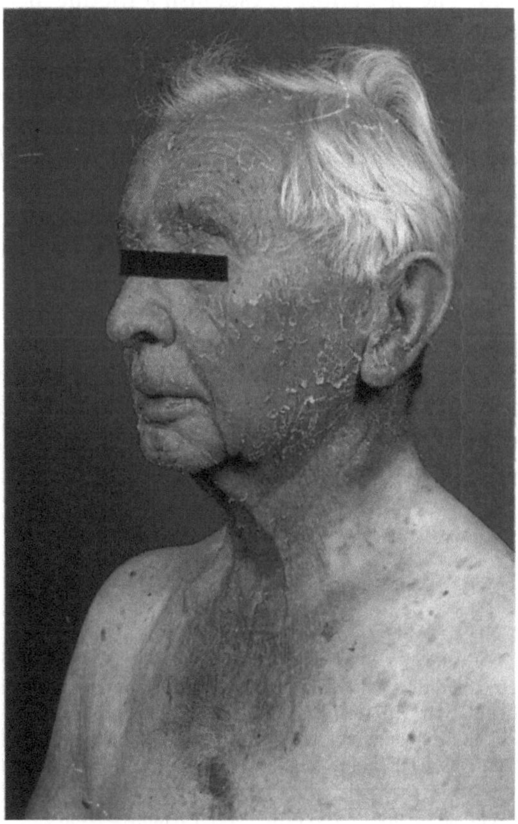

Fig. 5. Photoallergic dermatitis following intake of quinidine. Erythema, a dermal infiltrate, and scaling are the main features

Phototesting

Phototesting procedures in the work-up of a patient with suspected photosensitivity have been established previously [20, 21]. In a patient with alleged drug-induced photosensitivity, determination of the minimal erythema dose (MED) for UV-B and UV-A irridiation and provocative phototesting with UV-A and UV-B should be performed. The MED UV-B and UV-A are normal in patients with photoallergic dermatitis. Provocative UV-A phototesting may induce dermatitis in test areas of uninvolved skin, if the photosensitizer is present in the skin at the time of irradiation. This requires that a patient still be under medication. Lowered MEDs, photosensitivity to UV-A and/or UV-B, in terms of provoking spongiotic dermatitis in test areas in the absence of the photosensitizer, are features of persistent light reactivity and belong to the chronic actinic dermatitis disease spectrum [22].

Photopatch Test

The photopatch test is the method of choice to investigate suspected photosensitizers in a patient. Until the early 1980s photopatch testing was not standardized. The first effort to establish a routine method was initiated by the Scandinavian Photodermatitis Research Group in 1982 [23]. Following this example we coordinated 45 dermatological hospitals, including most major dermatological centers in West Germany, Austria, and Switzerland, in 1984 into a Photopatch Test Group [24]. The procedure was standardized with respect to: (a) test materials, concentration of test substances, and vehicles; (b) mode and schedule of application, irradiation, and reading; (c) evaluation of test reactions and their interpretation; and (d) irradiation source and exposure doses. The method is outlined in Table 1. The standard tray of test materials included 32 substances. These as well as test concentrations are shown in Table 2.

Recently, the first 1129 patients tested between 1985 and 1990 were evaluated [25]. Analyzing the test reactions with respect to their quality and time course, it was possible to establish reaction patterns which allowed distinction between phototoxic and photoallergic mechanisms in many patients. By this approach only 108 photoallergic test reactions in 83 patients, out of 2859 positive test reactions in 1129 patients, were identified.

Frequent photoallergens are listed in Table 3. Among the drugs, nonsteroidal anti-inflammatory agents and phenothiazines are most frequently identified as

Table 1. Method of photopatch testing.

Test materials applied via Finn Chambers to the back skin for 24 h
Irradiation with 10 J/cm^2 UV-A (320–400 nm)
Reading immediately and 24, 48, and 72 h later
Controls: Unirradiated patch test UV-A irradiation on untreated skin

Proposal of the Photopatch Test Working Group.

Table 2. Photopatch test substances.

Substance	Concentration[a] (%)
Tetrachlorsalicylanilide	0.10
Bromsalicylchloranilide	1.00
Tribromsalicylanilide	1.00
Buclosamide	5.00
Fentichlor	1.00
Hexachlorophene	1.00
Bithionol	1.00
Triclosan	2.00
Sulfonilamide	5.00
Chlorpromazine	0.10
Promethazine	1.00
Carprofen	5.00
Tiaprofenic acid	5.00
Quinidine	1.00
Musk ambrette	5.00
Musk mix	5.00
Perfume mix	8.00
6-Methylcoumarin	1.00
Paraaminobenzoic acid	5.00
Chlorothiazide	1.00
Furosemide	1.00
2-Hydroxy-4-methoxybenzophenone	2.00
3-(4-Methylbenzylidene)-camphor	5.00
4-Isopropyldibenzoylmethane	5.00
Cyclamate	1.25
Saccharin	0.40
Wood tar	3.00
Colophony	20.00
Balsam of Peru	25.00
Compositae mix	6.50
Tolbutamide	5.00
Thiourea	0.10

[a] In white petrolatum.

Table 3. Frequent photoallergens.

Nonsteroidal anti-inflammatory drugs	Tiaprofenic acid
	Carprofen
Phenothiazines	Promethazine
	Chlorpromazine
Disinfectants	Fentichlor
	Tetrachlorsalicylanilide
	Bithionol
Sunscreens	Eusolex 8020[a]
	Benzophenone
Fragrances	Musk ambrette[b]
	Perfume mixture[c]

[a] 4-Isopropyldibenzoylmethane.

[b] synthetic fragrance, mainly in men's perfumes.

[c] as recommended by the International Contact Dermatitis Research Group.

photoallergens. Topical agents gaining increasing importance as photoallergens are disinfectants, UV absorbers in sunscreens and other cosmetic products, and fragrances.

Evaluation of photopatch test results may often be difficult. Many nonspecific phototoxic reactions can occur, and distinction between phototoxic and photoallergic test reactions cannot always be made with certainty.

In addition, some seemingly photoallergic test reactions lack clinical relevance for the patient and, especially with systemic drugs, false-negative results may occur. This might be due to insufficient penetration of the test material through the stratum corneum barrier. It is also possible that only a metabolite of the drug acts as the photosensitizer. In the first case, modification of the photopatch test with application of the test materials to scarified skin might be useful. The procedure is known as the photoprick or photoscratch test [26]. The method is, however, not standardized and experience is scarce. If the drug has to be metabolized in order to create the photosensitizer, the only way to demonstrate photosensitivity to this drug is systemic photochallenge. This approach might also be helpful in evaluating the significance of an unexpectedly positive photopatch test reaction.

Systemic Photochallenge

In principle, the medication is administered in the usual way, and, at different time points thereafter, various test areas on noninvolved skin are irradiated with UV-A. The method is outlined in Table 3. If the skin is irradiated when the photosensitizing compound is present in the skin (this depends largely on the pharmacokinetics of the drug), a positive reaction is evoked which can be read on successive days depending on the time course of the reaction. Criteria for a positive result are erythema, infiltration, papulovesicles, and itching. Delayed pigmentation may be an indication of phototoxic or photoallergic reactions on a subclinical level. In this respect late readings, 1 or 2 weeks after the experiment, might be helpful.

Histopathologic examination of test reactions is a valuable aid in establishing a correct diagnosis. If a spongiotic dermatitis is revealed histopathologically, a photoallergic mechanism seems to be the most likely explanation and further suggests systemically induced photoallergy [27].

Conclusions

Drugs can induce both phototoxic and photoallergic reactions. The clinicopathologic features of these two types of systemic photosensitivity are usually distinct. Important newcomers among the photoallergic substances are nonsteroidal anti-inflammatory agents and, as topical agents, UV absorbers in sunscreens. Diagnostic procedures to identify photosensitizers are the photopatch test and systemic photoprovocation. Photopatch testing is currently being standardized and optimized. New developments include the photoprick or photoscratch tests; however, experience with these procedures is limited.

References

1. Frain-Bell W (1985) Cutaneous photobiology. Oxford University Press, Oxford, pp 125–152
2. Bernhard JD, Pathak MA, Kochevar IE, Parrish JA (1987) Abnormal reactions to ultraviolet radiation. In: Fitzpatrick TB, Eisen AZ, Wolff K, Freedberg IM, Austen KF (eds) Dermatology in general medicine. McGraw-Hill, New York, pp 1481–1507
3. Gollnick K (1968) Type II photooxygenation reactions in solution. Adv Photochem 6:1–122
4. Foote CS (1976) Photosensitized oxidation and singlet oxygen: consequences in biological systems. In: Pryor WA (ed) Free radicals in biology, vol 2. Academic, New York, pp 85–133
5. Dall'Acqua F (1986) Furocoumarin photochemistry and its main biological implications. In: Hönigsmann H, Stingl G (eds) Therapeutic photomedicine. Karger, Basel, pp 137–163
6. Kochevar IE (1987) Mechanisms of drug photosensitization. Photochem Photobiol 45:891–895
7. Schothorst AA, Suurmond D, deLuster A (1979) A biochemical screening test for the photosensitizing potential of drugs and disinfectants. Photochem Photobiol 29:531
8. Lim HW, Nowotny H, Gigli I (1983) Role of complement and polymorphonuclear cells in demethylchlortetracycline-induced phototoxicity in guinea pigs. J Clin Invest 71:1326–1335
9. Hasan T, Kochevar IE, McAuliffe DJ, Coopermann BS, Abdulah D (1984) Mechanism of tetracycline phototoxicity. J Invest Dermatol 83:179–183
10. Harris L, McKenna W, Rowland E, Krikler DM (1983) Side effects and possible contraindications of amiodarone use. Am Heart J 106:916–923
11. Hasan T, Kochevar IE, Abdulah D (1984) Amiodarone phototoxicity to human erythrocytes and lymphocytes. Photochem Photobiol 40:715–719
12. Korting HC, Kolz R, Schmoeckel C, Balda BR (1981) Amiodaronepigmentierung. Eine seltene, aber typische Medikamentnebenwirkung. Hautarzt 32:301–305
13. Miller RAW, McDonald ATJ (1984) Dermal lipofuscinosis associated with amiodarone therapy. Arch Dermatol 120:646–649
14. Waitzer S, Butany J, From L, Hanna W, Ramsay C, Downar E (1987) Cutaneous ultrastructural changes and photosensitivity associated with amiodarone therapy. J Am Acad Dermatol 16:779–787
15. Harber LC, Harris H, Baer RL (1966) Structural features of photoallergy to salicylanilides and related compounds. J Invest Dermatol 46:303–305
16. Harber LC, Harris H, Baer R (1966) Photoallergic contact dermatitis. Arch Dermatol 94:255–262
17. Kato S, Seki T, Katsumura Y et al. (1985) Mechanism for 6-methylcoumarin photoallergenicity. Toxicol Appl Pharmacol 81:295–301
18. Giudici PA, Maguire HC (1985) Experimental photoallergy to systemic drugs. J Invest Dermatol 85:207–209
19. Wirestrand L-E, Ljunggren B (1988) Photoallergy to systemic quinidine in the mouse. Acta Derm Venereol (Stockh) 68:41–47
20. Lehmann P, Hölzle E, von Kries R, Plewig G (1986) Lichtdiagnostische Verfahren bei Patienten mit Verdacht auf Photodermatosen. Zentralbl Hautkr 152:667–682
21. Hölzle E, Plewig G, Lehmann P (1987) Photodermatoses – diagnostic procedures and their interpretation. Photodermatol 4:109–114
22. Norris PG, Hawk JLM (1990) Chronic actinic dermatitis: a unifying concept. Arch Dermatol 126:376–378
23. Jansen CT, Wennersten G, Rysted I, Thune P, Brodthagen H (1982) The Scandinavian standard photopatch test procedure. Contact Dermatitis 8:155–158
24. Lehmann P (1990) Die Deutschsprachige Arbeitsgemeinschaft Photopatch-Test (DAPT). Hautarzt 41:295–297
25. Hölzle E, Neumann N, Hausen B, Przybilla B, Schauder S, Hönigsmann H, Bircher A, Plewig G (1991) Photopatch testing: a five-year experience of the German, Austrian and Swiss Photopatch Test Group. J Am Acad Dermatol (in press)
26. Schauder S (1990) Photodiagnostik: Der modifizierte intradermale Test im Vergleich zu anderen Verfahren zum Nachweis von phototoxischen und photoallergischen Arzneireaktionen. Z Hautkr 65:247–255
27. Lehmann P, Hölzle E, Plewig G (1988) Photoallergie auf Neotri und Kreuzreaktion auf Teneretic – Nachweis durch systemische Photoprovokation. Hautarzt 39:38–41

Angiotensin Peptides and Anaphylaxis *

K. Hermann[1], R. Rittweger[1], and J. Ring[2]

[1] Dermatologische Klinik und Poliklinik der Ludwig-Maximilians Universität München, Frauenlobstrasse 9–11, W-8000 München, Federal Republic of Germany
[2] Universitäts-Hautklinik und Allergie-Abteilung, Universitäts-Krankenhaus Eppendorf, Martinistrasse 52, W-2000 Hamburg 20, Federal Republic of Germany

Abstract

Angiotensin I and angiotensin II were measured in the plasma of patients with hymenoptera venom allergy (n = 50) and in controls (n = 21). The plasma concentrations of angiotensin I and angiotensin II were significantly lower in patients with hymenoptera venom allergy than in controls. (Angiotensin I, 9.52±0.62 vs 23.10±1.81 fmol/ml, $p<0.001$; angiotensin II, 2.84±0.16 vs 7.13±0.37 fmol/ml, $p<0.001$; mean±SEM). An inverse correlation between the plasma concentrations of angiotensin I and angiotensin II and the severity of clinical symptoms was observed. The immunoreactive material could be characterized on high performance liquid chromatography (HPLC) as Ile^5-angiotensin I, Ile^5-angiotensin II, and angiotensin II metabolites.

In human urine from healthy volunteers, angiotensin I and angiotensin II were detectable. Immunoreactive angiotensin I and angiotensin II could be characterized on HPLC as Ile^5-angiotensin I, Ile^5-angiotensin II, and angiotensin II metabolites. In patients suffering from anaphylactic reactions to drugs, food, or food additives, angiotensin I and angiotensin II were increased 2- to 12-fold in the urine after oral provocation (n = 15). The increase in the urine fractions was associated with clinical symptoms of anaphylaxis. However, oral provocation with a placebo failed to elicit anaphylactic symptoms or an increase in the levels of angiotensin I and angiotensin II (n = 7).

These findings suggest a possible involvement of angiotensin peptides in anaphylactic reactions.

Introduction

Anaphylaxis is a term which describes an acute generalized complex of symptoms which can affect cutaneous, cardiovascular, respiratory, or gastrointestinal functions. Anaphylactic reactions are immunologically mediated with an established role of IgE initiating the cascade of events. Mast cells or basophils carrying IgE on their cell membranes release vasoactive, chemotactic, and inflammatory medi-

* This work was supported by the Deutsche Forschungsgemeinschaft, Bonn, West Germany.

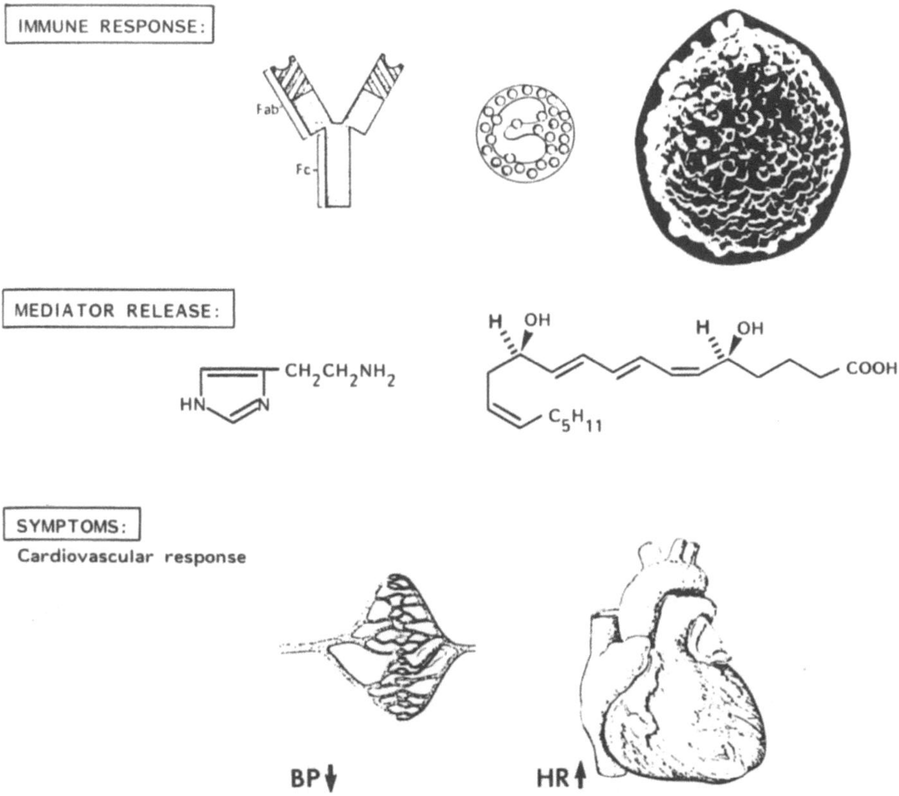

Fig. 1. The 3 steps involved in the manifestation of anaphylactic reactions. Independent of the participation of the immune systems, the release of vasoactive, chemotactic, or inflammatory mediators can induce clinical symptoms of anaphylaxis, such as impaired cardiovascular functions with a drop in blood pressure and a concomitant increase in heart rate as well as impaired respiratory, cutaneous, or gastrointestinal functions

ators after binding and bridging with allergens. The same symtoms in the absence of an antigen-antibody reaction are known as pseudo-allergic anaphylactoid reactions. Independent of the mechanism involved, the final step in the sequence of events that occurs during anaphylaxis is impaired function of the cutaneous, cardiovascular, respiratory, or gastrointestinal system (Fig. 1).

Anaphylaxis is a severe clinical problem in allergology. Clinical symptoms of anaphylaxis, with life threatening conditions, can occur in patients with hymenoptera venom allergy or in patients with adverse reactions to drugs, food, or food additives. An involvement of the immune system in anaphylactic reactions induced by hymenoptera venom has been established. However, there is no convincing correlation between the degree of immunological sensitization or skin test reactivity and the severity of clinical symptoms [6, 7]. The mechanisms involved in anaphylactoid reactions to drugs or food additives are still unclear but are most likely independent of the immune system. The patients are characterized by negative skin tests and a lack of specific antibodies against these agents. Based on history, skin tests, and in vitro tests, such as the releasability of histamine from leukocytes and the determination of immunological parameters, it is difficult to predict whether these patients will develop clinical symptoms of anaphylaxis after exposure to these agents.

The clinically relevant factors might therefore be found in the regulatory mechanisms counteracting the effects of vasoactive mediators to maintain homeostasis in blood pressure. Blood pressure, fluid, and electrolyte homeostasis are regulated by the renin angiotensin system (RAS). In addition, it has also been shown that the RAS is involved in conditions of stress and hemorrhage [3, 4]. This prompted us to study the putative role of angiotensin peptides in patients with anaphylactic reactions due to hymenoptera venom, drugs, food, or food additives.

Plasma Angiotensin in Hymenoptera Venom Allergy

It has been shown that anaphylactic reactions to hymenoptera venom are IgE mediated. Elevated levels of IgE to either bee or wasp venom have been identified in the serum of patients with hymenoptera venom allergy. Most of the patients show wheal and flare reactions in the skin prick test after application of bee or wasp venom. Basophil leukocytes, isolated from their blood, release histamine when incubated with bee or wasp venom in vitro [5, 6]. Despite these facts, prediction of the severity of the clinical symptoms after exposure to bee or wasp venom is still difficult. So far, no convincing correlation between the degree of immunological sensitization, as measured by RAST, skin test reactivity, or in vitro releasability of histamine from basophil leukocytes has been established [6]. This indicates that factors other than immunological parameters may be involved. It is possible to speculate that the patients possess a disturbance in their cardiovascular systems and are therefore unable to counteract the symptoms of anaphylaxis.

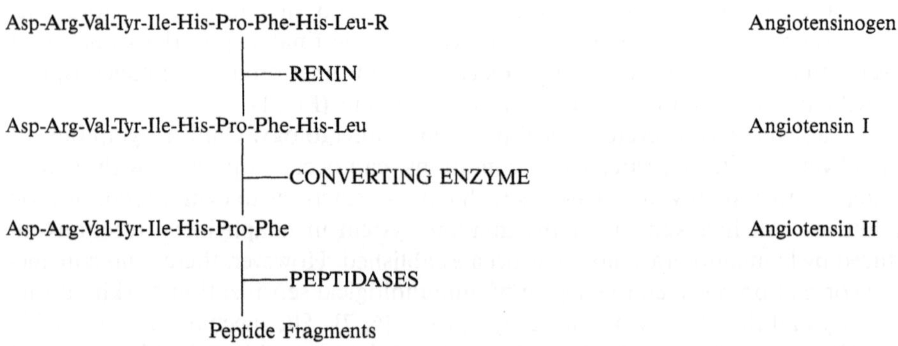

Fig. 2. Components of the renin angiotensin system

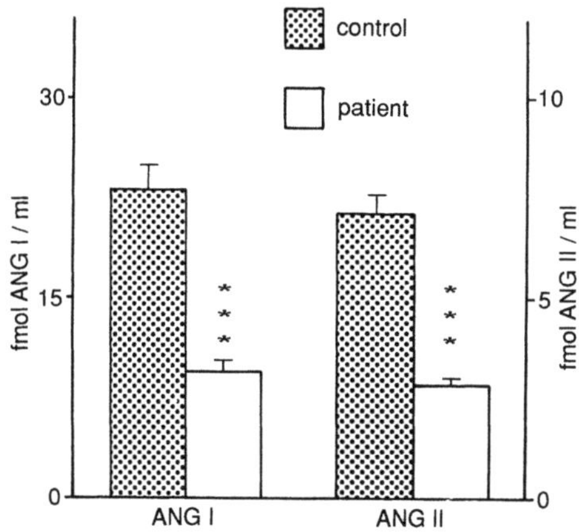

Fig. 3. Plasma concentrations of ANG I and ANG II in controls and patients with hymenoptera venom allergy. Patients with hymenoptera venom allergy showed significantly lower plasma concentrations of ANG I and ANG II than controls. Results are expressed as mean ± SEM in fmol peptide per ml; $***p<0.001$

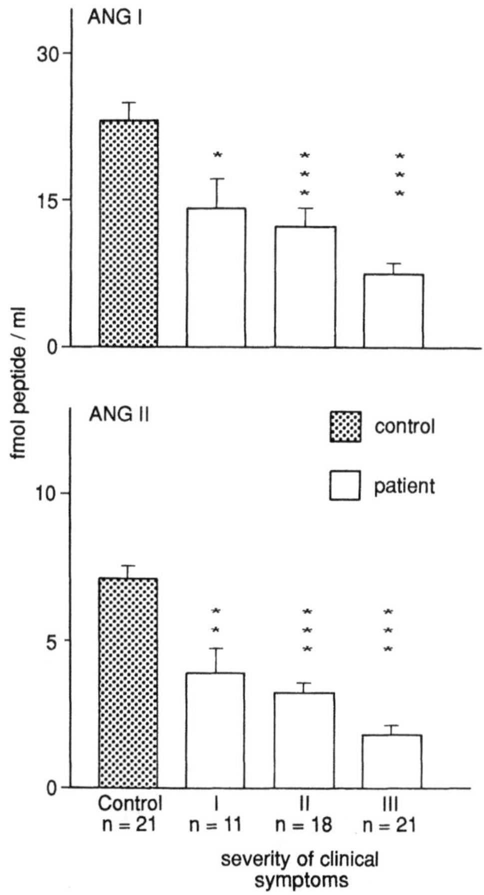

Fig. 4. Relation between the severity of clinical symptoms and the plasma levels of ANG I and ANG II in controls and patients with hymenoptera venom allergy. Results are expressed as mean ± SEM in fmol peptide per ml; $*p<0.01$, $**p<0.002$, $***p<0.001$

Normal cardiovascular function under physiological conditions is regulated by complex mechanisms including humoral and neuronal factors. One of these regulatory factors is the RAS. Angiotensin II (ANG II) is generated in a biochemical cascade, in which renin cleaves angiotensin I (ANG I) from the high molecular weight precursor angiotensinogen. ANG I is biologically inactive and needs to be activated by converting enzyme to form ANG II. ANG II is degraded by peptidases to biologically inactive fragments (Fig. 2) and is a potent vasoconstrictor. In addition, ANG II influences the activity of the central and peripheral sympathetic nervous system and stimulates the secretion of aldosterone from the adrenal gland.

The measurement of ANG I and ANG II in plasma of patients with hymenoptera venom allergy and controls revealed significant differences between both groups. Patients ($n = 50$) showed significantly lower plasma levels of ANG I and ANG II than controls ($n = 21$) (ANG I, 9.52 ± 0.62 vs 23.10 ± 1.81 fmol/ml, $p < 0.001$, ANG II, 2.84 ± 0.16 vs 7.13 ± 0.37 fmol/ml, $p < 0.001$; mean ± SEM) (Fig. 3). Compared to the controls, the concentrations of ANG I and ANG II in patients were inversely correlated with the severity of clinical symptoms. A significant reduction in the levels of ANG I and ANG II was noted with increased severity of clinical symptoms (Fig. 4). High performance liquid chromatography (HPLC) characterization of the immunoreactive ANG I and ANG II showed the presence of Ile⁵-ANG I, Ile⁵-ANG II, and ANG II metabolites (Fig. 5).

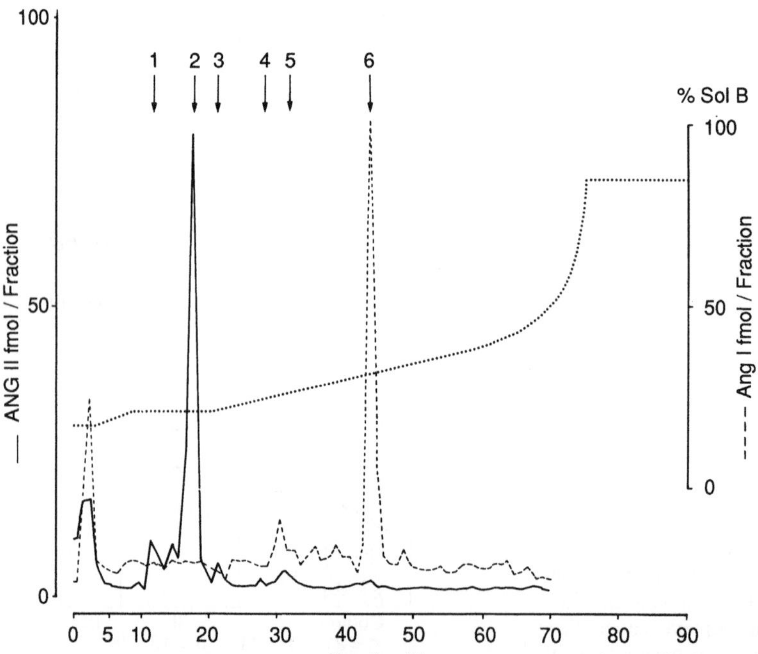

Fig. 5. HPLC characterization of ANG I and ANG II extracted from plasma on a reversed phase C_{18} column in an acetonitrile gradient. Ile^5-ANG I, Ile^5-ANG II, and ANG II metabolites were identified. *1*, Ile^1-ANG II$_{5-8}$tetrapeptide; *2*, Ile^5-ANG II; *3*, Ile^2-ANG II$_{4-8}$pentapeptide; *4*, Ile^3-ANG II$_{3-8}$hexapeptide; *5*, Ile^4-ANG III; *6*, Ile^5-ANG I

Urine Angiotensin in Anaphylactoid Reactions to Drugs, Food, and Food Additives

The diagnosis of allergic reactions with clinical symptoms of anaphylaxis associated with drugs, food, food additives, or other chemicals is still a major problem. Food allergies are IgE mediated as indicated by positive skin tests and the identification of specific antibodies in the patient's serum. In contrast, some drugs and other chemicals can induce anaphylactoid symptoms in the absence of an antigen-antibody reaction. The mechanisms of these reactions are by no means established and are therefore regarded as pseudo-allergic in origin. The symptoms mimic those of allergic reactions without evidence of immunological sensitization. Thus far, a reliable and reproducible diagnostic test does not exist. Since skin tests are mostly negative or not conclusive and specific antibodies can not be detected, the only approach for the diagnosis of this type of anaphylactoid reaction is the patient's history and provocation tests.

ANG II and its precursor ANG I are circulating plasma peptides involved in blood pressure control and regulation of water and electrolyte balance. So far, angiotensin peptides have been described in dog urine but, to our knowledge, not in human urine [2]. In order to avoid invasive diagnostic procedures, we decided to measure ANG I and ANG II in the urine of these patients as a biochemical parameter.

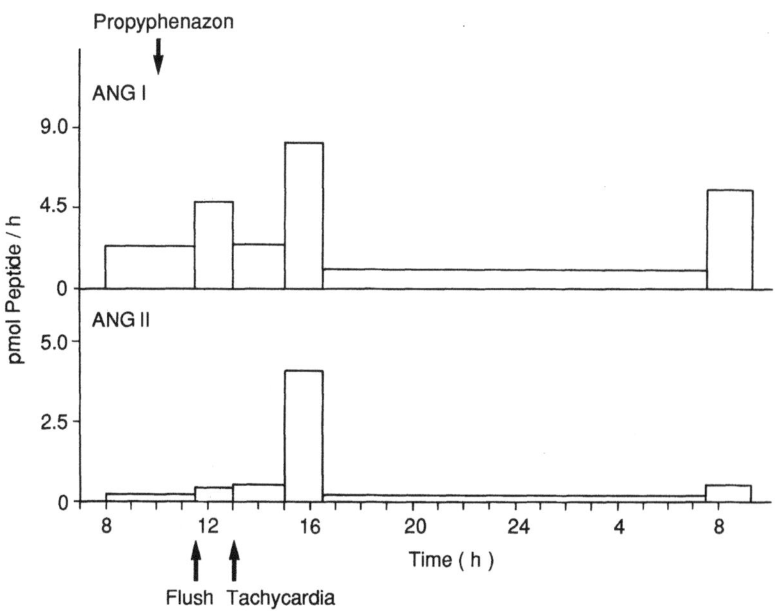

Fig. 6. Urinary excretion profile of ANG I and ANG II in a patient after oral provocation with propyphenazone. Within 2–3 h after the application of a single dose, the patient reported flush and tachycardia, which were associated with a marked increase in ANG I and ANG II in the subsequent urine fractions

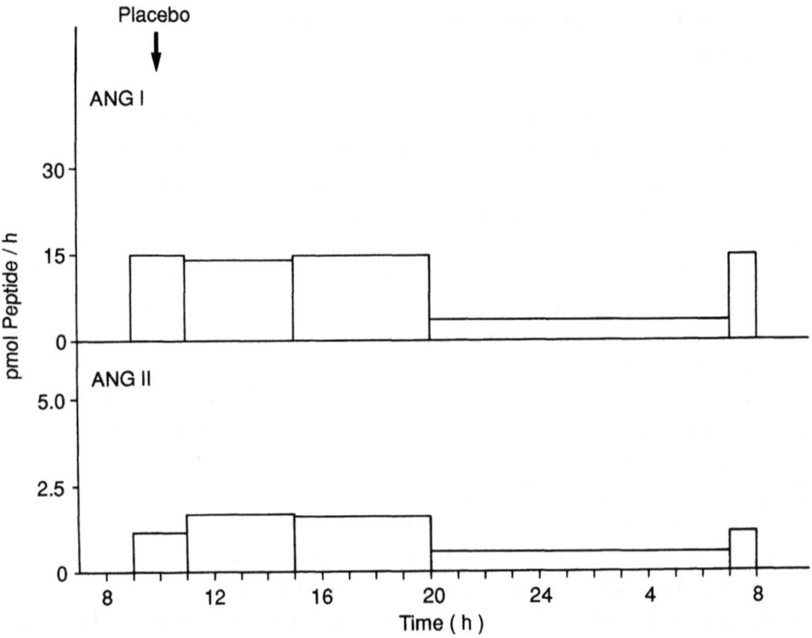

Fig. 7. Urinary excretion profile of ANG I and ANG II in a patient after oral provocation with a placebo. No anaphylactoid symptoms and no increase in ANG I or ANG II were observed

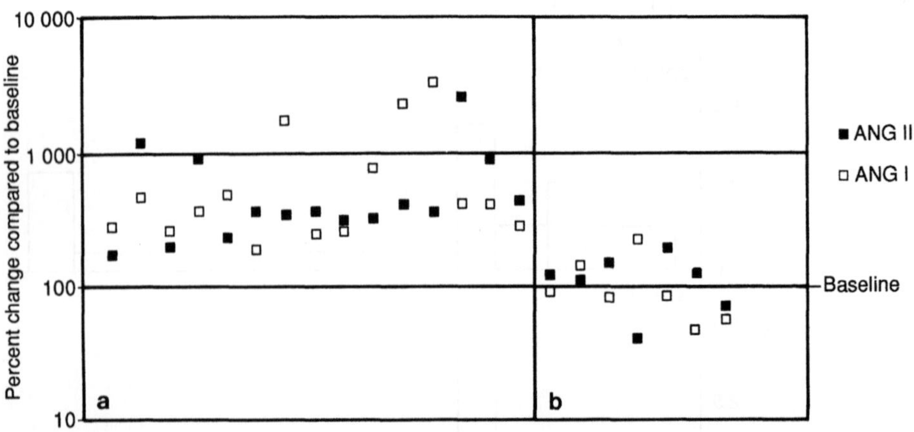

Fig. 8. **a** Increase in urinary excretion of ANG I and ANG II in patients with anaphylactoid symptoms after oral provocation ($n = 15$). **b** Urinary excretion of ANG I and ANG II in patients without anaphylactoid symptoms after oral provocation. No concomitant increase in ANG I and ANG II was noted ($n = 7$)

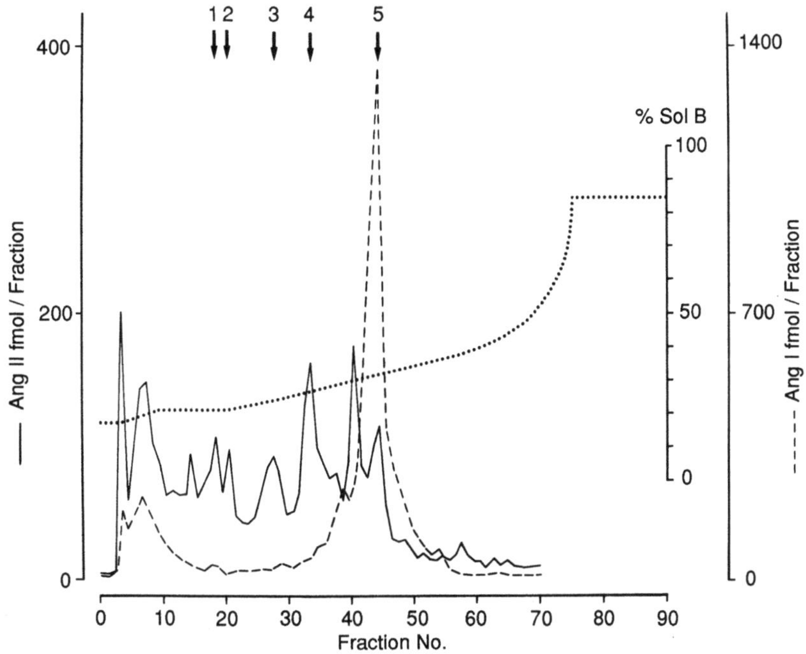

Fig. 9. HPLC characterization of ANG I and ANG II in urine on a reversed phase C_{18} column in an acetonitrile gradient. Ile-^{5}-ANG I, Ile^5-ANG II, and ANG III metabolites were identified. *1*, Ile^5-ANG II; *2*, Ile^2-ANG II$_{4-8}$pentapeptide; *3*, Ile^3-ANG II$_{3-8}$hexapeptide; *4*, Ile^4-ANG III; *5*, Ile^5-ANG I

In human urine from healthy volunteers, immunoreactive ANG I and ANG II were present. The average daily excretion of these peptides was 292.20 ± 62.50 pmol ANG I and 12.20 ± 2.50 pmol ANG II (mean ± SEM, $n = 14$).

The urinary excretion profile of ANG I and ANG II in a 33-year old man with a history of anaphylactoid reactions to propyphenazone is shown in Fig. 6. Within 2–3 h after the administration of propyphenazone, the patient reported flush and tachycardia. The latter was followed by a marked increase in ANG I and ANG II in the urine. By contrast, oral provocation with a placebo or a compound with no indication for anaphylactoid reactions in the patient's history failed to elicit anaphylactoid reactions or an increase in the urine levels of ANG I or ANG II (Fig. 7).

After oral provocation with drugs, food, food additives, or chemicals, ANG I and ANG II were elevated 2- to 12-fold in the urine of 15 patients. The increase in ANG I and ANG II was associated with clinical symptoms of anaphylaxis (Fig. 8 A). In seven patients without anaphylactoid reactions after oral provocation, no significant increase in ANG I or ANG II was found (Fig. 8 B).

Immunoreactive ANG I and ANG II were characterized on HPLC as Ile^5-ANG I, Ile^5-ANG II, and ANG II metabolites (Fig. 9).

Summary and Conclusions

Confirming data reported previously from our laboratory, patients with anaphylactic reactions to hymenoptera venom had significantly lower plasma levels of ANG I and ANG II than controls [1]. An inverse correlation between the plasma concentration of ANG I and ANG II and the severity of clinical symptoms was found in these patients – the lower the concentrations, the more severe the clinical symptoms.

After oral provocation of patients with anaphylactoid reactions to drugs, food, or food additives, ANG I and ANG II were increased 2- to 12-fold in the urine. The increase in ANG I and ANG II was associated with clinical symptoms of anaphylaxis. Oral provocation with a placebo or a compound with no indication for anaphylactoid reactions in the patient's history failed to elicit such a reaction or an increase in the urine levels of ANG I or ANG II.

One may tentatively speculate that patients with hymenoptera venom allergy have a disturbance in the RAS. This system seems to be down-regulated in these patients and thus unable to provide enough ANG II to counteract the symptoms of anaphylaxis. The increase in ANG I and ANG II in the urine of patients with anaphylactoid symptoms after oral provocation with drugs, food, or food additives may reflect a consumption of plasma ANG I or ANG II that is related to the clinical symptoms of anaphylaxis.

These findings may open new perspectives with regard to a possible role for angiotensin peptides in the sequence of events that occur during an anaphylactic reaction. The measurement of angiotensin peptides can be used as an objective parameter which may be helpful in the diagnosis and prediction of anaphylactic reactions.

Acknowledgements. The authors would like to thank Ms. Regina Böttcher, Michaela Koralka, Diana Ferino, Johanna Grosch and Ursula Wielert for their excellent technical assistance. ANG I and ANG II antibodies were generously provided by Dr. Ian M. Phillips, Department of Physiology, University of Florida, Gainesville, FL, USA. The editorial help of Ms. Pamla Decker is gratefully acknowledged.

References

1. Hermann K, Ring J (1990) Angiotensin und Insektengift-Anaphylaxie. Allergologie 13(1): S47–S48
2. Krol H, Villarreal D, Reams G, Bauer JH (1988) Renal metabolism and urinary excretion of angiotensin II. Clin Res 36(3):428A
3. Michailov ML, Schad H, Dahlheim H, Jacob ICM, Brechtelsbauer H (1987) Renin-angiotensin system responses of acute graded hemorrhage in dogs. Circ Shock 21:217–224
4. Proppe DW (1987) Control of plasma renin activity in heat-stressed baboons on varied salt intake. J Appl Physiol 62(4):1531–1537
5. Przybilla B, Ring J (1986) Hyposensibilisierungsbehandlung der Hymenopterengiftallergie: Aspekte der Indikationsstellung und Diagnose. Allergologie 9(1):S2–S10
6. Przybilla B, Ring J, Griesshammer (1989) Diagnostische Befunde bei Hymenopterengiftallergie. Allergologie 12(5):192–202
7. Ring J, Messmer K (1977) Incidence and severity of anaphylactoid reactions to colloid volume substitutes. Lancet 26:466–469

Granulocyte Mediator Release in Pseudo-allergic Reactions

W. Czech, E. Schöpf, and A. Kapp

Department of Dermatology, University of Freiburg, Hauptstrasse 7, W-7800 Freiburg i. Br., Federal Republic of Germany

Introduction

Acetylsalicylic acid (ASA) and other nonsteroidal anti-inflammatory drugs are among the most frequent causes of adverse drug reactions. The clinical symptoms often resemble allergy and consist of anaphylactic shock, bronchospasm, urticaria, and angioedema [8]. However, there is no evidence, that immune mechanisms, which are specific for the eliciting agent, are involved and therefore it has been suggested that such reactions should be designated as "pseudo-allergic reactions" (PAR) [9]. Besides their nonspecifity, PAR are distinguished from allergic reactions, by the fact that they occur at the first administration and thus do not need a sensitization phase, they are not transferable to other individuals of the same species, and they are not acquired but rather constitute a heriditary trait. There is evidence that the similarity of PAR and allergic reactions results from the fact that similar mediators and amplification systems are involved, for example, nonspecific release of histamine from mast cells or basophils [3] or activation of other granulocyte subsets; activation of thrombocytes [1]; activation of complement [7, 10]; or drug-induced influence on mononuclear cells resulting in altered release of cytokines. However, the pathogenesis of PAR remains unknown. Since skin tests are not reliable, the diagnosis relies on history and risky provocation tests. Therefore, the purpose of this study was to screen different leukocyte functions in order to establish in vitro test systems, thereby increasing our knowledge about the pathogenesis of PAR.

Methods

Patients and Controls

In vitro tests were performed on matched pairs (sex, age) consisting of patients with pseudoallergy to ASA, based on history and oral provocation tests, and healthy controls.

Polymorphonuclear Neutrophilic Granulocytes

Human polymorphonuclear neutrophilic granulocytes (PMN) were isolated from heparin-anticoagulated venous blood by ficoll gradient centrifugation followed by hypotonic lysis of red blood cells with NaCl. Cells were 98% PMN as judged by Pappenheim's stain and more than 95% viable by trypan blue exclusion [5].

Detection of Superoxide Production. Detection of superoxide was performed by measurement of the superoxide dismutase (SOD) inhibitable part of cytochrome C reduction as previously described [6]. PMN at a concentration of 10^7/ml were suspended in HEPES-buffered Hank's balanced salt solution (HBSS), containing 1 mg/ml BSA. PMN were distributed in 100 µl aliquots into 96 well, flat bottom tissue plates and preincubated with ASA (1000 µg/ml, 300 µg/ml, 100 µg/ml) at 37 °C for 15 min and subsequently covered with cytochrome C (120 µ*M* final concentration), in the presence or absence of SOD (200 µg/ml), and the stimuli phorbol myristate acetate (PMA) (10 µg/ml), granulocyte-macrophage colony-stimulating factor (GM-CSF) (10^3 U/ml), tumor necrosis factor (TNFα) (10^3 U/ml), or medium were added. Plates were incubated at 37 °C for 1 h. Absorbance was measured by an ELISA reader at 550 nm and results were expressed in n*M* cytochrome C reduced (= n$M\,^{\bullet}O_2^-$) per 10^6 PMN per well, after subtraction of absorbance for wells containing SOD.

Release of Peroxidase. Myeloperoxidase was measured as described previously [6]. PMN were suspended at a concentration of 5×10^6/ml in phosphate-buffered saline (PBS) containing 1 m*M* Ca^{2+} and Mg^{2+}. Assays were performed in 96 well, flat bottom tissue culture plates in the presence of 5 µg/ml cytochalasin B using 5×10^5 cells/well. After preincubation with ASA (1000 µg/ml, 300 µg/ml, 100 µg/ml) at 37 °C for 15 min *N* formyl-met-leu-phe (fmlp) (10^{-6} *M*) or medium was added and PMN were incubated at 37 °C for 1 h and centrifuged. Total cellular peroxidase activity was determined by addition of mixed alkyltrimethylammonium bromide (CETAB) (0.4%) to PMN. Supernatants were transferred and an indicator reagent consisting of o-phenylenediamine dihydrochloride (OPD) (0.5 mg/ml), hydrogen peroxide (0.1 m*M*), and CETAB (0.1%) in phosphate-citrate buffer (pH 5.5) was added. The reaction was stopped by acidification; the reaction product was measured at 492 nm in a Titertek Multiscan MCC. Results were expressed as percent of total content.

Lucigenin Dependent Chemiluminescence. Lucigenin dependent chemiluminescence (CL) [5, 6] represents a very sensitive measure of the release of reactive oxygen species (ROS) from PMN. Subsequently, for CL measurements PMN were suspended to a density of 5×10^6 cells/ml in HBSS (pH 7.4), containing lucigenin (2 m*M*), and BSA (1 mg/ml). Aliquots with 1×10^6 cells were preincubated with ASA (1000 µg/ml, 100 µg/ml) at 37 °C for 15 min. CL kinetic measurements were performed in a Biolumat LB 9505C (Berthold, Wildbad) after addition of the stimuli interleukin-5 (IL-5) (10^2 U/ml), TNFα (10^3 U/ml), PMA (10 ng/ml), or medium and the integral counts from a 0–60-min incubation interval were recorded.

Basophil Granulocytes

Histamine Release. Leukocytes were isolated from heparin-anticoagulated blood using a method described by Chodirker et al. [2] and suspended at a concentration of 2×10^6/ml in HBSS containing Ca^{2+} (0.7 *M*), glucose (2 mg/ml), and BSA (5 mg/ml). After preincubation of cells with one of the analgesic drugs, ASA (500 ng/ml), diclofenac (500 µg/ml), or indomethacin (5 µg/ml), or medium as a control at 37 °C for 15 min, spontaneous or anti-IgE (1 : 4000) (Behring-Werke, Marburg) stimulated histamine release was measured using a radioenzyme assay [4]. In order to determine total histamine content, the cell suspension was heated to 100 °C for 7 min. The concentration of histamine was calculated from a standard curve and results were expressed in ng/ml.

Eosinophil Granulocytes

Eosinophil Cationic Protein in Serum. For the measurement of eosinophil cationic protein (ECP) levels, 10 ml blood was collected and kept at room temperature for 60 min and then at 4 °C for another 30 min. After immediate centrifugation the serum was frozen at −70 °C. Measurements of ECP in serum were performed using a ECP radioimmunoassay (Pharmacia-LKB, Freiburg).

Statistical Analysis

For statistical analysis, Student's *t* test and the Mann-Whitney U test were used.

Results

Polymorphonuclear Neutrophilic Granulocytes

Production of Superoxide (n = 7). Release of superoxide spontaneously and upon stimulation with GM-CSF, TNF, and PMA did not significantly differ in patients and controls. Preincubation with ASA in different concentrations did not show significant influence on superoxide production in patients and controls (Table 1).

Release of Peroxidase (n = 13). In patients with PAR to ASA and controls no significantly different release of myeloperoxidase, either spontaneously or upon stimulation with fmlp, could be observed. Preincubation of PMN with various concentrations of ASA did not show a significant influence on release of peroxidase in patients and controls (Table 2).

Lucigenin-Dependent Chemiluminescence (n = 7). There was no significant difference in release of ROS detected by CL in patients and controls, either spontaneously or upon stimulation with IL-5, TNF or PMA. Neither in patients with

Table 1. Influence of preincubation (15 min, 37 °C) with ASA on production of superoxide by PMN spontaneously and upon stimulation with GM-CSF [10^3 U/ml], TNFα [10^3 U/ml], and PMA [10 ng/ml].

Stimulus	Patients	Controls
Medium control		
Medium	0.9±0.3	1.0±0.4
GM-CSF	3.5±0.8	2.6±0.6
TNFα	3.3±0.8	4.2±0.9
PMA	10.0±0.6	10.2±0.7
Preincubation: ASA (1000 µg/ml)		
Medium	0.2±0.1	0.4±0.2
GM-CSF	1.5±0.4	1.6±0.5
TNFα	2.7±0.5	2.5±0.4
PMA	8.1±0.4	7.4±0.4
Preincubation: ASA (300 µg/ml)		
Medium	0.6±0.2	0.8±0.4
GM-CSF	2.6±0.6	2.2±0.8
TNFα	3.7±0.7	3.6±0.9
PMA	8.8±0.5	10.0±0.4
Preincubation: ASA (100 µg/ml)		
Medium	0.5±0.2	0.6±0.4
GM-CSF	2.4±0.6	1.9±0.5
TNFα	2.9±0.6	3.1±0.5
PMA	8.8±0.7	9.0±0.3

Values represent mean ± SEM of $^{\bullet}O_2^-$ release in nM/10^6 PMN ($n = 7$).
ASA, acetylsalicylic acid; PMN, polymorphonuclear neutrophilic granulocytes; GM-CSF, granulocyte/macrophage colony-stimulating factor; TNFα, tumor necrosis factor α; PMA, phorbol myristate acetate.

PAR to ASA nor in healthy controls did preincubation with ASA significantly influence the release of ROS in vitro (Table 3).

Basophil Granulocytes

Histamine Release (n = 6). Patients with PAR to ASA and controls did not differ in spontaneous and anti-IgE induced histamine release in vitro. Neither ASA nor diclofenac and indomethacin, which often cross-react in PAR, significantly influenced histamine release in vitro (Fig. 1).

Eosinophil Granulocytes

ECP in Serum. ECP levels were measured in serum samples of patients with PAR to ASA ($n = 12$), atopic dermatitis (AD) ($n = 42$), psoriasis ($n = 32$), patients with a history of inhalant allergy ($n = 14$), and nonatopic healthy controls ($n = 31$). None of the patients with PAR suffered from symptomatic inhalant allergy or AD (Fig. 2). ECP levels were significantly increased in patients with PAR to ASA ($p \leq 0.01$) and AD ($p \leq 0.005$) in comparison to controls.

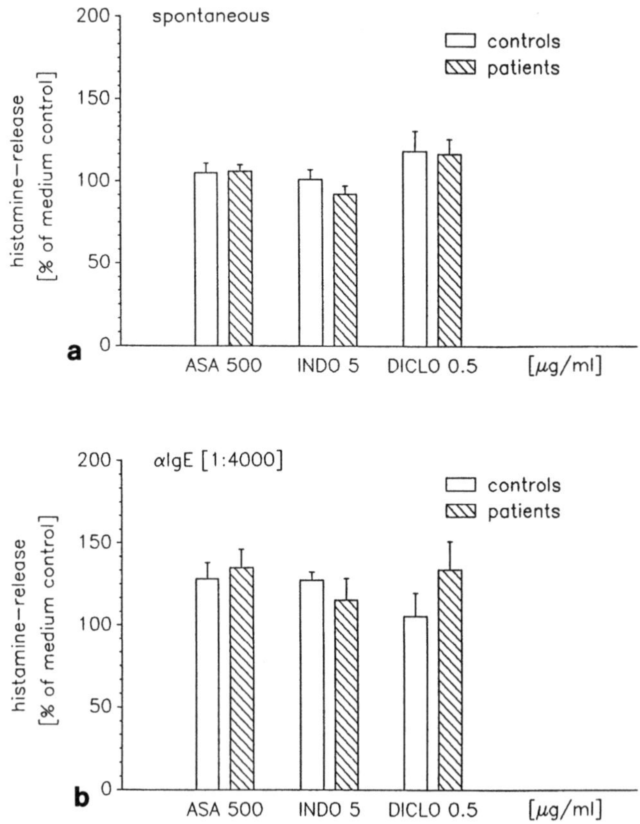

Fig. 1 a, b. Relative influence of preincubation (15 min, 37 °C) with ASA (500 μg/ml), indomethacin (5 μg/ml), and diclofenac (500 ng/ml) on **a** spontaneous and **b** anti-IgE (1 : 4000), induced histamine release. Values represent mean ± SEM of relative histamine release. Medium control = 100%; $n = 6$

Table 2. Influence of preincubation (15 min, 37 °C) with ASA on release of myeloperoxidase by PMN spontaneously and upon stimulation with fmlp [10^{-6} M].

Stimulus	Patients	Controls
Medium control		
Medium	9.3 ± 2.2	14.7 ± 3.4
Fmlp	69.2 ± 7.0	66.3 ± 4.4
Preincubation: ASA (1000 μg/ml)		
Medium	8.0 ± 1.7	11.4 ± 3.0
Fmlp	71.2 ± 6.8	70.2 ± 5.0
Preincubation: ASA (300 μg/ml)		
Medium	10.5 ± 2.4	12.2 ± 3.4
Fmlp	70.6 ± 6.7	68.8 ± 5.6
Preincubation: ASA (100 μg/ml)		
Medium	11.9 ± 2.6	11.0 ± 3.3
Fmlp	70.3 ± 6.1	66.7 ± 5.8

Values represent mean ± SEM % of total content ($n = 13$).
Fmlp, *N*-formyl-met-leu-phe.

Table 3. Influence of preincubation (15 min, 37 °C) with ASA on production of reactive oxygen species by PMN spontaneous and upon stimulation with IL-5 [10^2 U/ml], TNF [10^3 U/ml], and PMA [10 ng/ml].

Stimulus	Patients	Controls
Medium control		
Medium	13 ± 5	9 ± 2
Il-5	65 ± 17	58 ± 17
TNFα	293 ± 56	307 ± 49
PMA	1038 ± 97	1002 ± 129
Preincubation: ASA (1000 μg/ml)		
Medium	19 ± 7	10 ± 1
IL-5	85 ± 19	75 ± 16
TNFα	289 ± 53	346 ± 71
PMA	960 ± 167	761 ± 84
Preincubation: ASA (100 μg/ml)		
Medium	15 ± 7	7 ± 1
IL-5	83 ± 25	67 ± 16
TNFα	272 ± 38	395 ± 92
PMA	1051 ± 103	1159 ± 110

Values represent mean ± SEM × 10^{-6} of integral counts from a 0 – 60-min incubation interval ($n = 7$).

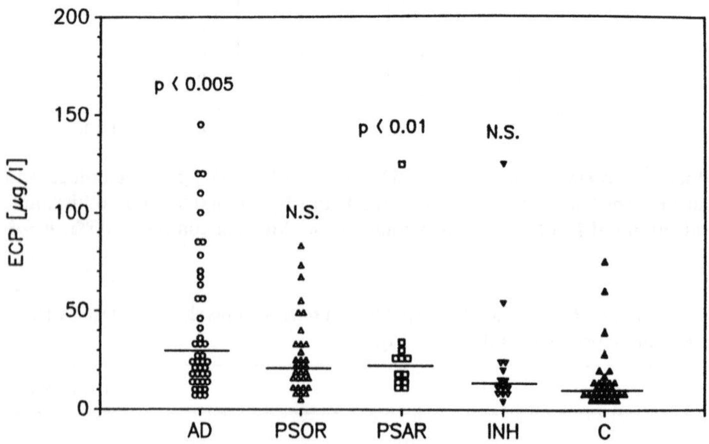

Fig. 2. ECP levels in serum of patients with pseudo-allergy to ASA (*PSAR*, $n = 12$), atopic dermatitis (*AD*, $n = 42$), psoriasis (*PSOR*, $n = 32$), patients with history of inhalant allergy (*INH*, $n = 14$) and nonatopic healthy controls (*C*, $n = 31$). Values represent mean ± SEM of ECP in μg/l

Summary and Conclusions

The pathogenesis of PAR to ASA and other nonsteroidal anti-inflammatory drugs is still unknown. Since diagnosis relies mainly on provocation tests, the purpose of this study was to establish procedures for in vitro diagnosis of PAR to analgesic drugs.

Different test systems were introduced including polymorphonuclear, basophil and eosinophil granulocytes as target cells.

In contrast to current opinion, a significant influence of ASA on the spontaneous or anti-IgE induced release of histamine by basophil leukocytes in vitro, as measured by a radioenzyme assay, could not be observed in patients with PAR to ASA and controls. Therefore, histamine release is not a suitable method for the diagnosis of PAR in vitro. A series of investigations were performed on PMN. Significantly, differences between patients and controls, as determined by preincubation of PMN with ASA, in production of superoxide, release of myeloperoxidase or ROS, either spontaneously or upon appropriate stimulation, could not be detected. These data clearly indicate that there is no evidence for an in vitro alteration of PMN response in patients with PAR.

However, in serum samples of patients with PAR to ASA and AD, elevated levels of ECP were detected. Therefore, it is tempting to speculate that the eosinophil could be a crucial target cell in pseudo-allergic reactions to analgesic drugs and further investigations are necessary to clarify its pathogenetic role in this disease.

References

1. Capron A, Ameisen JC, Joseph M, Auriault C, Tonnel AB, Caen J (1985) New functions for platelets and their pathological implications. Int Arch Allergy Appl Immunol 77:107–114
2. Chodirker WB, Bock GN, Vaughan JH (1968) Isolation of human PMN leukocytes and granules. Observation on early blood dilution and on heparin. J Lab Clin Med 71:9–19
3. Conroy MC, de Weck AL (1981) Effect of aspirin and indomethacin on histamine release from leukocytes of patients with suspected intolerance to aspirin. Int Arch Allergy Appl Immunol 66 [Suppl 1]:152–153
4. Fuhr N, Kownatzki E (1986) Inhibition of rat kidney histamine-n-methyltransferase by biogenic amines. Pharmacology 32:114–120
5. Kapp A, Luger TA, Maly FE, Schöpf E (1986) Granulocyte-activating mediators (GRAM): I. Generation by LPS-stimulated mononuclear cells. J Invest Dermatol 86:523–528
6. Kapp A, Zeck-Kapp G, Danner M, Luger TA (1988) Human granulocyte-macrophage colony stimulating factor: An effective direct activator of human polymorphonuclear neutrophilic granulocytes. J Invest Dermatol 91:49–55
7. König A, Schaub E, Voigtländer V, Virchow Ch, Rother U (1982) Zur Bedeutung des Komplementsystems beim Analgetika-Asthma. Allergologie 5:227–229
8. Mathews KP (1984) Clinical spectrum of allergic and pseudoallergic drug reactions. J Allergy Clin Immunol 74:558–566
9. Schlumberger HD (1980) Drug-induced pseudo-allergic syndrome as exemplified by acetylsalicylic acid intolerance. In: Dukor P, Kallos P, Schlumberger HD, West GB (eds) Pseudo-allergic reactions, pp 125–203
10. Voigtländer V, Hänsch G, Rother U (1981) Acetylsalicylic acid intolerance: a possible role of complement. Int Arch Allergy Appl Immunol [Suppl 1] 66:154–155

Photocontact Dermatitis and Persistent Light Reaction from Olaquindox in Piglet Feed

S. Schauder

Department of Dermatology, University of Göttingen, von-Siebold-Strasse 3, W-3400 Göttingen, Federal Republic of Germany

Introduction

Since the withdrawal of quindoxin from the EEC market in 1973 due to its carcinogenic properties in experimental animals, its derivatives *olaquindox* and *carbadox* have been used as antibiotic growth promoters in piglet feed (Fig. 1). Olaquindox was developed by Bayer and has been marketed since 1975 in 40 countries. In 1989 alone, 60 tons of olaquindox were sold in the Federal Republic of Germany. Piglet breeders, who mix olaquindox-containing premixes with the feed, expose themselves to the dust of this compound, which may induce allergic and photoallergic contact dermatitis [1, 2, 4].

In 1987, I discovered that chronic photosensitivity dermatitis with persistent light reaction follows photocontact dermatitis from olaquindox [7, 8]. Similar side effects were already known from quindoxin [10].

After the first report of my observation of olaquindox-induced skin reactions in *Top Agrar* (a journal for farmers) in September 1989, piglet breeders presented themselves in Göttingen and in other German departments of dermatology with similar symptoms [2, 5]. In Göttingen, nine patients, some of whom were misdiagnosed for years, were found to have photosensitivity dermatitis caused by olaquindox.

The purpose of this study is provide information about:

- history, clinical features, diagnostics, and treatment of nine patients with occupational photosensitivity from olaquindox;
- reaction of Bayer and the producers of olaquindox-containing premixes to my findings;
- effect on the diagnostic procedure recommended by the German, Austrian, and Swiss photopatch-test group.

Patients and Methods

Patients

During the years 1987 – 1990 nine piglet feeders with chronic photosensitivity dermatitis from olaquindox were seen. Duration of photosensitivity, history of

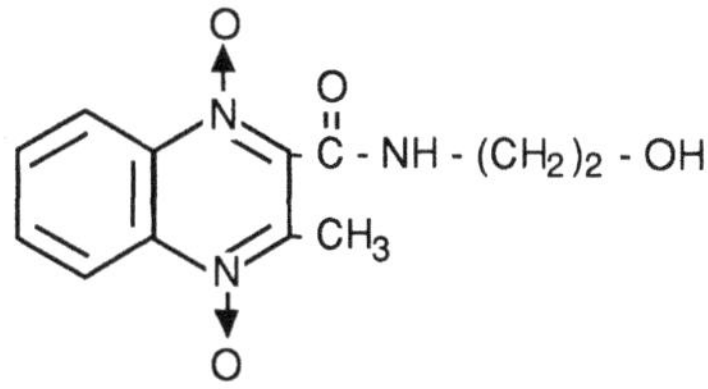

olaquindox
2 - [N - (2 - hydroxyethyl) - carbamoyl] - 3 - methyl - quinoxaline - 1,4 - dioxide

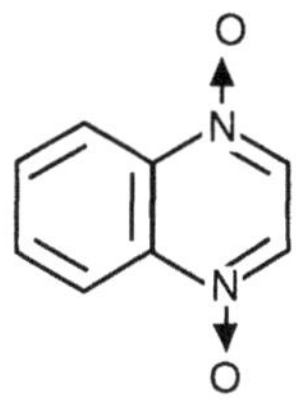

quindoxin
quinoxaline - 1,4 - dioxide

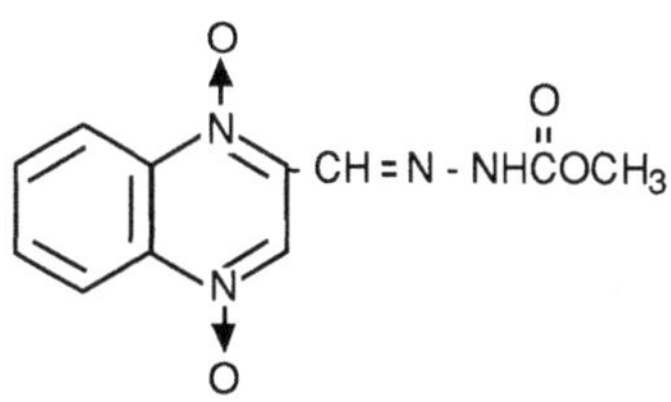

carbadox
2 - (2 - quinoxalinylmethylene) - hydrazine - carboxylic acid methyl ester 1,4 - dioxide

Fig. 1. Structural formulae of olaquindox, quindox, and carbadox

occupational and private contact to various substances, skin type, and atopic stigmata and signs were assessed. The clinical features varied from erythema and persistent papules to infiltrated plaques on light exposed skin, often with extension to nonexposed areas.

Phototest and Photopatch Test

Light sources: UV-B, Osram Ultra Vitalux 300 W (Osram, München); UV-A, UV-Test (Waldmann, Villingen-Schwenningen); Waldmann Bestrahlungskabine UV 1000 for 8-methoxypsoralen and ultraviolet A (PUVA); dosimetry, Centra UV-Meßgerät (Osram, München).

Test substances: Olaquindox (Bayer) 0.1% and 0.01% in white petrolatum; Carbadox (Pfizer) 0.5%, 0.1%, and 0.01% in white petrolatum; Sunscreen products and UV filters (Hermal, Reinbek); Photopatch test tray of the German, Austrian, and Swiss photopatch test group (Hermal); Material according to the *Deutsche Kontaktallergie Gruppe* (DKG) (Hermal) and occupational substances.

Procedure

Determination of the minimal erythema dose (MED) for each patient was made applying graded doses of UV-B (0.001 – 0.4J/cm^2 and UV-A (0.07 – 30 J/cm^2) to unexposed skin of the lower back. The MED UV-B and UV-A were determined as the least amount of irradiation needed to produce minimally perceptive erythema of the test site 24 h after irradiation.

Normally, the MED UV-B was at least 0.1 J/cm^2 (irradiation time 2 min) and MED UV-A was at least 20 J/cm^2 (irradiation time 48 min). The sites were observed up to 8 days after irradiation for evaluation of eczematous transformation.

Photopatch Test

Antigens (a – c) were applied in duplicate to the patient's midback using Finn chamber disks (Hermal). One series of patches was removed after 24 h, inspected, and irradiated with two-thirds of the MED UV-A. The other series was removed after 48 h and served as dark control. The irradiated set was read immediately and then 24, 48, and 72 h after irradiation. The nonirradiated set was evaluated 48, 72, and 96 h after application of the patches.

Reaction were recorded as follows: –, no reaction; 1 +, erythema; 2 +, erythema, edema; 3 + erythema, edema, papules, vesicles.

Photoallergy was diagnosed when the irradiated site was positive compared to a negative nonirradiated site.

Patch Test

Application of the antigens (d) and procedure were the same as for the nonirradiated set of the photopatch test.

Treatment

In seven patients, PUVA therapy was tried by irradiating the whole skin, usually three or four times a week, starting with very low UV-A doses which were slowly increased.

Results

After contact with olaquindox-containing premixes (Table 1), all patients first developed hand eczema (Fig. 2) and then photosensitive dermatitis of the arms, face,

Table 1. Olaquindox[a]-containing premixes employed by the patients.

Trade name	Producer
Bilactal Milchaustauschfutter	Schaumann
Biphosphoral-F-Mineralfutter	Schaumann
Blattivit 14 Mineralfutter für Schweine mit BAYO-N-OX	Höveler Kraftfutterwerke
Brockmann Bromin Mineralfutter	Brockmann
Brockmann Ferkelmarke	Brockmann
Gelita Amino-Mineralfutter	Gesellschaft für Tierernährung
Gelita S-Bayo-Mineralfutter	Gesellschaft für Tierernährung
Schaumann F-Mineralfutter für Ferkel	Schaumann
Tri-Phosphoral F-Mineralfutter	Schaumann
Tri-Lactal Ergänzungsfutter	Schaumann
Vitamiral 13-Mineralfutter	Westfälische Central-Genossenschaft
WCG Swina Ferkelaufzuchtfutter	Westfälische Central-Genossenschaft
Wülkamin Ferkelmineral F.B. Plus	Wuebken

[a] Meanwhile olaquindox has been removed from these premixes.

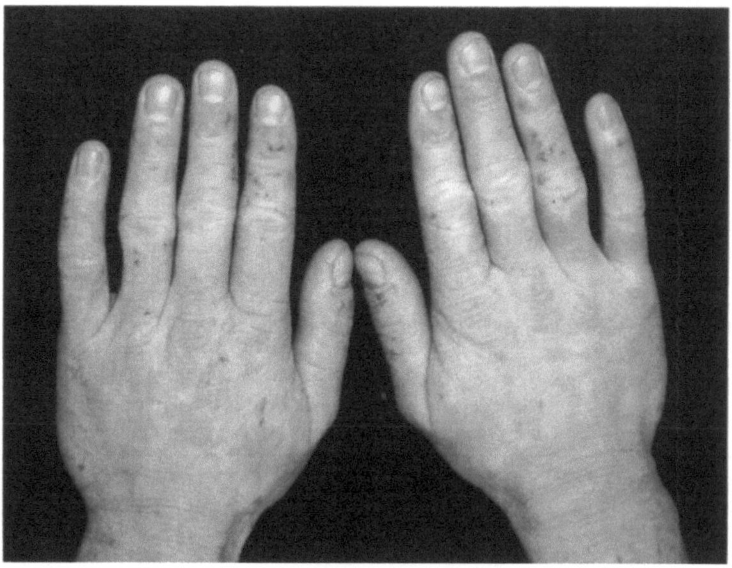

Fig. 2. Photocontact dermatitis from olaquindox affecting the hands (patient 3)

and neck (Fig. 3). Clinical data, first contact with olaquindox in premixes, beginning of photosensitivity, and time of diagnosis are summarized in Table 2.

Only patient 9 had features of atopic eczema, whereas patients 3–5 were misdiagnosed for years while not affected by this disease. The report on photosensitivity from olaquindox (patient 3) *Top Agrar* [7] prompted patients 4–9 to undergo examination in Göttingen.

Results of photopatch test and patch tests are shown in Table 3. Patients 1 and 3 developed additional (photo-)allergic reactions to UV filters (4-isopropyl-diben-

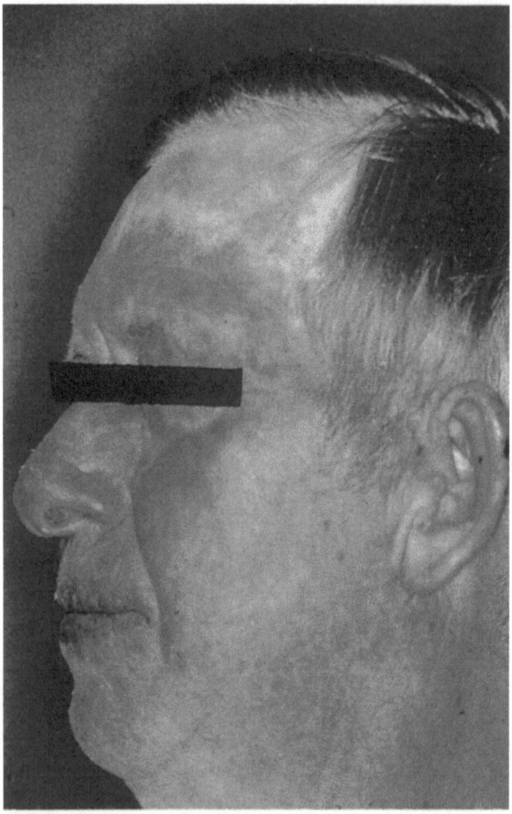

Fig. 3. Erythema and papules on the light-exposed areas of the face and the neck (patient 3). The forehead was covered by a cap

Table 2. Clinical data and history of photosensitivity in nine piglet breeders.

Patient	Sex	Age (years)	Atopic eczema	Skin type	First contact with olaquindox in premix	Beginning of photosensitivity (month/year)	Time of diagnosis (month/year)
1	M	75	no	II	–	5/1985	7/1987
2	F	61	no	II	2/1986	4/1988	3/1989
3	M	57	no	II	1/1986	8/1987	6/1989
4	M	29	no	II	9/1987	9/1987	11/1989
5	M	24	no	II	3/1987	5/1988	3/1990
6	M	50	no	IV	1/1987	3/1987	3/1990
7	F	36	no	II	7/1989	8/1989	4/1990
8	M	30	no	II	6/1985	5/1987	4/1990
9	M	28	yes	III	1/1984	7/1984	5/1990

zoylmethane, 4-*tert*.butyl-4′-methoxy-dibenzoylmethane, benzophenone-3, and 3-(4′-methylbenzylidene)-camphor) in commercial sunscreens they had used for light protection. Chlorpromazine elicited (photo-)allergic reactions in patients 8 and 9. They had stopped injecting this tranquilizer into pigs and piglets some years ago.

Table 3. Results of photopatch and patch tests.

Patient	Positive reactions	
	Photopatch tests	Patch tests
1	Olaquindox 0.01%[a] IDM Contralum ultra Creme (IDM, fragrance)	Fragrance mix, oak moss, chlorocresol compositae mix, feverfew, yarrow BDM, Anthélios Creme getönt (IDM, BDM, fragrance), ROC unsichtbarer Vollschutz 15, A+B (BDM)
2	Olaquindox 0.01%	Kathon CG
3	Olaquindox 0.01%	Furazolidone, BDM, MBC Anthélios Creme 11B-4A (IDM, B3) Contralum Ultra Creme (IDM, MBC) Ilrido Plus 15 Milch (BDM, MBC) ROC Sonnenblocker deckend LSF 15 (BDM, B3)
4	Olaquindox 0.01%	
5	Olaquindox 0.1%	Cobalt chloride, cobalt sulfate
6	Olaquindox 0.1%	Rubber mixes, neomycin sulfate, benzoic acid, formaldehyde, propylene glycol, potassium dichromate, cobalt chloride
7	Olaquindox 0.1%	Potassium dichromate, hexyl resorcinol
8	Olaquindox 0.1%, chlorpromazine[b]	Colophony, fragrance mix, rubber mixes
9	Olaquindox 0.1%	Chlorpromazine[b]

IDM, 4-isopropyl-dibenzoylmethane; BDM, 4-*tert.*butyl-4′-methoxy-dibenzoylmethane; B3, benzophenone-3; MBC, 3-(4′-methylbenzylidene)-camphor.
[a] Only the minimal concentration of olaquindox, which caused at least a 2+ reaction, is given. No reactions to olaquindox were seen in 25 controls. Photopatch tests with olaquindox-containing premixes elicit irritant reactions in controls and therefore should not be performed.
[b] No contact with chlorpromazine for several years.

Histopathology of a biopsy from the neck revealed acanthosis and a dermal infiltrate around blood vessels, which consisted predominantly of mononuclear cells (patient 3). In a biopsy from the test site of olaquindox (0.1%), 8 days after irradiation with UV-A, acantholysis with beginning blister formation and dense dermal infiltrates around blood vessels were found (patient 3).

MEDs for UV-A (Table 4) were decreased in eight out of nine piglet breeders before withdrawal of olaquindox.

Follow-up phototests in five patients, who had stopped using olaquindox, revealed persistent UV-A sensitivity. Tolerance to UV-A and UV-B slowly improved after withdrawal of olaquindox. PUVA therapy seems to have a beneficial effect.

Consequences and Conclusions

Bayer warns producers against adding olaquindox (800–1000 mg/kg) to premixes, but still advocates its usage in pellet form (15–50 mg/kg). Reports of adverse reactions to olaquindox-containing pellets have not been published so far.

Table 4. Minimal erythemal doses for UV-B and UV-A before and after withdrawal[a] of olaquindox.

	Interval (months)	Patient	Med UV-B J/cm^2	Med UV-A J/cm^2
First testing		1	0.075	1.7
Follow-up	8		0.12	6.0
First testing		2	0.15	28.0
Follow-up	–		n.d.	n.d.
First testing		3	0.6	2.3
Follow-up	5		0.1	7.0
Follow-up	10		0.15	>20.0
First testing		4	0.013	0.2
Follow-up	4		0.2	8.4
First testing		5	0.15	3.5
Follow-up	3		n.d.	>15.0
First testing		6	0.15	1.0
Follow-up	2		0.15	6.0
First testing		7	0.15	10.0
Follow-up	2		0.15	5.5
First testing		8	0.04	1.2
Follow-up	–		n.d.	n.d.
First testing		9	0.05	1.7
Follow-up	–		n.d.	n.d.

[a] Patient 7 was sold an "olaquindox-free" premix, which still contained this substance, as shown by analysis.

Since the patent of BAYO-N-OX (olaquindox) expired in 1985, only 25% percent of this compound is still sold by Bayer. All other manufacturers should also warn against olaquindox. By July 1990 all producers of premixes used by the patients had replaced olaquindox with tylosin, carbadox, etc. The photosensitizing potential of the latter, structurally related, antibiotic growth promoter has not yet been clarified.

My findings prompted the German, Austrian, and Swiss photopatch test group to recommend photopatch testing with olaquindox (0.1% in petrolatum/Hermal) for patients who have occupational contact with this substance and dermatitis of light-exposed skin.

Only chlorpromazine, a tranquilizer which is injected into piglets and pigs, induces similar occupational skin reactions in pig breeders [3, 9].

Early diagnosis is important. The sooner olaquindox is detected as the cause of photosensitivity, the sooner the persistent light reaction decreases. PUVA therapy improves tolerance to light. Ultraviolet-absorbing sunscreens often elicit additional (photo)allergic contact dermatitis (patients 1, 3, and ref. [5, 6]) and therefore should be avoided.

Industrial animal production not only endangers animals and consumers, but also farmers. Society should be willing to pay higher prices for meat produced under more natural conditions.

References

1. Bedello PG, Goitre M, Cane D, Roncarolo G (1985) Allergic contact dermatitis to BAYO-N-OX-I. Contact Dermatitis 12:284
2. Dunkel FG, Elsner P, Pevny I, Burg G (1990) Olaquindox-induziertes photoallergisches Ekzem und persistierende Lichtreaktion bei einem Schweinezüchter. 2. Allergologischer Workshop, 9. März 1990, Mainz
3. Ertle TC (1982) Beruflich bedingte Kontakt- und Photokontaktallergie bei einem Landwirt durch Chlorpromazin. Dermatosen 30:120
4. Francalanci S, Gola M, Georgini S, Muccinelli A, Sertoli A (1986) Occupational photocontact dermatitis from olaquindox. Contact Dermatitis 15:112
5. Hochsattel R, Gall H, Weber L, Kaufmann R (1991) Photoallergische Reaktion auf Olaquindox. Hautarzt 42:233–236
6. Schauder S, Ippen H (1988) Photoallergisches und allergisches Kontaktekzem durch Dibenzoylmethan-Verbindungen und andere Lichtschutzfilter. Hautarzt 39:435–440
7. Schauder S (1989) Photoallergie und extreme Lichtempfindlichkeit durch Olaquindox. Top Agrar 9:4
8. Schauder S (1989) Gefahren durch Olaquindox: Photoallergie, chronisch photosensitive Dermatitis und extrem gesteigerte Lichtempfindlichkeit beim Menschen, Hypoaldosteronismus beim Schwein. Dermatosen 37:183–185
9. Schauder S (1991) Aktinisches Retikuloid nach photoallergischem Kontaktekzem durch Chlorpromazin bei einem Schweinemäster. Dermatosen 39:12–17
10. Zaynoun S, Johnson BE, Frain-Bell W (1976) The investigation of quindoxin photosensitivity. Contact Dermatitis 2:343–352

Hyposensitization

Allergoids for Hyposensitization

J. Bousquet, A. Hejjaoui, and F.-B. Michel

Clinique des Maladies Respiratoires, CHU, Hopital l'Aiguelongue, Avenue du Major Flandre, 34059 Montpellier-Cedex, France

Abstract

Hyposensitization is widely used in the treatment of allergic diseases, but its side effects limit its use. Several attempts have been made to reduce the side effects of hyposensitization. Among them are the preparation of allergoids, formed by treating the native allergen with e.g. formaldehyde. Allergoids consist of molecules of various sizes, but a substantial proportion of them are made of polymers. Allergoids have mainly been prepared from pollens. Unfractionated allergoids are effective in the treatment of pollinosis, but they are not completely safe. High molecular weight allergoids are prepared by fractionating classical allergoids with a molecular sieve of 80 kDa. These preparations were found to be safe and effective and may represent one of the allergens of the future.

Introduction

In 1920, Ramon prepared a new vaccine by detoxifying the tetanus toxin with formaldehyde and heat. The resulting tetanus toxoid was found to immunize against the toxin and was devoid of the latter's severe side effects. Thus, the toxoid had a retained efficacy and was safe.

One of the major problems of hyposensitization is the occurrence of severe systemic side effects. Since 1935 many attempts have been made to increase the safety of allergens either by pyridine extraction or by adsorption on aluminium hydroxide or other delayed adjuvants. In 1970, Marsh et al. [1], following the first approach of Carter [19], prepared "allergoids" by submitting native allergens to formaldehyde and found that these preparations were immunogenic (retained immunogenicity) and probably safer than the native allergen (decreased allergenicity). Many other attempts were made, including the polymerization of allergens by glutaraldehyde or polyethylene glycol coupling. The term allergoid has been given to a wide variety of preparations; however, for clarity, in this article "allergoid" will refer only to formaldehyde-modified allergens.

Preparation and Analysis of Allergoids

Preparation

Ragweed, grass, and tree pollen allergoids have been prepared according to the two-step procedure of Marsh et al. [2]. The allergoid GOID is prepared from pollens of six different grass species (*Dactylis glomerata, Festuca elatior, Holcus lanatus, Lolium perenne,* and *Poa pratensis*). The methods of preparation and handling of the lyophilized allergen extract and the lyophilized GOID have been previously published in detail [2, 3]. Briefly, native allergens are dialyzed and incubated with formaldehyde at constant pH. A first incubation is done with 0.2 *M* formaldehyde for 14 days at 4 °C. Then, for the second incubation, the solution is diluted fourfold and incubated for 21 days at 32 °C. The resulting allergoid is dialyzed at 4 °C to remove formaldehyde and buffer salts. In some countries, GOID is adsorbed on aluminium hydroxide. High molecular weight allergoids have also been prepared [4] by separation with a preparative sephadex G100. Alle molecules with a molecular mass of over 85 kDa are pooled and lyophilized (HMW-GOID).

Evaluation of Allergenicity of Allergoids

The control of allergoids is rather difficult since it is impossible to determine if all relevant epitopes have been modified similarly. Thus, only global tests of allergenicity can be used. These often combine in vitro (RAST inhibition, IgG, histamine release assay) and in vivo (skin tests, nasal challenge) tests.

The first evaluation of allergenicity was done just after the first allergoids were prepared [5]. It was found that allergoids retained their capacity to induce guinea pigs to produce antibodies cross-reacting with the native allergen as measured by passive cutaneous anaphylaxis (PCA). The physicochemical properties of grass pollen allergoids were largely studied by Puttonen et al. [6], using chromatography procedures, and by Wihl et al. [8], using high performance liquid chromatography (HPLC). It was found that the human allergenicity of GOID was about 50–100 times less than that of the native allergen by in vivo tests and 1000 times by in vitro tests [7–9].

Comparison Between the Mixed Grass Pollen Allergens Used to Prepare Allergoids GOID and HMW-GOID

The native six grass pollen allergen mix and both allergoid preparations were tested in parallel to assess their molecular weight distribution and relative allergenicity [4]. The HPLC chromatogram of the three extracts showed that the native allergen and GOID consist mainly of molecules under 44 kDa, whereas HMW-GOID consists of larger molecules. By RAST inhibition it was observed that the in vitro allergenic activities of GOID and HMW-GOID were reduced by 1563- and 1054-fold, respectively, when compared to the native allergen. Skin tests results showed that the in vivo allergenic activities of GOID and HMW-GOID were reduced by 130- and 8500-fold, respectively, when compared to the native allergen. These studies suggest that HMW-GOID should be safer and at least as effective as GOID.

Efficacy and Safety of Allergoids

Methods evaluating the efficacy of immunotherapy include symptom medication scores, provocative challenges with soluble allergens or pollen grains, skin prick tests, and in vitro assays, such as the evolution of allergen-specific IgG [10]. However, there are very few studies comparing objective parameters with symptom medications scores during the pollen season and, except for nasal challenge with pollen grains [11, 12], the relevance of different tests is still a matter of debate.

Ragweed Pollen Allergy

Few double-blind, placebo-controlled studies have been performed with allergoids in individuals with ragweed pollen allergy [13, 14]. Norman et al. [13] compared allergoid, allergen, and placebo administered in a cluster regimen. They gave a high allergoid dose (50 times more antigen E in the allergoid group than in the allergen group) and observed a significant improvement of symptoms in both treated groups in comparison with placebo. However, owing to a high allergoid dose, many patients had a systemic reaction, indicating that unfractionated allergoids are not totally safe if large doses are given. The overall incidence of systemic reactions was similar in both treated groups. Meriney et al. [14] studied 20 patients, 10 receiving a placebo and 10 others the active treatment. They observed that patients receiving allergoid had significantly less symptoms during the ragweed pollen season and a significant increase of serum-specific IgG. No systemic reactions occurred in this group of patients.

Grass Pollen Allergy

Double-blind, placebo-controlled studies have shown that hyposensitization with formalinized allergoids is effective in controlling symptoms of grass pollen-induced rhinitis, conjunctivitis, and asthma [3, 4, 11, 12] (Fig. 1). Nasal challenge with grass pollen grains were performed in two studies [11, 12] with GOID or HMW-GOID. It was observed that the threshold dose of pollen grains inducing a positive challenge was significantly greater before hyposensitization, unchanged after treatment with placebo, and significantly increased after allergoid. There was a significant correlation between symptom scores during the pollen season and the nasal challenge result (Fig. 2). A significant increase in serum grass pollen-specific IgG or IgG1 and IgG4 was observed in all studies, but there was no significant correlation between the antibody level and clinical efficacy.

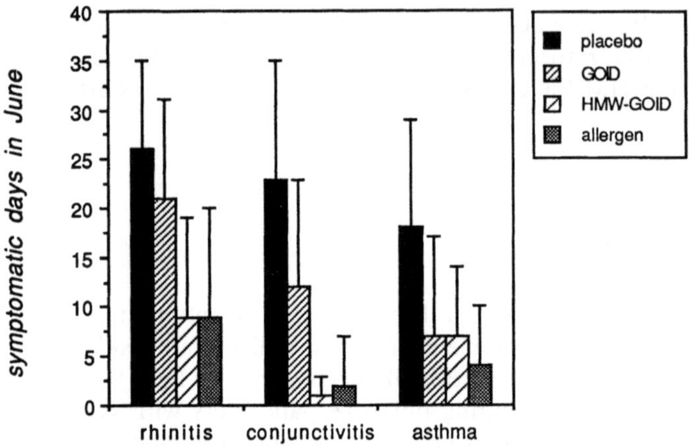

Fig. 1. Comparison of the efficacy of placebo, GOID, HMW-GOID and a standardized allergen extract in rhinitis, conjunctivitis, and asthma induced by grass pollens. [From 4]

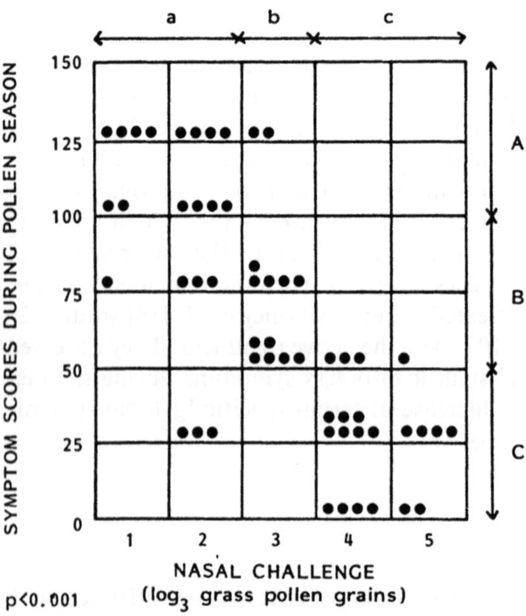

Fig. 2. Correlation between symptom scores during the pollen season and nasal challenge results. Statistical analysis by contigency table analysis. [From 12]

Two different preparations were used in these studies. The classical allergoid (GOID), prepared by the two-step procedure according to Marsh et al. [1, 2] was found to elicit more systemic reactions (SR) than HMW-GOID (4) (Fig. 3). Moreover, it was observed that the administration of GOID by a rush protocol elicited a high rate of SR, indicating that this mode of administration should not be used.

The dose of allergen to be administered during hyposensitization has not yet been completely determined. It has been demonstrated that low allergen dose, such as those given using the Rinkel method [20], are ineffective; thus, it was pro-

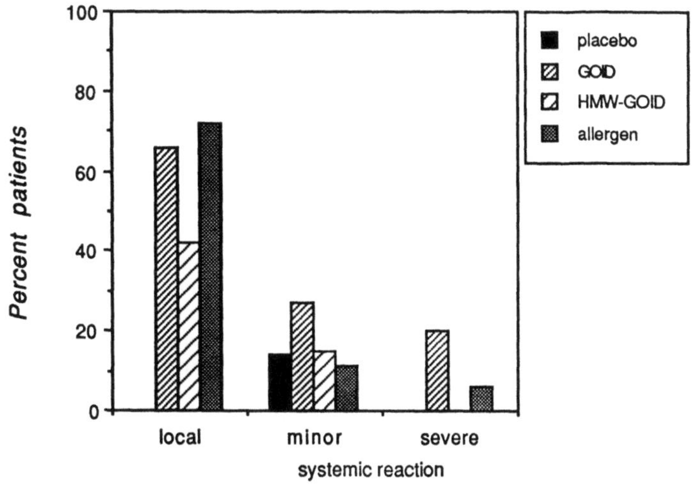

Fig. 3. Side effects induced by placebo, GOID, HMW-GOID, and a standardized allergen extract in pollen hyposensitization. [From 4]

posed that the highest tolerated dose be administered [15]. However, very high doses of allergens have induced an unacceptable rate of SR[14] (systemic reactions) leading to the concept of an "optimal dose" in which there is a balance between efficacy and safety. A double-blind, placebo-controlled study was carried out in 57 grass pollen allergic individuals comparing two doses of HMW-GOID and showed that when doses were increased five fold there was no improved efficacy in objective or subjective parameters. This suggests that the optimal dose is the smaller one since it is likely to be better tolerated [12].

Conclusions

Studies on grass pollen allergy with GOID and HMW-GOID confirm that allergoids are immunogenic since they decrease symptoms and end-organ reactivity to allergen and increase grass pollen IgG. However, GOID is not totally safe and the concept of "reduced allergenicity" proposed by Marsh et al. [1] was not completely correct. On the other hand, high molecular weight preparations are safe as shown in two studies with allergoids [4, 8] and in studies with polymerized glutaraldehyde-modified extracts [16–18]. Thus, "reduced allergenicity" is likely to be more a problem of polymerization than chemical treatment. In fact, both aldehydes may be effective in the preparation of high molecular weight preparations.

The future of allergoids is difficult to predict, as it is for hyposensitization as a whole. However, if epitopes can replace whole allergen extracts, it will become easier to prepare and control allergoids. They may then represent one of the immunologic treatments of the future for allergic diseases.

References

1. Marsh DG, Lichtenstein LM, Campbell DH (1970) Studies on "allergoids" prepared from naturally occurring allergens. I. Assay of allergenicity and antigenicity of formalinized rye group I component. Immunology 18:705–722
2. Marsh DG, Norman PS, Roebber M, Lichtenstein LM (1981) Studies on allergoids from naturally occurring allergens. III. Preparation of ragweed pollen allergoids by aldehyde modification in two steps. J Allergy Clin Immunol 68:449–459
3. Bousquet J, Hejjaoui A, Skassa-Brociek W, et al. (1987) Double-blind placebo controlled immunotherapy with mixed grass pollen allergoids. I. Rush immunotherapy with allergoids and standardized orchard grass pollen. J Allergy Clin Immunol 80:591–598
4. Bousquet J, Maasch H, Hejjaoui A, et al. (1989) Double-blind placebo controlled immunotherapy with mixed grass pollen allergoids. III. Comparison of an unfractionated allergoid, a fractionated allergoid and a standardized orchard grass pollen extract in rhinitis, conjunctivitis and asthma. J Allergy Clin Immunol 84:546–556
5. Haddad ZH, Marsh DG, Campbell DH (1972) Studies on "allergoids" prepared from naturally occurring allergens. II. Evaluation of allergenicity and assay of antigenicity of formalinized mixed grass pollen extracts. J Allergy Clin Immunol 49:197–209
6. Puttonen E, Maasch HJ, Pilström L (1982) Studies on allergen and allergoid preparations from purified timothy (*Phleum pratense*) pollen extracts. I. Physicochemical characteristics and binding to allergen-specific human IgE. Int Arch Allergy Appl Immunol 68:1–6
7. Puttonen E, Pilström L, Wahn U, Maasch HJ (1982) Studies on allergen and allergoid preparations from purified timothy (*Phleum pratense*) pollen extracts. II. Anaphylaxis studies in rats on histamine release from human leukocytes. Int Arch Allergy Appl Immunol 68:7–12
8. Wihl J-A, Pilström L, Maasch HJ (1985) Studies on allergen and allergoid preparations from purified timothy (*Phleum pratense*) pollen extracts. III. Comparative investigations by skin prick tests and nasal provocation tests. Int Arch Allergy Appl Immunol 76:162–167
9. Norman PS, Lichtenstein LM, Marsh DG (1981) Studies on allergoids from naturally occurring allergens. IV. Efficacy and safety of long-term allergoid treatment of ragweed hay fever. J Allergy Clin Immunol 68:460–470
10. Norman PS (1981) Immunotherapy. Prog Allergy 32:318–355
11. Bousquet J, Maasch H, Martinot B, Hejjauoi A, Wahl R, Michel FB (1988) Double-blind placebo controlled immunotherapy with mixed grass pollen allergoids. II. Comparison between parameters assessing the efficacy of immunotherapy. J Allergy Clin Immunol 82:439–446
12. Bousquet J, Hejjaoui A, Soussana M, Michel FB (1990) Double-blind placebo controlled immunotherapy with mixed grass pollen allergoids. IV. Comparison of the safety and efficacy of two dosages of high-molecular-weight allergoid. J Allergy Clin Immunol 85:514–522
13. Norman PS, Lichtenstein LM, Kagey-Sobotka A, Marsh DG (1982) Controlled evaluation of allergoids in the immunotherapy of ragweed hay fever. J Allergy Clin Immunol 70:248–260
14. Meriney DK, Kothari H, Chinoy P, Grieco MH (1986) The clinical and immunologic efficacy of immunotherapy with modified ragweed extract (allergoid) for ragweed hay fever. Ann Allergy 56:34–38
15. Bousquet J, Guérin B, Michel FB (1985) Clinical trials with standardized extracts. In: Brede HD, Stevens E (eds) Proceedings of the 3rd Paul-Ehrlich-Seminar on Regulatory Control and Standardization of Allergenic Extracts. Fischer, Stuttgart, pp 291–309
16. Metzger WJ, Patterson R, Zeiss CR, et al. (1976) Comparison of polymerized and unpolymerized antigen E for immunotherapy of ragweed allergy. N Engl J Med 295:1160–1165
17. Kelly JF, Zeiss CR, Suszko IM, Levitz D, Patterson R (1980) Polymerized whole ragweed: human safety and immune response. J Allergy Clin Immunol 65:50–56
18. Patterson R, Suszko IM, Bacal E, Zeiss CR, Kelly JF, Pruzansky JJ (1979) Reduced allergenicity of high molecular weight ragweed polymers. J Allergy Clin Immunol 63:47–50
19. Carter EB (1935) Detoxified pollen extract. To Abbott Laboratories: US Patent 2, 019, 808
20. Rinkel HI (1949) Inhalant allergy. III. The coseasonal application of serial dilution testing (titration). Ann Allergy 2:639–645

Hymenoptera Venom Allergy

B. Przybilla[1] and J. Ring[2]

[1] Dermatologische Klinik und Poliklinik der Ludwig-Maximilians-Universität, Frauenlobstrasse 9–11, W-8000 München 2, Federal Republic of Germany
[2] Hautklinik, Universitäts-Krankenhaus Eppendorf, Martinistrasse 52, W-2000 Hamburg 20, Federal Republic of Germany

Abstract

Immediate-type allergy to bee or wasp stings can be treated efficiently due to the availability of venom extracts. Basically, hyposensitization is indicated in all patients with IgE-mediated systemic (= anaphylactic) hypersensitivity reactions. Diagnostic procedures aim to specify the culprit insect and to prove IgE-mediated allergy. Basic diagnostics comprise history taking and skin threshold testing as well as RAST with hymenoptera venoms. Skin test and RAST results are influenced by several variables: reactivity, particularly in the RAST, is negatively correlated to the time interval elapsed since the last hypersensitivity reaction; negative or weakly positive results in the RAST are more frequent in wasp than in bee venom allergy; patients reacting to common aero-allergens in the prick test exhibit more frequently a higher reactivity to hymenoptera venoms than those without such reactions. There is a noteworthy increase of more severe reactions with the patient's age. In vitro diagnostics is completed by the basophil histamine release test (or basophil degranulation test) and the determination of specific IgG antibodies. There are several hyposensitization protocols which have been proven to be effective, rush hyposensitization on an in-patient basis still is the most advantageous. During the incremental treatment phase, systemic anaphylactic side effects may occur in a considerable number of patients, but usually these reactions are mild. Anaphylactic side effects are more frequent in patients with a history of a full shock than in those with milder sting symptoms. After 6 to 12 months of therapy the effect of hyposensitization should be evaluated by a sting challenge test. In our patients, 163 sting challenges caused only local reactions in 80%, in another 15% systemic symptoms were milder than prior to hyposensitization. In patients who continue to react systemically, an increase of the venom dose used for hyposensitization can improve the therapeutic effect. Repeated systemic reactions are a side effect in a small part of the patients, occurring particularly in bee venom allergy; in such cases individual modifications of the therapeutic procedure are necessary. If hyposensitization has been proven to be successful by sting challenge, it should be performed for three years. The protective effect of treatment seems to last for at least some time, the exact duration, however, is not yet known. Hyposensitization with venom extracts can be regarded as a major progress in allergology during recent years. However, a number of questions remains to be answered by further research, particularly with regard to diagnostics, therapy protocols and evaluation of efficacy.

Introduction

It has been more than 50 years since the use of bee venom [38] and more than 30 years since the use of wasp venom [39] were reported to be effective means of hyposensitization in individuals with anaphylactic reactions to hymenoptera stings. More recent research [12, 26, 35] has allowed the full development of this method.

The present routine use of venoms for diagnosis and treatment of hymenoptera venom allergy has to be regarded as one of the major advances of allergology in our time. Besides the beneficial clinical effects for the patient, the availability of these pure allergens has provided important findings on anaphylactic hypersensitivity and hyposensitization. However, scientific progress usually poses new problems, and this also holds true with regard to hymenoptera venom allergy.

The current status of the management of hymenoptera venom allergy, particularly with regard to hyposensitization, has been reviewed in recent papers [9, 40, 72, 79]. Here, we will focus on some issues concerning diagnosis and hyposensitization in hymenoptera venom allergy.

Relevance of Diagnostic Parameters

Diagnosis of IgE-mediated hymenoptera venom allergy is routinely based on patient history, skin tests with venoms, and determination of venom-specific IgE by RAST. These procedures may be supplemented by additional methods, such as basophil tests [59, 71, 81] or assessment of venom-specific IgG [27, 43, 54, 72]. The determination of the severity grade of the clinical reaction, the reactivity threshold to venom in the skin test, and the RAST class for venom permit some quantification, which has been used in scoring systems intending to balance the diagnostic findings [72, 74].

For severity grading, the scheme according to Mueller [46] is widely used. However, some details of this scale are complicated and arbitrary, and its application may yield equivocal results. The clear and easy to handle severity scale, published in the Lancet by Ring and Messmer in 1977 [65] (Table 1), is more appropriate and will be referred to here.

A number of studies in which untreated patients with previous systemic sting reactions underwent a diagnostic challenge sting have shown that none of the available diagnostic parameters allows one to predict with certainty the type of reaction to a re-sting [7, 16, 29, 53]. Furthermore, in these studies only 14%–38% [16, 53] of the patients again exhibited a systemic reaction. One could conclude from these results that diagnostic sting challenge is the best way to decide whether a patient needs hyposensitization. However, this procedure is, even if performed in an intensive care unit, potentially life threatening [3] and should not be used for routine purposes. Also, a sting challenge may act as a booster and lead to an increased risk during future stings.

The only valid criterion for starting venom hyposensitization is a previous, IgE-mediated, systemic sting reaction. Not only in the usual, immediate, anaphy-

Table 1. Grading of anaphylactic/anaphylactoid reactions. [After 65].

Severity grade	Skin	Gastrointestinal tract	Respiratory tract	Cardiovascular system
I	Pruritus Flush Urticaria Angioedema	No symptoms	No symptoms	No symptoms
II	Pruritus Flush Urticaria Angioedema (not mandatory)	Nausea Cramping	Rhinorrhea Hoarseness Dyspnea	Tachycardia Drop in BP Arrhythmia
III	Full shock			
IV	Cardiac and/or respiratory arrest			

lactic type of reaction, but, as reported recently, also in atypical, IgE-mediated, late-onset or serum sickness-like reactions may hyposensitization be helpful [63]. All diagnostic procedures beyond history taking aim to specify the culprit insect and to verify an IgE-mediated mechanism. Hyposensitization should be performed regardless of the severity grade, as patients presenting with a history of more severe sting symptoms report repeated sting reactions significantly more often than those with only one reaction (Fig. 1). Evidently, severity tends to increase with repeated reactions. It has been proposed that, in children with only mild systemic reactions, hyposensitization may not be necessary in view of the benign course of the disease in this age group [9, 68]. However, as a life threatening risk cannot be excluded in such children, it is safer to offer hyposensitization to these young patients, not least because of their overall substantial exposure to hymenoptera and the inherent uncertainties of children's anamnestic data.

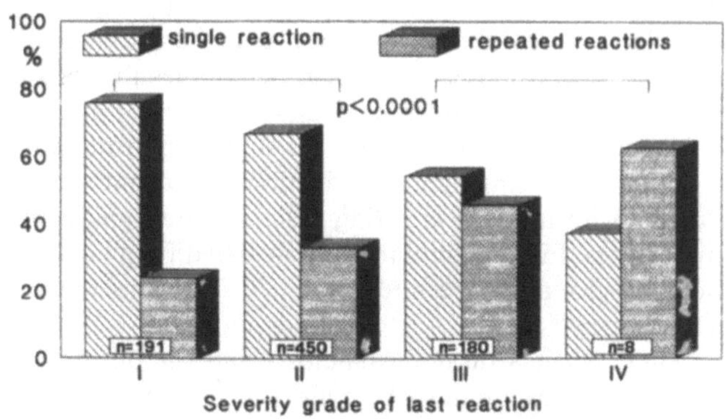

Fig. 1. Severity of sting reactions; single and repeated (≥2) reactions

Factors Influencing Diagnostic Parameters

When interpreting the results of venom skin tests and RASTs, it must be considered that they are influenced by a number of variables. Thus, it has been reported that the reactivity in the skin test [19, 23, 24] or RAST [17, 24, 44, 64] declines according to the time elapsed since the most recent hypersensitivity reaction. However, in a study on bee venom allergic patients, no such association has been found neither for the skin test nor the RAST results [2], and it has been reported that skin prick test results do not change significantly over a 3-year period [44]. In our patients, about 70% of whom were tested less than 1 year after their last sting reaction, only the RAST results, but not the reactivity thresholds in the prick test, were significantly negatively correlated to the time elapsed [60]. It seems that the results obtained in the skin test are more stable than those of the RAST.

Bee venom and vespid venom allergic patients differ with regard to the concentration of specific IgE against the respective venom. Positive RAST results have been reported in bee venom allergy in 70% – 100% [17, 42, 75], but only in 56% – 87.5% of vespid venom allergic patients [17, 23, 32]. In our patients, RAST classes 0 or 1 were present in 10.5% of 220 bee venom allergic individuals and in 31.3% of 163 vespid venom allergic subjects ($p<0.001$) [60]. No such difference between bee and vespid allergy was apparent when the reactivity thresholds in the skin test were compared [60].

An intriguing issue is the relationship of features of atopy to diagnostic parameters of hymenoptera venom allergy, which we have evaluated in a total of 501 patients [57]. Severity of sting reactions, skin test, and RAST reactivity to venoms were not significantly different in patients with or without a history of atopic diseases. An elevation of total serum IgE (≥100 kU/l) correlated to a higher frequency of RAST classes ≥2 ($p<0.01$), which can be explained by the contribution of specific IgE to total IgE, and to less severe reactions to hymenoptera stings ($p<0.05$). However, patients reacting less severely were also significantly younger, and this could explain the difference in reactivity to stings (see below). Furthermore, patients reacting in the prick test to at least one of three common aeroallergens (grass pollen, house dust mite, cat epithelia) had prick test thresholds ≤10 µg/ml and RAST classes ≥2 significantly ($p<0.05/p<0.01$) more often for hymenoptera venoms than did individuals with negative prick test results to these aeroallergens. Seemingly, prick test results to common aeroallergens reflect the individual IgE response, which also determines the magnitude of IgE production to venoms. The relationship of these features of atopy to diagnostic parameters of hymenoptera venom allergy are summarized in Table 2.

When discussing hyposensitization the patient's age must also be considered. Patients with more severe sting reactions are significantly older than those with milder ones (Fig. 2). Similarly, an increased frequency of more severe reactions in older age groups has been reported [37]. The older the patient, the more mandatory is therapy!

Thus, when a definite diagnosis and the decision on hyposensitization are made, the following must be considered: routine diagnostic parameters, time interval elapsed since the precedent sting reaction, culprit insect (bee or vespid), "atopy status", and the age of the patient. For example, a 55-year-old individual

Table 2. Relationship of features of an atopic status to diagnostic parameters of hymenoptera venom allergy. [From 54].

Features of atopy	Severity of sting reactions	Reactivity to venoms	
		Skin test	RAST
Positive history of atopic disease(s)	∅	∅	∅
Elevated total IgE (≥100 kU/l)	↓	∅	↑
Positive prick test reactions to aeroallergens[a]	∅	↑	↑

↓/∅/↑, decreased/not different/increased compared to patients without the respective feature.
[a] At least one 1+ reaction to grass pollen, cat epithelium, or house dust mite.

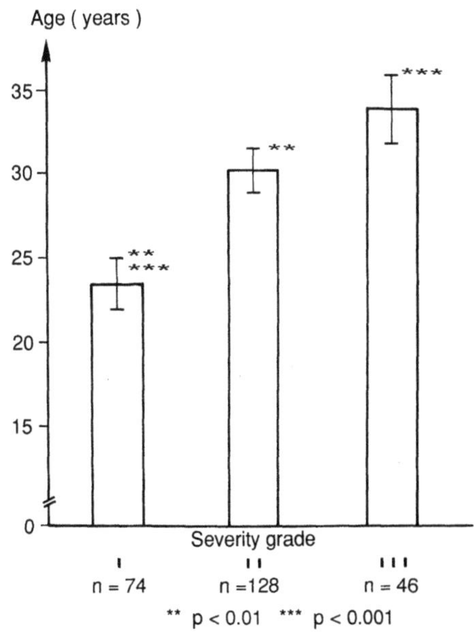

Fig. 2. Severity of sting reactions and patients' age

with a history of a severity grade II reaction to a yellow jacket sting 1 year ago, a negative skin test with common aeroallergens, a negative hymenoptera venom RAST, and only a weak skin test reaction to vespid venom may be at a much higher risk when re-stung than a 14-year-old individual with a severity grade II reaction due to a bee sting 3 months ago, a positive prick test reaction to grass pollen, and a high reactivity in the skin test and RAST with bee venom.

Tolerance of Rush Hyposensitization

The aim of hyposensitization is to give maximum protection with a minimum of serious side effects. In general, aqueous venom preparations are used. Only a few studies have dealt with hyposensitization using monomethoxy polyethylene glycol (mPEG)-modified honeybee venom [49, 52] or vespid venom adsorbed to aluminum hydroxide [45]; mPEG-modified preparations were somewhat better tolerated but less effective than aqueous solutions; alum adsorbed venom may allow some prolongation of the injection intervals during maintenance therapy. However, at present no definite clinically relevant advantages of these modifications are apparent. The routine maintenance dose of aqueous preparations usually is 100 µg, which, after the incremental phase, is administered every 4 weeks. Higher doses may be useful in case of increased exposure [47] or failure of routine treatment (see below).

There are numerous protocols for venom hyposensitization. Their nomenclature is somewhat confusing, e. g., there are "rush", "rapid", "slow rush", "modified rush", "semi-rush", "classical", "slow", "cluster", or "step" venom hyposensitizations [6, 9, 18].

However, only two principle forms of therapy should be distinguished, according to the manner in which the maintenance dose is reached: in "rush" hyposensitization this involves injections administered continuously over one to several days. The other approach, "conventional" hyposensitization, involves injections given at intervals through several weeks to months. Protocols in use can be assigned to one of these two principle methods or a combination of both.

As hymenoptera venom allergy is a life threatening disease, only systemic reactions during hyposensitization should be regarded as serious side effects. In general, "slower" protocols cause less side effects than rush hyposensitization [9, 66]; however, in representative studies, the percentage of patients exhibiting at least one systemic reaction during the incremental treatment phase evidently is not simply related to the respective procedure (Table 3). There are many variables which may influence the occurrence of systemic side effects, and to our knowledge, there does not exist any controlled study aiming to compare rush and conventional hyposensitization with regard to side effects.

Overall, rush hyposensitization on an inpatient basis still seems the most advantageous procedure: protection is achieved rapidly; side effects, if they occur,

Table 3. Frequency of systemic side effects during the incremental phase of hymenoptera venom hyposensitization.

Author	*n*	Treatment courses	
		Systemic reactions (%)	Protocol
Small et al. [70]	13	0	C
Nataf et al. [50]	52	1.9	R
Bäurle and Schwarz [4]	70	2.9	R
Chipps et al. [13]	44	6.8	C
Golden et al. [18]	64	15.6	C
Nüßlein et al. [51]	77	26.0	R
Przybilla et al. [58]	290	37.6	R
Thurnheer et al. [73]	21	38.1	R
	21	38.1	C
Yunginger et al. [83]	20	80.0	R

C, conventional; R, rush.

can be treated safely; and treatment is also possible during the months when insects are flying. We have used a protocol according to which incremental venom doses are administered up to four times daily [58], reaching the maintenance dose of 100 μg after an average of 9 treatment days. Systemic side effects during 290 hyposensitization courses were as follows [58]: There were systemic reactions in 37.6%. Usually, these reactions were mild (19.0%, severity grade I; 18.3%, severity grade II); in only one patient did full shock develop, which was quickly reversed with adequate treatment. Systemic side effects started in more than 60% of those reacting at venom doses ≥10 μg. Treatment with bee or vespid venom did not differ with regard to the occurrence of systemic adverse effects. Of 84 patients, 47.6% with a history of a full shock due to insect stings exhibited systemic reactions during rush hyposensitization as compared to 27% of 37 patients with a history of disseminated skin symptoms only ($p < 0.05$). In comparison to the severity grade of the most severe precedent sting reaction, symptoms during rush hyposensitization were less severe in 86.5% and more severe in only 1.5%. In bee venom allergy, patients with a high reactivity to bee venom in the skin test (threshold concentration ≤10 μg/ml) had a significantly greater frequency of systemic reactions during rush hyposensitization than those with a lower reactivity (50.7% vs 30.5%; $p < 0.01$); such a relationship was not found in vespid venom allergic individuals. No relation between RAST classes and the occurrence of systemic side effects was evident.

Control of Therapeutic Efficacy

Parameters of reactivity to venoms, as evaluated in the skin test or in vitro, change during hyposensitization. It is beyond the scope of this article to deal with these effects in detail. The important point to make is that there is no test parameter which would permit one to determine the success of treatment. This is not surprising. Since before hyposensitization there is no parameter predicting the type of reaction when the patient is restung, why should there be any in the treated patient? In particular, the assumption of a positive relation between the titer of venom-specific IgG and protection, put foreward for some time [25, 31, 67, 76, 80], can no longer be maintained. In our patients, the development of levels of venom-specific IgG during hyposensitization and the levels before a challenge sting did not differ in individuals with and without systemic symptoms resulting from this procedure [55] (Fig. 3). In a recent study, there was an even higher concentration of venom-specific IgG in patients reacting to a challenge sting than in those not reacting [47].

A sting challenge test is the only method for assessing the effect of venom hyposensitization. When such testing was done with single insect stings in treated patients, complete protection, that is the absence of a systemic reaction, was found in about 80%–100% (Table 4). We perform a challenge test 6–18 months after reaching the maintenance dose. Sting challenge should not be done immediately after the incremental phase of rush hyposensitization, as there could be a nonspecific refractory state, nor immediately before discontinuation of

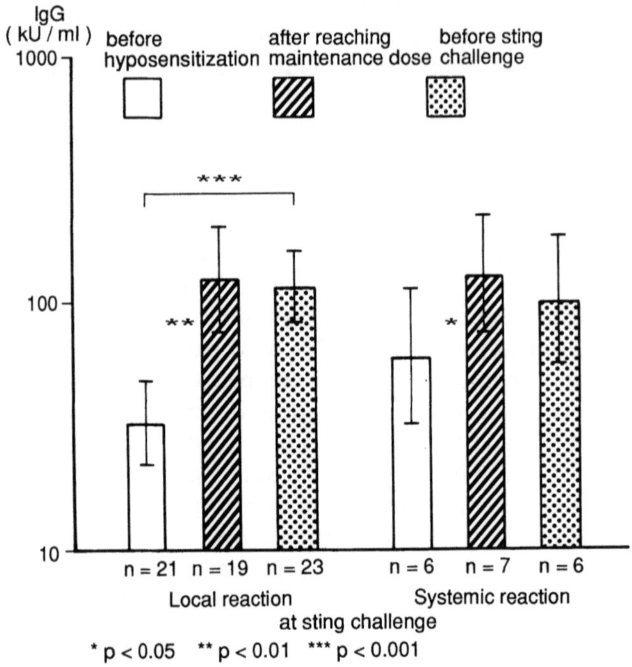

Fig. 3. Specific IgG antibodies in bee venom hyposensitization

Table 4. Control of efficacy of venom hyposensitization by sting challenge.

Author	Challenges (*n*)	Systemic reactions (*n*)	Protected (%)
Golden et al. [18]	56 (4)[a]	0	100
Chipps et al. [13]	40	1	97.5
Nüßlein et al. [51]	62 (12)[a]	2	96.8
Hunt et al. [26]	18	1	94.4
Kästner et al. [30]	83	5	94.0
Przybilla et al. [58]	163	32	80.4
Hoffman et al. [25]	25	5	80.0
Müller et al. [47]	67	15	77.6

[a] Field stings included in total number.

therapy, as it may act in a different way than venom injections and, at the worst, cause resensitization.

Among 157 of our patients challenged in this way, close to 80% no longer reacted systemically to the sting, and about 15% had less severe reactions than in their history (Table 5) [58]. The outcome of the sting challenge was related to the following clinical features [58]: patients with skin reactions only, due to the challenge sting, were significantly younger than those with more severe symptoms (33.4±2.9 years vs 44.3±3.7 years; $p<0.05$); the occurrence of systemic reactions at the challenge test was positively correlated to the occurrence of systemic side

Table 5. Severity grade of 157 sting challenge reactions in relation to prior sting reactions[a]. [From 58]. Reactions above the dotted lines were at challenge less severe than in history.

Severity grade of challenge reaction	Total (%)	History of sting reactions (%)			
		Severity grade			
		I	II	III	IV
Local reaction	78.9	12.1	38.8	25.4	2.6
I	13.4	1.3	8.3	3.8	0
II	5.8	0	2.6	2.6	0.6
III	1.9	0	0	1.9	0
Total	100	13.4	49.7	33.7	3.2

[a] Most severe reaction reported.

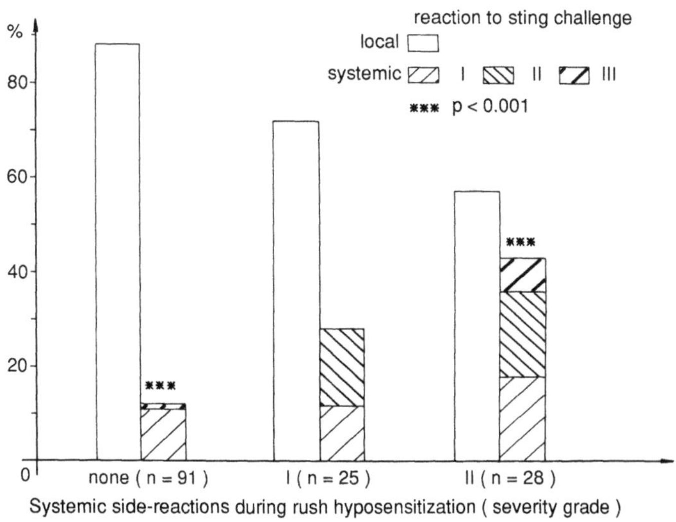

Fig. 4. Reaction to sting challenge in relation to side effects of rush hyposensitization. [After 58]

effects during rush hyposensitization (Fig. 4); patients with a history of a full shock to previous insect stings also had a tendency toward more severe reactions (≥ severity grade II) at the challenge test.

Treatment Failures

Sting challenge testing is of eminent practical importance as, in patients still systemically reacting, therapeutic efficacy can be improved in many cases by increasing the venom dose used for hyposensitization every 4 weeks or by reducing the time interval between injections of the usual dose of 100 μg [36, 41, 55] (Ta-

Table 6. Results of hymenoptera venom hyposensitization with increased[a] maintenance doses in patients not protected by treatment with 100 μg/4 weeks. [From 55].

Patient	Venom	Severity grade of sting challenge reaction	
		Before dose increase	After dose increase
1	Bee	I	III
2	Bee	I	Local reaction
3	Vespid	I	Local reaction
4	Vespid	I	Local reaction
5	Vespid	II	Local reaction
6	Vespid	III	Local reaction

[a] 150 or 200 μg/4 weeks.

ble 6). The routine use of an increased venom dose of 200 μg may be more effective than the 100 μg dose [11, 47]. However, this "double" dose cannot be recommended generally, as it is expensive and necessary only in a small number of patients.

Repeated and sometimes severe systemic reactions occur in a few patients as serious side effects. They may start during the incremental phase or maintenance therapy and may hamper continuation of treatment substantially. For yet unknown reasons, they seem to be much more frequent in bee venom than in vespid venom allergy [66a]. There are a number of factors which may facilitate these reactions and thus should be looked for. These comprise concomitant sensitizations to other allergens, focal infections, thyroid disease, inadvertent administration of drugs not allowed during hyposensitization (e.g., beta blockers, nonsteroidal antiinflammatory agents), or mastocytosis. If exclusion of such factors is unproductive, an increase of the venom dose per time unit up to 400 μg/4 weeks [10] may be helpful, and pretreatment with antihistamines or mast cell blockers before venom injections may be tried. However, if in some patients, despite these measures, it is not possible to reach the regular maintenance dose of 100 μg/4 weeks, then treatment should be continued with the highest dose tolerated. Such patients have to be regarded as being at an increased risk when re-stung. In bee venom allergic patients with repeated systemic reactions, hyposensitization may be facilitated, at least temporarily, by the administration of beekeeper γ-globulin, which is rich in bee venom-specific IgG. This experimental treatment has been shown to improve the tolerance and possibly also the effectiveness of hyposensitization [8, 28, 34, 48, 56, 82].

Duration of Hyposensitization

How long should venom hyposensitization be performed? It has been suggested that a substantially decreased reactivity in the skin test, a negative RAST (or basophil degranulation test), or an increase of venom-specific IgG may indicate protection and thus permit discontinuation of treatment [1, 14, 15, 20–22, 43,

Table 7. Frequency of systemic sting challenge reactions after discontinuing venom hyposensitization.

Author	Hyposensitization (years)		Re-stung patients (n)	Systemic reactions (%)
	Duration	Discontinued		
Golden et al. [20]	5–8	1	29	0
Golden et al. [21]	5–8	2–5	74	3 (–10)
Schuberth et al. [69]	≥5	1	27	7
Urbanek et al. [78]	4–7	1	29	3
		2	14	14
Berchtold et al. [5]	3	1	37	20
	4–11	1	53	21

61, 73, 77]. However, after hyposensitization, there seemingly is no skin test or in vitro test parameter which could predict with certainty the type of future sting reaction [21, 62, 69].

Lifelong venom hyposensitization is probably the only procedure guaranteeing lifelong protection, but it is inconvenient to the patient, expensive, and possibly risky with regard to potential long-term effects of allergen administration. Thus, it has been widely accepted that treatment should be performed only for limited periods of time. At present, we stop after 3 years if the success of hyposensitization has been proven by a sting challenge performed as described above. In a few exceptional patients, a longer therapy may be considered if there is an extremely high exposure or other individual risks, possibly also including a history of severe previous sting reactions [33].

Patients in whom hyposensitization has been stopped are at some risk of developing systemic reactions again when re-stung. However, as can be seen from a few available studies in which sting challenges were performed after some years off therapy, the frequency of systemic reactions is rather low and does not substantially exceed that found at challenges performed during hyposensitization (Table 7). Sting challenges in patients off treatment raise some concern about the possibility of resensitization. Although this risk seems to be small, the procedure should not be used for routine purposes. Rather, patients should try to avoid reexposure to insect stings as much as possible.

If systemic insect sting reactions recur, hyposensitization has to be started from the beginning.

Final Remarks

Hymenoptera venom allergy can now be treated efficiently in most patients; however, many questions remain, especially with regard to diagnostics, treatment protocols, and evaluation of efficacy. A most intriguing issue is the evident dissociation between immunological test parameters and clinical reactivity, which poses practical problems and raises questions with regard to the concept of allergic diseases. Hymenoptera venom allergy surely will stay a field of intense and exciting scientific research.

References

1. Barde SH, Georgitis JW, Mauriello PM, Reisman RE (1983) Fall in serum venom-specific IgE (vIgE) as a criterion for discontinuation of venom immunotherapy (VIT). J Allergy Clin Immunol 71:141
2. Bar-Sela S, Shalit M, Kalbfleisch JH, Fink JN (1983) The relative value of skin tests and radioallergosorbent test in the diagnosis of bee sting hypersensitivity. J Allergy Clin Immunol 72:690–694
3. Bauer CP (1986) Stichprovokationen zur Diagnostik von Insektengift-Allergien? Allergologie 9:S14
4. Bäurle G, Schwarz W (1983) Hymenopterengift-Allergie. Stellenwert des allergenspezifischen IgG bei der Therapie. Dtsch Med Wochenschr 108:1351–1355
5. Berchtold E, Helbling A, Müller U (1989) Allergy to honeybee stings: results of sting challenge (CH) 1 year after discontinuation of venom immunotherapy (VIT). Allergologie 12 (Kongreßausgabe, Abstracts):90
6. Bernstein DI, Mittman RJ, Kagen SL, Korbee L, Enrione M, Bernstein IL (1989) Clinical and immunologic studies of rapid venom immunotherapy in hymenoptera-sensitive patients. J Allergy Clin Immunol 84:951–959
7. Blaauw PJ, Smithuis LOMJ (1985) The evaluation of the common diagnostic methods of hypersensitivity for bee and yellow jacket venom by means of an in-hospital insect sting. J Allergy Clin Immunol 75:556–562
8. Bousquet J, Fontes A, Robinet-Lévy M, Aznar R, Ménardo JL, Michel FB (1984) Combination of active and passive immunization in honey bee venom (HBV) immunotherapy. J Allergy Clin Immunol 73:108
9. Bousquet J, Müller UR, Dreborg S, Jarisch R, Malling H-J, Mosbech H, Urbanek R, Youlten L (1987) Immunotherapy with hymenoptera venoms. Position paper of the Working Group on Immunotherapy of the European Academy of Allergy and Clinical Immunology. Allergy 42:401–413
10. Bousquet J, Ménardo JL, Velasquez G, Michel FB (1988) Systemic reactions during maintenance immunotherapy with honey bee venom. Ann Allergy 61:63–68
11. Bousquet J, Knani J, Velasquez G, Ménardo JL, Guilloux L, Michel FB (1989) Evolution of sensitivity to hymenoptera venom in 200 allergic patients followed for up to 3 years. J Allergy Clin Immunol 84:944–950
12. Busse WW, Reed CE, Lichtenstein LM, Reisman RE (1975) Immunotherapy in bee-sting anaphylaxis. Use of honeybee venom. JAMA 231:1154–1156
13. Chipps BE, Valentine MD, Kagey-Sobotka A, Schuberth KC, Lichtenstein LM (1980) Diagnosis and treatment of anaphylactic reactions to hymenoptera stings in children. J Pediatr 97:177–184
14. Clayton WF, Reisman RE, Georgitis JW, Wypych JI, Arbesman CE (1983) Effect of prolonged venom immunotherapy on serum venom-specific IgE and IgG. Clin Allergy 13:301–307
15. Dietschi R, Wüthrich B, Marti-Wyss S, Cuhat J (1987) Der Basophilen-Degranulationstest (BDT) als Verlaufsparameter einer Hyposensibilisierung mit Hymenopterengiften. Schweiz Med Wochenschr 117:1728–1735
16. Engel T, Heinig JH, Weeke ER (1988) Prognosis of patients reacting with urticaria to insect sting. Results of an in-hospital sting challenge. Allergy 43:289–293
17. Glowania HJ (1981) Ergebnisse des RAST und des Hauttestes in der Diagnose von Bienen- und Wespengiftallergien. Berichtsband RAST 2:173–178
18. Golden DBK, Valentine MD, Kagey-Sobotka A, Lichtenstein LM (1980) Regimens of hymenoptera venom immunotherapy. Ann Intern Med 92:620–624
19. Golden DBK, Valentine MD, Kagey-Sobotka A, Lichtenstein LM (1982) Prevalence of hymenoptera venom allergy. J Allergy Clin Immunol 69:124
20. Golden DBK, Addison BI, Gadde J, Kagey-Sobotka A, Valentine MD, Lichtenstein LM (1989) Prospective observations on stopping prolonged venom immunotherapy. J Allergy Clin Immunol 84:162–167
21. Golden DBK, Kwiterovich KA, Kagey-Sobotka A, Valentine MD, Lichtenstein LM (1989) Discontinuing venom immunotherapy (VIT): determinants of clinical reactivity. J Allergy Clin Immunol 83:273

22. Graft DF, Schuberth KC, Kagey-Sobotka A, Kwiterovich KA, Niv Y, Lichtenstein LM, Valentine MD (1984) The development of negative skin tests in children treated with venom immunotherapy. J Allergy Clin Immunol 73:61–68
23. Grant JA, Rahr R, Thueson DO, Lett-Brown MA, Hokanson JA, Yunginger JW (1983) Diagnosis of *Polistes* wasp hypersensitivity. J Allergy Clin Immunol 72:399–406
24. Harries MG, Kemeny DM, Youlten LJF, McK Mills M, Lessof MH (1984) Skin and radioallergosorbent tests in patients with sensitivity to bee and wasp venom. Clin Allergy 14:407–412
25. Hoffman DR, Gillman SA, Cummins LH, Kozak PP, Oswald A (1981) Correlation of IgG and IgE antibody levels to honey bee venom allergens with protection to sting challenge. Ann Allergy 46:17–23
26. Hunt KJ, Valentine MD, Sobotka AK, Benton AW, Amodio FJ, Lichtenstein LM (1978) A controlled trial of immunotherapy in insect hypersensitivity. N Engl J Med 299:157–161
27. Jarisch R (1980) Die Bienengiftallergie (Modell einer IgE-mediierten Soforttypallergie). Wien Klin Wochenschr [Suppl] 122:3–27
28. Jarisch R (1981) Passive immunotherapy in bee venom-allergic patients. Arch Dermatol Res 270:230
29. Kampelmacher MJ, van der Zwan JC (1987) Provocation test with a living insect as a diagnostic tool in systemic reactions to bee and wasp venom: a prospective study with emphasis on the clinical aspects. Clin Allergy 17:317–327
30. Kästner H, Kalveram KJ, Forck G (1984) Immunstatus von hyposensibilisierten Insektengiftallergikern nach dreijähriger Behandlung. Berichtsband RAST 4:181–185
31. Kemeny DM, MacKenzie-Mills M, Harries MG, Youlten LJF, Lessof MH (1983) Antibodies to purified bee venom proteins and peptides. II. A detailed study of changes in IgE and IgG antibodies to individual bee venom antigens. J Allergy Clin Immunol 72:376–385
32. Kleinhans D (1979) Diagnostik der Insektentoxinallergie (Biene, Wespe) mit dem Radio-Allergo-Sorbens-Test. Berichtsband RAST 1:16–22
33. Lantner R, Reisman RE (1989) Clinical and immunologic features and subsequent course of patients with severe insect-sting anaphylaxis. J Allergy Clin Immunol 84:900–906
34. Lessof MH, Sobotka AK, Lichtenstein LM (1977) Protection against anaphylaxis in hymenoptera-sensitive patients by passive immunization. Monogr Allergy 12:253–256
35. Lichtenstein LM, Valentine MD, Sobotka AK (1974) A case for venom treatment in anaphylactic sensitivity to hymenoptera sting. N Engl J Med 290:1223–1227
36. Lichtenstein LM, Valentine MD, Sobotka AK (1979) Insect allergy: the state of the art. J Allergy Clin Immunol 64:5–12
37. Lockey RF, Turkeltaub PC, Baird-Warren IA, Olive CA, Olive ES, Peppe BC, Bukantz SC (1988) The hymenoptera venom study I, 1979–1982: demographics and history-sting data. J Allergy Clin Immunol 82:370–381
38. Lotter G (1939) Sensibilisierung für Bienengift durch Typhus-Antitoxin und Desensibilisierung mit Forapin. MMW 86:330–331
39. Loveless MH (1962) Immunization in wasp-sting allergy through venom-repositories and periodic insect stings. J Immunol 89:204–215
40. Malling HJ (ed) (1988) Immunotherapy. Position paper. Prepared by the Immunotherapy Subcommittee of the European Academy of Allergology and Clinical Immunology. Allergy [Suppl 6] 43
41. Ménardo JL, Bousquet J, Delair L, Michel FB (1984) Treatment failures during maintenance therapy in honey bee venom allergy. J Allergy Clin Immunol 73:188
42. Miyachi SM, Lessof MH, Kemeny DM (1979) Evaluation of bee sting allergy by skin tests and serum antibody assays. Int Arch Allergy Appl Immunol 60:148–153
43. Mokry L, Wüthrich B, Dietschi R (1985) Zur kausalen Behandlung der Hymenopterenstichallergie. Klinische Erfahrungen und serologische Verlaufskontrolle (spezifische IgE- und IgG-Antikörper) bei Hyposensibilisierung mit Bienen- und Wespengift. Schweiz Rundsch Med 74:1005–1016
44. Mosbech H, Christensen J, Dirksen A, Søborg M (1986) Insect allergy. Predictive value of diagnostic tests: a three-year follow-up study. Clin Allergy 16:433–440
45. Mosbech M, Malling HJ, Biering I, Bôwadt H, Søborg M, Weeke B, Löwenstein H (1986) Immunotherapy with yellow jacket venoms. A comparative study including 3 different extracts, one adsorbed to aluminium hydroxide and two unmodified. Allergy 41:95–103
46. Mueller HL (1966) Diagnosis and treatment of insect sensitivity. J Asthma Res 3:331–333

47. Müller UR, Helbling A, Bischof M (1989) Predictive value of venom-specific IgE, IgG and IgG subclass antibodies in patients on immunotherapy with honey bee venom. Allergy 44:412–418
48. Müller UR, Morris T, Bischof M, Friedli H, Skarvil F (1986) Combined active and passive immunotherapy in honeybee-sting allergy. J Allergy Clin Immunol 78:115–122
49. Müller UR, Rabson AR, Bischof M, Lomnitzer R, Dreborg S, Lanner Å (1987) A double-blind study comparing monomethoxy polyethylene glycol-modified honeybee venom and unmodified honeybee venom for immunotherapy. I. Clinical results. J Allergy Clin Immunol 80:252–261
50. Nataf P, Guinnepain MT, Herman D (1984) Rush venom immunotherapy: a 3-day program for hymenoptera sting allergy. Clin Allergy 14:269–275
51. Nüßlein H, Köstler C, Glück H, Baenkler HW, Kalden JR (1984) Diagnostik und Therapie der Bienen- und Wespengiftallergie. Therapiewoche 34:421–427
52. Öhman S, Björkander J, Dreborg S, Lanner Å, Malling H-J, Weeke B (1986) A preliminary study of immunotherapy with a monomethoxy polyethylene glycol modified honey bee venom preparation. Allergy 41:81–88
53. Parker JL, Santrach PJ, Dahlberg MJE, Yunginger JW (1982) Evaluation of hymenoptera-sting sensitivity with deliberate sting challenges: inadequacy of present diagnostic methods. J Allergy Clin Immunol 69:200–207
54. Przybilla B, Ring J (1986) Hyposensibilisierungsbehandlung der Hymenopterengiftallergie: Aspekte der Indikationsstellung und Dosierung. Allergologie 9:S2–S10
55. Przybilla B, Ring J, Baruth J (1984) Beziehung zwischen dem Erfolg einer Hyposensibilisierungsbehandlung mit Insektengiftextrakten und der Konzentration spezifischer Antikörper der Klasse IgG (sIgG). Berichtsband RAST 4:169–176
56. Przybilla B, Ring J, Galosi A, Geursen RG, Stickl HA (1986) Bee venom immunoglobulin for prophylaxis of anaphylactic reactions during bee venom immunotherapy (rush hyposensitization). Immunol Allergy Pract 8:107–111
57. Przybilla B, Ring J, Grießhammer B (1987) Atopy and hymenoptera venom allergy (HVA). J Allergy Clin Immunol 79:233
58. Przybilla B, Ring J, Grießhammer B, Braun-Falco O (1987) Schnellhyposensibilisierung mit Hymenopterengiften. Verträglichkeit und Therapieerfolg. Dtsch Med Wochenschr 112:416–424
59. Przybilla B, Ring J, Wielgosch J (1988) Der Basophilen-Histamin-Freisetzungstest als diagnostische Methode bei Hymenopterengift-Allergie. Hautarzt 39:662–670
60. Przybilla B, Ring J, Grießhammer B (1989) Diagnostische Befunde bei Hymenopterengiftallergie. Zur Bedeutung von Anamnese, Hauttest und RAST. Allergologie 12:192–202
61. Randolph CC, Reisman RE (1986) Evaluation of decline in serum venom-specific IgE as a criterion of stopping venom immunotherapy. J Allergy Clin Immunol 77:823–827
62. Reisman RE, Lantner R (1989) Further observations of stopping venom immunotherapy: comparison of patients stopped because of a fall in serum venom-specific IgE to insignificant levels with patients stopped prematurely by self-choice. J Allergy Clin Immunol 83:1049–1054
63. Reisman RE, Livingston A (1989) Late-onset allergic reactions, including serum sickness, after insect stings. J Allergy Clin Immunol 84:331–337
64. Reisman RE, Arbesman CE, Lazell M (1979) Observations on the aetiology and natural history of stinging insect sensitivity: application of measurements of venom-specific IgE. Clin Allergy 9:303–311
65. Ring J, Messmer K (1977) Incidence and severity of anaphylactoid reactions to colloid volume substitutes. Lancet 1:466–469
66. Rzany B, Rosenkranz A, Wekkeli M, Hippmann G, Götz M, Jarisch R (1990) Systemische Nebenwirkungen der spezifischen Immuntherapie mit Insektengiften. Allergologie 13:S63–S65
66a. Rzany B, Przybilla B, Jarisch R, Aberer W, Dietschi R, Wüthrich B, Bühler B, Frosch P, Rakoski J, Kiehm M, Kuhn W, Urbanek R, Ring J (1991) Clinical characteristics of patients with repeated systemic reactions during specific immunotherapy with hymenoptera venoms. A retrospective study. Allergy 46:251–254
67. Schuberth KC, Golden DBK, Kagey-Sobotka A, Valentine MD, Lichtenstein LM (1981) Evaluation and treatment of insect-sting allergy. In: Ring J, Burg G (eds) New trends in allergy. Springer, Berlin Heidelberg New York, pp 260–268
68. Schuberth KC, Graft DF, Kagey-Sobotka A, Kwiterovich KA, Szklo M, Lichtenstein LM, Valentine MD (1983) Do all children with insect allergy need venom therapy? J Allergy Clin Immunol 71:140

69. Schuberth KC, Kwiterovich KA, Kagey-Sobotka A, Lichtenstein LM, Valentine MD (1987) Discontinuing venom immunotherapy in skin test positive children. J Allergy Clin Immunol 79:126
70. Small P, Barrett D, Biskin N (1983) Venom immunotherapy – a critical evaluation of in vitro techniques. Ann Allergy 50:256–259
71. Sobotka AK, Valentine MD, Benton AW, Lichtenstein LM (1974) Allergy to insect stings. I. Diagnosis of IgE-mediated hymenoptera sensitivity by venom-induced histamine release. J Allergy Clin Immunol 53:170–184
72. Studiengruppe Insektengift-Allergie der Arbeitsgemeinschaft Dermatologische Forschung (1989) Richtlinien für die Diagnose und Behandlung von Überempfindlichkeitsreaktionen auf Bienen- und Wespenstiche. Allergologie 12:43–45
73. Thurnheer U, Müller U, Stoller R, Lanner A, Hoigné R (1983) Venom immunotherapy in hymenoptera sting allergy. Comparison of rush and conventional hyposensitization and observations during long-term treatment. Allergy 38:465–475
74. Urbanek R (1979) Neue Konzepte der Behandlung von Insektengiftallergien. Derm Beruf Umwelt 27:44–48
75. Urbanek R, Karitzky D (1981) Insektengift-Allergie im Kindesalter. Hyposensibilisierung: Indikation und Therapie mit Insektengift-Extrakten. Allergologie 4:56–59
76. Urbanek P, Krauss U, Ziupa J, Smedegard G (1983) Venom-specific IgE and IgG antibodies as a measure of the degree of protection in insect-sting-sensitive patients. Clin Allergy 13:229–234
77. Urbanek R, Kuhn W, Forster J (1984) Prolonged venom immunotherapy: specific IgE and IgG antibodies as criteria for discontinuation of treatment. J Allergy Clin Immunol 73:188
78. Urbanek R, Forster J, Kuhn W, Ziupa J (1985) Discontinuation of bee venom immunotherapy in children and adolescents. J Pediatr 107:367–371
79. WHO/IUIS Working Group (1989) The current status of allergen immunotherapy (hyposensitisation). Allergy 44:369–379
80. Wüthrich B, Arrendal H, Lanner A (1981) Antikörper-Antwortmuster (spezifische IgE und IgG) von Insektenstich-Allergikern unter Immuntherapie mit Giftpräparaten. Schweiz Med Wochenschr 111:1756–1765
81. Wüthrich B, Dietschi R, Berlinger F, Marti-Wyss S, Cuhat J (1987) Der Basophilen-Degranulationstest in der Diagnostik der Hymenopterengift-Allergie. Schweiz Med Wochenschr 117:1333–1341
82. Yunginger JW, Santrach PJ (1979) Treatment failures following honeybee venom immunotherapy: use of passive immunization. J Allergy Clin Immunol 63:179
83. Yunginger JW, Paull BR, Jones RT, Santrach PJ (1979) Rush venom immunotherapy program for honeybee sting sensitivity. J Allergy Clin Immunol 63:340–347

Safety of Hyposensitization

J. Rakoski, B. Jessberger, C. Szliska, and E. Vocks

Dermatologische Klinik Technische Universität München, Biedersteinerstraße 29,
W-8000 München 40, Federal Republic of Germany

Abstract

Specific hyposensitization is a well-established therapy for IgE-mediated allergic rhinitis, asthma bronchiale, and insect venom allergies. In 0.1% – 1% of therapies, serious side effects have to be treated. Fatalities following hyposensitization are known from the literature. We analyzed these data to find out the most important risk factors.

In the last 2 years national and international organizations of allergologists have published recommendations for safe hyposensitization. We performed prospective studies following these guidelines and found serious side effects from hyposensitization in 1.1% of 448 patients. There were 8372 injections of respiratory ailments and insect venom allergies within 18 months. All side effects were successfully treated without requiring hospitalization in an intensive care unit.

Introduction

Specific hyposensitization is an established therapy for IgE-mediated allergic rhinitis, asthma bronchiale, and allergies to insect venoms. The efficacy of hyposensitization was shown by placebo-controlled studies with pollens (grasses, ragweed), house dust mites [12], and insect venoms [6].

The side effects of hyposensitization have been studied in countless prospective and retrospective studies [14]. These studies are often not comparable with each other. We chose studies involving more than 100 patients and more than 1000 injections with different inhalant allergens and bee and wasp venoms (Table 1). The studies provided data about the ratio of side effects to injections. The risk of a systemic side effect is about 0.9% per injection.

The most important fact from all these reports seems to be that, in all published controlled prospective and retrospective studies, no deaths following hyposensitization occurred.

Table 1. Adverse reactions in controlled therapy studies: systemic side effects in hyposensitization.

Author	Year	Allergen	Patients (*n*)	Injections	% Side effects/ Injection
Tipton	1982	Grasses	59	1859	1.5
Glowania	1986	Grasses	91	1177	1.4
Vervloet	1980	Inhalants	19739	151994	0.1
Greenberg	1986	Inhalants	628	20588	0.25
Nelson	1985	Inhalants	416	20645	0.3
Jarisch	1988	Inhalants + venoms	884	14141	0.5
Rakoski et al. [11]	1986	Inhalants	378	7736	0.87
Müller	1981	Venoms	100	4141	1.8
Nataf	1984	Venoms	52	2340	0.37
Rakoski et al. [11]	1986	Venoms	146	2790	0.89

Hyposensitization and Fatalities

The British Committee on Safety of Medicine (CSM) reported on deaths caused by hyposensitization in the U.K. In West Germany 22 patients died from hyposensitization between 1981 and 1990 (G. Siefert 1988, personal communication). The circumstances of the fatalities were not mentioned in either publication. Siefert mentioned only that in five patients the main causes of death were medical circumstances not related to hyposensitization. There were 16 deaths due to malpractice as a result of intravasation and insufficient treatment of shock. The CSM reported 14 fatalities due to the administered therapy itself (Table 2).

These data also showed that the risk is higher in mite therapy than in pollen therapy. We analyzed detailed data from four publications reporting on 8 patients (Table 3) [1, 5, 8, 10]. All patients (11–70 years) were treated for respiratory aller-

Table 2. Allergens and fatalities. [From 3].

Allergen	Therapies administered	Deaths
Mite	138000	7
Pollen	720000	2
Mixed extracts	592000	5

Table 3. Possible causes of shock.

Study	*n*	Wrong	Contact with allergen	Infection or asthma	High sensitivity	No supervision
Lockey et al. [18]	24	7	9	1	9	2
Haffner [5]	3	1	–	3	1	1
Chaumont et al. [1]	1	–	1	–	–	–

Table 4. Treatment measures for anaphylactic shock.

Study	*n*	Adrenalin	Antihistamines	Theophylline	O_2	Cortisone	Volume
Lockey et al. [8]	18	11		4	8	9	3
Haffner [5]	3	2	1		3	3	
Chaumont et al. [1]	1		1			1	

gies; most were asthmatics. Of the 28 patients, 9 were treated with the wrong dose, 10 patients had contact with a relevant allergen, and 10 were very sensitive to the allergens of the treatment. Three patients left after the injection and thus were without medical supervision. The therapy of anaphylactic shock is summarized in Table 4; none of the patients were treated accordingly [11].

Conclusions

National and international organizations of allergologists have published guidelines and advice for hyposensitization therapy. We have summarized these recommendations in Tables 5 and 6.

Before a patient can be treated by hyposensitization, sufficient diagnosis is necessary in order to determine all of his or her sensitivities and allergies. If hyposensitization is appropriate and if the allergens are available for injection, then the patient must be carefully instructed about the procedure. The therapy must be performed by a physician who is also able to treat anaphylactic shock.

Before the injection, it is necessary to take a short history about the general health of the patient, the status of the disease to be treated (including medication), and tolerance of the last injection at the end of hyposensitization. After the injection, the physician must monitor the patient for 30 min and be prepared to treat partial or full shock if necessary.

Table 5. Checklist before therapy: guidelines for hyposensitization.

Sufficient diagnostic measures
Suitable patient
Suitable allergens by indicated therapy
Instruction of patient

Table 6. Most important points during therapy: guidelines for hyposensitization.

Possibility for treatment of shock
Right dose
Therapy only by the physician
Monitoring of the patient for 30 min

Table 7. Controlled study (18 months): side effects in 494 patients after 8372 injections.

	Inhalant allergen injections ($n = 5882$)	Insect venom injections ($n = 2790$)
Local reactions	284 (5.1%)	no data
Conjunctivitis/rhinitis	20 (0.35%)	2 (0.07%)
Pruritus	13 (0.23%)	3 (0.1%)
Urticaria	10 (0.23%)	8 (0.28%)
Asthma	15 (0.26%)	0 (0.0%)
Cardiovascular	5 (0.08%)	12 (0.43%)

Following these guidelines, we treated 494 patients, with allergies to inhalants and insect venoms, with a total of 8372 injections (Table 7). We treated systemic advanced reactions in 0.9% of the patients. After treatment, we monitored the patients for approximately 1–2 h.

References

1. Chaumont SG, Mangin P, Lugnier AJ (1980) Choc anaphylatique mortel au cours d'un traitement de désensibilisation par Allergene. Soc Med Leg 297–400
2. Creticos PS, van Metre TE, Modiney MR, Rosenberg GL, Norman PS, Adkinson NR Jr (1984) Dose response of IgE and IgG antibodies during ragweed immunotherapy. J Allergy Clin Immunol 73(1/1):94–104
3. CSM-Update (1986) Br Med J 293:948
4. Düngemann H (1975) Zur Therapie des Heuschnupfens. Inf Arzt 3(6):1–11
5. Haffner HT (1986) Letale Komplikationen bei Desensibilisierungsbehandlungen. Aspekte zur Untersuchung und rechtsmedizinischen Begutachtungen. Zentralbl Haut Geschlechtskr 151:302–310
6. Hunt KJ, Valentine MD, Sobotka AK, Benton AW, Amodio FJ, Lichtenstein LM (1978) A controlled trial of immunotherapy in insect hyposensitivity. N Engl J Med 299:157
7. Hupke U (1988) Änderungen der Konzentration Allergen spezifischer IgG- und IgE-Antikörper. Dissertation, Technical University of Munich
8. Lockey R, Benedict L, Turteltaub P, Bukantz S (1987) Fatalities from immunotherapy and skin testing. J Allergy Clin Immunol 76:660–667
9. Mietke T (1986) Therapiekontrolluntersuchungen bei Gramineae-Allergikern. Dissertation, Technical University of Munich
10. Rands D (1980) Anaphylactic reaction to desensitization of allergic rhinitis and asthma. Cleve Med J 281:848
11. Rakoski J, von Mayenburg J, Lagally G (1986) Untersuchungen am Risiko der spez. Hyposensibilisierungsbehandlung mit Inhalationsallergenen und Insektengiften. Doppelinjektionen und Einzelinjektionen. Allergologie 9:398–401
12. Sörensen H (1973) Den kliniske värdi af hyposensibilisiering ved asthma bronchiale og rhinitis allergica. Ugeskr Laeger 138(44):2703–2707
13. Von Mayenburg J, Düngemann H, Rakoski J, Stix E (1981) Ergebnisse einer 3jährigen Hyposensibilisierung mit L-Tyrosin-Pollen Allergoid. Allergologie 1:36–42
14. Wekkeli M, Rosenkranz A, Hippmann G, Jarisch R, Götz M (1989) Systemische Nebenwirkungen bei der Immuntherapie allergischer Erkrankungen – eine vergleichende Studie. Wien Klin Wochenschr 101(19):639–652

Trends in the Use of Specific Immunotherapy

A. Rosendahl Lassen[1], L. Jacobsen[1], and U.G. Svendsen[2]

[1] ALK Laboratories, Bøge Allé 10–12, 2970 Hørsholm, Denmark
[2] Pulmonary Department, KAS, Gentofte County Hospital, Niels Andersensvej 65, 2900 Hellerup, Denmark

Introduction

The introduction of standardized extracts has led to a better approach to specific immunotherapy. Thanks to improved extract quality, it has become possible to transfer results from clinical research and experience into clinical practice. Previously, lack of standardization was a main source of dubious results and the lack of success of specific immunotherapy (SIT).

SIT is an effective treatment of IgE-mediated diseases and, when the treatment is performed with extracts of relevant composition and potency, the rate of efficacy is high. Previous success rates of 60%–70% are today being surpassed by success rates of >90%, including SIT for allergens previously regarded as less effective, such as cat hair and dander and house dust mites [2, 3, 11].

Success rate is sometimes defined as the number of studies in which the conclusion was in favor of immunotherapy; at other time, success rate is defined as the frequency of treated patients who benefited from the treatment with respect to either clinical, paraclinical, or immunological parameters. In this chapter success rate is defined as the frequency of patients who have improved with respect to clinical parameters and target organ sensitivity.

Present State

Several studies performed with standardized extracts have shown that the symptom and medication scores in treated patients are significantly lower than in untreated controls (Fig. 1, Table 1 and 2). In this context it must be remembered that immunotherapy often is compared with a so-called placebo group. However, the placebo group also receives concomitant symptomatic medication and is therefore not a group without treatment. Therefore, symptoms and medication should always be included in the evaluation of the clinical effect.

SIT with standardized extract has proven efficient in treatment of both rhinitis caused by tree, grass, and weed pollens and house dust mites (Table 1) [8] and asthma caused by pollens, animal hair and danders, especially cat and house dust mites (Table 2). The effect of SIT for treatment of pollen asthma in patients suffering from both rhinitis and asthma is very good. This has been shown by

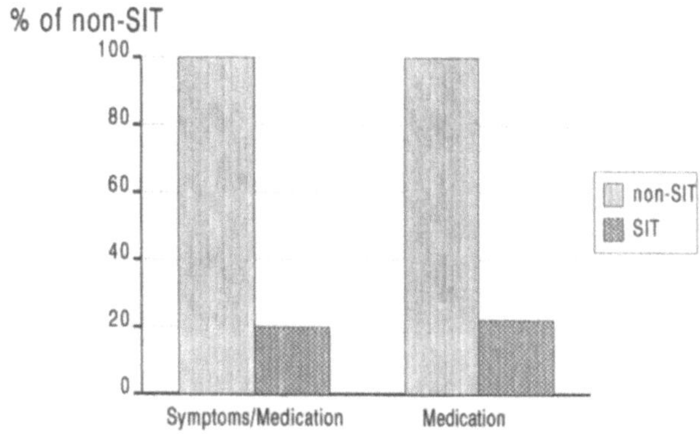

Fig. 1. Reduction in medication. SIT reduced the need of concomitant medication by 78% – 80% according to Østerballe [15] (*left*) and Rak et al. [7] (*right*)

Østerballe [15] and has recently been confirmed [6], These results indicate that successful immunotherapy is better obtained if treatment is initiated before the asthma disease has progressed too far.

Besides short-term improvement in clinical and paraclinical parameters, immunotherapy offers a long-term effect. This was described by Mosbech et al. [5] and Østerballe [15] and has recently been confirmed in a follow-up study of patients who received SIT to tree pollens 5 years earlier (Wihl, personal communication). None of the treated patients developed asthma symptoms during the period of SIT, and the total number of patients with asthma symptoms or in the need of asthma medication were still reduced 5 years after termination of SIT (Fig. 2).

The study by Hedlin et al. [3] demonstrates that SIT can affect not only the sensitivity to allergens, but also the nonspecific hyperreactivity which is a prominent feature in asthma. The tolerance to histamine is thus increased in 90% of patients receiving immunotherapy with cat allergens (Fig. 3).

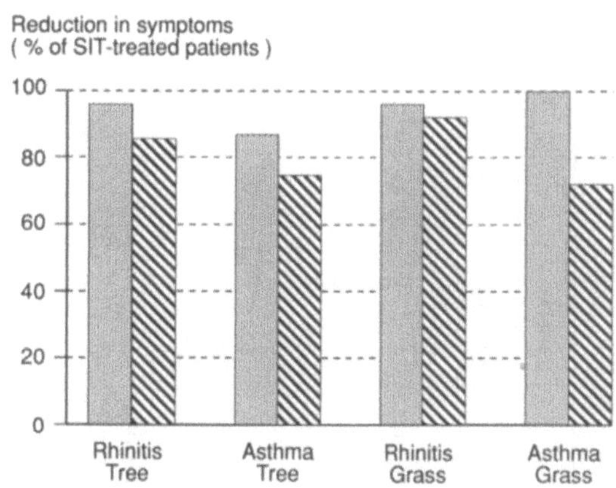

Fig. 2. The short- and long-term effects of SIT. Patients were evaluated subjectively after 3 years (*stippled bars*) of active treatment [6, 15] and 5 years after termination of SIT ([5]; Wihl, personal communication; Mosbech, personal communication). The majority of the patients still benefited from the treatment after 5 years follow-up (*hatched bars*)

Table 1. Results of four rhinitis SIT studies using pollen allergens.

Allergen	Patients		Controlled	Dose (SQ-E)		Challenge			Clinical effect		Reference
	Included	Evaluated		Aim	Actual	Group	Rate	Method	Effect	Method	
Tree (*Alnus, Corylus, Betula*)	53	34	+	100000	76000	↓ *	97%	NPT, 3 years	97%	Subjective evaluation	Nüchel-Petersen et al. [6] Wihl et al. [14]
Grass (*Phleum*)	40	39	+	100000	70000	↓ *		NPT, 3 years	97%	Subjective evaluation	Mosbech et al. [5] Østerballe [15, 16]
Weed (*Artemisia*)	24	11	+	100000	84000	↓ $p = 0.053$	89%	CPT, 2 years	↓ $p<0.059$	Medication	Svendsen et al. [9]
Tree/grass (*Betula/Phleum*)	24	13	+	100000	95000	↓ ***					
Grass (*Phleum*)	40	21	+	100000	92000	↓ **		CPT, 1 year	↓ *** ↓ *** ↓ ***	Subjective symptom and medication scores	Varney et al. [12]

SIT, specific immunotherapy; SQ-E, SQ-units; NPT, nasal provocation test; CPT, conjunctival provocation test.
* $p<0.05$; ** $p<0.01$; *** $p<0.001$; ↓, reduction in sensitivity.

Table 2. Results of nine asthma SIT studies using various allergens.

Allergen	Patients		Con-trolled	Dose (SQ-E)		Challenge			Clinical effect		Reference
	Included	Evaluated		Aim	Actual	Group	Rate	Method	Effect	Method	
Tree (*Alnus, Corylus, Betula*)	26	20	+	100000	76000				87%	Subjective evaluation	Nüchel-Petersen et al. [6] Wihl et al. [14]
Grass (*Phleum*)	7	7	+	100000	70000				100%	Subjective evaluation	Østerballe [15]
Dog	27	15	+	100000	80000	↓ n.s. ↓ *	67% 80%	BPT, 1 year CPT, 1 year	73%	Subjective evaluation	Valovirta et al. [10]
Cat	22	22	+	326000	214000	↓ **	91%	BPT, 1 year	Not done		van Metre et al. [11]
Dog/cat	29	14	+	100000	80000	↓ *	64%	BPT, 9 months	Not done		Bertelsen et al. [1]
Cat		16	+			↓ ***	94%	BPT, 3 years	71%	Global	
	40			100000	70000					assess-	Hedlin et al. [3]
Dog		14	+			↓ *	70%	BPT, 3 years	45%	ment	
House dust mites	24	24	+	60000	45000	↓ **		BPT, 1 year	Not done		Wahn et al. [13]
House dust mites	80	48	+	100000	100000	↓ **	95%	BPT, 2 years	Not yet published		Haugaard et al. [2]

SIT, specific immunotherapy; n.s., not significant; SQ-E, SQ-units; BPT, bronchial provocation test; CPT, conjunctival provocation test.
*$p<0.05$; **$p<0.01$; **$p<0.001$; ↓, reduction in senstitivity.

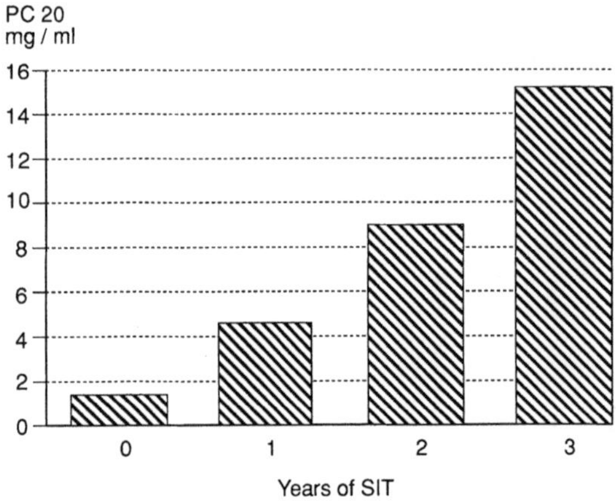

Fig. 3. The year by year development in nonspecific hyperreactivity in cat sensitive asthmatic patients receiving SIT. A highly significant reduction in sensitivity is observed (90%; $p<0.001$) [3]. PC20, concentration of histamine eliciting at 20% fall in FEV_1 (forced expiratory volume in 1 second)

Future Trends

J. Bousquet (personal communication) has proposed a new view on asthma in which worsening of asthma is described in three phases:

- First, the early stage, at which the allergic reaction (bronchospasm) is the prominent feature.
- A second phase in which inflammation becomes a more prominent part of the symptoms.
- A third phase, in which irreversible tissue damage takes place. At this stage neither pharmacological treatment nor SIT is beneficial to the patient.

Based on the view of Bousquet, it is evident that treatment of asthma should concentrate on preventing this irreversible destruction. There is increasing interest in evaluating whether SIT could affect inflammatory cells.

It was elegantly demonstrated by Rak et al. [7] that seasonal increases in eosinophil and neutrophil chemotactic activity in bronchoalveolar lavage and in blood could be abolished by immunotherapy, indicating an inhibition of inflammation. Similarly, reduction in serum neutrophil chemotactic activity following SIT was observed by McHugh and Ewan [4].

Future Perspectives

Even though more investigations are needed, it seems likely that SIT might improve the prognosis of patients with asthma. Some data also indicate that immunotherapy might prevent the development of asthma in patients suffering from rhinitis.

It seems that the optimum treatment of allergic patients with true IgE-mediated diseases involves SIT. Furthermore, treatment should be initiated earlier in order to make the most of its preventive potential.

It is likely that future research will concentrate on mechanisms, particularly those of inflammation and the role of immunotherapy in preventing inflammation and destruction. In the future, there should be a better selection of patients who can benefit from SIT and clearer indications for therapy. In this way the clinical effects of SIT can be greatly improved.

References

1. Bertelsen A, Andersen JB, Christensen J, Ingemann L, Kristensen T, Østergaard P Aa (1989) Immunotherapy with dog and cat extracts in children. Allergy 44:330–335
2. Haugaard L, Dahl R, Jacobsen L (1989) A dose-response study of immunotherapy in asthmatica. XIV Congress of the European Academy of Allergy and Clinical Immunology, Berlin (West), 17–22. Allergologie. Sondernummer B1366 E
3. Hedlin G, Graff-Lonnevig V, Heilborn H, Lilja G, Norrlind K, Pegelow K-O, Sundin B, Løwenstein H Immunotherapy with cat and dog dander extracts. V. Effects of 3 years of treatment. J Allergy Clin Immunol (to be published)
4. McHugh SM, Ewan PW (1989) Reduction of increased serum neutrophil chemotactic activity following effective hyposensitization in house dust mite allergy. Clin Exp Allergy 19:327–334
5. Mosbech H, Østerballe O (1988) Does the effect of immunotherapy last after termination of treatment. Allergy 43:523–529
6. Nüchel-Petersen B, Janniche H, Munch EP, Wihl JÅ, Böwadt H, Ipsen H, Løwenstein H (1988) Immunotherapy with partially purified and standardized tree pollen extracts. Allergy 43:353–362
7. Rak S (1988) Bronchial hyperresponsiveness and cellular and humoral factors involved in allergic inflammation during pollen season. Thesis, University of Gothenburg, Sweden
8. Ewan P, Alexander MM, Snape C, Ind PW, Agrell B, Dreborg S (1988) Effective hyposensitization in allergic rhinitis using a potent partially purified extract of house dust mite. Clin Allergy 18:501–508
9. Svendsen UG, Heinig J, Frølund L, Jacobsen L, Lassen AR (1989) The effect of immunotherapy on specific and concomitant mugwort pollen allergy in a double blind study. XIV Congress of the European Academy of Allergy and Clinical Immunology, Berlin (West), 17–22. Allergologie. Sondernummer B1366 E
10. Valovirta E, Koivikko A, Vanto T, Viander M, Ingemann L (1984) Immunotherapy in allergy to dog: A double-blind clinical study. Ann Allergy 53:85–88
11. Van Metre TE, Marsch DG, Adkinson NF, Kagey-Sobotka A, Khattignavong A, Norman PS, Rosenberg GL (1988) Immunotherapy for cat asthma. Allergy Clin Immunol 82:1055–1068
12. Varney V, Gaga M, Frew AJ, Aber VR, Kay AB, Durham SR (1991) Usefulness of immunotherapy in patients with severe summer hay fever uncontrolled by antiallergic drugs. Br Med Journal 302:265–269
13. Wahn U, Schweter C, Lind P, Løwenstein H (1988) Prospective study on immunologic changes induced by two different Dermatophagoides pteronys sinus extracts prepared from whole mite culture and mite bodies. J All Clin Immunol 82:360–370
14. Wihl JÅ, Ipsen H, Nüchel-Petersen B, Munch EP, Janniche H, Løwenstein H (1988) Immunotherapy with partially purified and standardized tree pollen extracts. Allergy 43:363–369
15. Østerballe O (1982) Immunotherapy with grass pollen major allergens. Allergy 37:379–388
16. Østerballe O (1982) Nasal and skin sensitivity during immunotherapy with two major allergens 19, 25 and partially purified extract of timothy grass pollen. Allergy 37:169–177

Autoimmune Diseases

Autoantibodies Provide Insights into Antigens Driving Autoimmunity*

E. M. Tan

W. M. Keck Autoimmune Disease Center, The Scripps and Research Institute, La Jolla, CA 92037, USA

Abstract

Autoantibodies to intracellular, predominantly nuclear and nucleolar, antigens occur in systemic autoimmune diseases such as systemic lupus erythematosus, scleroderma, Sjogren's syndrome, and dermatomyositis/polymyositis. In addition to their clinical importance as diagnostic markers, these autoantibodies have been used to characterize the structure and function of their cognate antigens. Many of these have been shown to be subunits of multicomponent subcellular particles involved in essential cell functions, such as DNA replication, transcription, splicing, and translation. Autoantibodies have also been used to demonstrate that some of the autoepitopes are higher ordered conformational structures, such as tertiary and quaternary structures which are composed of discontinuous amino acid sequences. Autoepitopes also include active sites engaged in important functions or in binding to other molecules. These findings provide important insights into the biological processes driving the autoimmune response.

Introduction

A special characteristic of certain systemic autoimmune diseases, such as systemic lupus erythematosus (SLE), scleroderma, mixed connective tissue disease, Sjogren's syndrome, and dermatomyositis/polymyositis, is an immune response manifested by the presence of antibodies to intracellular antigens which are normally inaccessible to the immune system [1]. These antigens may be localized in various cell compartments, such as the nucleoplasm, nuclear matrix, nucleolus, and cytoplasm. Another characteristic of these autoantigens is that they are highly conserved in evolution and include DNA, histones, and proteins which are present in all cell types and in many divergent species and are engaged in important or essential cell functions. The biological events which evoke these unusual immune responses and the relationship of antibodies to clinical symptoms have been of continuing interest to investigators in basic and clinical biology for many years.

*This is publication #6473-MEM supported by National Institutes of Health grants AR32063 and AI31540.

Antigens Are Subunits of Multicomponent Subcellular Particles

SLE has been regarded as the prototype systemic autoimmune disease because of the exuberance of autoantibodies. A partial list of antibodies detected in the sera of patients with lupus is shown in Table 1 and includes antibodies to double-strand DNA, singlestrand DNA, histones, and several nonhistone nuclear proteins complexed with RNA to form small ribonucleoprotein (snRNP) particles. A patient with lupus will have an average of three to four of these autoantibodies present simultaneously in the circulation. Multiple species of autoantibodies are also present in the sera of patients with scleroderma (Table 1), but they are of different specificities from lupus and the antigens appear to be predominantly nucleolar in location. The latter are Scl-70, RNA polymerase 1, fibrillarin, and PM-Scl. For the past three decades there has been an active interest in elucidating the nature of antinuclear antibodies. Immunofluorescence analysis has provided the key pieces of information and, to date, it continues to be an important analytical tool. Since tissue culture cells or tissue sections are used as antigen substrates in immunofluorescence, a broad spectrum of intracellular antigens are available for reaction with antibodies. In addition, since the antigens are present in their "native" states, certain autoantibodies which are reactive with native epitopes are more

Table 1. Subcellular particles or functional domains are characteristic antigenic targets in systemic autoimmune disease.

Designation of autoantigen	Molecular features	Subcellular particles or functional domain
Systemic lupus erythematosus		
Native DNA	Double-strand DNA	Nucleosome
Denatured DNA	Single-strand DNA	Nucleosome
Histones	H1, H2A, H2B, H3, H4	Nucleosome
Sm	Proteins 28, 29, 16, and 13 kDa complexed with U1, U2, U4, U5, U6 small nuclear RNAs	Small nuclear ribonucleoprotein (snRNP)
Nuclear RNP	Proteins 70, 33, and 22 kDa complexed with U1 snRNA	snRNP
SS-B/La	Protein 48 kDa, complexed with RNA pol III transcripts	La-RNPs
SS-A/Ro	Proteins 60, 52 kDa complexed with Y1 – Y5 RNAs	Associated with La-RNPs
PCNA	Protein 36 kDa subunit of DNA polymerase delta	Replisome
Scleroderma		
Scl-70	100 kDa DNA topoisomerase I	Fibrillar center (FC) of nucleolus
RNA polymerase I	Proteins 210 to 11 kDa subunits of RNA pol I	FC of nucleolus
Fibrillarin	34 KDa protein of U3 RNP	Dense fibrillar component (DFC) of nucleolus
PM-Scl	Subunit proteins of 110 – 20 kDa	Granular component (GC) of nucleolus
Centromere antigens	Proteins 17, 80, and 140 kDa of kinetochore	Primary constrictions of condensed chromosomes

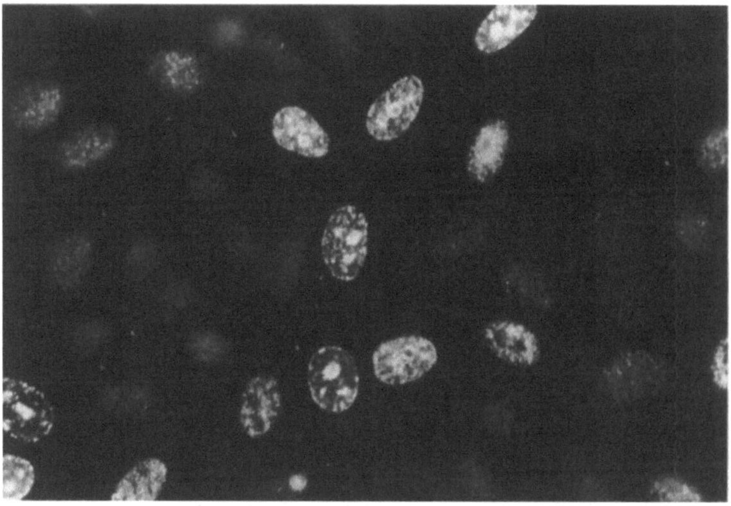

Fig. 1. Immunofluorescence distribution of proliferating cell nuclear antigen (PCNA) on tissue culture cell line HEp-2. The outstanding feature is the varied pattern of PCNA distribution, with some nuclei showing a high concentration and others with barely detectable PCNA. The cells showing high concentration of the antigen also demonstrate varied patterns of distribution

readily detectable by this method. Many intracellular particles and organelles are targets of recognition by autoantibodies and can be visualized fluorescently as different structural sizes and shapes distributed in different cell compartments. Figure 1 depicts the localization of the nuclear protein proliferating cell nuclear antigen (PCNA) in a human epithelial cell line, HEp-2. PCNA is present in the nucleoplasm and nucleoli of some cells, but is absent or present in trace amounts in other cells. Another feature is the different pattern of PCNA distribution in cells which show a higher abundance of this protein. The immunofluorescence localization of PCNA in the nucleoplasm or nucleolus is identical to areas showing uptake of isotope-labeled thymidine in autoradiography. Thus, PCNA is a protein which is localized in areas of DNA replication. Several studies have shown that PCNA is the auxiliary protein of DNA polymerase δ, – a polymerase engaged in synthesis of DNA at the replication fork [2–4]. As shown in Table 1, many intracellular antigens have been found to be subunits of multicomponent intracellular particles. The antigens, double-strand DNA, single-strand DNA, and histones are components of the nucleosome. Sm and nuclear RNP are subunits of snRNP particles which are involved in splicing of precursor mRNA. The SS-A/Ro and SS-B/La antigens are subunits of the La-RNPs and PCNA is a subunit of particles involved in DNA replication. In scleroderma, many antigens are associated with the nucleolus and have been localized by immunoelectron microscopy in fibrillar centers, dense fibrillar components, and granular components of the nucleolus.

One of the central questions in clinical immunology, especially in the study of systemic autoimmune diseases, is the reason(s) for the multiplicity of autoantibodies in these diseases. The recent molecular characterization of nuclear antigens has provided key pieces of information, showing that many intracellular antigens are subunits of larger particles. Subcellular particles, such as snRNPs, are composed of several different protein species complexed with several different RNA species. The U snRNPs, which react with anti-Sm and anti-RNP antibodies, assemble at the splice junctions of precursor mRNA in an ordered fashion to excise introns and ligate cut ends of exons thus forming mature mRNA. The autoantibodies designated anti-Sm and anti-nuclear RNP, which were initially characterized immunologically, have been shown to be directed at several different proteins of U1, U2, and U4–U6 snRNPs. Anti-Sm antibodies react with at least four proteins of 29, 28, 16, and 13 kDa and the anti-RNP with three proteins of 70, 33, and 22 kDa. Collectively, these and other data show that intracellular particles composed of multisubunit components play important roles in driving the autoimmune response.

Immunogenic Subcellular Particles Are Involved in Essential Functions

The involvement of antigens in important and essential biological functions of the cell has been described above with relationship to DNA replication (PCNA) and in pre-mRNA splicing (Sm and nuclear RNP). Other antigens are components of subcellular particles involved in transcription. RNA polymerase 1, an antigen recognized by some patients with scleroderma [5], is localized in the fibrillar centers of the nucleolus and is involved in transcription of ribosomal genes. SS-B/La is a 48 kDa protein which is the target of antibodies in patients with lupus and Sjogren's syndrome [6, 7]. This protein is involved in RNA polymerase II function, including termination of pol III transcription [8]. In dermatomyositis and polymyositis, some autoantibodies are directed against transfer RNA synthetases involved in the aminoacylation of histidyl, threonyl, and alanyl transfer RNAs [9–11].

Autoepitopes Are Frequently Higher Ordered Conformational Structures

Insights into the structure of epitopes recognized by naturally occurring autoantibodies have been obtained from the study of recombinant products of cDNA clones which encode PCNA. The strategy was to produce deletion mutants of PCNA cDNA and to analyze the reactivity of recombinant proteins both by immunoprecipitation of transcription/translation products and by western blotting of fusion proteins [12]. As a preliminary approach, 15-mer synthetic peptides which spanned the entire sequence of full-length protein were used in an ELISA to determine reactivity of two murine monoclonal antibodies raised against purified PCNA and a rabbit polyclonal antibody raised against an N-terminal synthetic peptide. These experimentally induced antibodies reacted with the expected synthetic peptides (Fig. 2), the rabbit polyclonal antiserum reacting with peptide 2 and the murine monoclonal antibodies with peptide 12. These experimentally

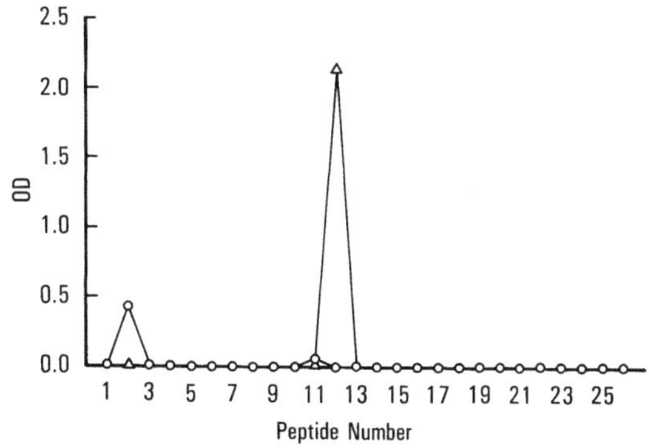

Fig. 2. Some 26 synthetic peptides were constructed consisting of 15 amino acid residues per peptide and spanned the entire length of PCNA. The peptides were constructed to overlap partially with one another. *Open circles* demonstrate the activity of rabbit polyclonal antiserum raised against an amino terminal peptide. It reacted only with peptide 2 (residues 11–24) in this ELISA system. Two murine monoclonal antibodies raised against PCNA reacted selectively only with peptide 12. Fourteen human lupus antisera to PCNA were tested against the synthetic peptides and none of the 14 reacted. [From 12]

induced antibodies were highly specific in the ELISA, reacting with single synthetic peptides and showing no cross-reactivity with other peptides. In contrast, none of 14 human SLE sera, which had been shown by immunodiffusion and immunofluorescence to react with PCNA, showed any reaction with the 26 synthetic peptides tested. These 26 synthetic peptides of 15 residues each spanned the entire continuous sequence of PCNA and were constructed to overlap with one another, so that any sequence of six continuous residues would be represented. This study demonstrated that none of 14 lupus autoantibodies were reactive with any region of PCNA which consisted of six linear continuous amino acid residues. Deletion mutants of PCNA were constructed as shown in Fig. 3. In vitro protein products (IVPs) 1–6 represented in vitro transcription/translation products and fusion proteins (FPS) 1–13 represented fusion products of deletion mutants generated by restriction enzymes. Experimentally induced antibodies, i.e., rabbit polyclonal antibody to N-terminal peptide and two murine monoclonal antibodies induced by immunization with purified PCNA, reacted by both immunoprecipitation and western blotting with the expected protein products. The 14 lupus sera demonstrated a variety of reactivities, summarized in Table 2. All 14 human sera immunoprecipitated the full-length translation product IVP 1 but had different reactivities with truncated products. In western blotting nine human sera failed to react with any of the fusion proteins, whereas five others were reactive in different patterns. In general, the lupus sera could be divided into four subgroups, as depicted in Table 2. By a process of deduction analysis, the epitopes recognized by the 14 human lupus sera could be mapped as illustrated in Fig. 3.

This analysis, taken together with the total lack of reactivity of human autoantibodies with synthetic peptides, demonstrates the striking difference between epitopes recognized by induced antibodies and by natural autoantibodies. Epitopes recognized by human autoantibodies comprise higher ordered confor-

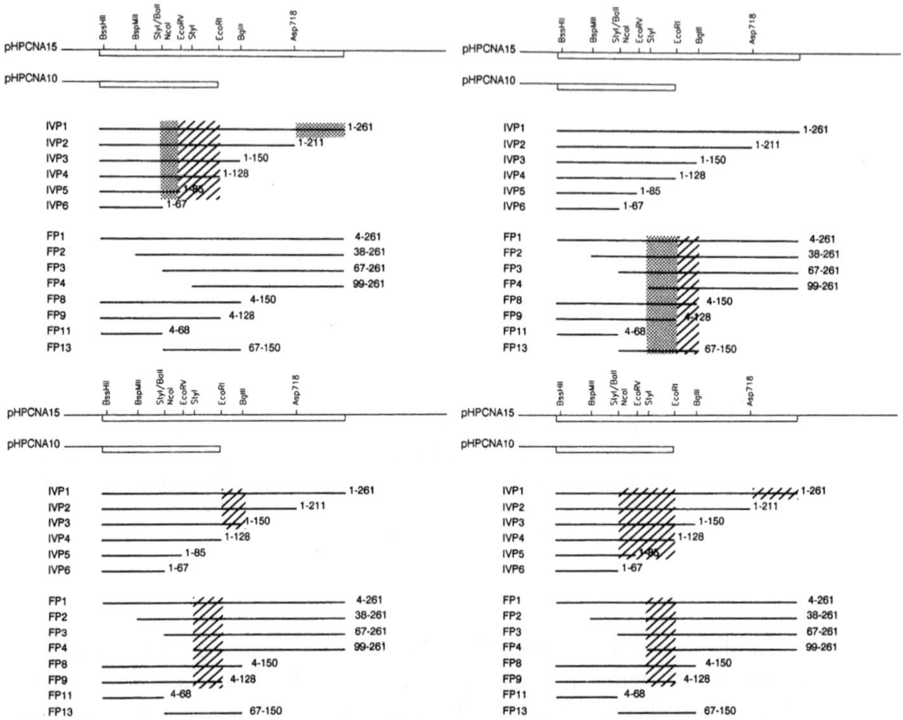

Fig. 3. Epitope mapping of reactive regions in PCNA deduced by subtraction analysis of data derived from immunoprecipitation and western blotting (see Table 3). SLE group II sera (*top left*) were reactive only by immunoprecipitation and the regions necessary for reactivity could be localized to the *stippled* and *hatched* areas. SLE group III sera (*top right*) were nonreactive with truncated translation products but were reactive with FPs and the regions necessary for reactivity were mapped to the *shaded areas*. The reactivities of group IVA are shown in *bottom left* and group IVB in *bottom right* of the figure and they incorporate properties of both group II and group III. [From 12]

mational structures which are not represented in the synthetic peptides nor in many protein products constructed from deletion mutants of DNA. This type of conformational structure may be formed by amino acid residues from two or more regions of the molecule that are brought into proximity with one another by protein folding (tertiary conformation) or by a conformation which is induced by the binding of the antigen with other molecules (quaternary conformation). These observations emphasize the special features of some "native" epitopes recognized by autoantibodies.

Autoepitopes Are Frequently Active Sites

The conserved characteristic of epitopes recognized by natural autoantibodies suggests that these epitopes could be related to structures which have been preserved in evolution in order to subserve important or perhaps essential structural

Table 2. Immunoreactivity of in vitro protein products (IVP) and fusion proteins (FP) of PCNA.

Protein product	AA sequence	Reactivity with antibodies															
		RABab	MoAb 19A2	SLE I					SLE II				SLE III			SLE IV A NE	SLE IV B FL
				AI	YK	MI	KU	JO	CR	OK	CA	EB	PT	AK	YO		
IVP immunoprecipitation																	
IVP 1	1 – 261	+	+	+	+	+	+	+	+	+	+	+	+	+	+	+	+
IVP 2	1 – 211	+	+	–	–	–	–	–	+	–	–	–	–	–	–	+	–
IVP 3	1 – 150	+	+	–	–	–	–	–	+	–	–	–	–	–	–	+	–
IVP 4	1 – 128	+	–	–	–	–	–	–	+	+	+	+	–	–	–	–	+
IVP 5	1 – 85	+	–	–	–	–	–	–	–	+	+	+	–	–	–	–	+
IVP 6	1 – 67	+	–	–	–	–	–	–	–	–	–	–	–	–	–	–	–
FP immunoblotting																	
FP-1	4 – 261	+	+	–	–	–	–	–	–	–	–	–	+	+	+	+	+
FP-2	38 – 261	–	+	–	–	–	–	–	–	–	–	–	+	+	+	+	+
FP-3	67 – 261	–	+	–	–	–	–	–	–	–	–	–	+	+	+	+	+
FP-4	99 – 261	–	+	–	–	–	–	–	–	–	–	–	+	+	+	+	+
FP-8	4 – 150	+	+	–	–	–	–	–	–	–	–	–	+	+	+	+	+
FP-9	4 – 128	+	+	–	–	–	–	–	–	–	–	–	–	+	+	+	+
FP-11	4 – 68	+	–	–	–	–	–	–	–	–	–	–	–	–	–	–	–
FP-13	67 – 150	–	+	–	–	–	–	–	–	–	–	–	–	+	–	–	+

AA, amino acid; SLE, systemic lupus erythematosus.

or functional roles in the biology of the cell. Two studies were especially revealing in showing that epitopes recognized by autoantibodies play important functional roles.

Certain patients with polymyositis produce antibodies to threonyl-tRNA synthetase. The reaction of natural autoantibody was compared with an antibody induced by immunization of rats with purified threonyl-tRNA synthetase [13]. The human autoantibody reacted with the native but not with the denatured form of synthetase. This was demonstrated in immunoblots in which SDS treated and gel electrophoresed threonyl-tRNA synthetase was analzyed by the standard western blotting technique. The human antibody was not reactive with this form of synthetase; however, if the synthetase was not subjected to western blotting but was directly applied to cellulose nitrate in a dot blot assay, human antibody was fully reactive. In contrast, the experimentally induced rat antibody to threonyl-tRNA synthetase was reactive in both western blots and dot blots. This study suggested that the epitope recognized by human antibody was at least conformational in nature and the conformation was lost in the western blotting procedure. This conclusion received further support in a functional assay in which human autoantibody was able to inactivate threonyl-tRNA synthetase, whereas the rat antibody was inactive.

Experiments with PCNA also illustrated the functional nature of the epitope recognized by naturally occurring antibodies [14]. Human antibody was capable of neutralizing DNA polymerase δ function, based on its ability to inhibit the activity of PCNA which is required by pol δ for nucleotide chain synthesis in template/primer systems containing high template/primer ratios (poly(dA)/oligo(dT); 2:1). The rabbit polyclonal antibody and murine monoclonal antibodies to PCNA described above were unable to inhibit this function. These two studies emphasize the important feature that epitopes on autoantigens recognized by naturally occurring antibodies frequently include the active or functional sites of these proteins. In contrast, experimentally induced antibodies appear to recognize different antigenic sites on these proteins, some of which appear to be denatured regions of the target molecules.

Conclusion

The study of autoantibodies occurring in certain systemic autoimmune diseases has provided insights into some important details of the autoimmune process. It is now apparent that the antigens which drive the autoimmune response are subunits of multicomponent subcellular particles. These particles are involved in essential cellular functions which include DNA replication, transcription, precursor mRNA splicing, translation, and cell division. An analysis of epitopes recognized by autoantibodies shows that some of these epitopes are higher ordered conformational structures which are at least tertiary or quaternary in nature. These conformational structures could be induced by protein folding or by intermolecular binding of the antigen with other proteins or nucleic acids. Finally, autoepitopes are frequently the active sites of the proteins which may be involved in function or in binding with other subunit components of the particle.

These data indicate that in vivo immunogen in certain systemic autoimmune diseases is an *activated* subcellular particle engaged in cell function. Immune responses made against this particle can be directed at several epitopes in one subunit and at several subunits in the same particle. An important topic to address in future studies is the identities of the stimuli which lead to the activation of cell functions regulated by such particles. All varieties of stimuli should be considered, including those which are endogenous or exogenous and physiologic or nonphysiologic, since the activation of normal functions, such as DNA replication, transcription, splicing, translation, and cell division, is regulated by complex pathways and influenced by normal or aberrant mechanisms.

References

1. Tan EM (1989) Antinuclear antibodies: diagnostic markers for autoimmune diseases and probes for cell biology. Adv Immunol 44:93–151
2. Mathews MB, Bernstein RM, Franze BR Jr, Garrels JI (1984) Identity of the proliferating cell nuclear antigen and cyclin. Nature 309:374–376
3. Tan CK, Castillo C, So AG, Downey AM (1986) An auxiliary protein for DNA polymerse delta from fetal calf thymus. J Biol Chem 261:12310–12316
4. Prelich G, Stillman B (1988) Coordinated leading and lagging strand synthesis during SV40 DNA replication in vitro requires PCNA. Cell 53:117–126
5. Reimer G, Rose KM, Scheer U, Tan EM (1987) Autoantibody to RNA polymerase I in scleroderma sera. J Clin Invest 79:65–72
6. Chan EKL, Tan EM (1987) Human autoantibody-reactive epitopes on SS-B/La are highly conserved in comparison with epitopes recognized by murine monoclonal antibodies. J Exp Med 166:1627–1640
7. Chambers JC, Kenan D, Martin BJ, Keene JD (1988) Genomic structure and amino acid sequence domains of the human La autoantigen. J Biol Chem 263:18043–18051
8. Gottlieb E, Steitz JA (1989) Function of the mammalian La protein influences both the accuracy and the efficiency of RNA polymerase III transcription in vitro. EMBO J 8:841–850
9. Rosa MD, Hendrick JP Jr, Lerner MR, Steitz JA, Reichlin M (1983) Mammalian $tRNA^{His}$-containing antigen is recognized by the polymyositis-specific antibody anti-Jo-1. Nucleic Acids Res 11:853–870
10. Mathews MB, Reichlin M, Hughes GR, Bonsi RM (1984) Anti-threonyl-tRNA synthetase, a second myositis-related autoantibody. J Exp Med 160:40–44
11. Bunn CC, Bernstein RM, Mathews MB (1986) Autoantibodies against alanyl-tRNA synthetase and $tRNA^{Ala}$ co-exist and are associated with myositis. J Exp Med 163:1281–1291
12. Huff JP, Roos G, Peebles CL, Houghten R, Sullivan KF, Tan EM (1990) Insights into native epitopes of proliferating cell nuclear antigen using recombinant DNA protein products. J Exp Med (in press)
13. Dang CV, Tan EM, Traugh JA (1988) Myositis autoantibody reactivity and catalytic function of threonyl-tRNA synthetase. FASEB J 2:2376–2379
14. Tan CK, Sullivan K, Li X, Tan EM, Downey KW, So AG (1987) Autoantibody to the proliferating cell nuclear antigen neutralizes the activity of the auxiliary protein for DNA polymerase delta. Nucleic Acids Res 15:9299–9308

The Diagnostic Significance of Antinuclear Antibodies

M. Meurer

Department of Dermatology, Ludwig-Maximilians-Universität, Frauenlobstrasse 9–11, W-8000 München 2, Federal Republic of Germany

Abstract

The production of autoantibodies reactive with various cellular constituents is the immunological hallmark of systemic connective tissue diseases (CTD). The fine specifities of autoantibodies have proved to be very useful in establishing a diagnosis and in helping to formulate therapeutic strategies.

The autoantibodies can be classified into two major groups: (1) those found in particular CTD (anti-topoisomerase I, -centromere, -dsDNA, -Sm, -Jo1, -PM/Scl, -fibrillarin, -RNA-polymerase I, -Mi2) can be defined as disease-specific and were designated as marker antibodies and (2) those associated with certain clinical features observed in various CTD (anti-Ro/SSB, -LA/SSA, -U1RNP, -histone, -cardiolipin) can be defined as symptom-specific.

Clinical examples for the first group of disease-specific autoantibodies (Ab) are: anti-dsDNA-Ab in systemic lupus erythematosus, anti-topoisomerase I-Ab in diffuse systemic scleroderma as well as anti-Jo1-Ab in patients with polymyositis and interstitial lung fibrosis.

Symptom-specific is the association of anti-Ro/SSA-Ab with light-sensitive cutaneous lupus erythematosus or with systemic scleroderma and Sjögren syndrome and the association of anti-cardiolipin-Ab with recurrent abortions and arterial and venous thromboses.

New studies implicate that the formation of certain autoantibodies is influenced by different MHC class II antigens: a particularly strong association seems to exist between anti-PM/Scl-Ab or anti-Jo1-Ab and HLA-DR3 in patients with distinct scleroderma subsets. Thus, genetic factors seem to be involved in the autoimmune process underlying CTD and may explain the clinical and autoantibody heterogeneity in defined disease subsets.

Introduction

This article deals with the utility of antinuclear antibodies as diagnostic markers of certain autoimmune diseases. In this context the term antinuclear antibodies (ANAs) will be used as a generic description of different autoantibodies which are targeted – as described in detail by M. Tan (see p. 363) – at nuclear, nucleolar or cytoplasmic antigens.

In 1948, with the description of the lupus erythematosus (LE) cell test by Hargraves et al. [1], a serologic method for the diagnosis of systemic lupus erythematosus (SLE) became for the first time available. It is known today that the LE cell test covers only one of many ANAs that can appear in inflammatory connective tissue diseases such as localized scleroderma (LS), cutaneous systemic scleroderma (SSc), dermatomyositis (DM), and mixed connective tissue disease (MCTD). In recent years it has become increasingly clear that these autoimmune diseases are distinguished by different autoantibodies or sets of ANAs which characterize each disease with its own serologic profile.

Detection of ANA

For routine purposes, indirect immunofluorescence microscopy (IIF) and double immunodiffusion (DI) are reliable methods of detecting ANAs [2].

For the IIF test, smears of epithelial cell cultures serve as antigen substrates. HEp-2 cells cultured from human pharynx carcinoma are the ones most widely used. These mitotic, active cells enable one to see the antibody binding to various cell compartments much better than animal tissue substrates which have been used up to now.

Depending upon the density and distribution of the antigens in these cell compartments, ANA produce either a homogeneous or a finely or coarsely speckled nuclear pattern. Moreover, in HEp-2 cells ANA can be traced which react only with the nucleoli or with the centromere region of chromosomes in resting or mitotic cells. These antibodies are directed against structural proteins of the kinetochore, on which the microtubules of the spindle apparatus set in metaphase.

Not all ANA of diagnostic relevance produce characteristic binding patterns in the IIF test and must therefore be demonstrated with other methods. Normally, the Ouchterlony test, in which precipitating antibodies against U1-RNP, Sm, Jo-1, La(SSB), Scl-70 or PM-Scl can be demonstrated, has proven to be optimal. Extracts of rabbit or calf thymus cell nuclei (ENA) are mostly used as antigen substrate. Antibodies against Ro(SSA) can be traced by immunodiffusion with the help of human spleen extracts, but do not react with HEp-2 cells in routine IIF tests. Antibodies against double-stranded DNA are mostly detected in IIF on *Crithidia luciliae.*

Lately, immunodiffusion tests have been complemented by more sensitive enzyme-linked immunoassays (ELISA) for the detection of antibodies against histones, single-stranded or native DNA and Ro(SSA) antigens. Western blot immunoprecipitation is more precise; with this method the protein composition of some nuclear antigens, especially of the nonhistone RNA-protein complexes U1-RNP, Sm, Ro(SSA) and La(SSB), can be analyzed. Specific ribonucleic acids, which bind to these antigenic protein complexes, can be characterized by immunoprecipitation of radiolabeled cell extracts with ANAs isolated from patients sera [3].

Diagnostic Relevance of ANAs

Systemic Lupus Erythematosus

SLE is characterized by a heterogeneous and polyclonal antibody response with an average of three different circulating antibodies present simultaneously in one patient [4]. By IIF, almost all patients with SLE show ANAs in high titers, often with homogeneous nuclear fluorescence pattern (Fig. 1a). Highly specific for SLE are antibodies against double-stranded DNA, which in acute disease states are present in about 60%–90% and anti-Sm-antibodies which can be demonstrated in 10%–30% of SLE patients, mostly together with antinuclear RNP antibodies [5].

Besides antinative DNA and anti-Sm antibodies, autoantibodies to ribosomal RNP can be detected in less than 10% of SLE patients. In immunoblotting, these autoantibodies recognize three ribosomal phosphoproteins of approximate molecular weights of 38000, 16000, and 15000; in the IIF test on HEp-2 cells, these antibodies produce a distinct cytoplasmic staining [6]. Antiribosomal RNP antibodies were found in one study to be serologic markers for psychoses secondary to SLE and longitudinal studies of antibody activity revealed that anti-r-RNP levels increase before and during the active phase of psychosis [7].

Subacute Cutaneous Lupus Erythematosus

Subacute cutaneous lupus erythematosus, a clinical subtype of LE, is characterized by disseminated, plaquelike or anular erythematosquamous lesions which heal without scarring. Patients with SCLE frequently show increased light sensitivity and arthralgias, whereas other organ manifestations of SLE are only rarely present. More than 90% of SCLE patients are ANA-positive; ANA titers are usually very high without showing a uniformly characteristic binding pattern. Antibodies to the cytoplasmic Ro(SSA) antigen detected by immunodiffusion or other methods are regarded as serologic marker of SCLE [8]; they can be found in 60% – 80% of such patients and are associated in about half of the cases with anti-La(SSB) antibodies. The majority of these patients is rheumatoid factor-positive and shows the histocompatibility locus antigen (HLA) haplotype B8/DR3 [9].

An important feature which should be considered by the clinician in interpreting the significance of ANAs in SLE – or other immune diseases – is the combination in which they can be detected [10]; for example, the presence of both anti-Ro(SSA) and anti-La(SSB) antibodies in patients who fulfill established clinical criteria for SLE indicates a more benign course of the disease with a later onset and a lower frequency of renal involvement and polyserositis. In other SLE patients, however, antibodies to Ro(SSA) may be found in combination with anti-DNA or anti-Sm antibodies but without anti-La(SSB); in these cases, a more progressive disease course with multiple organ involvement has been observed [11].

A very interesting feature of the Ro(SSA) and La(SSB) antibody system is its association with atrioventricular heart block and with skin rashes in infants born of mothers who carry these antibodies [12]. There are several reports showing that the maternally transferred antibodies are directly involved in the pathogenesis of cardiac and cutaneous manifestations of neonatal LE [13]. Antibodies to La(SSB) and/or Ro(SSA) may be also found in those rare cases of SLE that are associated with inherited deficiencies of the complement protein C2 or C4 [14].

Chronic Discoid LE

About 70% of the patients with disseminated chronic discoid LE but only 25% with cutaneous LE limited to the face, neck, or skull have ANAs when tested by routine immunofluorescence methods. The immunofluorescent binding patterns of such ANAs are not characteristic, and precipitating antibodies against defined antigens such as nuclear RNP or Ro(SSA) are present in only 10% – 20% of patients with chronic discoid LE. Patients with chronic discoid LE and antibodies against Ro(SSA) may be "ANA negative" when tested by routine screening and may develop arthralgia/arthritis and Sjögren's syndrome in rare cases [2].

Systemic Scleroderma

The detection and characterization of circulating antibodies have become important tools for the diagnosis of scleroderma and for defining subsets of the disease. Their involvement in the pathogenesis of systemic scleroderma, however, is still questionable [15].

By routine methods ANAs can be found in the sera of more than 95% of patients with systemic scleroderma [15]. The antibody titers can be very high but in general do not show any correlation with disease activity. By indirect immunofluorescence on HEp-2 cells, three characteristic fluorescence patterns can be distinguished: a nucleolar stain (Fig. 1 b), a centromere stain (Fig. 1 c) and a finely speckled nuclear stain combined with nucleolar staining produced by antibodies against DNA topo-isomerase 1 (Scl-70 antigen).

Diffuse Systemic Scleroderma

Antinucleolar antibodies are mostly seen in patients with diffuse scleroderma (dSSc) and are rarely seen in other connective tissue diseases. Several antigens reacting with antinucleolar antibodies have been characterized: low molecular weight (4–6S) ribonucleic acid (RNA), a novel nucleolar 7–2 ribonucleoprotein, and a basic protein with an M_r of 34000 termed fibrillarin, which is associated with nucleolar U3-RNA [16]. These antifibrillarin antibodies produce a distinct "clumpy" nucleolar staining (Fig. 1 b); they were recently described to characterize a subtype of scleroderma patients with widespread telangiectasias, diffuse scleroderma and pulmonary involvement [17]. Antinucleolar antibodies producing a distinct speckled nucleolar pattern are directed against the RNA polymerase I-complexes localized in the fibrillar regions of nucleoli [18]. Another class of antinucleolar antibodies producing homogeneous nucleolar staining and additional

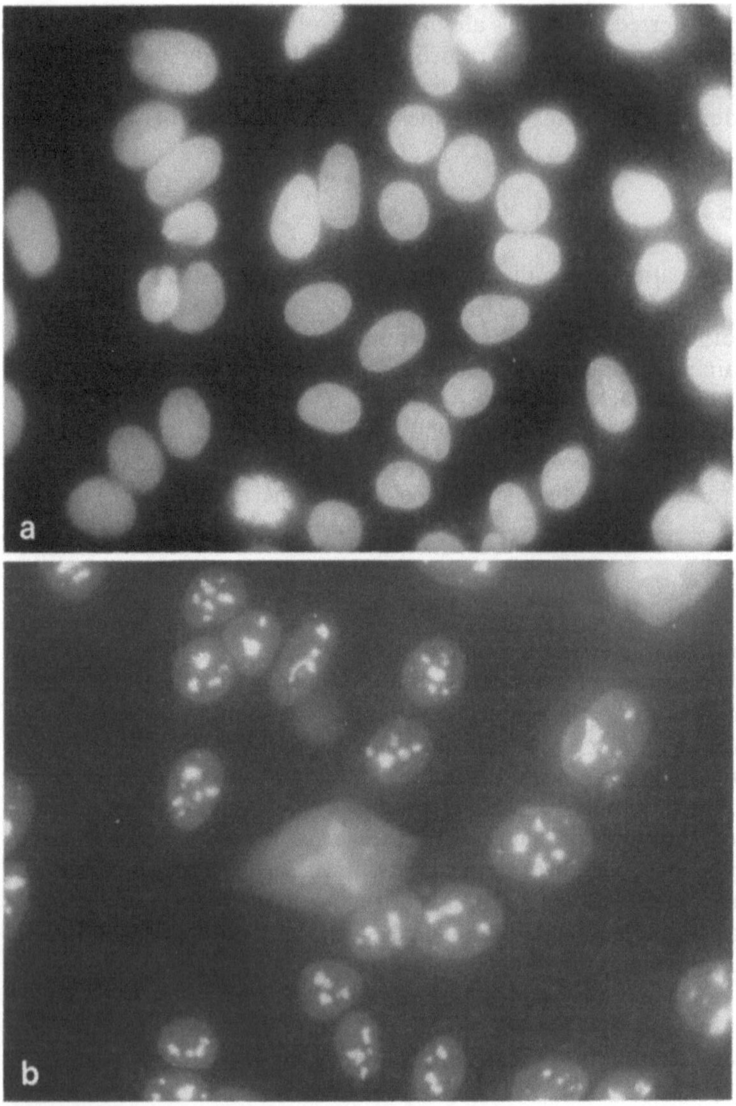

Fig. 1a, b

Fig. 1a–d. Pattern of circulating ANAs in connective tissue diseases. Indirect immunofluorescence on HEp-2 cells. (Serum dilution 1:40; fluorescein isothiocyanate [FITC]-antihuman IgG diluted 1:20 in phosphate-buffered saline; magnification, ×160). **a** Homogeneous nuclear staining with pronounced reaction of condensed chromatin in mitotic cells; **b** nucleolar clumpy staining reaction of antibodies with nucleolar fibrillarin (U3-RNP); **c** nuclear centromere staining: the antibodies clearly recognize kinetochore proteins in interphase and metaphase chromosomes; **d** nuclear speckled pattern: reaction of antibodies with the nuclear matrix protein U1-RNP

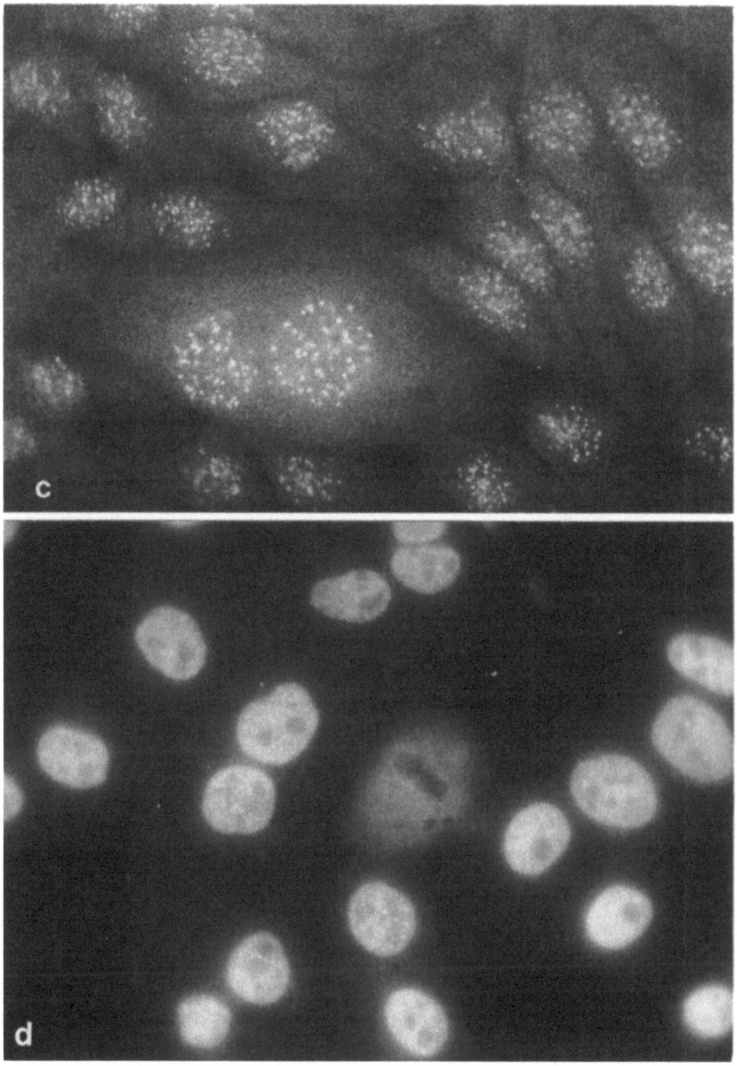

Fig. 1c, d

weak staining of the nucleoplasm is directed against the PM-Scl antigen, which contains a group of 11 possibly preribosomal proteins with an M_r of 20000–110000 [18]. Scleroderma patients with anti-PM-Scl-antibodies show a high incidence of dermatomyositis-like skin changes associated with polymyositis [19]. In addition patients with this subgroup of polymyositis-scleroderma overlap syndrome may have a nondeforming and nonerosive arthritis and rheumatoid factor, usually in lower concentrations. In a recent report [19], the striking association of class II MHC antigens HLA-DR3 and HLA-DR3/4 with the immune response against PM-Scl was demonstrated. Association with an HLA-class II antigen not implicated in other scleroderma variants indicates that the polymyositis-scleroderma overlap syndrome defined by anti-PM-Scl is clinically and immunologically distinct.

By immunodiffusion antibodies to the nuclear enzyme DNA topoisomerase I (Scl-70 antigen) can be detected in about 30% – 50% of sera from patients with scleroderma [15]. Scl-70 antibodies are highly specific for systemic scleroderma and were only occasionally found in patients with related disorders such as polymyositis or Raynaud's syndrome. They are more frequent in patients with diffuse scleroderma where they may be present in 60% of the patients. The occurrence of anti-Scl-70 antibodies indicates a more progressive and more severe course of the disease in such patients [20, 21]. Scl-70-positive sera may also contain other antibodies such as anti-Ro(SSA) antibodies. The presence of both Scl-70 antibodies and anticentromere antibodies in one patient is rare and may predict severe disease [22]. A close association between HLA-DR5 and anti-DNA-topoisomerase I in patients with scleroderma was reported [19].

Limited Systemic Scleroderma

Anticentromere antibodies can be detected in 12% to 43% of all patients with systemic scleroderma, mostly in patients with a limited or acroscleroderma (lSSc) or with the CREST variant of scleroderma. In most studies pulmonary fibrosis and restrictive lung disease were found to be less frequent in anticentromere antibody-positive patients compared to anticentromere antibody-negative patients [20, 21]. However, in a small percentage of cases, anticentromere antibodies can be associated with severe pulmonary hypertension and with gastrointestinal involvement [22]. Anticentromere antibodies are also present in 10% – 15% of patients with primary biliary cirrhosis, of whom about half have some evidence of limited scleroderma [23]. In other connective tissue diseases, anticentromere antibodies are very rare. They are present, however, in about 20% of patients with idiopathic Raynaud's disease or Raynaud's syndrome as a prodrome of systemic scleroderma where they may be detected several years prior to the onset of other scleroderma symptoms [24]. Findings of a significant association of anticentromere antibodies with the presence of at least one of the HLA-alleles DR1, DR4 or DR8 suggest that genetic factors may be also important in the expression of these autoantibodies [19].

Localized Scleroderma

Antinuclear antibodies have been reported in 30% – 80% of patients with localized scleroderma [25, 26]; they are usually present in low titers and do not produce specific binding patterns when tested by indirect immunofluorescence on tissue-cultured cells. Only very rarely, autoantibodies specific for systemic scleroderma such as anticentromere or anti-Scl-70 antibodies can be found in localized scleroderma. In these cases one has to exclude the possibility of coexistent systemic and localized scleroderma. ANA seem to be more frequent in patients with generalized morphea or with linear scleroderma involving the subcutaneous tissue and the muscles [25]. However, no convincing correlation can be drawn between the presence of ANA and possible organ involvement in localized scleroderma. In addition, it has been reported that sera from patients with localized scleroderma may contain antibodies to single-stranded DNA in about 60% of cases [26].

Dermatomyositis and Polymyositis

Antinuclear antibodies can be detected in about 60% – 80% of patients with DM or polymyositis (PM) [27]. When detected by indirect immunofluorescence, titers are usually very high, but no specific binding patterns can be discerned. By immunodiffusion or immunoblotting with soluble cell extracts a family of precipitating antibodies was identified that was found to be highly characteristic for PM or DM, respectively [28]. These autoantibodies target as antigen certain species of transfer RNA synthetases: histidyl-tRNA synthetase (50 kDa = Jo-1), threonyl-tRNA synthetase (80 kDa) and alanyl-tRNA synthetase (110 kDa). Anti-Jo-1 antibodies were described in approximately 25% of patients with polymyositis; many of these myositis patients also have associated interstitial lung fibrosis [29]. A second myositis-related autoantibody was identified by immunodiffusion using calf or rabbit thymus extracts as antigen source. The antibody recognizes the Mi-2 antigen, which consists of two proteins of 61 and 53 kDa [30]. Structure and function of this nuclear antigen are yet unknown. Antibodies to Mi-2 were so far found only in patients with dermatomyositis. The sensitivity of this serologic marker, however, is low since only 10% – 30% of DM patients are positive for anti-Mi-2 [30]. The diagnostic significance of antibodies against the nucleolar PM-Scl antigen for the polymyositis-scleroderma overlap syndrome has already been discussed.

Mixed Connective Tissue Disease

Mixed connective tissue disease (MCTD) is a clinical overlap syndrome which was initially recognized on the basis of autoantibodies against nuclear RNP [31]. These autoantibodies can be demonstrated by indirect immunofluorescence on HEp-2 cells through their characteristic nuclear binding pattern (Fig. 1 d). The antibody can be more precisely defined by western blot techniques: antinuclear RNP antibodies immunoblot the 70-kDa protein of the nuclear matrix and the 33-kDa (A protein) and the 22-kDa protein (C protein) of U1-RNP; in contrast to SLE sera, patients with MCTD, however, do not recognize the B-, D-, or E-core proteins of U1-RNP [32]. The lack of this anti-Sm specificity in MCTD sera is highly diagnostic. Yet not all patients with restricted antinuclear RNP autoimmune response clinically have MCTD. When using established clinical criteria, about 40% – 50% of patients with antinuclear RNP antibodies may have classical LE or systemic scleroderma without any evidence of clinical overlap [33].

Conclusion

In order to characterize the relationship between clinical diagnosis or symptoms and the specificity of ANAs, these autoantibodies can be classified into two major groups: (1) those found in a particular disease entity can be designated as marker antibodies, and (2) those associated with certain clinical expressions or distinct clinical subgroups can be defined as symptom specific.

Marker ANAs include antibodies against topoisomerase I (antitopo I/Scl-70) and various nucleolar antigens in diffuse systemic scleroderma, centromere antibodies in limited systemic scleroderma, double-stranded DNA antibodies and anti-Sm antibodies in SLE, anti-Jo-1 antibodies in PM and anti-Mi-2 antibodies in DM. Symptom-specific ANAs include antibodies to the La(SSB) and/or Ro(SSA) antigens; they can be found in distinct subtypes of LE with limited systemic involvement such as in SCLE or in LE with Sjögren's syndrome or in neonatal LE with congenital heart block; antinuclear RNP antibodies (anti-U1-RNP) and anti-PM-Scl antibodies are associated with certain clinical overlap syndromes and antiribosomal RNP antibodies were reported to be more frequent in SLE patients with psychosis.

References

1. Hargraves MM, Richmond H, Morton R (1948) Presentation of two bone marrow elements: the "tart" cell and the "L.E." cell. Mayo Clin Proc 23:25–28
2. Meurer M, Bieber T (1987) Immunhistologische und serologische Diagnostik von Autoimmunerkrankungen der Haut. Hautarzt 38:S59–S68
3. Tan EM, Chan EKL, Sullivan F, Rubin RI (1988) Antinuclear antibodies (ANAs): diagnostically specific immune markers and clues toward the understanding of systemic autoimmunity. Clin Immunol Immunopathol 47:121–141
4. Notman DD, Kurata N, Tan EM (1975) Profiles of antinuclear antibodies in systemic rheumatic diseases. Ann Intern Med 83:464–469
5. Van Venrooij WJ (1987) Autoantibodies against small nuclear ribonucleoprotein components. J Rheumatol 14 [Suppl]:78–82
6. Francoeur AM, Peebles CL, Heckmann KJ, Lee JC, Tan EM (1985) Identification of ribosomal protein autoantigens. J Immunol 135:2378
7. Bonfa E, Golombek SJ, Kaufman LD, Skelly S, Weissbach H, Brot N, Elkon KB (1987) Association between lupus psychosis and anti-ribosomal protein antibodies. N Engl J Med 317:265–271
8. Deng JS, Sontheimer RD, Gilliam JN (1984) Relationship between antinuclear and anti-Ro/SS-A antibodies in subacute cutaneous lupus erythematosus. J Am Acad Dermatol 11:494–499
9. Maddison PJ, Isenberg DA, Goulding NJ, Leddy J, Skinner RP (1988) Anti La(SSB) identifies a distinctive subgroup of systemic lupus erythematosus. Br J Rheumatol 27:27–31
10. Tan EM (1989) Antinuclear antibodies: diagnostic markers for autoimmune diseases and probes for cell biology. Adv Immunol 44:93–151
11. Wasicek CA, Reichlin M (1982) Clinical and serological differences between systemic lupus erythematosus patients with antibodies to Ro versus patients with antibodies to Ro versus patients with antibodies to Ro and La. J Clin Invest 69:835–843
12. Buyon JP, Ben-Chetrit E, Karp S, Roubey RAS, Pompeo L, Reeves WH, Tan EM, Winchester R (1989) Acquired congenital heart block. Pattern of maternal antibody response to biochemically defined antigens of the SSA/Ro-SSB/La system in neonatal lupus. J Clin Invest 84:627–634
13. Litsey SE, Noonan JA, O'Connor WN, Cottrill CM, Mitchell B (1985) Maternal connective tissue disease and congenital heart block. Demonstration of immunoglobulin in cardiac tissue. N Engl J Med 312:98–100

14. Meyer O, Hauptmann G, Tappeiner G, Ochs HD (1985) Genetic deficiency of C4, C2 or C1q and lupus syndromes. Association with anti-Ro(SS-A) antibodies. Clin Exp Immunol 62:678–684
15. Krieg T, Meurer M (1988) Systemic scleroderma. Clinical and pathophysiological aspects. J Am Acad Dermatol 18:457–481
16. Reimer G, Steen VD, Penning CA, Medsger TA, Tan EM (1988) Correlates between autoantibodies to nucleolar antigens and clinical features in patients with systemic sclerosis (scleroderma). Arthritis Rheum 31:525
17. Kurzhals G, Krieg T, Meurer M, Reimer G (1990) Clinical association of autoantibodies to fibrillarin with diffuse scleroderma and disseminated telangiectasia. J Am Acad Dermatol 23:832–836
18. Reimer G, Raska I, Tan EM, Scheer U (1987) Human autoantibodies: probes for nucleolus structure and function. Virchows Arch B 54:131–143
19. Genth E, Mierau R, Genetzky P, von Mühlen CA, Kaufmann S, von Wilmowsky H, Meurer M, Krieg T, Pollmann HJ, Hartl PW (1990) Immunogenetic associations of scleroderma-related antinuclear antibodies. Arthritis Rheum 33:657–665
20. Meurer M, Scharf A, Luderschmidt Ch, Braun-Falco O (1985) Zentromerantikörper und Antikörper gegen Scl-70-Nucleoprotein bei progressiver systemischer Sklerodermie. Diagnostische und prognostische Bedeutung. Dtsch Med Wochenschr 109:8–14
21. Weiner ES, Earnshaw WC, Senecal JL, Bordwell B, Johnson P, Rothfield NF (1988) Clinical associations of anticentromere antibodies and antibodies to topoisomerase I. A study of 355 patients. Arthritis Rheum 31:378–385
22. Jarzabek-Chorzelska M, Blaszczyk M, Kolacinska-Strasz Z, Chorzelski T, Jablonska S, Maul GG (1990) Antikinetochore and antitopoisomerase I antibodies in systemic scleroderma: comparative study using immunoblotted recombinant antigens, immunofluorescence, and double immunodiffusion. Arch Dermatol Res 282:76–83
23. Makinen D, Fritzler MJ, Davis P, Sherlock S (1983) Anticentromere antibodies in primary biliary cirrhosis. Arthritis Rheum 26:914–917
24. Kallenberg CGM, Pastoor GW, Wouda AA III (1982) Anticentromere antibodies in patients with Raynaud's phenomenon: clinical significance of anticentromere antibodies. Ann Rheum Dis 41:282–287
25. Do Vale E, Gerstmeier H, Meurer M, Krieg T, Braun-Falco O (1987) Spektrum antinukleärer Antikörper bei zirkumskripten Formen der Sklerodermie. Dtsch Med Wochenschr 111:1922–1927
26. Falanga V, Medsger TA, Reichlin M (1987) Antinuclear and anti-single-stranded DNA antibodies in morphea and generalized morphea. Arch Dermatol 123:350–353
27. Meurer M, Hausmann-Martinez-Pardo G, Braun-Falco O (1989) Das Spektrum antinukleärer und antizytoplasmatischer Antikörper bei Dermatomyositis und Polymyositis-Overlap-Syndromen. Hautarzt 40:623–629
28. Bunn CC, Bernstein RM, Mathews MB (1986) Autoantibodies against analyl-tRNA synthetase and tRNA Ala coexist and are associated with myositis. J Exp Med 163:1281–1291
29. Bernstein RM, Morgan SH, Chapman J, Bunn CC, Mathews MB, Turner-Warwick M, Hughes GRV (1984) Anti-Jo-1 antibody: a marker for myositis with interstitial lung disease. Br Med J 289:151–152
30. Targoff IN, Reichlin M (1985) The association between Mi-2 antibodies and dermatomyositis. Arthritis Rheum 28:796–803
31. Sharp GC, Irwin W, Tan EM, Gould G, Holman HR (1972) Mixed connective tissue disease – an apparently distinct rheumatic disease syndrome associated with a specific antibody to an extractable nuclear antigen (ENA). Am J Med 52:148–159
32. Petersson I, Wang G, Smith E, Wigzell H, Hedfors E, Horn J, Sharp GC (1986) The use of immunoblotting and immunoprecipitation of (U) small nuclear ribonucleoproteins in the analysis of sera of patients with mixed connective tissue disease and systemic lupus erythematosus. Arthritis Rheum 29:986
33. Combe B, Rucheton M, Graafland H, Jussiez V, Brunel C, Sany J (1989) Clinical significance of anti-RNP and anti-Sm autoantibodies as determined by immunoblotting and immunoprecipitation in sera from patients with connective tissue diseases. Clin Exp Immunol 75:18–24

The Anticardiolipin Syndrome – A Clinical Study*

P. A. Reyes-López, J. M. Casanova, and M. C. Amigo

Instituto Nacional de Cardiologia "Ignacio Chávez", Juan Badiano núm. 1 Secc. XVI Tlalpan. México, D. F. C. P 14080 Mexico

Abstract

Although the presence of serum antibodies against phospholipid moeities were known since 1906, and its pathogenic potential was suggested in the 50's when acquired coagulopathies were recognized, only in 1983 using highly sensitive assays for electronegative phospholipids a specific clinicopathologic entity, characterized by recurrent venous and arterial thrombosis, thrombocytopenia and fetal loss was described as the antiphospholipid antibody syndrome (APAS).

Two forms of it have been accepted: one associated with autoimmune disease: systemic rheumatic diseases or hematological cytopenic processes; another one, not associated with any specific disease, is called "primary" antiphospholipid antibody syndrome (PAPs).

We search for APA in our patients, using the ELISA described by Loizu, adapted to recognize IgG isotype. We identify 14 patients with PAPs, 11 systemic lupus erythematosus patients with circulating APA, and 25 patients with a miscellaneous array of clinical diagnosis who had circulating APA.

In the first group high titer IgG APA was universal, 69% had false-positive VDRL, 50% lupus anticoagulant but ANA were positive at low titer, only in one case. Thrombocytopenia occurred in 77%, thrombosis, arterial in 62%, venous 54% and 87% of pregnancies finished in abortion, up to 7 consecutives in some women. Clotting abnormalities, central and peripheral nervous system disease, and heart valves and vessels abnormalities were very common. No renal disease nor articular complaints were noticed.

Lupus patients with APA often represent an oligosymptomatic disease, with certain features, such as livedo reticularis and malleolar ulceration, with increased frequency. The third group did not show special characteristics.

The PAPs represents a definitive diagnostic category. Its recognition is important because steroid therapy is not always required, in contrast antiplatelet drugs could be the main therapeutic maneuver.

It is possible that the presence of APA in SLE defines a subgroup within this disease. Therapeutic implications can be also derived in this case.

The miscellaneous group is not well defined, because our practice is in a cardiologic reference center, an overrepresentation of heart diseases is obligatory,

* This work was supported partially by grant from CONACYT A128CCOE 900909 (SA-7).

however, there is a possibility that some valvular diseases are related to the presence of APA, and not simply a coincidental finding. This aspect needs further study.

Introduction

It has been known for many years that syphilis can induce antibodies that bind cardiolipin, an anionic diphosphatidylglycerol. The standard nontreponemal tests for syphilis use tissue extracts or a mixture of cardiolipin, neutral phosphatidylcholine, and cholesterol, i.e., the V.D.R.L. antigen [1]. In the 1950s a "biologically false positive" test for syphilis [2] was recognized along with an acquired circulating anticoagulant, first called "lupus anticoagulant", a misnomer still in use [3, 4].

These serologic aberrations often occur together in patients with increased frequencies of recurrent thrombosis [5], recurrent spontaneous abortion and intrauterine death [6], pulmonary hypertension [7], thrombocytopenia [8], and neurologic disease [9]. By 1983 a solid phase radioimmunoassay to recognize antiphospholipid antibodies was available [10]. A little later a more convenient sold phase immunoenzyme assay [11] allowed the recognition of a "family" of autoantibodies against cardiolipin and other anionic or zwitterionic phospholipids. The clinical relevance of these antiphospholipid antibodies (APA) is a result of the demonstration of their presence not only in syphilis and systemic lupus erythematosus (SLE), but also in a variety of infections, autoimmune and drug-induced disorders, and in a certain proportion of other patients and healthy individuals [12–15].

Clinical and Immunological Background

The oldest tests used to recognize APA are the standard tests for syphilis, i.e., the Wassermann test and similar complement fixation tests, the V.D.R.L. (flocculation) test, and the rapid plasma reagin (agglutination) test. These recognize preferentially IgM. Syphilitic serum usually is strongly positive, but it contains low levels of IgG. Although these antibodies bind cardiolipin [16, 17], they are different from APA produced in other conditions. Reagin does not cause anticoagulant activity [18, 19] and no correlation exists between the binding to cardiolipin-coated plates and V.D.R.L. titer [20, 21]. Binding to V.D.R.L. antigen is always greater and there is no cross-reactivity with other anionic phospholipids [22]. The "new" APA, IgG, IgM, and IgA recognize epitopes in anionic phospholipids with a chain of at least 14 carbon atoms and are able to react with laminar or hexagonal phospholipid structures [23]. Since APA bind to a variety of phospholipids that have in common only a phosphodiester group, the latter has been proposed as the epitope for APA. This concept may explain many immunochemical and clinical characteristics of APA through cross-reactivity [24–26]; however, it is only weakly supported by results of work with cross-reactive DNA-monoclonal antibodies made in mouse-mouse hybridomas [27, 28], in human-human hybridomas [29], or in polyclonal systems in rabbits [30, 31]. The polyclonal APA found in humans with SLE or other clinical conditions have a relatively restricted specificity, in contrast to the polyspecificity shown by monoclonal antibodies, exactly the opposite of what might be expected [32]. In addition, analysis of IgG subclasses and light chain distribution in sera of 60 patients with SLE showed that all IgG subclasses of APA were present and λ- exceeded κ-light chains. In the anti-DNA group of antibodies, IgG1 and IgG3 were predominant κ- and exceed λ-light chains [33]. Therefore, the epitopes for APA, the response to phospholipids, and the cross-reactivity reactions need further study. There is agreement in regard to differentiating reagin from APA. The latter are accepted as antibodies which bind negatively charged phospholipids.

In the clinic APA are detected as acquired anticoagulant activity in phospholipid-dependent clotting assays or as antibodies in an ELISA using cardiolipin-coated plates. The results of these two tests are not parallel. It is recommended that both be performed in order to identify as many cases as possible.

Associated clinical features have been identified mainly in retrospective studies. A recent textbook summarizes the information [34]: of the more than 800 patients whose plasma contained lupus-anticoagulant activity, about 25%–36% had a history of venous or arterial thrombosis, and, in patients with anticardiolipin antibodies of the IgG isotype, the frequency of thrombosis may exceed 50% in those with moderate or high antibody levels. The hemostatic profile is characterized first by thrombocytopenia, a well-known complication in patients with lupus-anticoagulant activity and a frequent feature in those with anticardiolipin IgG. In addition, it is very common to demonstrate a prolonged partial thromboplastin time not corrected by fresh normal plasma. Fetal loss is also a common finding.

All these data were sufficient to postulate the existence of a clinical entity, "antiphospholipid syndrome" [35]. This syndrome may overlap with other autoimmune disorders, in particular SLE. Thus, some patients with few or no manifestations of SLE could be classified as having primary antiphospholipid syndrome (PAPS), and those who fulfilled accepted SLE criteria [36] had what was referred to as secondary PAPS. There are also patients with other diseases who have APA, complicating further the concept and boundaries of the syndrome.

Our aim in this article is to address two questions: Do the presence of IgG anticardiolipin antibodies make up a distinctive disease in clinical terms? What are the clinical features associated with this entity? In other words, we wish to set up a clinical profile of PAPS.

Methods and Patients

The Presence of APA

The ELISA recommended was standardized in our laboratory [37, 38]. Briefly, cardiolipin (Sigma Chemical Co., St. Louis, MO, USA) dissolved in ethanol was adsorbed onto plastic trays (Nunc Inc.) under vacuum; free, unreacted sites were blocked with fetal calf serum; and diluted human serum was added. After incubation and extensive washing, goat Ig specific for Fc-human IgG, followed by rabbit IgG specific for Fc-goat IgG coupled to peroxidase were added. The reaction was stopped, visualized with orthophenylenediamine and hydrogen peroxide, and read at 490 nm in an automatic photometer (MicroELISA reader, Dynatech Inc., Baltimore, MD, USA).

The use of antigen-negative wells to correct for nonspecific binding, serial dilution of high and medium-positive and -negative samples, and triplicate readings of each sample improved the reproducibilitiy of the assay.

From 114 healthy donors (72 men and 42 women) with a mean age of 26.5 years, a discrimination point at 0.203 OD units was determined. This point included 5 SD to the mean.

Patients

Sera collected from clinics were sent to us without information regarding diagnosis. After processing 200 samples, we selected values above the discrimination point; hospital charts were retrieved and the patient histories reviewed.

It was possible to distinguish three groups of patients: in group I, there were 15 patients with manifestations such as those described in PAPS; group II consisted of 10 SLE patients who easily fulfilled the classification criteria [36]; in group III there were 25 patients with miscellaneous diagnoses: 7 with rheumatic heart disease and cardiac surgery for valve prosthesis in the past, 6 with ischemic disease (2 having had myocardial infarction), 5 with systemic arterial hypertension, 2 with type II diabetes mellitus, 1 each with Takayasu's arteritis, congenital heart disease, retinal vasculitis and livedo reticularis, gout, and 1 with positive antinuclear antibodies (ANA) without a final diagnosis (Table 1).

Table 1. Demography of patients with circulating IgG APA.

	Group I	Group II	Group III
Patients (*n*)	15	10	25
Sex F (*n*)	12	7	20
F:M ratio	4:1	2.3:1	4:1
Age (mean ± SD/median)	36.7 ± 15.3/32	34.5 ± 14.9/27	48.2 ± 16.2/49
Range	18–78	13–55	19–77
Diagnosis [a]	PAPS	SLE	Miscellaneous

[a] In group I initial diagnoses were not correct in 13 patients. PAPS refers to our final diagnosis. Group III diagnoses are mentioned in the text. All patients were Mexican and racially homogeneous. APA, antiphospholipid antibodies.

Results

Relevant clinical features in these 50 patients are summarized in Tables 2 and 3. Thrombosis was very common among group I patients. It was widely distributed and severe and involved venous and arterial trees with vena cava obstruction in two patients. These patients also had deep leg vein thromboses, a finding present in six more patients. Probably as a consequence of venous thrombosis, half of the patients developed pulmonary thromboembolism.

Table 2. Clinical features in patients with circulating IgG APA (I).

	Primary APAS (group I)		SLE and APA (group II)		Miscellaneous and APA (group III)	
	n 15	(%)	*n* 10	(%)	*n* 25	(%)
Thrombosis						
Venous	8	(53)	2	(20)	0	
Arterial	9	(60)	0		4	(16)
Both	7	(47)	0		0	
Obstetric disease						
Abortion	8	(80)	0		3	(15)
Hemocytopenic disease						
Thrombocytopenia	11	(73)	3	(30)	3	(12)
Leukopenia	3	(20)	5	(50)	5	(20)
Hemolytic anemia	1	(6)	0		0	

APA, antiphospholipid antibodies.

Table 3. Clinical features in patients with circulating APA (II).

	Primary APAS (group I) *n* 15	SLE and APA (group II) *n* 10	Miscellaneous and APA (group III) *n* 25
Skin/vascular			
Raynaud's	2	6	0
Leg ulcers	2	2	0
Mucous ulcers	2	5	0
Livedo reticularis	5	5	1
Heart			
Mitral valve	3	2	7
Aortic valve	4	1	6
Tricuspid valve	3	1	1
Pulmonary valve	4	0	0
Nervous system			
Convulsive disorder	6	0	2
Vascular headache	4	3	3
Neuropathy	4	0	0

APA, antiphospholipid antibodies.

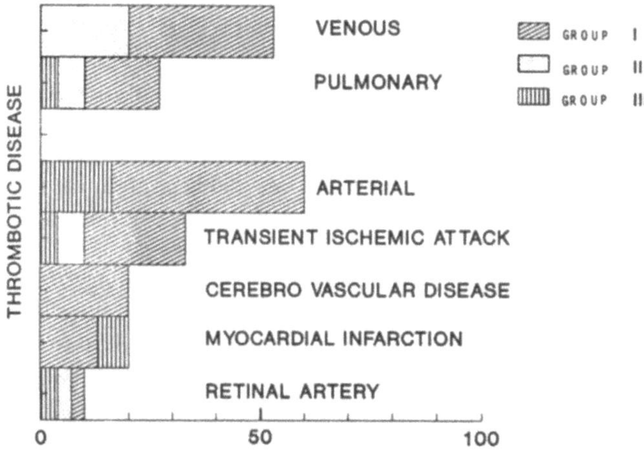

Fig. 1. Thrombotic disease in patients with circulating IgG-antiphospholipid antibodies expressed as percentage of patients with primary antiphospholipid syndrome (group I), systemic lupus erythematosus (group II), and miscellaneous (group III)

Arterial disease in this group caused mesenteric insufficiency, retinal artery obstruction, transient ischemic attacks, cerebrovascular disease, and myocardial infarction in young people without risk factors (Fig. 1). Transient ischemic attacks preceeded the cerebrovascular disease in three patients; two other patients had, besides the cerebrovascular disease, extensive thrombotic disease affecting arteries and veins.

Thrombosis also affected group II and III; neither its frequency nor its severity was similar to the manifestations in group I. Only two SLE patients had deep leg vein thrombosis: one developed pulmonary thrombotic disease, and only one had transient ischemic attacks. In group III no venous thrombosis was seen, four patients had arterial disease, and five myocardial infarction; only one suffered pulmonary thrombosis. These patients were older and predisposing conditions cannot be ruled out (Fig. 1).

Spontaneous abortion or intrauterine death was reported by 8/10 women in the first group. Two of them had seven consecutive and the others five consecutive spontaneous abortions. A patient developed acute myocardial infarction 4 days after the abortion. In contrast, only 3/20 women in group III reported obstetric abnormalities in the past. Hematologic features, thrombocytopenia, autoimmune hemolytic anemia, and leukopenia usually were not clinically manifested, although in some patients it was present when laboratory tests were done.

Thrombocytopenia defined as a platelet count of less than 100×10^9 platelets/L occurred most frequently. It was present in 11 patients within group I and 3 each in groups II and III. In contrast, leukopenia was more common in SLE (five patients) and less common in other. Autoimmune Coombs reactive anemia was present in a single patient in group I as Evans syndrome. The coincidence of thrombocytopenia and leukopenia was observed in all groups with similar frequencies. Vascular abnormalities were detected in the three groups. Systemic hypertension was present in nine group III patients: seven in group I, another with Sneddon syndrome, and another with SLE.

Primary pulmonary hypertension was limited to two group I and two group II patients. Livedo reticularis, Raynaud's phenomenon, and leg or mucosal ulcers were detected in group I and II patients almost exclusively. Neurological and heart involvement were conspicuous. A sensory-motor peripheral neuropathy occurred in four patients in group I and was debilitating in one patient. Within the same group, transverse myelitis was present in one patient and multifocal demyeliniza-tion and Devic's syndrome in another.

Cerebrovascular or cerebellar disease secondary to multiple infarction or occlusive disease was common in all groups. The same was true for vascular headache. However, severe cases of cerebrovascular disease were limited to group I patients; two had Gerstmann syndrome and the other two had dementia. Chorea occurred in a patient from group III.

Heart disease was frequent in group I. Conventional cardiovascular physical examination disclosed 11 patients with organic heart murmurs; heart failure was present on admission in two patients and one required urgent mitral valve commisurotomy. Heart valve disease affected both heart chambers, with left side disease predominating.

Mitral valve dysfunction was identified in 12 patients, 7 from group III, 3 from group I, and 2 SLE patients. Aortic valve with regurgitation, stenosis, or both occurred in 11 patients (6 from group III, 4 from group I, and 1 with SLE). The tricuspid valve was regurgitant in five patients, three from group I; this group had the only patient with pulmonary valve dysfunction (Table 3).

A valve disease index, the product of the number of patients in each group multiplied by the number of affected valves, gave a value three times higher in

Table 4. Heart valve disease in patients with APA.

Valve disease	Group I	*n*	Group II	*n*	Group III	*n*
Mitral	Regurgitation	1	Regurgitation	1	Regurgitation + stenosis	4
	Regurgitation + stenosis	2	Regurgitation + stenosis	1	Stenosis	2
					Prolapse	1
Aortic	Regurgitation	2			Stenosis	3
	Stenosis	1	Thickening	1	Regurgitation + stenosis	2
	Both	1				
					Regurgitation	1
Tricuspid	Regurgitation	3	Regurgitation	1	Regurgitation	1
Pulmonary	Regurgitation	2				
	Stenosis	2				
Number of affected patients	10/15		2/10		10/25	
Diseased valves	14		4		14	
Diseased valves index	1.55		1.0		0.56	

Table 5. Combination thrombocytopenia and heart valve disease in patients with APA.

		Group I	Group II	Group III
Thrombocytopenia	Present	9	0	0
and valve disease	Absent	6	10	25
Confidence interval[a]		35–87	0–28	0–14
		$p<0.05$	NS	
			$p<0.05$	

[a] Comparing groups I and II; $p<0.05$, groups II and II; ns; groups I and III, $p<0.05$.

group I than in group III. This is important because group III is made up of cardiac patients. Therefore, even taking into consideration the selection bias inherent in the hospital, PAPS patients had relatively more valve disease (Table 4).

Combined thrombocytopenia and valve disease were present only in one patient from group I. Group II and group III patients had either thrombocytopenia or valve disease but not both (Table 5).

In addition to clinical data, differences in laboratory findings were also significant. Hemostasis and autoantibody patterns separate clearly the three groups (Fig. 2). Prolonged partial thromboplastin time was the most common abnormality; ten patients in group I had this finding, but only two in group II and one in group III had this feature. With regard to presence of plasma anticoagulant activity, the "lupus anticoagulant" was not identified in a single patient within group III. In contrast, it was present in three of nine patients tested in group I as well as in two of ten patients with SLE.

False-positive V.D.R.L. was observed with decreasing frequency from group I to group III. Rheumatoid factors (RFs) and ANAs were an almost exclusive feature of group II patients.

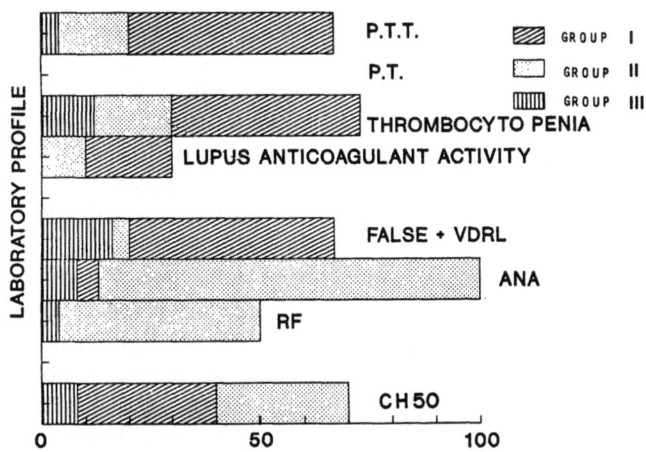

Fig. 2. Laboratory features in patients with circulating IgG-antiphospholipid antibodies expressed as percentage of patients with primary antiphospholipid syndrome (group I), systemic lupus erythematosus (group II), and miscellaneous (group III)

By definition all patients had IgG APA, in group I, 13 of them showed high titers with a mean of 1.2 OD units. In contrast high titer IgG was the exception in other groups; the means were 0.26 and 0.34 OD units in groups II and III, respectively.

Conclusions

The presence of IgG APA is a serologic characteristic more commonly seen in females, and it is possible to distinguish three clinical settings in regard to the antibody levels and range of clinical manifestations. The most numerous APA-positive patients (Group III) are relatively old people, with low or moderate IgG APA levels without plasma-anticoagulant activity, and with few a clinical manifestations of thrombotic disease, cytopenia, or obstetric complications. In these patients the presence of the antibody could be incidental.

Patients with SLE had low or moderate levels of IgG APA. A certain proportion of these patients, about 40% in several series, developed clinical manifestations which are, to some extent, different from those present in SLE without APA. The presence of recurrent thrombosis, thrombocytopenia, and Coombs reactive hemolytic anemia, which can be expressed together as Fishers Evans syndrome, livedo reticularis, and leg ulcers, are characteristic of SLE patients with APA [39–42]. As expected, in this study patients who belonged to group II had increased frequencies of these features, along with mucosal ulcers, Raynaud's phenomenon, leukopenia and, of course, non-organ specific autoantibodies (the lupus-related findings).

A third cluster of patients had predominantly high levels of IgG APA. They had a syndrome which included as prominent features extensive and severe thrombotic disease of veins and arteries; occlusive vascular disease of the central nervous system, perhaps with the vasa nervorum affected in some patients; and involvement of other vessels. Hemocytopenic disease, with thrombocytopenia as the major component was also present, although usually not clinically overt. Sexually active females suffered obstetric complications which were the third most frequent component of the syndrome. Skin and vascular abnormalities, neurologic complaints not necessarily due to obstructive disease, and heart disease with valve dysfunction were also part of the clinical entity. Some authors have described a clinical picture similar to the one reported here (Table 6). These series were collected in Europe and in our country; no major differences exist, supporting the concept that PAPS is a clinical entity of its own.

We accept that our series is biased since it was collected in a cardiology center; therefore, the relatively high proportion of thromboembolic events, and especially the valvular heart disease, could be overrepresented; however, in the current literature there are many reports of SLE patients with APA who had heart disease and some of them required valve prostheses [43–46]. These reports originate in developed countries where rheumatic fever is not prevalent and infectious endocarditis was ruled out with appropriate studies. In Mexico rheumatic fever is still a public health problem, although in continuous decline; a comment on this point is obligatory.

Table 6. Comparison of clinical features in primary antiphospholipid antibodies syndrome in several series.

	Alarcón-Segovia $n = 9$	Asherson $n = 70$	Mackworth $n = 20$	Present $n = 15$
Sex ratio F:M	8:1	2:1	9:1	4:1
Age (mean)	25.6	38.5	32.7	36.7
Thrombosis n (%)				
Venous	6	38 (54)	7 (35)	8 (53)
Arterial	5	31 (44)	5 (25)	9 (60)
Pulmonary TE	–	18 (47)[a]	4 (57)[a]	4 (50)[a]
TIA	–	15 (21)	2 (10)	5 (33)
AMI	–	5 (7)		2 (13)
Abortion	4	24 (55)	12 (80)[b]	8 (80)[b]
Cytopenia				
Thrombocytopenia	4	32 (46)	6 (30)	11 (73)
Hemolytic anemia		3 (4)	–	1 (6)
Laboratory findings				
IgG APA[c]		41 (59)	14 (70)	12 (80)
aPTT (prolonged)	8	–	–	10 (67)
False-positive VDRL	5	17 (33)	5 (25)	10 (67)
Lupus anticoagulant				3 (30)

Pulmonary TE, pulmonary thromboembolic disease; TIA, transient ischemic attacks; AMI, acute myocardial infarction.
[a] This percentage was related to venous thrombosis.
[b] Considering married females.
[c] Titers higher than 5SD. Lupus anticoagulant in the present series was assayed in only nine patients.

Among group I patients four recalled a recurrent pharyngitis during their childhood; however, no clear picture of rheumatic fever was suggested by history and an elevated Antistreptolysine 0 (AS0) titer was not recorded. The pattern of valve involvement is not the same one usually seen in typical cases of rheumatic heart disease; damage of the pulmonary valve is extremely rare in children with rheumatic fever and also very rare in adults with rheumatic heart disease [47, 48].

The combination of thrombocytopenia and heart valve dysfunction has not been described in rheumatic heart disease as far as we know. It is timely to point out that 30% – 50% of young adults, with heart valve dysfunction diagnosed as chronic rheumatic heart disease, do not have evidence of rheumatic fever in their history. Perhaps PAPS should be included as a cause of chronic heart valve dysfunction in the differential diagnosis of rheumatic heart disease.

The lack of a formal demonstration of a cause and effect relationship between APA and cellular or tissue damage, prevents a general acceptance of PAPS as a clinical entity. Several studies address the issue of the pathogenesis of PAPS as a consequence of circulating APA, which have been shown to be thrombogenic and to have an in vitro effect on endothelial cells [49–51]. Contradictory data from other laboratories and questionable extrapolation of in vitro findings to human disease prevent any strong conclusions [52–54]. The broad interest in APA by investigators from a wide range of disciplines will perhaps solve the pathogenesis issue in a near future. In the meantime, clinicians must be able to identify PAPS patients in order to avoid unnecessary treatment with prolonged use of steroid or immunosuppressive agents.

In our patients, as in other series, recurrent thrombosis was best treated with oral anticoagulants and drugs that inhibit platelet aggregation. The use of aspirin and low doses of prednisone improved pregnancy outcome in two of our patients who delivered normal babies; however, our experience is anecdotal.

It is likely that APA and its clinical correlates will be a subject for clinical and research immunologists for some time. May their work finally shed light on this fascinating disease.

Acknowledgement. The authors gratefully acknowledge the help of J. L. Bañales, J. L. Fuziwara, and L. Galindo.

References

1. Larsen SA, Bradford LL (1986) Serodiagnosis of syphilis. In: Rose NR, Friedman H, Fahey JL (eds) Manual of clinical immunology, 2nd edn. American Microbiological Society, Washington DC, p 425
2. Moore JE, Mohr CF (1952) Biologically false positive serologic tests for syphilis: type, incidence and cause. JAMA 150:467
3. Conley CL, Hartmann RC (1952) A hemorrhagic disorder caused by circulating anticoagulant in patients with disseminated lupus erythematosus. J Clin Invest 31:621
4. Boxer M, Ellmann L, Carvalho A (1976) The lupus anticoagulant. Arthritis Rheum 19:1244
5. Mueh JR, Herbst KD, Rapaport SI (1980) Thrombosis in patients with the lupus anticoagulant. Ann Intern Med 92:156
6. Nilsson IM, Astedt B, Hedner V, et al. (1975) Intrauterine death and circulating anticoagulant. Acta Med Scand 197:153
7. Asherson RA, Mackworth-Young CG, Boey M, et al. (1983) Pulmonary hypertension in systemic lupus erythematosus. Br Med J 287:1024
8. Schleider MA, Nachman RL, Jaffe EA, et al. (1976) A clinical study of the lupus, anticoagulant. Blood 48:499
9. Fullford KWM, Catterall RD, Delhanty JJ, et al. (1972) A collagen disorder of the nervous system presenting as multiple sclerosis. Brain 95:373
10. Harris EN, Gharavi AE, Boey ML, et al. (1983) Anticardiolipin antibodies: detection by radioimmunoassay and association with thrombosis in systemic lupus erythematosus. Lancet 2:1211
11. Loizu S, McGrea JD, Rudge AC, et al. (1985) Measurement of anticardiolipin antibodies by an enzyme-linked immunosorbent assay (ELISA): standardization and quantitation of results. Clin Exp Immunol 62:738
12. Harris EN, Gharavi AE, Hughes GRV (1985) Antiphospholipid antibodies. Clin Rheum Dis 11:591
13. Sontheimer RD (1987) The anticardiolipin syndrome. A new way to slice and old pie, or a new pie to slice? Arch Dermatol 123:590
14. Amigo MC (1987) El síndrome anticardiolipina y su relación a los padecimientas cardiovasculares. Arch Inst Cardiol Mex 57:349
15. Harris EN (1989) Anticardiolipin antibodies and autoimmune diseases. Curr Opin Rheumatol 1:215
16. Costello PB, Green FA (1986) Reactivity patterns of human anticardiolipin and other antiphospholipid antibodies in syphilitic sera. Infect Immun 51:771
17. Harris EN, Gharavi AE, Loizu E, et al. (1985) Cross reactivity of antiphospholipid antibodies. J Clin Lab Immunol 59:393

18. Johannson EA, Lassus A (1974) The occurrence of circulating anticoagulants in patients with syphilitic and biologically false positive antilipoidal antibodies. Ann Clin Res 6:105
19. Shoenfeld Y (1980) Circulating anticoagulant and serological tests for syphilis. Acta Derm Venereol (Stockh) 60:356
20. Koike T (1984) Antiphospholipid antibodies and biological false positive serological tests for syphilis in patients with systemic lupus erythematosus. Clin Exp Immunol 56:193
21. Colaco CB, Male DK (1985) Antiphospholipid antibodies in syphilis and a thrombotic subset of SLE: distinct profiles of epitope specificity. Clin Exp Immunol 59:449
22. Gharavi AE, Harris EN, Ashershon RA, et al. (1987) Anticardiolipin antibodies: isotype distribution and phospholipid specificity. Ann Rheum Dis 46:1
23. Rauch J, Tannenbaum M, Tannenbaum H, et al. (1986) Human hybridoma lupus anticoagulants distinguish between lamellar and hexagonal phase lipid systems. J Biol Chem 261:9672
24. Guarnioni M, Eisner D (1974) A DNA antigen that reacts with antisera to cardiolipin. Biochem Biophys Res Commun 58:347
25. Colaco BC, Elkon KB (1985) The lupus anticoagulant. A disease marker in ANA negative lupus that is cross-reactive with autoantibodies to ds DNA. Arthritis Rheum 28:67
26. Rauch J, Tannenbaum H, Stollar BD, et al. (1984) Monoclonal anticardiolipin antibodies bind DNA. Eur J Immunol 14:529
27. Lafer FM, Rauch J, Andrezejewski C, et al. (1981) Polyspecific monoclonal lupus autoantibodies reactive with both polynucleotides and phospholipids. J Exp Med 153:897
28. Koike T, Tomiska M, Kumassai A (1984) Specificity of mouse hybridoma antibodies to DNA. II. Phospholipid reactivity and biological false positive serological test for syphilis. Clin Exp Immunol 57:345
29. Shoenfeld Y, Rauch J, Massicotte H, et al. (1983) Polyspecificity of monoclonal lupus autoantibodies produced by human-human hybridomas. N Engl J Med 308:414
30. Filat D, Zlotnick AY, Fischell R (1986) Evaluation of the cross-reaction between anti DNA and anticardiolipin antibodies in SLE and experimental animals. Clin Exp Immunol 65:269
31. Smeenk RJT, Lucassen WAM, Swaak TJG (1987) Is anticardiolipin activity a cross-reaction of anti DNA or a separate entity? Arthritis Rheum 30:607
32. Emien W, Pistky DS, Taylor RP (1986) Antibodies to DNA: a perspective. Arthritis Rheum 29:1417
33. Gharavi AE, Harris EN, Lockshin MD, et al. (1988) IgG subclass and light chain distribution of anticardiolipin and anti DNA antibodies in SLE. Ann Rheum Dis 47:286
34. Harris EN, Hughes GRV (1989) Antiphospholipid antibodies. In: McCarty DJ (ed) Arthritis and allied conditions, 11th edn. Lea and Febiger, Philadelphia, p 1068
35. Hughes GRV (1983) Thrombosis, abortion, cerebral disease and the lupus anticoagulant. Br Med J 287:1088
36. Tan EM, Cohen AS, Fries JF, et al. (1982) The 1982 revised criteria for classification of systemic lupus erythematosus. Arthritis Rheum 25:1271
37. Harris EN, Gharavi AE, Patel SP, et al. (1987) Evaluation of the anticardiolipin antibody test: report of an international workshop held 4 april 1986. Clin Exp Immunol 68:215
38. Bañales JL, González-Ortega ME, Clark P, et al. (1989) Anticuerpos anticardiolipina. Significado clínico y límites del método. Arch Inst Cardiol Mex 59:393
39. Alarcón-Segovia D, Deleze M, Oria C, et al (1989) Antiphospholipid antibodies and the anitiphospholid syndrome in SLE. A prospective analysis of 500 consecutive patients. Medicine (Baltimore) 68:353
40. Asherson RA, Kamastha MA, Gil A, et al. (1989) Cerebrovascular disease and antiphospholipid antibodies in SLE, lupus-like disease, and the primary antiphospholipid syndrome. Am J Med 86:391
41. Hatron PY, Bouchez B, Wattel A, et al. (1986) Chorea, systemic lupus erythematosus, circulating lupus anticoagulant. J Rheumatol 13:991
42. Love PE, Santoro SA (1990) Antiphospholipid antibodies: anticardiolipin and the lupus anticoagulant in SLE and in non-SLE disorders. Prevalence and clinical significance. Ann Intern Med 112:682
43. Ansari A, Larson P, Bates HD (1985) Cardiovascular manifestations of SLE: current perspective. Prog Cardiovasc Dis 27:431

44. Stratton KV, Chatham WW, Reveille JD, et al. (1988) Clinically significant valvular heart disease in SLE. Am J Med 85:645
45. Galve E, Candell-Riera J, Pigran C, et al. (1988) Prevalence, morphologic types and evolution of cardiac valvular disease in SLE. N Engl J Med 319:817
46. Chartash EK, Lans DM, Paget SA, et al. (1989) Aortic insufficiency and mitral regurgitation in patients with SLE and the antiphospholipid syndrome. Am J Med 86:407
47. Disciascio G, Taranta A (1980) Rheumatic fever in children. Am Heart J 99:635
48. Guadalajara JF (1984) Fiebre reumática. In: Guadalajara JF (ed) Cardiologia 3rd edn. Mendez, México, p 527
49. Carreras LO, Vermylen JG (1982) "Lupus" anticoagulant and thrombosis – possible role of inhibition of prostacyclin formation. Thromb Haemost 48:28
50. Angles-Cano E, Sultan I, Clauvel JP (1979) Predisposing factors to thrombosis in SLE. J Lab Clin Med 94:313
51. Carion R, Tobelem G, Belluci S, et al. (1988) Effect of lupus anticoagulant on antithrombogenic properties of endothelial cells – inhibition of thrombomodulin-dependent protein C activation. Thromb Haemost 60:54
52. Hasselar P, Derksen RHWM, de Groot PG (1988) Thrombosis associated with antiphospholipid antibodies cannot be explained by effects on endothelial cells and platelet prostanoid synthesis. Thromb Haemost 59:80
53. Francis RB, McGhee WG, Feinstein DI (1988) Endothelial dependent fibrinolysis in subjects with the lupus anticoagulant and thrombosis. Thromb Haemost 59:412
54. Deleze M, Oria CV, Alarcón-Segovia D (1988) Occurrence of both hemolytic anemia and thrombocytopenia purpura (Evan's syndrome) in SLE. Relationship to antiphospholipid antibodies. J Rheumatol 15:611

Antibodies to Basement Membrane Antigens

S. Kàrpàti and T. Krieg

Dermatologische Klinik der Ludwig-Maximilians-Universität München, Frauenlobstrasse 9–11, W-8000 München 2, Federal Republic of Germany

Abstract

The dermo-epidermal basement membrane zone has a complex structure on the ultrastructural level. Several of its protein components have been isolated and identified. Collagen IV forms the structural scaffold and is found in the lamina densa; laminin which has important cell binding functions is mainly located in the lamina lucida. Nidogen is another glycoprotein isolated from the basement membrane zone which also contains a heparan sulfate proteoglycan. Collagen VII is the molecular constituent of the anchoring fibrils. In addition, several other components are present in the basement membrane zone, which are not characterized in detail. Some of them have been identified as antigens in bullous diseases with circulating antibodies. These include the bullous pemphigoid, Herpes gestationis, cicatricial pemphigoid and the epidermolysis bullosa acquisita. In other diseases, e.g., dermatitis herpetiformis Duhring, linear IgA-dermatosis binding of circulating antibodies have been correlated to distinct morphological structures within the basement membrane zone. The exact clinical nature of the antigen, however, has not yet been determined. Identification of antigens in patients with bullous diseases has therefore not only helped to establish diagnosis of many diseases but in addition provided insight into the structure and composition of the basement membrane zone as well as into basic mechanisms of cellular adhesions.

Functions of the Basement Membrane

Although the basement membrane (BM) is a very thin structure, it has to fulfill a large variety of different functions. It supports the cytoskeleton, separates different tissue compartments, acts as a filtration barrier, and controls the migration of cells [1]. The BM acts also as a receptor for cell membranes and modulates many cellular functions. It forms a scaffold for tissue repair and plays a key role in the regulation of morphogenesis and wound healing. In the skin the BM is present around blood vessels, nerves, and at the dermo-epidermal junction where it separates the epidermis from the underlying stroma.

Structure of the BM

The BM accounts for a very small percentage of the total extracellular matrix and its components are highly insoluble. Therefore, for a very long time, is was difficult to obtain sufficient information about the chemical nature of the molecules contributing to its structure. This problem was overcome by the discovery of a tumor that produces large amounts of BM, by developments in molecular biology, and by the identification of autoimmune diseases which are characterized by circulating autoantibodies [4] directed against distinct proteins of the BM. They include Goodpasture's syndrome, some aspects of Chagas' disease, and several blistering diseases, such as bullous pemphigoid, herpes gestationis, epidermolysis bullosa acquisita (EBA), and probably also dermatitis herpetiformis [2]. In some of these diseases the antigens have already been identified on the molecular level, in others they are still unknown.

The complexity of the BM zone becomes even more obvious with high power electron microscopy. One can distinguish the lamina lucida and the lamina densa. The epidermal cells attach to the lamina lucida by hemidesmosomes. Filaments extend from the attachment site through the BM, and anchoring fibrils connect the BM with the underlying connective tissue (Fig. 1).

Molecular Constituents of the BM

During the last 10 years several of the molecular constituents of the BM have been defined and characterized [1–3]. *Collagen type IV* is present in all BMs and represents the structural scaffold [4]. *Heparan sulfate proteoglycans* are exclusively found in BM and the same is true for the glycoproteins *nidogen* and *laminin. Collagen type VII* is found only in the dermo-epidermal junction zone, along with *kalinin*, a recently characterized molecule (Dr. R.E. Burgeson, personal commu-

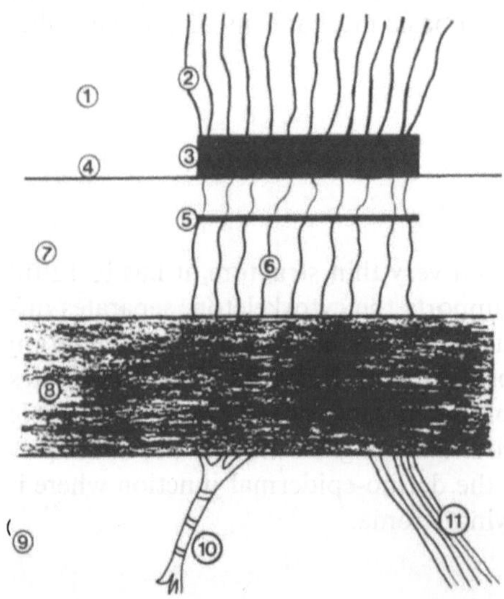

Fig. 1. The skin basement membrane zone. *1*, Lower portion of basal keratinocyte; *2*, tonofilaments; *3*, attachment plaque of hemidesmosome; *4*, plasma membrane; *5*, subbasal dense plate; *6*, anchoring filaments; *7*, lamina lucida; *8*, lamina densa; *9*, superficial dermis; *10*, anchoring fibrils; *11*, microfibrillar bundles

Table 1. Components of the basement membrane zone.

Collagen IV		Collagen VII
Heparan sulfate proteoglycan		Kalinin
Nidogen/entactin		Integrins
Laminin		Bullous pemphigoid antigen
	Fibronectin	
	BM-40	

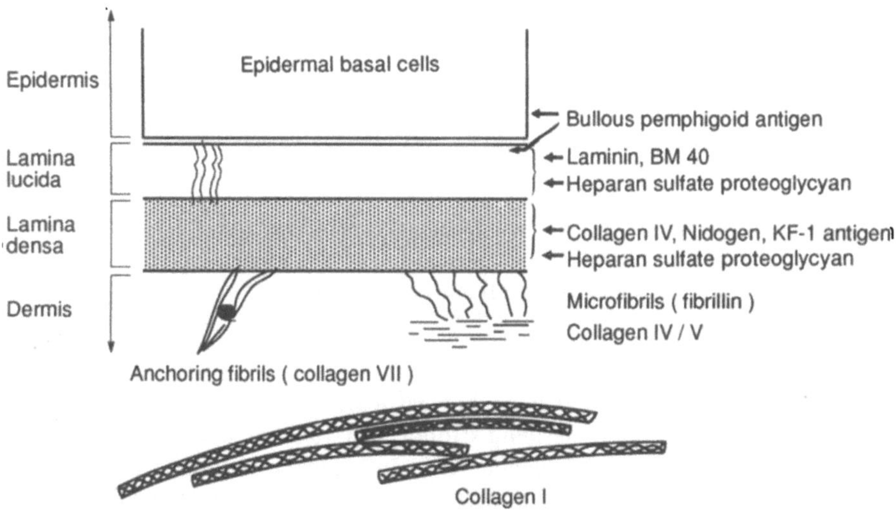

Fig. 2. Molecular constituents of the skin basement membrane zone

nications). *Integrins* probably are incorporated into attachment sites of keratinocytes, where the *bullous pemphigoid antigen* is also found. *Fibronectin* and a smaller glycoprotein, *BM-40*, are not exclusively found in BM but are present also in interstitial connective tissue (Table 1, Fig. 2).

Different Functions of BM Proteins

The chemical isolation and characterization of these molecular constituents of the BM zone allow one to exactly determine the different functions of BM proteins. Laminin is self-aggregating and can bind to other BM proteins. It also binds to cells and can modulate many cellular activities, such as adhesion and differentiation. Some structural domains within this large glycoprotein have even been shown to contain epidermal growth factor (EGF)-like sequences and to act as growth factors [6]. Nidogen interacts with laminin but it also binds to collagen IV and proteoglycans and has a high affinity for calcium. It therefore plays an important role in providing cohesion to the macromolecular organization of different BM proteins. Collagen IV can act as a cell binding protein, but its main

Table 2. Biological functions of basement membrane proteins.

Laminin	
	Self-aggregation and binding to other BM proteins
	Cell adhesion and modulation of cellular activities
	Growth factor
Nidogen	
	Binding to collagen IV, laminin, and proteoglycan
	Cell adhesion
	Calcium binding
Collagen IV	
	Self-assembly and mechanical scaffold for anchoring of other BM proteins
	Cell adhesion
Collagen VII	
	Anchoring of the BM to the underlying stroma
BM-40	
	Calcium binding
	Binding to collagen IV
Kalinin	
	Hemidesmosomal link between collagen VII and keratinocytes?

function probably is to serve as a mechanical scaffold for the BM. Collagen VII connects the BM with the underlying stroma. BM-40 is the major calcium-binding protein and interacts with collagen IV. Its biological role within the BM, however, has not yet been determined in detail. Kalinin strongly binds to collagen VII and seems to act as a link between anchoring fibrils and keratinocytes (Table 2).

Ultrastructural Distribution of BM Proteins

The isolation of BM proteins has led to production of specific antibodies, which have been used in indirect immunoelectron microscopy to assign molecules to distinct structures. Laminin is mainly located in the lamina lucida; collagen IV is found in the lamina densa, along with nidogen and heparan sulfate proteoglycan. Collagen VII was identified as the major structural component of the anchoring fibrils [6, 7].

Different Aspects of Autoimmune Diseases Related to the BM Zone

The organ-specific expression of BM proteins has important clinical implications since it explains the localization of certain diseases. The bullous pemphigoid antigen, kalinin, and collagen VII are specific for stratified epithelium. Type IV collagen is found in all BM, where it is present in a three-dimensional network [2, 3] built up by individual molecules with well-known structures (Fig. 3). Two α_1 and

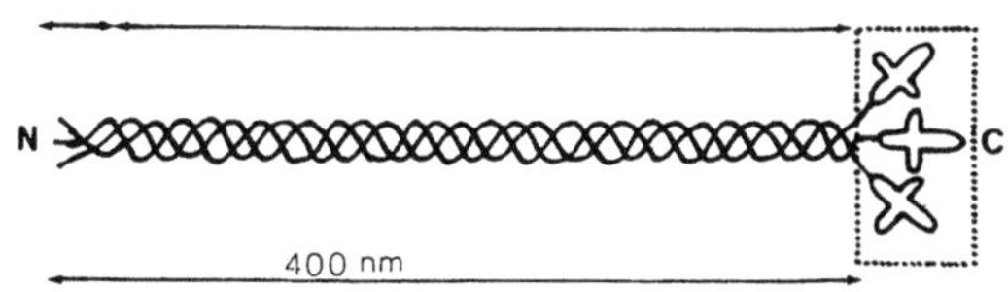

Fig. 3. Structure of collagen IV molecule

one α_2 chains form a long triple helical domain with large nonhelical domains at both ends. In the glomerular BM and in the lung collagen IV molecules can contain an additional polypeptide chain, α_3. This chain is also incorporated into the NC-1 domain, and it has been shown that, under these conditions, the NC-1 domain serves as an antigen in an autoimmune disease. Thus, due to the tissue-specific expression of the α_3 chain, Goodpasture's syndrome typically has lung involvement and proliferative glomerulonephritis [8, 9] (Tables 3, 4).

In EBA antibodies bind to anchoring fibrils; in patients with bullous pemphigoid and herpes gestationis, antibodies bind to the very upper part of the lamina lucida. In contrast, in cicatricial pemphigoid, antibodies bind to the lower part of the lamina lucida; in this disease the blisters leave scars (Fig. 4).

Collagen type VII can also be involved in autoimmune diseases. Since it was localized to anchoring fibrils and is only found in the dermo-epidermal junction zone, it is not surprising that the clinical symptoms of this disease include the development of blisters on exposed body sites. Using immunoelectron microscopy the immune complexes were localized to beneath the lamina densa.

Table 3. Autoimmune diseases with circulating antibodies directed against basement membrane components.

Goodpasture's syndrome
Bullous pemphigoid
Herpes gestationis
Cicatricial pemphigoid
Epidermolysis bullosa acquisita
Chagas' disease

Table 4. Basement membrane antigens in autoimmune diseases.

Disease	Antigen
Goodpasture's syndrome	α_3 (IV) Collagen (NC-1)
Bullous pemphigoid Herpes gestationis Cicatricial pemphigoid	180- or 230-kDa Hemidesmosomal protein $\beta_4\alpha_6$ Integrin?
Epidermolysis bullosa acquisita	Collagen VII
Chagas' disease	Laminin

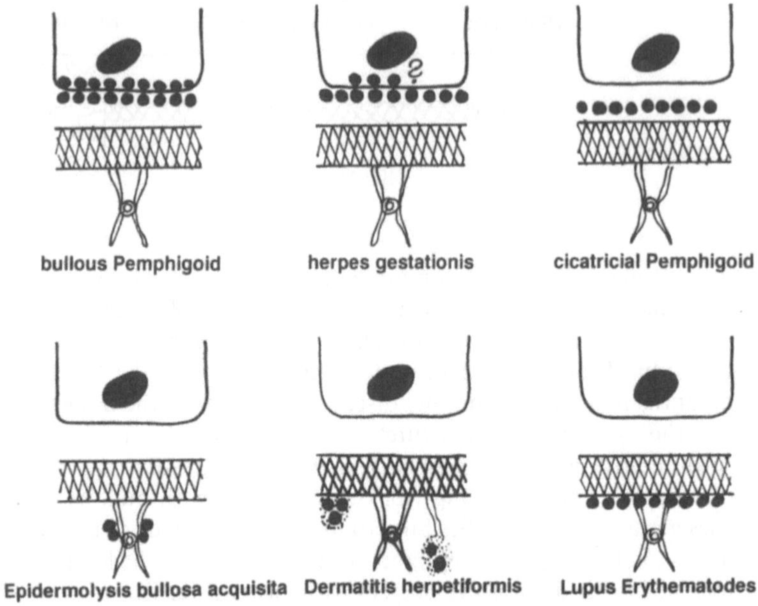

Fig. 4. Distribution of tissue-bound immunoglobulins along the BM zone in different autoimmune diseases

Immunoblotting of BM extract and incubation with sera from patients with EBA revealed two bands, one with a molecular mass of 290 kDa and another with a mass of 140 kDa [10]. A few years later, type VII collagen was described, and purified antibodies could be used for indirect immunoelectron microscopy. On skin the pattern of staining was very similar to that obtained from EBA skin. The molecular structure of collagen VII was then elucidated. It has a very long triple helical and at the end a large globular domain (Fig. 4). This NC-1 domain binds to the lamina densa, the molecules aggregate head-to-head, and the NC-1 domains of the other molecules bind to the anchoring plaques in the dermis. This NC-1 domain of collagen VII is identical to the EBA antigen [11].

The bullous pemphigoid antigen has already been well characterized and has a molecular mass of 230 kDa; it was found to be a polypeptide from the hemidesmosomal plaque of keratinocytes. In addition a sequenced clone was found to recognize a 9-kb mRNA species. Additional proteins with molecular masses of 180 kDa, 200 kDa, and 160 kDa were separated, and recognized by bullous pemphigoid antibodies. It is not clear yet whether this might reflect a heterogeneity of the disease or whether the smaller proteins represent breakdown products of the original 230-kDa protein [12].

In herpes gestationis, interestingly, similar 180-kDa and 230-kDa polypeptides were recently described to be the antigens. These 180-kDa and 230-kDa proteins were identical to those identified by bullous pemphigoid serum.

Also in cicatricial pemphigoid a recent publication described antigens with molecular masses of 230 and 180 kDa similar to bullous pemphigoid antigen [13].

Dermatitis herpetiformis (DH) is usually associated with a latent celiac disease. In these patients no circulating antibodies against the skin have been detected, but most have IgAs that bind to reticular structures of the jejunum, esophagus, and other organs with a reticular network. These so-called anti-endomysium, anti-reticulin, or anti-jejunal antibodies are very characteristic for celiac disease and can be detected in the diseased small bowel of DH patients. The granular IgA staining under the BM and in the papillary dermis detected in DH, but not in celiac skin, most likely represents immune complex aggregates deposited partly along anchoring fibers, elastic microfibrillar bundles, and collagen fibers, but were also found separated from any structural elements. The anchoring fibrils, elastic microfibrils, and collagen fibers do not stain for IgA (Fig. 5). The IgA aggregates in DH papillary skin may recognize a still unknown skin antigen (DH factor) or be deposited without specific antigenic binding.

Laminin has a typical cross-like structure. It is composed of three short arms and one long arm, has various structural domains, and carries several sugar residues. One of these residues, galactosyl-α_1-α_3-galactose, was found to be recognized by antisera from patients with Chagas' disease. These antibodies are generated against similar carbohydrate epitopes present on the surface of the parasites which are responsible for the disease. The antibodies react with laminin in blood vessels, muscles, and peripheral nerves. They are therefore thought to be involved in some of the degenerative changes observed in these patients [14].

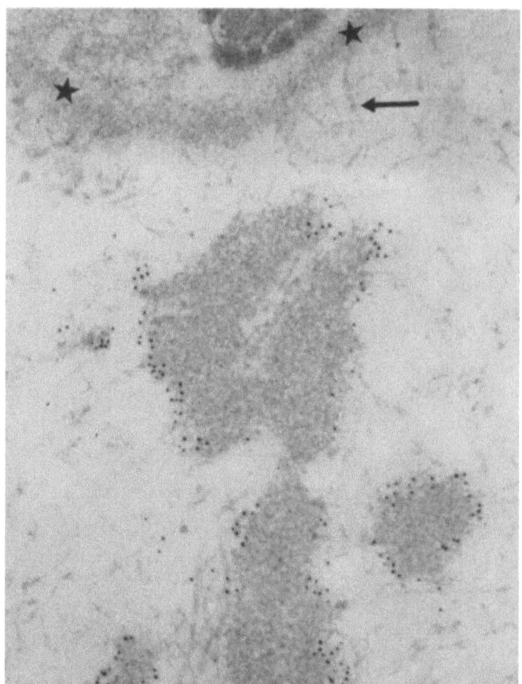

Fig. 5. Dermatitis herpetiformis (DH) skin by ultrastructural immunogold microscopy. IgA-positive aggregates (DH bodies) under the BM zone (*stars*). The anchoring fibrils (*arrow*) are unlabeled (×89320)

References

1. Timpl R, Dziadek M (1986) Structure, development and molecular pathology of basement membranes. Int Rev Exp Pathol 29:1–112
2. Timpl R (1989) Structure and biological activity of basement membrane proteins. Eur J Biochem 180:487–502
3. Martin GR, Timpl R, Müller PK, Kühn K (1985) The genetically distinct collagens. Trends Biochem Sci 10:285–287
4. Yurchenco PD, Furthmayr H (1984) Self assembly of basement membrane collagen. Biochemistry 23:1839–1850
5. Panayotou G, End P, Aumailley M, Timpl R, Engel J (1989) Domains of laminin with growth-factor activity. Cell 56:93–101
6. Sakai LY, Keene DR, Morris NP, Burgeson RE (1986) Type VII collagen is a major structural component of anchoring fibrils. J Cell Biol 103:1577–1586
7. Keene DR, Sakai LY, Lunstrum GP, Morris NP, Burgeson RE (1987) Type VII collagen forms an extended network of anchoring fibrils. J Cell Biol 104:611–621
8. Butkowski RJ, Langeveld JPM, Wieslander J, Hamilton J, Hudson BG (1987) Localization of the Goodpasture epitope to a novel chain of basement-membrane collagen. J Biol Chem 262:7874–7877
9. Saus J, Wieslander J, Langeveld JP, Quinones S, Hudson BG (1988) Identification of the Goodpasture antigen at the alpha3 (IV) chain of collagen IV. J Biol Chem 263:13374–13380
10. Woodley DT, Briggaman RA, O'Keefe EJ, Inman AO, Queen LL, Gammon WR (1983) Identification of skin basement membrane autoantigen in epidermolysis bullosa acquisita. N Engl J Med 16:1007–1013
11. Woodley DT, Burgeson RE, Lunstrum G, Bruckner-Tuderman L, Reese M, Briggaman RA (1988) Epidermolysis bullosa acquisita antigen is the globular carboxyl terminus of type VII procollagen. J Clin Invest 81:683–687
12. Stanley JR, Tanaka T, Mueller S, Klaus-Kovtun V, Roop D (1988) Isolation of cDNA for bullous pemphigoid antigen by use of patient's autoantibodies. J Clin Invest 82:1864–1870
13. Bernard P, Prost C, Lecerf V, Intrator L, Combemale P, Bedane C, Roujeau JC, Revuz J, Bonnetblanc JM, Dubertret L (1990) Studies of cicatricial pemphigoid autoantibodies using immunoelectron microscopy and immunoblot analysis. J Invest Dermatol 94:630–635
14. Towbin H, Rosenfelder G, Wieslander J, Avila JL, Rojas M, Szarfman A, Esser K, Nowack H, Timpl R (1987) Circulating antibodies to mouse laminin in Chagas' disease and normal individuals recognize terminal galactosyl (alpha1–3)-galactose epitopes. J Exp Med 166:419–432

Contact Dermatitis

Genetics of Contact Allergy*

J. Karvonen and S. Silvennoinen-Kassinen

Department of Dermatology and Department of Medical Microbiology, University of Oulu, 90220 Oulu, Finland

Abstract

For the development of contact allergy both the presence of an allergen and a genetical susceptibility are essential. Susceptibility to allergic sensitization varies between individuals. Most are easily sensitized with potent allergens like dinitrochlorbenzene (DNCB) or poison ivy while some are not.

It has been shown with inbred mice and guinea pig strains that susceptibility to contact sensitivity is genetically controlled. The mode of inheritance seems to be dominant and the genes controlling the development of contact sensitivity are, in most cases, linked with major histocompatibility complex (MHC) genes. Such immune response (Ir) genes have been demonstrated in several animals.

In humans individual differences in susceptibility to contact sensitivity also exist. Family studies have shown that parents sensitized to DNCB or other allergens are more likely to have children susceptible to contact allergy than parents who are not easily sensitized. A twin study based on data from the Danish Twin Register showed a significant difference between the concordance rates for nickel allergy among monozygotic vs dizygotic twins.

It has been surprising and disappointing for researchers that in humans no clear-cut associations between contact sensitivity and HLA antigens have been found, although several studies have been published on both class I and class II antigens. However, a recent study using restriction fragment length polymorphism analysis of class II HLA genes could demonstrate a significant association between an HLA-DQA fragment and nickel allergy. This may be the first evidence for the presence of an Ir gene controlling contact allergy in humans.

Introduction

The susceptibility to contact allergy varies. Most persons easily develop allergy after contact with superallergens like dinitrochlorbenzene (DNCB) while about 5% are highly resistant even after repeated exposures. In the same way repeated

* This study was supported by grants from the Finnish Allergy Research Foundation and the Paulo Foundation.

contact with poison ivy leads to allergy in most but not in all individuals. Genetic predisposition is not the only but perhaps the most probable explanation for these individual differences.

Animal Studies

It has been shown with inbred guinea pig strains that some strains easily develop contact allergy to DNCB, metal compounds, and other chemicals while other strains are resistant [1, 2]. The disposition to contact allergy seems to be dominantly inherited in guinea pigs [3]. In most cases the genetic control of contact allergy is linked with the major histocompatibility complex (MHC) in guinea pigs [4] and in mice [5]. An immune response (Ir) gene controlling the development of nickel allergy has been located on the right margin of the I-A area in the MHC in mice [6]. Thus, there is strong evidence for an important role of MHC-linked Ir genes in the development of contact allergy in animals.

Classical Genetic Studies in Humans

In 1967 Walker et al. [7] published a study in which they had sensitized 301 individuals in 91 families to DNCB and nitrosodimethylaniline. It was shown that children whose parents were sensitized became sensitized at a higher rate than did children whose parents were not sensitized. If both parents were sensitized the risk of the child getting sensitized was greater than if only one of the parents was sensitized. In a Danish twin study on nickel allergy 1546 female twin pairs were questioned and 115 pairs with possible nickel allergy were patch-tested [8]. The concordance rate was significantly higher among monozygotic than dizygotic twins.

HLA Studies in Humans

The MHC linkage of contact allergy in animals made HLA studies in humans interesting. The important role of class II HLA antigens in the presentation of antigens to T cells increased the hopes of HLA investigators. Altogether more than ten studies of possible HLA associations of contact allergies have been published. However, the results have been disappointing. Although some weak associations have been found in some studies, the conclusion of all data is that there are no significant associations between HLA-A, B, C, or DR antigens and contact allergy [9]. Restriction fragment length polymorphism analysis is a new method which can be used to increase the power of the analysis of polymorphism of HLA genes. With this method it was recently shown that nickel allergy is associated with a *Taq*I HLA-DQA restriction fragment. This fragment occurred in 67% of nickel-allergic patients compared with 31% of controls [10]. If this first report can be verified in further studies, it obviously is the first evidence of an Ir gene controlling contact allergy in humans. The location of this possible gene near the HLA-DQ area is exactly what could be expected from the results of studies in mice.

Polymorphism of the T Cell Receptor

Other polymorphisms than HLA might also be important in the study of the genetics of allergy. The polymorphism of T cell receptors is one possibility. We have recently shown that cells activated during a nickel-allergic reaction carry mainly α and β T cell receptors. The nickel-specific cells do not predominantly use any of the β chain variables $V\beta5$, $V\beta6$, or $V\beta8$ [11]. We have also analyzed the T cell receptor β chain haplotypes and found no difference in the haplotype frequencies between nickel-allergic and control individuals (Silvennoinen-Kassinen et al., unpublished results). Thus, in these limited studies, we have not found any associations between T cell receptor polymorphism and nickel allergy.

Conclusion

Contact allergy clearly has a genetic background. Genes controlling contact allergy are within the MHC in many animals and possibly also in humans. The role of T cell receptors in the genetics of contact allergy is worth further study.

References

1. Chase MW (1941) Inheritance in guinea pigs of the susceptibility to skin sensitization with simple compounds. J Exp Med 73:711
2. Levine BB, Ojeda A, Benacerraf B (1963) Studies on artificial antigens. III. The genetic control of the immune response to hapten poly-L-lysine conjugates in guinea pigs. J Exp Med 118:953
3. Polak L, Barnes JM, Turk JL (1968) The genetic control of contact sensitization to inorganic metal compounds in guinea-pigs. Immunology 14:707
4. Geczy AF, DeWeck AL (1975) Genetic control of sensitization to structurally unrelated antigens and its relationship to histocompatibility antigens in guinea pigs. Immunology 28:331
5. Schulz LD, Bailey DW (1975) Genetic control of contact sensitivity in mice: effect of H-2 and non H-2 loci. Immunogenetics 1:570
6. Ishii N, Ishii H, Ono H, Horiuchi Y, Nakajima H, Aoki I (1990) Genetic control of nickel sulfate delayed-type hypersensitivity. J Invest Dermatol 94:673
7. Walker FB, Smith PD, Maibach HI (1967) Genetic factors in human allergic contact dermatitis. Int Arch Allergy 32:453
8. Menne T, Holm NV (1983) Hand eczema in nickel sensitive female twins. Genetic predisposition and environmental factors. Contact Dermatitis 9:289

9. Karvonen J, Silvennoinen-Kassinen S, Ilonen J, Jakkula H, Tiilikainen A (1984) HLA antigens in nickel allergy. Ann Clin Res 16:211
10. Olerup O, Emtestam L (1988) Allergic contact dermatitis to nickel is associated with a *Taq* I HLA-DQA allelic restriction fragment. Immunogenetics 28:310
11. Silvennoinen-Kassinen S, Ikäheimo I, Kauppinen M, Karvonen J (1990) Cell surface markers of nickel induced 7-day lymphocyte blasts in nickel sensitive subjects. 20th Annual Meeting of the European Society for Dermatological Research, June 9–12, Turin

Atopy and Contact Allergy

F. Enders[1], B. Przybilla[1], and J. Ring[2]

[1] Dermatologische Klinik und Poliklinik, Ludwig-Maximilians-Universität, Frauenlobstrasse 9–11, W-8000 München 2, Federal Republic of Germany
[2] Hautklinik, Universitäts-Krankenhaus Eppendorf, Martinistrasse 52, W-2000 Hamburg 20, Federal Republic of Germany

Abstract

Impairment of cellular immunity is one of the characteristic immunological features found in patients with atopic eczema. For example, in vitro there are decreased lymphocyte responses to stimulation with mitogens and antigens. In vivo sensitization studies with neoantigens (e. g., dinitrochlorobenzene) have disclosed a clearly reduced reactivity in patients with atopic eczema compared to controls. This leads to the assumption that there may be a reduced frequency of allergic contact sensitization in patients with atopic eczema. However, the pertinent literature on the prevalence of allergic contact sensitization in patients with atopic eczema does not allow one to draw definite conclusions. The results are contradictory, reporting lower, equal, and higher sensitization rates in atopic eczema. Interpretation is hampered by methodological flaws, as most of the studies are retrospective and often without adequate controls. When comparing patients with atopy to nonatopic individuals, we did not find a difference with regard to the overall reactivity rate to compounds of the patch test standard series; however, there were differences when the frequency of reactions to individual compounds was considered. Thus, there was a significantly higher frequency of contact sensitization to nickel sulphate (15.2%/10.0%), potassium dichromate (5.9%/4.3%), and thiuram mix (4.2%/2.6%) in atopics than in nonatopics. In contrast, contact allergy to balsam of Peru (5.3%/6.7%), wool alcohols (2.9%/4.3%), neomycin (2.4%/3.5%), and parabens (0.8%/2.1%) was significantly less frequent in atopics than in nonatopics. However, as atopics were younger than nonatopics, these findings may be explained at least in part by the age difference. Current knowledge suggests that atopy does not protect against allergic contact sensitization. Further studies are necessary to clarify the relationship between contact allergy and atopy.

Introduction

Impairment of cellular immunity is one of the characteristic immunological features found in patients with atopic eczema [3, 32]. As allergic contact eczema is due to a cellular immune reaction, considerable controversy still exists as to the frequency and role of allergic contact sensitivity in the patient with atopic eczema.

Whether contact sensitivity in atopic eczema patients is less frequent than in nonatopics has been a matter of particularly intense discussion. During the last three decades, many investigations concerning the frequency of allergic contact sensitivity in patients with atopic eczema have been done; nonetheless, we are still unable to draw definite conclusions. It has not yet become clear if the prevalence of contact sensitivity in the individual with atopic eczema is equal, increased, or decreased compared to individuals without atopy.

Immunological Aspects

The immunological aspects of the atopic trait (tendency to develop atopic eczema, allergic rhinitis, and allergic bronchial asthma) have been studied for many years. During the past few years, considerable attention has been paid to the basic physiological abnormalities in atopic eczema, e.g., disturbances of the immune system, changed pharmacological reactivity, and disturbances of epidermal functions [33, 35].

An immunological basis of atopic eczema is suggested by a number of characteristic features. With regard to cellular immunity, various abnormalities were found, e.g., decreased proliferation of lymphocytes in response to antigens and mitogens in vitro, a decreased number of mature T lymphocytes in the peripheral blood, a T suppressor cell deficiency, a decreased natural killer cell activity, a dysfunction of monocytes and neutrophils, an increase in the number of IgE binding B lymphocytes, and a decrease of delayed-type skin test reactions [8–10, 17, 36].

Humoral immunity in atopic eczema is characterized especially by an increased IgE immune response, and a temporary IgA deficiency and increased IgG4 levels have been reported [10, 22, 25]. As a sequel to the increased IgE response, patients with atopic eczema often exhibit positive prick test reactions to common environmental aeroallergens and food antigens.

A defect of cell-mediated immunity has been noted in up to 80% of patients with atopic eczema. Clinically, this corresponds to an increased susceptibility to viral infections (herpes simplex, human papilloma, vaccinia, or molluscum contagiosum) and to an increased incidence of dermatophyte and *Staphylococcus aureus* infections [5, 19].

In addition, a number of studies have shown that atopic patients are more difficult to sensitize to dinitrochlorobenzene (DNCB) than control subjects [16, 20, 30]. Furthermore, patients with severe atopic eczema are more difficult to sensitize to DNCB than patients with only mild skin lesions [37].

Jones et al. [23] reported the results of patch testing with *Rhus* antigen (poison ivy) in atopic eczema patients and age-matched controls: only 15% of atopic eczema patients had positive reactions to *Rhus* antigen as opposed to 61% of controls. Repeated testing of subjects who were negative at the first test revealed that one-third of the controls had become sensitized by the initial test, whereas only 6% of patients with atopic eczema had converted to a positive reaction. This points to a decreased tendency of patients with atopic eczema to become sensitized.

Other studies have demonstrated that patients with atopic eczema also exhibit reduced delayed hypersensitivity responses to intradermal skin tests using "recall" antigens, e.g., microbial antigens such as mumps, tuberculin, trichophytin or monilial extracts [16, 20, 29].

Reactions to Common Contact Allergens

All these findings suggest a reduced reactivity of the T cell system in atopics. Thus, it is not surprising that a decreased response to contact allergens of the common environment in patients with atopic eczema, or generally in atopy, is often discussed. However, the prevalence of allergic contact sensitivity in atopic eczema patients remains controversial. There are studies claiming lower, equal, and higher sensitization rates in atopic eczema patients than in controls, the frequency of positive patch test reactions being 15%–46% in atopic eczema patients and 30%–52% in controls (Table 1).

Our Findings

From 1978 to 1983 and in 1987 a total of 2021 patients with an atopic diathesis were tested with a standard series (Table 2); 87% of these had atopic eczema, 13% suffered from respiratory atopic disease (allergic rhinitis and/or allergic bronchial asthma). During the same period a total of 9837 nonatopic individuals (the complementary group to the atopics out of all patients tested) were patch-tested with the same material. The age distribution of these patients is given in Table 3. Test-

Table 1. Reactions to standard contact allergens in the patch test.

Investigator	Atopics		Nonatopics	
	Tested (n)	Positive reactions (%)	Tested (n)	Positive reactions (%)
Epstein et al. [15]	100	28		
Cronin et al. [11]	233	26	4000[a]	40
Bandmann et al. [2]	130	15		
Breit [6]	101	37	1226	49
Lisi and Simonetti [26]	61	25		
Marghescu [28]	129	40	4480	51
Brunner et al. [7]	1539	38	8515	37
Blondeel et al. [4]	935	40	3427	51
Huber et al. [21]	65	46	78	30
Pürschel and Ditrich [31]	1303	29		
De Groot [13]	214	37	285	52

[a] 233 atopics and 3767 nonatopics.

Table 2. Patch testing with a standard series of test substances.

Nickel sulphate	5% pet	Thiuram mix[c]	1% pet
Fragrance mix[a,h]	16% pet[i]	Mafenide	10% pet
Balsam of Peru	25% pet	Parabens[d]	15% pet
Cobalt chloride	1% pet	Gentamicin sulphate	20% pet
Potassium dichromate	0.5% pet	PPD mix[e]	0.6% pet
Wool alcohols	30% pet	Mercuric chloride	0.1% pet
Caine mix[b]	7% pet	Turpentine peroxide	0.3% pet
p-Phenylendiamine	1% pet	Epoxy resin	1% pet
Formaldehyde	2% H_2O	Phenylmercury borate	0.0025% pet
Neomycin sulphate	20% pet	Mercapto mix[f]	1% pet
Benzocaine	5% pet	Ethylenediamine[h]	1% pet
Colophony	20% pet	Naphthyl mix[g]	1% pet
Clioquinol	5% pet	Petrolatum	100%

[a] Cinnamic alcohol 2%; cinnamic aldehyde 2%; eugenol 2%; amylcin alcohol 2%; hydroxy-citronellal 2%; geraniol 2%; isoeugenol 2%; oak moss 2%.
[b] Benzocaine 5%; amethocaine hydrochloride 1%; cinchocaine 1%.
[c] Tetramethylthiuram disulfide 0.25%; tetramethylthiuram monosulfide 0.25%; tetramethylthiuram disulfide 0.25%; dipentamethylenethiuram disulfide 0.25%.
[d] Methyl-, 3%; ethyl-, 3%; butyl-, 3%; propyl-, 3%; benzyl-*p*-hydroxybenzoate 3%.
[e] Phenylcyclohexyl-p-phenylenediamine 0.25%; isopropylaminodiphenylamine 0.1%; diphenyl-*p*-phenylenediamine 0.25%.
[f] Mercaptobenzothiazole 0.25%; *N*-cyclohexylbenzothiazylsulfonamide 0.25%; morpholinylmercaptobenzuothiazole 0.25%; dibenzothiazyl disulphide 0.25%.
[g] Phenyl-β-naphthylamine 0.5%; di-β-naphthyl-*p*-phenylenediamine 0.5%.
[h] Tested since August 1982.
[i] 1982/83 16%; 1987 8%.

Table 3. Age of patients tested.

	<11	11–20	21–30	31–40	41–50	51–60	61–70	>70	Total
Atopics[a]	2.3%	16.1%	25.7%	20.1%	16.0%	10.5%	5.9%	3.4%	100%
Nonatopics[b]	0.9%	9.2%	18.0%	18.4%	16.8%	15.8%	11.4%	9.5%	100%

[a] $n = 2021$.
[b] $n = 9837$.

ing was performed according to suggestions of the International Contact Dermatitis Research Group (ICDRG). Statistical analysis was done with the chi-square test.

In comparing the patients with atopy to the nonatopic individuals no difference with regard to the overall reactivity rate to compounds of the standard series was found. At least one positive reaction was seen in 40.4% of the atopics and in 39.7% of the nonatopics. However, there were differences when the frequency of reactions to various compounds were considered. Comparing atopics to nonatopics, there was a significantly higher frequency of contact sensitization to nickel sulphate (15.2%/10.0%) and thiuram mix (4.2%/2.6%). In contrast, contact allergy to other compounds was significantly less frequent in atopics than in

Table 4. Patch testing with a standard series.

	Positive reactions (% of n)					
	Total		Males		Females	
	Atopics ($n = 2021$)	Nonatopics ($n = 9837$)	Atopics ($n = 598$)	Nonatopics ($n = 3917$)	Atopics ($n = 1423$)	Nonatopics ($n = 5920$)
Nickel sulphate	15.2	10.0***	5.2	2.8**	19.5	14.9***
Fragrance mix[a]	9.5	9.2	9.0	9.5	9.9	8.9
Potassium dichromate	5.3	4.3	4.8	5.5	5.4	3.6
Cobalt chloride	5.5	4.7	4.2	2.9	6.1	5.9
Balsam of Peru	5.3	6.7*	4.5	6.3	5.7	7.3*
Formaldehyde	4.2	3.5	3.5	3.2	4.4	3.6
Thiuram mix	4.2	2.6***	3.0	2.5	4.6	2.6***
p-Phenylenediamine	3.4	4.3	2.7	4.5*	3.7	4.1
Wool alcohols	2.9	4.3**	2.8	3.7	2.9	4.6**
Colophony	2.7	2.8	3.3	2.5	2.5	3.0
Neomycin	2.4	3.5*	1.8	3.3*	2.7	3.6
Caine mix[b]	2.2	4.5***	1.5	4.7***	2.5	4.5***
Gentamicin	1.5	1.6	1.8	1.5	1.3	1.7
Benzocaine	1.3	3.1***	1.2	3.4**	1.4	2.9**
PPD mix[b]	1.3	1.2	1.3	1.8	1.3	0.8
Clioquinol	1.1	2.8***	1.5	3.2*	1.0	2.5***
Parabens	0.8	2.1***	0.5	1.7*	1.0	2.3**

*$p = 0.05$; **$p = 0.01$; ***$p = 0.001$.
[a] Tested since August 1982: 1003 atopics (267 male, 736 female), 3057 nonatopics (1207 male, 1850 female).
[b] See Table 2.

nonatopics (balsam of Peru, 5.3%/6.7%; wool alcohols, 2.9%/4.3%; neomycin, 2.4%/3.5%; benzocaine, 1.3%/3.1%; parabens, 0.8%/2.1%) (Table 4).

Reactivity Rates in Atopics and Nonatopics

When trying to interpret these results, one has to consider that, in our study, the atopics tested were younger than the nonatopics. The finding of different reaction rates, e.g., to nickel, wool alcohols, benzocaine, or parabens, may be explained at least in part by this age bias [14]. However, in a prospective and age-matched study Huber et al. [21] did not find a significant difference with regard to the prevalence of contact sensitivity in atopics compared to nonatopics. Furthermore, like us they found a significantly different frequency of nickel sensitivity in patients with atopic eczema (28%) compared to the control group (6%) [21]. Lammintausta et al. [24] also reported no significant difference with regard to the patch test reactivity rate when atopics and nonatopics engaged in wet work in a hospital were compared.

The reason for the increased frequency of nickel sensitivity in patients with atopic eczema, also found in other studies [20, 27, 34, 38, 39], may be due to an increased permeability of the stratum corneum in atopics. An easy penetration of nickel ions in patients with atopic eczema has been shown [12, 18].

With regard to the increased frequency of reactions to thiuram mix, it can be assumed that atopics come into contact with rubber more readily than others by using gloves to protect their hands at the working place or at home. Similar results showing a higher frequency of reaction to rubber components in this patient group have already been reported [1].

Taken together, current knowledge of the frequency of positive patch test reactions in atopics suggests that atopy does not protect against allergic contact sensitization, and it may even facilitate sensitization to some compounds.

Future Aspects

The wide range of results found in different studies is probably due to the different criteria used. Interpretation is also hampered by methodological flaws since most of the studies were retrospective and often without adequate controls.

Some pertinent parameters which may influence the results profoundly are the definition of atopy (or atopic eczema), the composition of the control group, the selection of patients for patch testing, sex and age of patients tested, the selection and preparation of allergens, the number of allergens, and the patch test procedure (e.g., exposure and reading times).

A major problem is the definition of atopy or atopic eczema. As there is not yet any definite marker, one will have to rely on characteristic and reproducible criteria. However, to carry out a reasonable study, only a few criteria should be used.

It is as difficult to define the control group. Should it comprise all patients complimentary to those defined as atopics? Or, should it be a special subgroup selected on the basis of other positive criteria? Besides being age-matched to the atopics, the controls should also be matched according to profession or any other important criteria.

Further studies are necessary to clarify the relationship between contact sensitivity and atopy. Prevalence data on contact allergy in atopy are important, as they will hopefully allow recognition of exposures that are especially risky for these individuals.

References

1. Bandmann HJ, Agathos M (1980) Die atopische Handdermatitis. Dermatosen 28:110–113
2. Bandmann HJ, Breit R, Leutgeb C (1972) Kontaktallergie und Dermatitis atopica. Arch Dermatol Forsch 244:332–334
3. Blaylock WK (1976) Atopic dermatitis: diagnosis and pathobiology. J Allergy Clin Immunol 57:62–79
4. Blondeel A, Achten G, Dooms-Goossens A, Buekens P, Broeckx W, Oleffe J (1987) Atopie et allergie de contact. Ann Dermatol Venereol 114:203–209

5. Braun-Falco O, Plewig G, Wolff HH (1984) Dermatologie und Venerologie. Springer, Berlin Heidelberg New York
6. Breit R (1981) Positive Epikutantestreaktionen bei Dermatitis atopica. Hautarzt [Suppl 5] 32:147–148
7. Brunner R, Przybilla B, Ring J, Enders F (1987) Epikutantestergebnisse bei atopischen und nichtatopischen Patienten. Allergologie 10:427
8. Butler M, Atherton D, Levinsky RJ (1982) Quantitative and functional deficit of suppressor T cells in children with atopic eczema. Clin Exp Immunol 50:92–98
9. Byrom NA, Timlin DM (1979) Immune status in atopic eczema: a survey. Br J Dermatol 100:491–498
10. Chiarelli F, Canfora G, Verrotti A, Amerio P, Morgese G (1987) Humoral and cellular immunity in children with active and quiescent atopic dermatitis. Br J Dermatol 116:651–660
11. Cronin E, Bandmann HJ, Calnan CD, Fregert S, Hjorth N, Magnusson E, Maibach HI, Malten H, Meneghini CJ, Pirilä V, Wilkinson DS (1970) Contact dermatitis in the atopic. Acta Derm Venereol (Stockh) 50:183–187
12. Dahl MV (1983) Some aspects of atopic dermatitis. Arch Dermatol 119:237–242
13. De Groot AC (1990) The frequency of contact allergy in atopic patients with dermatitis. Contact Dermatitis 22:273–277
14. Enders F, Przybilla B, Ring J, Burg G, Braun-Falco O (1988) Epikutantestung mit einer Standardreihe. Hautarzt 39:779–786
15. Epstein S, Mohajerin AH, Marshfield W (1964) Incidence of contact sensitivity in atopic dermatitis. Arch Dermatol 90:284–287
16. Forsbeck M, Hovmark A, Skog E (1976) Patch testing, tuberculin testing and sensitization with dinitrochlorobenzene and nitrosodimethylaniline of patients with atopic dermatitis. Acta Derm Venereol (Stockh) 56:135–138
17. Frajman M, Gonzalez L, Alvarado A, Yock J (1987) Cellular immunity and IgE levels in atopic patients. Allergy 42:81–84
18. Gloor M, Wagner L (1985) Nichtimmunologische Funktionsstörungen der Haut beim Neurodermitiker. Zentralbl Haut Geschlechtskr 150:505–509
19. Hanifin JM (1988) Atopic Dermatitis. In: Middleton E, Reed CE, Ellis EF, Adkinson NF, Yunginger JW (eds) Allergy: principles and practice. Mosby, St Louis, pp 1403–1428
20. Hovmark A (1975) An in vivo and in vitro study of cell mediated immunity in atopic dermatitis. Acta Derm Venereol (Stockh) 55:181–186
21. Huber A, Fartasch M, Diepgen TL, Bäurle G, Hornstein OP (1987) Auftreten von Kontaktallergien beim atopischen Ekzem. Dermatosen 35:119–123
22. Ishizaka K (1976) Cellular events in the IgE antibody response. Adv Immunol 23:1–52
23. Jones HE, Lewis CW, McMarlin SL (1973) Allergic contact sensitivity in atopic dermatitis. Arch Dermatol 107:183–187
24. Lammintausta K, Kalimo K, Havu VK (1982) Contact allergy in atopics who perform wet work in hospital. Dermatosen 30:184–189
25. Leung DYM, Geha RS (1986) Immunoregulatory abnormalities in atopic dermatitis. Clin Rev Allergy 4:67–86
26. Lisi P, Simonetti S (1985) Contact sensitivity in children and adults with atopic dermatitis – a chronological study. Dermatologica 171:1–7
27. Malten KE (1971) Nickel-allergic contact dermatitis and atopy. Dermatologica 142:113–116
28. Marghescu S (1985) Patch test reactions in atopic patients. Acta Derm Venereol [Suppl] 114:113–116
29. McGeady SJ, Buckley RH (1975) Depression of cell-mediated immunity in atopic eczema. J Allergy Clin Immunol 56:393–406
30. Palacios J, Fuller EW, Blaylock WK (1966) Immunological capabilities of patients with atopic dermatitis. J Invest Dermatol 47:184–490
31. Pürschel W, Ditrich O (1989) Neurodermitis atopica und Kontaktallergie. Allergologie 12:203–208
32. Ring J (1983) Was ist Atopie? In: Braun-Falco O, Burg G (eds) Fortschritte der praktischen Dermatologie und Venerologie, vol 10. Springer, Berlin Heidelberg New York, pp 103–111
33. Ring J (1988) Angewandte Allergologie (2. Aufl). MMV Vieweg, München

34. Rudzki E, Grzywa Z (1975) Contact sensitivity in atopic dermatitis. Contact Dermatitis 1:285–287
35. Schöpf E (1979) Immunologie und Pathogenese der atopischen Dermatitis. In: Braun-Falco O, Wolff HH (eds) Fortschritte der praktischen Dermatologie und Venerologie, vol 9. Springer, Berlin Heidelberg New York, pp 87–94
36. Stingl G, Gazze LA, Czarnecki N, Wolff K (1981) T cell abnormalities in atopic dermatitis patients: imbalances in T cell subpopulations and impaired generation of con A-induced suppressor cells. J Invest Dermatol 76:468–473
37. Uehara M, Sawai T (1989) A longitudinal study of contact sensitivity in patients with atopic dermatitis. Arch Dermatol 125:366–368
38. Vestey JP, Gawkrodger DJ, Wong WK, Buxton PK (1986) An analysis of 501 consecutive contact clinic consultations. Contact Dermatitis 15:119–125
39. Zacher KD, Ippen H (1984) Das Nickel-Ekzem bei jungen Mädchen. Dermatosen 32:46–54

Neutrophil-Activating Peptide 1/Interleukin 8

M. Sticherling, E. Bornscheuer, J.-M. Schröder, and E. Christophers

Department of Dermatology, University of Kiel, Schittenhelmstrasse 7, W-2300 Kiel, Federal Republic of Germany

Introduction

In recent years different cytokines have been claimed to play a role in initiation and perpetuation of the eczematous tissue reaction. Among these factors is the neutrophil activating peptide 1/interleukin-8 (NAP-1/IL-8) [1]. This 72 amino acid peptide and variants thereof are produced by a number of different cell types, e.g., monocytes, endothelial cells [2], and fibroblasts [3]. Apart from its main target cell, the neutrophil, NAP-1/IL-8 was also shown to exert chemotactic activity on lymphocytes [4]. As numerical and functional changes have been observed with these cells in eczema IL-8 may well play a role in this disease entity.

With monoclonal anti-NAP-1/IL-8 antibodies at hand [5], immunohistological examination of the tissue distribution of NAP-1/IL-8 can be performed. Such studies on psoriasis vulgaris revealed an inverse relation between immunoreactivity and the inflammatory state [6]. We have now tested contact eczema and atopic dermatitis for NAP-1/IL-8 immunoreactivity.

Material and Methods

Monoclonal anti-NAP-1/IL-8 antibodies were produced by immunization of mice with NAP-1/IL-8 purified from stimulated human monocytes. They detect the genuine 72 amino acid peptide NAP-1/IL-8 and truncated forms thereof, i.e., endothelial cell-derived NAP (ENAP, 69 amino acids) and fibroblast-derived NAP (FINAP, 77 amino acids) as shown by ELISA and western blot [5]. They do not or only slightly cross-react with related peptides from the β-thromboglobulin family. Furthermore, no reactivity with a peptide with melanoma growth stimulatory activity (MGSA) nor with keratins was shown.

Biopsies were taken under local anesthesia after written consent from 15 patients with contact eczema, 5 patients with positive patch test reactions, and 7 patients with atopic eczema. Normal skin was obtained from patients undergoing plastic reconstructive surgery and was used as controls. Biopsies were quick frozen in liquid nitrogen and stored at $-70\,°C$ until processing.

For immunohistology cryostat tissue sections were fixed in acetone and incubated with primary antibody. Appropriate dilutions of monoclonal antibodies,

Table 1. Distribution pattern of NAP-1/IL-8 immunoreactivity with monoclonal antibody 52E8 in different disease entities and normal skin.

Skin disorder	Distribution pattern		
	Homogeneously positive	Focally negative	Homogeneously negative
Acute contact eczema	+	+	+
Positive patch test reactions	+	–	–
Atopic eczema	+	+	+
Psoriasis vulgaris	+	+	+
Normal skin	+	–	–

which are contained in culture supernatants (RPMI 1640, 8% fetal calf serum), were determined in advance. Staining was performed using the avidin-biotin peroxidase technique (ABC kit, Vector Labs) and diaminobenzidine or amino-ethylcarbazol as substrate.

Results

Using the monoclonal anti-NAP-1/IL-8 antibody 52E8, three patterns of immunoreactivity could be observed in contact eczema, positive patch test reactions, and atopic eczema. Pattern 1 showed a homogeneous staining over the entire course of epidermis as in normal skin. This was observed in sparsely infiltrated eczema. Pattern 2 consisted in focally decreased immunoreactivity which could be found above dense dermal infiltrates or beneath parakeratosis. Pattern 3 demonstrated almost no staining in biopsies with inflammatory infiltrates, distinct acanthosis, and parakeratosis. Interestingly, spongiotic intraepidermal vesicles are always negative, including the keratinocytes which surround or underlie the vesicles. Cells of the acrosyringium and hair follicles are always positive even in areas of decreased epidermal immunoreactivity.

Conclusions

As shown in this study NAP-1/IL-8 immunoreactivity could be correlated with the inflammatory state of eczematous tissue, with a distinct decrease in epidermal immunoreactivity above dermal infiltrates, beneath parakeratosis and around spongiotic vesicles. Altogether, no obvious difference in immunoreactivity could be detected between contact eczema and atopic eczema.

The results obtained are similar to those for psoriasis vulgaris, in which an inverse relationship was also detected between immunoreactivity and the inflammatory state of the tissue. Accordingly, the results indicate a relation to inflammatory processes as such rather than to special disease entities.

The existence of NAP-1/IL-8 in both psoriatic and eczematous lesions has been substantiated by the purification of considerable amounts of biologically active peptide from scaling material of both diseases [7].

References

1. Matsushima K, Oppenheim JJ (1989) Interleukin 8 and MCAF: Novel inflammatory cytokines inducible by IL-1 and TNF. Cytokine 1:2–13
2. Schröder JM, Christophers E (1989) Secretion of novel and homologous neutrophil activating peptides by LPS-stimulated human endothelial cells. J Immunol 142:244–251
3. Schröder JM, Sticherling M, Henneicke HH, Preissner WC, Christophers E (1990) IL-1α or TNFα stimulate release of three NAP-1/IL-8-related neutrophil chemotactic proteins in human dermal fibroblasts. J Immunol 144:2223–2232
4. Larsen CG, Andersen AO, Appella E, Oppenheim JJ, Matsushima K (1989) The neutrophil activating protein (NAP-1) is also chemotactic for T-lymphocytes. Science 243:1464–1466
5. Sticherling M, Schröder JM, Christophers E (1989) Production and characterization of monoclonal antibodies against neutrophil activating peptide NAP/IL-8. J Immunol 143:1628–1634
6. Sticherling M, Bornscheuer E, Schröder JM, Christophers E (1991) Localization of NAP-1/IL-8 immunoreactivity in normal and psoriatic skin. J Invest Dermatol 96:26–30
7. Schröder JM, Christophers E (1990) Determination of IL-8-related cytokines in the stratum corneum of chronic as well as acute inflammatory skin diseases. J Invest Dermatol 95:488

A Simple Method To Determine Permeation Resistance of Polymer Gloves

A. Rothe[1] and H. Hoffmann[2]

Zentralinstitut für Arbeitsmedizin, Abteilung Spezielle Noxen, Nöldnerstrasse 40/42, O-1134 Berlin, Federal Republic of Germany
[2]Bootsbau Berlin GmbH i. G. (former Yachtwerft Berlin), Müggelseedamm 40–70, O-1162 Berlin, Federal Republic of Germany

Introduction

The only effective measure to prevent occupational contact dermatitis is to avoid completely contact with allergens. Therefore, wearing polymer gloves is often recommended. However, its protective effect is at best temporarily limited and depends both on the materials used and the noxious agents [2, 4, 10–13, 16]. Furthermore, in view of the hundreds of sensitizing chemicals there is generally a lack of exact information about specific penetration resistance of the various types of gloves [9]. The only exception to the rule seems to be the 4 H[(R)] chemicals and permeation list of Safety 4 (Lyngby, Denmark) [5, 15].

The aim of this contribution is to demonstrate the efficiency of a forgotten but simple in vitro method to evaluate permeation resistance of polymer gloves.

Materials and Methods

Two out of four highly specialized racing boat builders fell ill while working with a new epoxy resin system after a very short exposure time. Therefore, it was necessary to find adequate protective gloves.

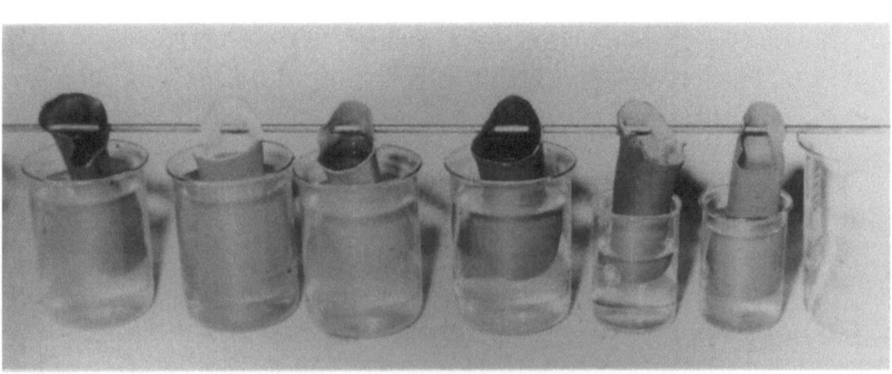

Fig. 1. Experimental setup for analyzing penetrating substances in polymer gloves

Table 1. Agents and their identification.

Allergens	Indicator system
Novolac epoxy resin (containing reactive diluent)	Solvent red 25
1,4-Butanediol diglycidyl ether (reactive diluent) [6]	Iodine (A)
	Iodide starch reagent (M)
4,4′-Diamino-3,3′-dimethyldicyclohexylmethane isophorone diamine	pH Paper (M)
Acetone	Sodium nitroprusside (M)
Methylene chloride	Solvent red 25 (A)

M, medium; A, penetrating substances.

Table 2. Polymer gloves.

Item	Material	Origin
Oil resistant rubber glove ASK no. 820a	Nitril-butadiene Rubber latex	East Germany
Oil resistant rubber glove ASK no. 822a	Nitril butadiene Rubber latex	East Germany
Household rubber glove no. 821a	Latex	East Germany
Polyethylene gloves (PE)	Polyethylene	Switzerland
Camatril-Velour	Nitril rubber	
"Double grip" 432	Polyvinylchloride (PVC)	Great Britain
Multipurpose glove ASK no. 811	Chloroprene	East Germany

According to Liebscher's method [8], cut-off fingers of gloves of various types, filled with the chemical in question, were put into an aqueous medium. To make the first traces of the penetrating substance (PS) visible, sensitive indicator reagents were added to the medium and/or to the PS (Fig. 1). Penetration times were then registered. Materials are listed in Tables 1 and 2.

Results

Penetration resistance of the various types of gloves are shown in Figs. 2, 3, and 4. Acetone and methylene chloride penetrated all gloves within no more than 30 min. The limiting factor concerning permeation resistance was 1,4-butanediol diglycidyl ether. This substance is a known allergen [6]. Both with regard to resistance against epoxy resin chemicals and its wearing qualities, the nitril glove 820a was selected as the protective glove. The experimental findings were confirmed by patch testing one of the sensitized individuals using the glove material as a barrier between the patch test substance and the skin.

It was recommended to use the glove only once and for no longer than 3.5 h. The sensitized boat builder continued to work without complaints. Since then no further report of contact dermatitis has been received.

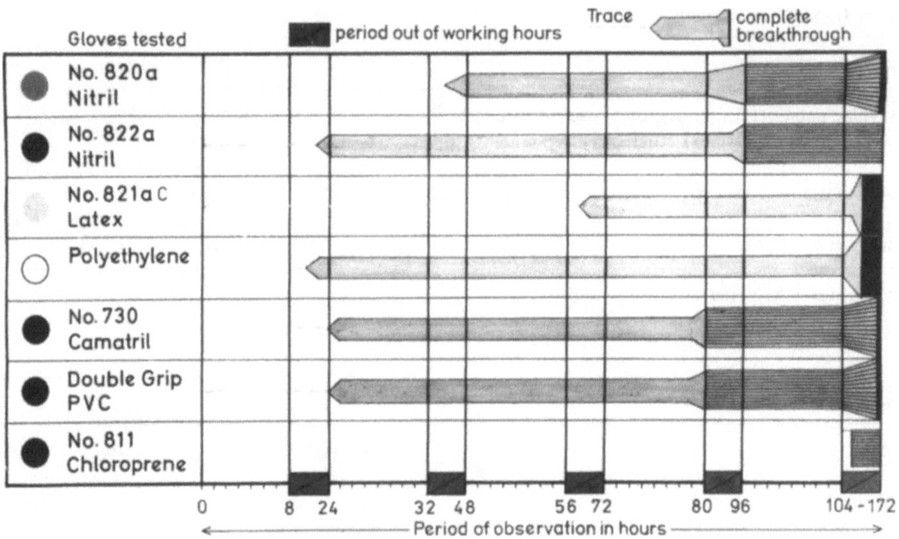

Fig. 2. Penetration time of the novolac epoxy resin

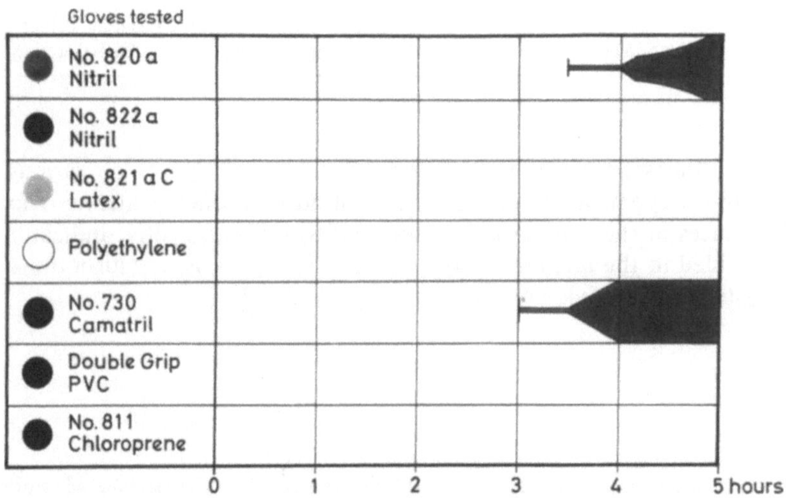

Fig. 3. Penetration time of the alkaline hardener

Conclusions

Without doubt Liebscher's method to evaluate permeation resistance of polymer gloves [8] cannot replace technically demanding and very modern methods, which were developed to exactly and scientifically investigate the permeability of polymer gloves [3, 5, 7, 14]. However, the method presented here provides sufficiently

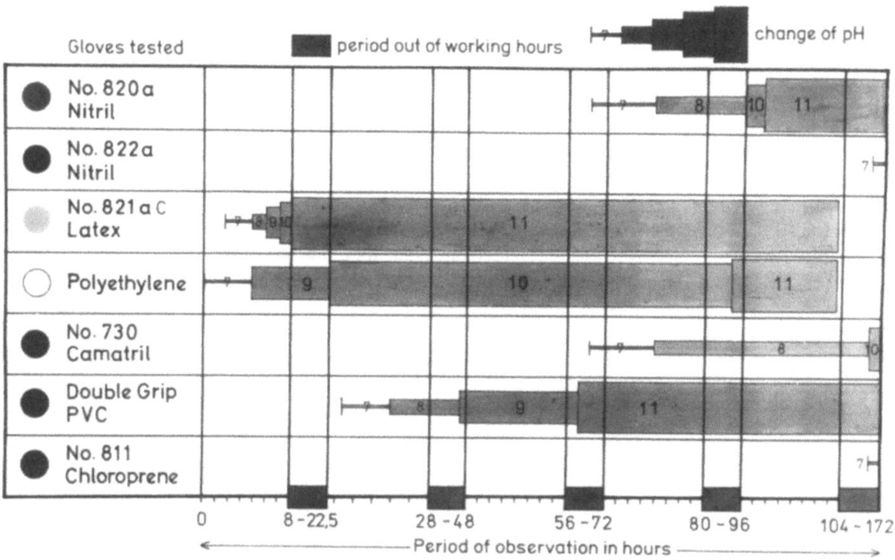

Fig. 4. Penetration time of 1,4-butanediol diglycidyl ether

reliable practical information about the protective effectiveness of polymer gloves. Since the permeation lists published by the producers of polymer gloves usually provide information about a limited number of chemicals, in vitro methods such as Liebscher's are occasionally required. This method is cheap and very easy to manage; thus, it can also be used in a small factory laboratory. If it is necessary to carry out such an examination, it is advisable to collaborate with a dermatologist experienced in the field of occupational dermatology.

References

1. Berardinelli SP, Hall R (1985) Site-specific whole glove chemical permeation. Am Ind Hyg Assoc J 46:60–64
2. Blanken R, Nater JP, Beenhoff E (1987) Protection against epoxy resins with glove material. Contact Dermatitis 16:46–47
3. Forsberg K, Baniadis S (1986) The permeation of multi-component liquids through new and pre-exposed glove material. Am Ind Hyg Assoc J 47:189–193
4. Fregert S, Tegner E (1972) Patch test reaction to a contaminant on rubber gloves. Contact Dermatitis Newsl 13:350
5. Henriksen HR, Petersen HJS (1986) Bedre Handsker mod epoxy og andre kemikalier (Better gloves against epoxy and other resins). Arbejdsmiljøfondet, Copenhagen
6. Jolanki R, Estlander T, Kanerva L (1987) Contact allergy to an epoxy reactive diluent: 1,4 butanediol diglycidyl ether. Contact Dermatitis 16:87–92
7. Krüger E (1989) Untersuchungen zur Penetration der Körperschutzmittel durch verschiedene Pestizide. Report, Symposium of CMEA countries, Bratislava, 1989
8. Liebscher J (1969) Zur Frage der Verhütung von Lösungsmittelschäden der Haut durch zweckmäßige Arbeitsschutzmittel. Dissertation, Humboldt University, Berlin

9. Mehlem P (1987) Persönliche Schutzausrüstungen. In: Dicke W, Mehlem P (eds) Alles über Hautschutz, Hautreinigung, Hautpflege. Wirtschaftsverlag NW, Verlag für neue Wissenschaft, Bremerhaven 58–67
10. Moursiden HT, Faber O (1973) Penetration of protective gloves by allergens and irritants. Trans St. John's Hosp Derm Soc 59:230–234
11. Pegum JS, Medhurst FA (1971) Contact dermatitis from penetration of rubber gloves by acrylic monomer. Br J Dermatol 2:141–143
12. Pegum JS (1979) Penetration of protective gloves by epoxy resin. Contact Dermatitis 5:281–283
13. Roed-Petersen JA (1989) New glove material protective against epoxy and acrylate monomer. In: Frosch PJ, Dooms-Goosens A, Lachapelle J-M, Rycroft RJG, Scheper RJ (eds) Current topics in contact dermatitis. Springer, Berlin Heidelberg New York, pp 603–606
14. Weber T, Berenci G (1972) Über die Permeabilität der Schutzhandschuhe für verschiedene Pflanzenschutzmittel. Int Arch Arbeitsmed 30:23–30
15. Chemische Fabrik Stockhausen (1990) 4 H Chemikalienschutzliste. 4 H Safety 4 you
16. Williams JR (1979) Permeation of glove materials by physiologically harmful chemicals. Am Ind Hyg Assoc J 40:877–882

Age Dependence and Regional Anatomical Variability of Cutaneous Irritation

K.-P. Wilhelm*[1,2], A.B. Cua[1], and H.I. Maibach[1]

[1] Department of Dermatology, School of Medicine, University of California, San Francisco, CA, USA
[2] Department of Dermatology, Medizinische Universität zu Lübeck, Ratzeburger Allee 160, W-2400 Lübeck, Federal Republic of Germany

Abstract

Exogenous dermatoses can be of allergic or irritant type or a combination of both. Although irritant dermatitis is at least as common as allergic contact dermatitis, relatively little is known about its pathophysiology. In the present study the age dependence and regional anatomical variability of cutaneous irritation was investigated for the model irritant sodium lauryl sulphate (SLS) in two age groups of human volunteers (25.9±1.4, mean±SEM, $n = 7$ and 74.6±1.9, $n = 8$).

The experiment involved application of 400 µl of SLS (0.25%) for 24 h under occlusion to ten different anatomical locations; forehead, upper arm, volar and dorsal aspects of the forearm, postauricular region, palm, abdomen, upper back, thigh, and ankle. The irritant reactions were quantified by transepidermal water loss (TEWL) measurements and with visual scores. Nontreated symmetrical anatomical regions served as controls.

SLS induced a mild erythematous reaction and significant TEWL increase on most regions tested except for the palm. Irritant reactions were significantly stronger on most anatomical locations in the young population as assessed by both visual evaluation and TEWL measurements. SLS irritation showed marked anatomical variability in both age groups. The thigh showed the strongest reaction with a 4.8-fold and 3.7-fold increase in TEWL in the young and aged group, respectively. In contrast, the palm was most resistant, with no erythematous response or TEWL increase in either age group.

Introduction

Exogenous dermatoses can be of allergic or irritant type or a combination thereof. Although irritant dermatitis is at least as common as allergic contact dermatitis [1], relatively little is known about its pathophysiology. The objective of the present study was to investigate the age dependence and regional anatomical variability of cutaneous irritation.

* KPW was supported by a postdoctoral fellowship provided by the Deutsche Forschungsgemeinschaft (DFG) which is gratefully acknowledged.

Methods

Study Population. Seven young (25.9±1.4 yrs; mean±SEM) and eight aged (74.6±1.9) females volunteered after signing a written informed consent form. This study adhered to the recommendations given in the Revised Declaration of Helsinki (Tokyo, 1985) and was approved by the University of California-San Francisco Committee on Human Research.

Treatment. The volunteers were treated with 400 μl of 0.25% sodium lauryl sulphate (SLS) (Dupenol C, Du Pont, Wilmington, DE), which was applied for 24 h using an occlusive polypropylene chamber (Hilltop Laboratory, Cincinatti, OH) to ten different anatomical locations: forehead, upper arm, dorsal and volar aspects of the forearm, postauricular region, palm, abdomen, upper back, thigh, and ankle. Nontreated symmetrical sites served as controls.

Measurements. Transepidermal water loss (TEWL) was measured with an Evaporimeter (EP1, ServoMed, Stockholm, Sweden) 24 h after removal of SLS. The probe was held in place perpendicular to the skin surface until a stable TEWL value was established (for approximately 30 sec). Skin temperature was measured using a thermistor (Tele-Thermometer, Yellow Springs Instruments, OH). TEWL values were corrected to a standard skin reference temperature of 30 °C as described by Mathias et al. [2]. Before measurements were taken, all the volunteers had rested at invariant ambient conditions (20 °–23 °C, 40%–49% relative humidity).

Erythema was graded according to a five point visual scale: 0, no reaction; 0.5, equivocal; 1, slight, spotty erythema; 2, mild to moderate uniform erythema; 2, intense erythema; 4, intense redness with edema.

Capacitance as a measure of stratum corneum hydration was measured in duplicate using a capacitance meter (Corneometer CM 820 PC, Courage and Khazaka, Cologne, FRG).

Statistics. To compare differences between the age groups a two-tailed *t* test for unpaired data was used. All statistical tests were done with a statistical software package (Stat View II, Abacus Concepts, Berkeley, CA) on a personal computer (Apple Macintosh SE 30, Apple Cupertino, CA).

Results and Discussion

A significant anatomical variation in SLS irritation was observed in both age groups (Table 1, Fig. 1). In aged individuals the strongest reactions were observed on the forehead and on the postauricular region, whereas on the palm, ankle, dorsal aspect of the forearm, and the thigh no visible reactions were elicited (Table 1). In the young population, in contrast, only the palm was resistant to SLS-induced erythema and the thigh showed the strongest erythematous response. Magnusson and Hersle, in contrast, found the upper back more reactive than the

Table 1. Visual scores.

Region	Young	Old
Forehead	0.50 ± 0.19 (57.1)	0.44 ± 0.26 (37.5)
Upper arm	0.86 ± 0.24 (85.7)	0.38 ± 0.16 (50.0)
Volar forearm	0.93 ± 0.23 (85.7)	0.13 ± 0.08[a] (25.0)
Dorsal forearm	0.64 ± 0.18 (71.4)	0.00 ± 0.00[a] (0.0)
Postauricular	0.50 ± 0.15 (71.4)	0.44 ± 0.18 (50.0)
Palm	0.00 ± 0.00 (0.0)	0.00 ± 0.00 (0.0)
Abdomen	0.86 ± 0.26 (71.4)	0.13 ± 0.08[a] (25.0)
Upper back	0.86 ± 0.24 (85.7)	0.19 ± 0.13[a] (25.0)
Thigh	1.36 ± 0.37 (100.0)	0.00 ± 0.00[a] (0.0)
Ankle	0.14 ± 0.09 (28.6)	0.00 ± 0.00 (0.0)

Visual scores 24 h after removal of SLS. Given are means ± 1 SEM; in parenthesis, the percentage of the study population showing erythema graded 0.5 or higher. Regional variability in SLS irritation was particularly evident in the young age group where the thigh showed the highest reactivity in contrast to the palm where no erythematous reaction was noted.

[a] Mean score significantly lower in the aged group ($p \leq 0.05$).

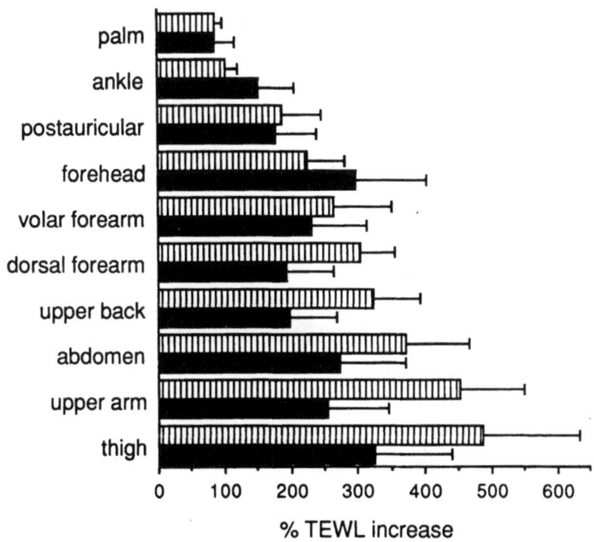

Fig. 1. Relative increase in transepidermal water loss (*TEWL*) 24 h after application of SLS (in percent of untreated controls) on 10 anatomical regions in young (*hatched bars*) and aged (*solid bars*) volunteers (mean ± SEM, $n = 7-8$ volunteers). TEWL increase on SLS-treated skin was statistically significant ($p \leq 0.05$) on all anatomical regions except for the palm and the ankle. Differences were not significant between the age groups

forearm and the thigh after challenge with a different irritant, benzalkonium chloride [3]. Dimethyl sulfoxide whealing was higher on the forehead than on the back and on the forearm [4]. Feldman and Maibach showed that the permeability of hydrocortisone was significantly higher on the forehead than on the back and lowest on the forearm [5]. However, in the present study we obtained the highest erythema

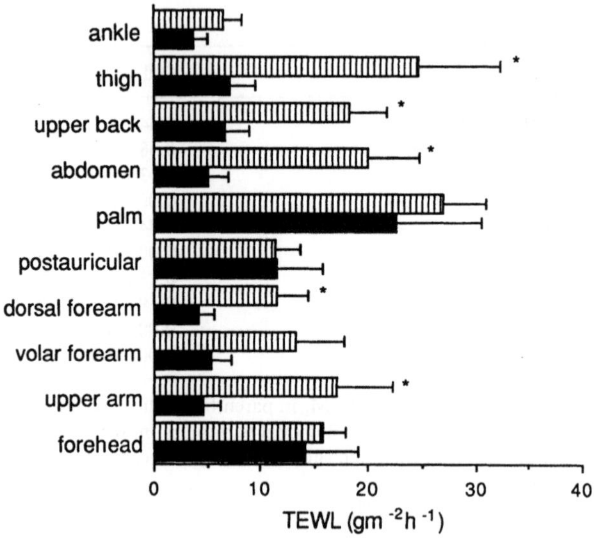

Fig. 2. Transepidermal water loss (*TEWL*) 24 h after application of SLS on 10 anatomical regions in young (*hatched bars*) and aged (*solid bars*) volunteers (mean ± 1 SEM, $n = 7-8$ volunteers); *, significant difference between the age groups ($p \leq 0.05$)

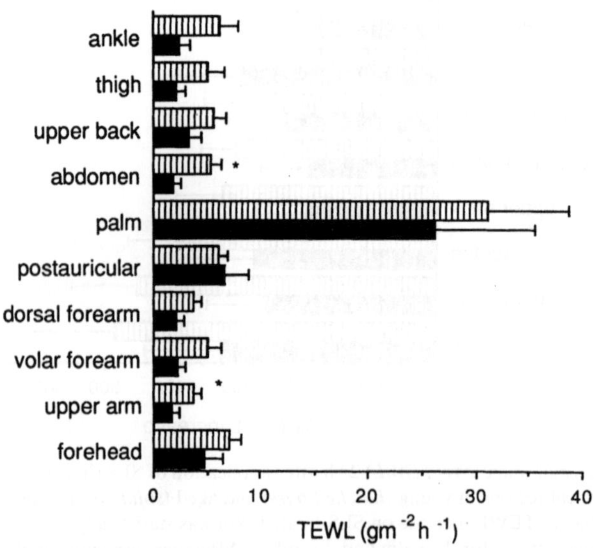

Fig. 3. Transepidermal water loss measurements (*TEWL*) on 10 nontreated anatomical regions in young (*hatched bars*) and aged (*solid bars*) volunteers (mean ± 1 SEM, $n = 7-8$ volunteers); *, significant difference between the age groups ($p \leq 0.05$)

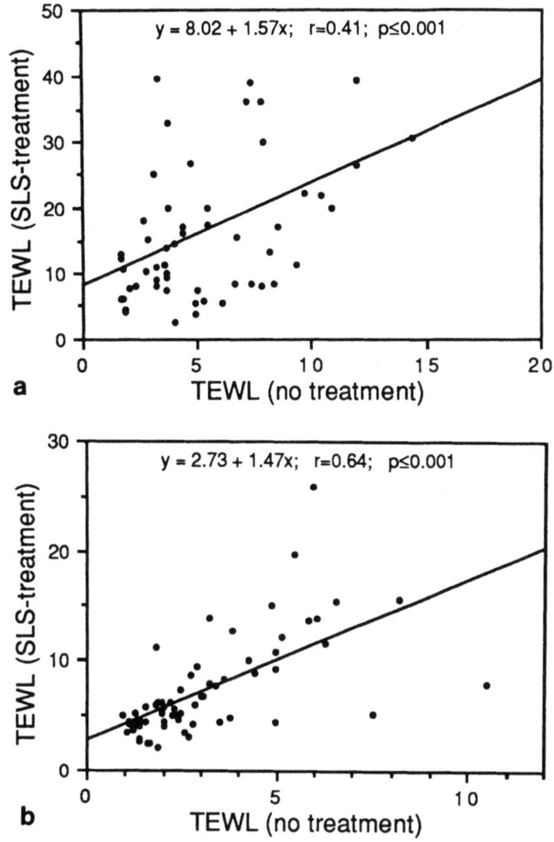

Fig. 4a, b. A significant linear correlation exists between TEWL of untreated skin and TEWL of SLS-irritated skin in **a** young and **b** aged volunteers. Measurements were taken at nine different anatomical locations; $n = 7-8$ volunteers. Note different scales

scores for the thigh and only moderate irritation on the forehead (Table 1). These differences in the regional susceptibility to cutaneous irritation may be best explained by distinctly different pathophysiological pathways for diverse irritants [6].

A significantly smaller susceptibility to SLS irritation in aged rather than in young individuals was suggested by visual scores (Table 1) and TEWL measurements (Fig. 2). This is in agreement with earlier studies by Coenraads et al., who found a decreased susceptibility to croton oil irritation with age [7]. Frosch et al. demonstrated that whealing after dimethyl sulphoxide also significantly decreased with age [4]. A less efficient barrier in the young population, as demonstrated by higher TEWL baseline values in this study (Fig. 3), and/or a comprised cutaneous blood vessel network and a reduced inflammatory response in the elderly [8, 9] might explain our findings. The relevance of baseline TEWL as an indicator for an individual's susceptibility to SLS irritation is controversial [10, 11]. In the present study, the SLS-induced increase in TEWL was linearly correlated with the TEWL of untreated skin in both age groups (Fig. 4), suggesting that the degree of barrier damage was related to barrier function before exposure. The correlation, however, was stronger in the aged population. Capacitance measurements did not show significant differences between the age groups or between irritated and control skin (data not shown). The results of the present study emphasize the importance of age distribution and anatomical region in experimental studies on irritant dermatitis.

We suspect that as a broader depth of data becomes available, these fundamental observations may be put to clinical use by age specific pharmacologic cutaneous dosing, as is now increasingly the case with oral and parenteral medications.

References

1. Andersen KE, Benezra C, Burrows D et al. (1987) Contact dermatitis. A review. Contact Dermatitis 16:55–78
2. Mathias CGT, Wilson DM, Maibach HI (1981) Transepidermal water loss as a function of skin surface temperature. J Invest Dermatol 77:219–220
3. Magnusson B, Hersle K (1965) Patch test methods. II. Regional variations of patch test response. Acta Derm Venereol 45:257–261
4. Frosch PJ, Duncan S, Kligman AM (1980) Cutaneous biometrics I. The response of human skin to dimethyl sulphoxide. Br J Dermatol 102:263–274
5. Feldman RJ, Maibach HI (1967) Regional variation in percutaneous penetration of 14-C cortisol in man. J Invest Dermatol 48:181–183
6. Patrick E, Maibach HI, Burkhalter A (1985) Mechanisms of chemically induced skin irritation. Toxicol Appl Pharmacol 81:476–490
7. Coenraads PJ, Bleumink E, Nater JP (1975) Susceptibility to primary irritants. Contact Dermatitis 1:377–381
8. Tagami H (1971/72) Functional characteristics of aged skin. 1. Percutaneous absorption. Acta Dermatol (Kyoto) 66/67:19–21
9. Balin AK, Pratt LA (1989) Physiological consequences of human skin aging. Cutis 43:431–436
10. Wilhelm KP, Maibach HI (1990) Factors predisposing to cutaneous irritation. Dermatol Clin 8:17–22
11. Tupker RA, Coenraads PJ, Pinnagoda J, Nater JP (1989) Baseline transepidermal water loss (TEWL) as a prediction of susceptibility to sodium lauryl sulphate. Contact Dermatitis 20:265–269

Immediate-Type Reactions to Rubber Products: IgE Mediated?

T. Fuchs [1], R. Wahl [2], and J. Geier [1]

[1] Department of Dermatovenerology I, Georg-August-Universität, W-3400 Göttingen, Federal Republic of Germany
[2] Allergopharma, J. Ganzer KG, Department of Research and Development of Allergen Extracts, W-2057 Reinbek, Federal Republic of Germany

Introduction

Contact urticaria (CU), often associated with severe anaphylactic reactions to latex products is being increasingly reported [1, 2, 4–8, 10, 13, 14]. Atopic patients and medical personnel are mainly affected. In most cases, an IgE-mediated allergy to natural latex has been demonstrated, especially by investigation of serum-specific IgE (RAST). The aim of the present study is to present own diagnostic data which includes different in vivo and in vitro methods.

Methods

16 patients with CU to different latex products were investigated as follows (see Table 1):

- Rub test, scratch and patch test with liquid latex (Semperit, Austria), different latex gloves, pure corn starch (Bio sorb) and talcum.
- Scratch and patch test with thiuram mix, mercapto mix, PPD mix, and, in particular cases, with various other rubber chemicals (Trolab-Hermal, FRG); concentration and vehicle according to the recommendations of the International Contact Dermatitis Research Group (ICDRG). Patch tests were performed with Finn chambers with an exposure time of 48 h.
- Scratch test with a self-prepared aqueous extract of latex gloves (Peha-taft), incubated at room temperature 2–40 h.
- Skin prick tests with pollen and other inhalant allergens (ALK, Denmark; Allergopharma, FRG).

Sera of patients 1–10 were measured by RAST using latex allergen disks from Pharmacia, self-prepared glove (Peha-taft) allergen disks, and the glove material directly. Allergen disks were prepared by using an extract of gloves, which were incubated overnight at 4 °C in Cocas solution (0.5% NaCl + 0.25% $NaHCO_3$ without phenol). The solution was lyophilized, the lyophilisate was dissolved in doubly distilled water, a protein determination made [5], and the extract was used for preparation of the allergen disks. Using the glove material directly [5], small particles were cut from a glove and the sera were incubated with these particles. The results were compared to data obtained with a nonallergic control pool serum ($n = 154$).

Table 1. Immediate-type reactions to rubber products: clinical data, skin test, RAST.

Patient	Symptoms and source	Liquid latex	Rubber chemicals	Latex gloves	Scratch test with glove extract (incubated in water)	RAST latex Pharmacia		RAST latex[b] Allergopharma		Atopy
						% binding 1.61[a]	class 0[a]	% binding 1.82[a]	class 0[a]	
1, age 30 ♀ nurse	CU, hand dermatitis: Latex gloves	Neg. (s)	Neg. (s), pos. (p): thiram mix	Neg. (s), Pos. (p)	Neg. (20 h)	0.29	0	1.18	0	Atopic dermatitis, pollinosis
2, age 23 ♀ medical technician	CU: Latex gloves	Pos. (s)	Neg. (s, p)	Pos. (s)	Pos. (2 h)	0.44	0	1.41	0	Pollinosis, dyshydrotic hand dermatitis
3, age 49 ♀ cleaner	Quincke edema: Cofferdam Latex gloves, suction device	Pos. (s)	Neg. (s), pos. (p): TMTD, TETD, TMTM, MBT, ZDC	Pos. (s, p)	Pos. (6 h)	18.21	3	10.50	2	–
4, age 36 ♀ anaesthesiologist	CU, hand dermatitis: Latex gloves	Pos. (s, p)	Neg. (s, p)	Pos. (s, p)	Neg. (16 h)	1.03	0	1.38	0	Pollinosis, mite allergy
5, age 20 ♀ nurse	CU, rhinitis, conjuctivitis: Latex gloves	Pos. (s)	Neg. (s, p)	Pos. (s)	Pos. (20 h)	0.31	0	1.62	0	Mite allergy
6, age 33 ♀ housewife	CU: Latex gloves	Pos. (s)	Neg. (s, p)	Pos. (s)	Pos. (3 h)	0.38	0	2.42	0	Pollinosis
7, age 36 ♀ instr. nurse	CU, rhinitis, conjunctivitis, asthma: Latex gloves	Neg. (s)	Neg. (s, p)	Pos. (s)	Pos. (18 h)	3.04	1	4.12	1	Pollinosis, mite allergy
8, age 33 ♂ gynecologist	CU, hand dermatitis: Latex gloves	Pos. (s)	Neg. (s, p)	Pos. (r, p)	–	0.43	0	0.24	0	–

9, age 33 ♀ nurse – intensive care unit	CU, rhinitis, conjunctivitis, asthma: Latex gloves	Pos. (s)	Neg. (s, p)	Pos. (s)	Pos. (24 h)	3.11	1	6.81	2	Pollinosis
10, age 30 ♂ surgeon	CU: Latex gloves	Pos. (r)	Pos. (s): TMTD	Pos. (r)	Pos. (3 h)	1.79	0	1.31	0	–
11, age 50 ♀ chemical technican	CU, rhinitis: Latex gloves	Pos. (s)	Pos. (s): mercapto mix, PPD mix	Pos. (s)	Pos. (24 h)	<0.35[c]	0	–	–	Pollinosis
12, age 28 ♂ mechanic	CU, quincke edema, dermatitis: spondylolisthesis Latex gloves, rubber electrodes	Pos. (s)	Pos. (p): TMTD, TMTM, DOD, electrodes (black)	Pos. (s)	–	<0.35[c]	0	–	–	–
13, age 21 ♀ medical assistant	CU: Latex gloves, condoms	Pos. (r)	Neg. (s, p)	Pos. (r)	Pos. (10 h)	<0.35[c]	0	–	–	Pollinosis
14, age 38 ♀ sales woman (meat)	CU, quincke edema, anaphylactic shock (narcosis): Latex gloves, condoms	Pos. (s)	Neg. (s, p)	Neg. (s)	Pos. (40 h) Oxford tubus	0.98[c]	2	–	–	Pollinosis, atopic dermatitis, animal allergy
15, age 28 ♂ medical student	CU: Latex gloves	Pos. (r)	Neg. (s, p)	Pos. (r)	Neg. (22 h)	–	–	–	–	Atopic dermatitis, cat allergy
16, age 49 ♀ nurse	CU: Latex gloves	Pos. (s)	Neg. (s, p)	Pos. (r)	Neg. (24 h)	–	–	–	–	–

Neg., negative; pos., positive; r, rub test; s, scratch test; p, patch test; CU, contact urticaria.
[a] Nonallergic control pool serum. [b] Glove extract. [c] PRU/ml.

Sera of patients 11–15 were measured by RAST using latex allergen disks (Pharmacia, FRG) in the RAST laboratory at the University of Göttingen.

For the determination of the molecular weight of the IgE specificities ("allergens") of the glove extract, sera of patients 1–7 (1 : 5 diluted) were investigated by Western blot [3]. The same extract as for the preparation of the allergen disks was used.

For the determination of the isoelectric points of the IgE specificities ("allergens") of the glove extract, sera of patients 1–10 (1 : 5 diluted) were investigated by immunoprint [11]. The same extract as for Western blot was used.

Results and Discussion

Most patients investigated were atopic (11/16). Besides anaphylactic reactions, five patients showed signs of hand dermatitis [14]. In 14 of 16 patients (87.5%), the tests with liquid latex in different dilutions and with the incriminating gloves led to positive reactions. The allergen(s) seemed in part to be water soluble, as mentioned earlier [9]. Of 14 patients, 10 (71.4%) revealed positive reactions to the self-prepared glove extract. The incubation time is seemingly insignificant. In two patients, positive reactions to tetramethylthiuram disulfide (TMTD, thiram), tetramethylthiuram monosulfide (TMTM), 4,4′-dihydroxydiphenyl (DOD), mercapto mix, and p-phenylenediamine mix (PPD mix = "black rubber mix") were considered as possible sole or contributing factors to the development of CU [2, 14]. Corn starch (Bio-sorb) and talcum were negative in all patients. Of 14 sera, 10 (71.4%) showed RAST class 0. This differs from other reports, in which positive RASTs are stated more often. By using glove material directly, the result obtained with serum 3 was positive (not shown).

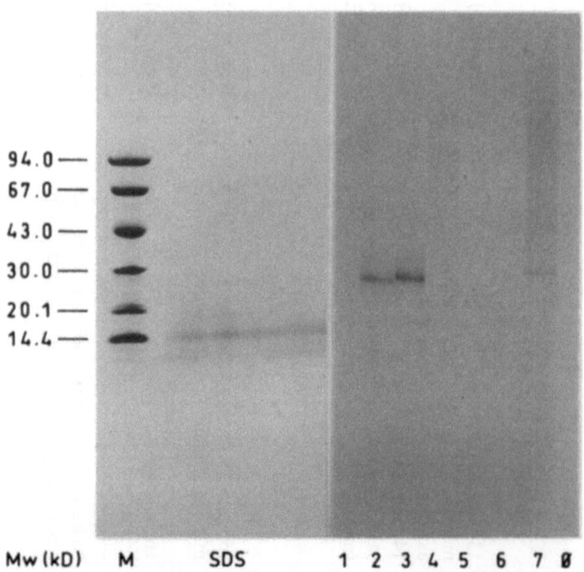

Fig. 1. SDS-PAGE (*left*) and Western blot (*right*) using the glove extract and sera of patients 1–7. *O*, nonallergic control pool serum; *M*, marker protein

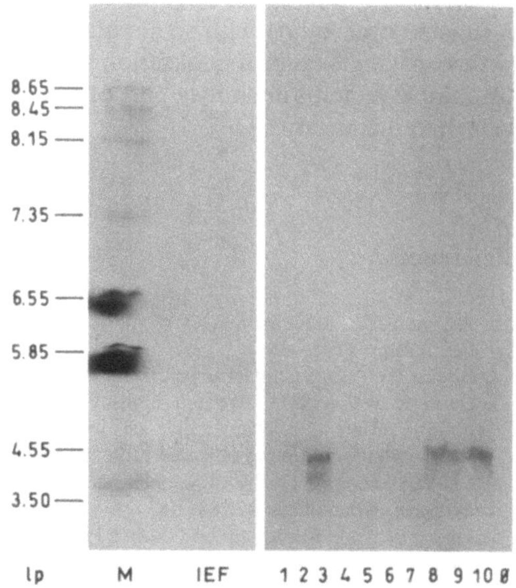

Fig. 2. IEF (*left*) and immunoprint (*right*) using the glove extract and sera of patients 1–10. *O*, nonallergic control pool serum; *M*, marker protein

Figure 1 shows the SDS-PAGE and the Western blot of the extract. By SDS-PAGE, protein bands of ≦14 kDa, and approximately 28 kDa can be seen. By Western blot, sera of patients 2, 3, and 7 detected the 28 kDa protein as an allergen. This differs from the results of Morales et al. [9], Turjanmaa [13] and Slater [12], who presumed a 10 kDa polypeptide and a 14 kDa protein, respectively, to be the major allergens of latex.

By isoelectric focusing (IEF) (Coomassie blue staining) no protein bands could be detected. By immunoprinting in sera of patients 3, 6, 8, 9, and 10, allergen bands in an pH range between 3.8 and 4.55 were observed. This shows that radiostaining (immunoprint) is more sensitive than Coomassie blue staining (Fig. 2).

Conclusions

Skin tests are reliable when performed by experienced individuals and carry practically no risk. Rubber chemicals (TMTD etc.) seem to be a cause of anaphylactic reactions and should be routinely tested. It is desirable to have a standardized latex extract available, which should be included in the standard series of inhalant and contact allergens.

With sera of only four patients, positive RAST classes were measured using different latex allergen disks. Using the glove particles directly, positive results were obtained in patient 3. Although sera 2, 8, and 10 showed RAST class 0, allergen bands could be seen by immunoblot. It is to be presumed that in this case the immunoblot is more sensitive than the RAST.

From our data, it seems obvious that there are mechanisms, other than those that are IgE mediated (5), that are responsible for the clinical picture. It is supposed that the allergen(s) of gloves is (are) water soluble. By using glove particles, incubated over 2 days with serum and [^{125}I] anti IgE, a positive result compared with nonallergic control pool serum was obtained. This shows either that the water soluble proteins are only a part of the allergenic proteins or that they were not extracted quantitatively.

References

1. Axelsson JGK, Johansson SGO, Wrangsjö K (1987) IgE-mediated anaphylactoid reactions to rubber. Allergy 42:46–50
2. Belsito DV (1990) Contact urticaria caused by rubber. Dermatol Clin 8:61–66
3. Burnette WM (1981) "Western blotting": electrophoretic transfer of proteins from sodium dodecyl sulfate – polyacrylamide gels to unmodified nitrocellulose and radiographic detection with antibody and radioiodinated protein. Anal Biochem 112:195–203
4. Ehl W, Hartjen A, Thiel C, Aulepp H, Fuchs E (1988) Latex-Allergien als IgE-vermittelte Sofortreaktionen. Allergologie 11:182–187
5. Frosch PJ, Wahl R, Bahmer FA, Maasch HJ (1986) Contact urticaria to rubber gloves is IgE-mediated. Contact Dermatitis 14:241–245
6. Geier J, Fuchs Th (1990) Kontakturtikaria durch Gummihandschuhe. Z Hautkr 65:267–272
7. Jäger D, Baur X, Kleinhans D, Schulte C, Tauer I (1989) Identification of latex allergens. Allergologie 12: Proceedings XIVth Congress of the EAACI, Abstracts, p 20
8. Kleinhans D (1984) Contact urticaria to rubber gloves. Contact Dermatitis 10:124–125
9. Morales C, Basomba A, Carreira J, Sastre A (1989) Anaphylaxis produced by rubber glove contact. Case reports and immunological identification of the antigens involved. Clin Exp Allergy 19:425–430
10. Nutter AF (1979) Contact urticaria to rubber. Br J Dermatol 101:597–598
11. Peltre G, Lapeyre J, David D (1982) Heterogeneity of grass pollen allergens (*Dactylis glomerata*) recognized by IgE antibodies in human patients sera by a new nitrocellulose immunoprint technique. Immunol Lett 5:127–131
12. Slater JE (1990) Human antibody response to rubber proteins. Ann Allergy 64:93
13. Turjanmaa K (1987) Incidence of immediate allergy to latex gloves in hospital personnel. Contact Dermatitis 17:270–275
14. Turjanmaa K, Reunala T (1989) Latex-contact urticaria associated with delayed allergy to rubber chemicals. In: Frosch PJ, Dooms-Goosens A, Lachapelle J-M, Rycroft RJG, Scheper RJ (eds) Current topics in contact dermatitis. Springer, Berlin Heidelberg New York, pp 460–464
15. Wahl R, Geissler W, Maasch HJ (1985) Comparison of classical lowry, modified lowry and a dye-binding assay for the estimation of protein in allergen extracts and influence of different parameters on the modified lowry assay. Biol Chem Hoppe-Seyler 366:979–984

Mite Allergy

The Storage Mite Story *

S. G. O. Johansson[1], M. van Hage-Hamsten[1], E. Johansson[1], and A. Wirén[2]

[1] Department of Clinical Immunology, Karolinska Hospital, 10401 Stockholm, Sweden
[2] Swedish Agriculture University, 75007 Uppsala, Sweden

Abstract

When allergists in the beginning of the 1960s started to question that house dust was one defined allergen some of them initiated microscopic investigations of house dust samples. They noticed that house dust samples often contained a great variety of mite species, and that in many cases non-pyroglyphid mites were dominating. These mites are now often referred to as storage mites. However, since dust samples from private homes most consistently contained pyroglyphid mites, the *Dermatophagoides* mites were given the highest priority and the storage mites were somewhat forgotten. Since then extensive work have been performed on the isolation, characterization and clinical importance of *Dermatophagoides* allergens.

The interest in storage mites as allergens was increased some years ago when it was discovered that allergy to storage mites was an important problem in certain occupational settings, e.g. farming. Today, we have information about sensitization to approximately 10 species of storage mites. The most important storage mites are *Lepidoglyphus destructor*, *Glycyphagus domesticus*, *Tyrophagus putrescentiae* and *Acarus siro*. In Brazil and other South American countries and probably also in south eastern USA, *Blomia* is an important mite.

The possibility of allergenic similarities between house dust mites and storage mites is an important question that has been addressed in several investigations. The reported results vary from a high degree of similarity to almost no allergenic cross-reactivity at all. As far as *Lepidoglyphus* is concerned it does contain unique allergens and depending on the primary sensitization the patients develop a more or less specific allergy to this mite genus.

In many countries and environments allergy to mites is most important and it is now generally accepted that many species of mites are of clinical significance. Although *Dermatophagoides* probably are the dominating mites in most house

* This work was supported by the Swedish Work Environment Fund (project no. 83-1182), the Swedish Medical Research Council (grant no. 16X-105), the Swedish Asthma and Allergy association, the Konsul Tore Nilsson Foundation, the Konsul Th C. Berghs Foundation, and the Karolinska Institute.

dust samples, several species of storage mites are equally important in other environments. In addition, since the degree of allergenic cross-reactivity between storage mites and house dust mites is limited, it is important to consider both kinds of mites for diagnosis and immunotherapy in most cases of suspected mite allergy.

Introduction

In the beginning of the 1960s Voorhorst et al. [39] noticed the occurrence in house dust of pyroglyphid and non-pyroglyphid mites. They concentrated their efforts on studies of mites belonging to the genus *Dermatophagoides*, which were shown to be the major source of allergen in house dust. It was shown that *Dermatophagoides pteronyssinus* was the predominant mite species encountered in houses in northern Europe and *Dermatophagoides farinae* in North America. However, others found that in many damp houses non-pyroglyphid mites represented a higher proportion of the total mite population than classical house dust mites [31]. Since non-pyroglyphid mites were most often found in food and grain stores, barns, and similar locations, they became known as storage mites.

Recent studies have shown that several species of storage mites can be found in farming environments [14, 18], and studies from Scotland [7], Finland [33], Sweden [35], and Denmark [17] have shown that storage mites might be important respiratory allergens. Storage mites are found in many parts of the world, especially where the climate is temperate and large quantities of cereal grain are grown and stored [29, 30]. Moreover, the bedding of house pets is commonly infested by storage mites and they can also cause problems for horseback riders when stables become infested with mites.

Acarological Relationships

Some 40000 species of acari (ticks and mites) are thought to exist [26]. Mites compose a wide range of families. Among the various classifications used, Fig. 1 shows a scheme that is accepted by most acarologists [21]. Both non-pyroglyphid and pyroglyphid mites belong to the suborder Astigmata. It might be expected that species within the same family would be allergenically more closely related than species belonging to different families. However, the allergenic properties of the respective mite species are not necessarily linked to their taxonomic position.

The most important storage mites are *Lepidoglyphus destructor*, *Acarus siro*, *Glycyphagus domesticus*, and *Tyrophagus putrescentiae*. The dominating mite in South America is a non-pyroglyphid mite of the genus *Blomia*, which includes *Blomia tropicalis*, *Blomia kulagini*, and *Blomia freemani*. *Tyrophagus putrescentiae* used to be a serious problem in Japan where it infested the tatami mats regularly used in traditional Japanese housing.

Subclass Suborder	Family	Genus	Species
Acari—Astigmata	Acaridae	Acarus	Acarus siro
			Acarus farris
		Tyrophagus	Tyrophagus putrescentiae
			Tyrophagus longior
	Glycyphagidae	Lepidoglyphus	Lepidoglyphus destructor
		Glycyphagus	Glycyphagus domesticus
		Gohieria	Gohieria fusca
		Blomia	Blomia kulagini
			Blomia tropicalis
	Chortoglyphidae	Chortoglyphus	Chortoglyphus arcuatus
	Pyroglyphidae	Dermatophagoides	Dermatophagoides pteronyssinus
			Dermatophagoides farinae
		Euroglyphus	Euroglyphus maynei

Fig. 1. The acarological relationship between different storage and house dust mites

Allergenic Cross-Reactivity

Storage mites are taxonomically distinct from house dust mites. Evidence of cross-reactivity between *D. farinae* and several storage mite species has been reported by Miyamoto et al. [23]. On the other hand, both Wraith et al. [42] and Agha and Gnanasakthy [1] failed to show any correlation between positive skin prick test (SPT) reactions to the house dust mite *D. pteronyssinus* and four storage mites. A recent study confirmed that there is no significant correlation between house dust mites (*D. pteronyssinus* and *D. farinae*) and storage mites (*A. siro*, *T. putrescentiae* and *L. destructor*) [20]. Based on RAST inhibition studies, we reported in 1987 that there is no allergenic cross-reactivity between non-pyroglyphid and pyroglyphid mites [36]. These data were later confirmed in vivo by bronchial challenges [37]. Georges et al. [12] also reported a lack of cross-reactivity between two house dust mites and four storage mites. These results were based on RAST results from 60 asthmatic children. By using immunodiffusion, however, Green and Woolcock [13] found that *T. putrescentiae* and *D. farinae* have at least one antigen in common. Furthermore, *T. putrescentiae* and *D. farinae* have been characterized by crossed immunoelectrophoresis (CIE) and crossed radioimmunoelectrophoresis (CRIE). The two mites were shown to share two antigenic and allergenic determinants and two determinants were also shared by *T. putrescentiae* and *D. farinae* feces [3]. In a review article Ford and Platts-Mills [10] recently concluded that patients exhibiting positive skin tests to both pyroglyphid and non-pyroglyphid mites generally appear to do so because of multiple sensitizations to the different species rather than because of cross-reactive antibodies.

We have also studied the allergenic cross-reactivity between the non-pyroglyphid mites *L. destructor* and *B. kulagini* in two different countries, Brazil and Sweden.

The results from the RAST inhibition studies suggest that *L. destructor* and *B. kulagini* share some allergenic components, but they also seem to lack some allergenic determinants in relation to each other. However, this apparent deficiency of allergen(s) is dependent on where the subject has been sensitized. If we had investigated only the Swedish farmers with respect to allergenic cross-reactivity between *L. destructor* and *B. kulagini*, our conclusions would have been that *L. destructor* is the important mite, having all major allergens, and that *B. kulagini* is not important since it seems to lack the major allergenic determinants of *L. destructor* and does not reveal any major allergens of its own. In contrast, if only the subjects from Brazil had been studied, the conclusion would have been the reverse: *B. kulagini* is the important mite and *L. destructor* is just cross-reacting [38]. Our findings demonstrate the difficulties inherent in studying allergenic cross-reactivity in human systems. For definition and detailed mapping of allergenic epitopes, monoclonal antibodies are probably a useful [6] but laborious approach.

Although there may be as many as 20 mite species that are of major importance, it is essential to establish which species is the main provoker of IgE-mediated sensitization in each region and in each environment. Further epidemiological and immunological studies concerning allergy to mites are therefore needed in various parts of the world.

Allergy to Storage Mites

Allergy to insect material and mites was noted early on in farming populations. The first allergic disorder attributed to mites was an outbreak of "epidemic asthma" in grain workers. The cause was the predatory mite *Pyemotes ventricosus* which feeds on the larvae of insects that live on infested grain and straw [2]. Immediate hypersensitivity to grain dust was shown to be common in 1974 by Warren et al. [40]. The authors concluded that grain dust may, among other things, contain a large number of mites, such as *L. destructor*, and that this mite species might be an important antigenic component of grain dust. A recent report on grain elevator workers from Denmark stated that storage mite allergens appear to be the most important among those tested [27]. In the past few years several species of storage mites have also been shown to cause IgE-mediated sensitization among rural workers, who to a varying extent develop asthma, rhinitis, or conjunctivitis when exposed to barn dust. In the first report Davies et al. [8] concluded that *L. destructor* was likely to be involved in the recurrent nocturnal asthma in one farmer after exposure to grain dust. IgE-mediated respiratory allergy to storage mites has since been shown to be common both in Scotland, the UK, Finland, and Denmark [4, 7, 16, 17, 33].

Allergic sensitization to storage mites in non-farming populations has been reported from Japan [23], Southeast Asia [41], Hong Kong [11], New Guinea [13], and many of the farming countries in Europe, such as France [12, 15], England [22, 42], Denmark [20], and the Netherlands [32] (Fig. 2).

We have studied the prevalence of IgE-mediated hypersensitivity to respiratory allergens, including mites, in a rural population of Gotland, a Swedish island in

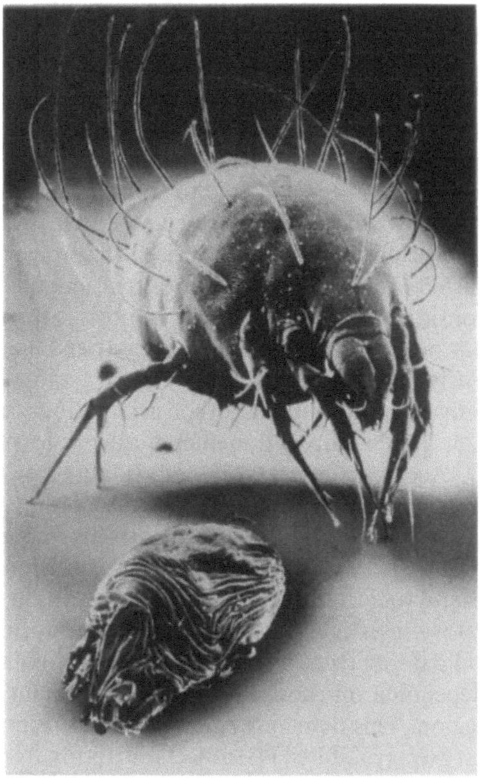

Fig. 2. Scanning electron microscopy pictures of *G. domesticus* (*top*) and *E. maynei* (*bottom*) illustrating the differences in size

the Baltic sea. A total of 2578 (91%) participants, age 15–65 years and mainly occupied with farming, answered a questionnaire. Of 460 selected farmers, 440 (96%) participated in a medical examination. From a clinical point of view the storage mite *L. destructor* was the main mite sensitizer with a prevalence of allergy (e.g., symptoms when handling stored hay or grain and a positive RAST) of 6.2% [35]. By bronchial provocation tests we established that *L. destructor* gives rise to asthma [37]; *D. pteronyssinus* was the second important mite (5.2%). However, besides the common house dust mite, *D. pteronyssinus*, other house dust mites, e.g., *Euroglyphus maynei* are also important (Fig. 2). We have recently studied the clinical and allergenic relationships between these two mite species. We concluded that both species have unique allergen(s), but *E. maynei* seems to be deficient in some allergenic determinants of *D. pteronyssinus* [34]. From a clinical point of view *E. maynei* should not be overlooked as the causative allergen when investigating subjects with suspected allergy to house dust.

Socioeconomic Aspects

It has been proposed that allergy to the house dust mite is the most widespread and prevalent allergy in the world. In addition, it is obvious that one has to consider allergy to many more species of non-pyroglyphid and pyroglyphid mites. Depending on the climate and the social situation allergy to storage mites occur as a house dust or occupational allergy.

IgE-mediated occupational allergy among farmers appears to be a problem of far greater importance than farmer's lung. In contrast to what one would have expected, the main allergens seem to be mites. It might be speculated that the clinical importance of allergy to storage mites is underestimated in other parts of the world. We have recently calculated that if only 3% of the nearly 56 million farmers worldwide [9] were sensitized to storage mites, it would account for 1.7 million sufferers, and the cost of both treatment and allergen control measures would be considerable [19]. Accurate diagnosis is therefore important to prevent those without occupational asthma being advised inappropriately to change or leave work. Early detection is mandatory since symptoms become aggravated with time. Not only farmers, but also other occupations, e.g., grain handlers [5, 27] and bakers [25, 28] develop IgE-mediated allergy to storage mites.

Access to extracts of high quality constitutes a prerequisite for widespread treatment by hyposensitization. Accordingly, all storage mite extracts should be characterized and the major antigens and allergens isolated to allow preparation of purified extract prior to treatment. Monoclonal antibodies may prove to be a useful tool in future characterization studies. Further results of clinical and laboratory investigations among larger groups of farmers should be done in order to validate the treatment. Hyposensitization should include different mite species, depending on those that are the dominant sensitizers in a particular country or region. This demands epidemiological surveys and inventories of the acarofauna on farms inhibited by subjects suffering from allergic respiratory disease. Furthermore, methods to measure the level of airborne storage mite allergens and thus the risk of developing asthma are required.

References

1. Agha M, Gnanasakthy A (1981) A cluster analysis of the effects of storage mites as allergens in relation to certain occupations and living conditions. Clin Allergy 11:499–504
2. Ancona G (1923) Asma epidemico da "Pediculoides ventricosus". Policlinico 30:45–70
3. Arlian LG, Geis DP, Vyszenski-Mohler DL, Bernstein IL, Gallagher JS (1984) Cross antigenic and allergenic properties of the house dust mite *Dermatophagoides farinae* and the storage mite *Tyrophagus putrescentiae*. J Allergy Clin Immunol 74:172–179
4. Blainey AD, Topping MD, Ollier S, Davies RJ (1988) Respiratory symptoms in arable farmworkers: role of storage mites. Thorax 43:697–702
5. Blainey AD, Topping MD, Ollier S, Davies RJ (1989) Allergic respiratory disease in grain workers: the role of storage mites. J Allergy Clin Immunol 84:296–303
6. Chapman MD (1988) Allergen specific monoclonal antibodies: new tools for the management of allergic disease. Allergy [Suppl 5] 43:7–14
7. Cuthbert OD, Brostoff J, Wraith DG, Brighton WD (1979) "Barn allergy": asthma and rhinitis due to storage mites. Clin Allergy 9:229–236
8. Davies RJ, Green M, Schofield NMcC (1976) Recurrent nocturnal asthma after exposure to grain dust. Am Rev Respir Dis 114:1011–1019
9. Food and Agricultural Organization (1984) UN Production Yearbook. 38:63–74

10. Ford AW, Platts-Mills TAE (1987) Standardized extracts, dust mite, and other arthropods (inhalants). Clin Rev Allergy 5:49–73
11. Gabriel M, Cunnington AM, Allan WGL, Pickering CAC, Wraith DG (1982) Mite allergy in Hong Kong. Clin Allergy 12:157–171
12. Georges P, Delvigne A, de Montis G (1987) RAST et Acariens des denrées entreposées. Allerg Immunol 19:393–397
13. Green WF, Woolcock AJ (1978) *Tyrophagus putrescentiae*: an allergenically important mite. Clin Allergy 8:135–144
14. Griffiths DA, Wilkin DR, Southgate BJ, Lynch SM (1976) A survey of mites in bulk grain stored on farms in England and Wales. Ann Appl Biol 82:180–184
15. Hardel PJ, de Lajudie JP, Portal B, Ville G, Guilloux L, d' Athis P (1986) L'allergie à *Tyrophagus putrescentiae* et à *Lepidoglyphus destructor* dans une population d'adultes jeune asthmatiques. Allerg Immunol 18:25–32
16. Ingram CG, Jeffrey IG, Symington IS, Cuthbert OD (1979) Bronchial provocation studies in farmers allergic to storage mites. Lancet 2:1330–1332
17. Iversen M, Korsgaard J, Hallas T, Dahl R (1990) Mite allergy and exposure to storage mites and house dust mites in farmers. Clin Exp Allergy 20:211–219
18. Jeffrey IG (1976) A survey of the mite fauna of Scottish farms. J Stored Prod Res 12:149–156
19. Johansson SGO, van Hage-Hamsten M, Kurvits J (1987) Storage mite allergy in farmers. Pract Allergy Immunol 4:83–86
20. Korsgaard J, Dahl R, Iversen M, Hallas T (1985) Storage mites as a cause of bronchial asthma in Denmark. Allergol Immunopathol 13:143–149
21. Krantz GW (1970) A manual of acarology. OSU, Corvallis
22. Maunsell K, Wraith DG, Cunnington AM (1968) Mites and house dust allergy in bronchial asthma. Lancet 1:1267–1270
23. Miyamoto T, Oshima S, Mizuno K, Sasa M, Ishizaki T (1969) Cross-antigenicity among six species of dust mites and house dust antigens. J Allergy 44:228–238
24. Morrow Brown H, Filer JL (1968) Role of mites in allergy to house dust. Br Med J 3:646–647
25. Musk AW, Venables KM, Crook B, Nunn AJ, Hawkins R, Crook GDW, Graneek BJ, Tee RD, Farrer N, Johnson DA, Gordon DJ, Darbyshire JH, Newman-Taylor AJ (1989) Respiratory symptoms, lung function, and sensitization to flour in a British bakery. Br J Ind Med 46:636–642
26. Nathanson ME (1969) Arthropods and allergy. J Asthma Res 7:55–63
27. Revsbech P, Andersen G (1987) Storage mite allergy among grain elevator workers. Allergy 42:423–429
28. Revsbech P, Dueholm N (1990) Storage mite allergy among bakers. Allergy 45:204–208
29. Sinha RN (1963) Stored product acarology in Canada. Adv Acarol 1:70–88
30. Sinha RN (1964) Mites of stored grain in Western Canada – ecology and methods of survey. Proc Entomol Soc Manitoba 20:19–33
31. Spieksma FTM, Spieksma-Boezeman MIA (1967) The mite fauna of house dust with particular reference to the house dust mite *Dermatophagoides pteronyssinus*. Acarologia 9:226–241
32. Spieksma FTM, Voorhorst R (1969) Comparison of skin reactions to extracts of house dust, mites, and human skin scales. Acta Allergol (Copenh) 24:124–146
33. Terho EO, Husman K, Vohlonen I, Rautalahti M, Tukiainen H (1985) Allergy to storage mites of cow dander as a cause of rhinitis among Finnish dairy farmers. Allergy 40:23–26
34. Van Hage-Hamsten M, Johansson SGO (1989) Clinical significance and allergenic cross-reactivity of *Euroglyphus maynei* and other non-pyroglyphid and pyroglyphid mites. J Allergy Clin Immunol 83:581–589
35. Van Hage-Hamsten M, Johansson SGO, Höglund S, Tüll P, Wirén A, Zetterström O (1985) Storage mite allergy is common in a farming population. Clin Allergy 15:555–564
36. Van Hage-Hamsten M, Johansson SGO, Johansson E, Wirén A (1987) Lack of allergenic cross-reactivity between storage mites and *Dermatophagoides pteronyssinus*. Clin Allergy 17:23–31
37. Van Hage-Hamsten M, Ihre E, Zetterström O, Johansson SGO (1988) Bronchial provocation studies in farmers with positive RAST to the storage mite *Lepidoglyphus destructor*. Allergy 43:545–551
38. Van Hage-Hamsten M, Machado L, Barros MT, Johansson SGO (1990) Comparison of clinical significance and allergenic cross-reactivity of the storage mites *Blomia kulagini* and *Lepidoglyphus destructor* in Sweden and Brazil. Allergy 45:409–417

39. Voorhorst R, Spieksma-Boezeman MIA, Spieksma FTM (1964) Is a mite (*Dermatophagoides* sp.) the producer of the house dust allergen? Allerg Asthma 10:329–334
40. Warren P, Cherniack RM, Tse KS (1974) Hypersensitivity reactions to grain dust. J Allergy Clin Immunol 53:139–149
41. Woolcock AA, Cunnington AM (1980) The allergenic importance of house dust and storage mites in asthmatics in Brunei, S.E. Asia Clin Allergy 10:609–615
42. Wraith DG, Cunnington AM, Seymour WM (1979) The role and allergenic importance of storage mites in house dust and other environments. Clin Allergy 9:545–561

House Dust Mites in German Homes

U. Wahn, S. Lau-Schadendorf, B. Ehnert, and A. Weber
Universitätsklinik, Heubnerweg 6, W-1000 Berlin 19, Federal Republic of Germany

Abstract

IgE-mediated hypersensitivity reactions to dust mite allergens are quite common in the atopic population. They may contribute to allergic airway diseases as well as to the degree of inflammation in atopic dermatitis patients.

In the past, the presence of the house dust mite was documented by microscopy of house dust samples. Since a number of allergenic molecules (Der p I, Der p II, Der f I, Der f II) have been identified as major allergens, purified and used for the production of monoclonal and monospecific antibodies, quantitative measurements of allergens by ELISA or RIA technique have become possible. Our knowledge of the prevalence of mite allergens in houses and their significance for atopic patients has considerably increased after these techniques had been used.

In Germany both, *Dermatophagoides pteronyssinus* and *Dermatophagoides farinae* allergens are almost equally important, the presence of one mite being not related to the other. In the majority of individual homes there are seasonal variations in mite allergens with a peak in the fall period. These variations are more pronounced in *D. pteronyssinus* allergens. Certain indoor conditions like coal heating obviously influence mite growth. Atopic children living in an environment with more than 2000 ng/g dust mite allergens have a significantly higher risk to become sensitized and develop IgE-antibodies to mites than children living in houses with less than 400 ng/g dust mite allergens.

Allergic reactions to proteins from house dust mites play an important role in various atopic diseases in childhood and adulthood. *Dermatophagoides pteronyssinus* and *Dermatophagoides farinae* are of major significance as allergen sources [1–6]. Their major allergens have been biochemically characterized and purified. At least for the group I allergens, Der p I and Der f I, heat labile glycoproteins with a molecular mass of approximately 24 kDa, mite feces appear to be the major source of allergen [7]. Group I allergens of *Dermatophagoides pteronysssinus* and *Dermatophagoides farinae* have close physical, chemical and immunochemical homologies [8–12]. The availability of purified environmental allergens and the production of non-cross-reacting monoclonal or affinity-purified monospecific antibodies directed to these allergens as research tools are an important prerequisite for studies on the relationship between allergen exposure in human immune response.

We tried to answer the following questions:

1. Which of the mites are present in German houses?
2. Are there seasonal variations in indoor mite allergen concentrations?
3. Is there a dose-response relationship between allergen exposure and sensitization?
4. How efficacious are certain elimination procedures?

Dust Collection, Extraction and Allergen Enzyme-Linked Immunoadsorbent Assay

Dust samples were collected in new dust bags using a vacuum cleaner, and mattresses and carpets were vacuumed for 5 min. Dust bags were placed into plastic bags, mailed to our laboratory and kept at 4 °C until analysis. Dust extracts were produced by agitation for 3 h at room temperature 1:5 (wt/vol) in 0.125 mol/l of ammonium hydrogen carbonate containing 0.1% sodium azide. After centrifugation, the supernatants were filtered through a filter 220 nm in diameter (Millex GV, Millipore Ltd., Harrow, Middlesex, UK) and stored at −20 °C. Precoated polystyrene microtiter trays and reagents for sandwich enzyme-linked immunosorbent assay (ELISA) were obtained from ALK (Copenhagen, Denmark). For assay of Der p I, plates coated with monoclonal, non-cross-reacting antibodies and horseradish peroxidase conjugated, species specific rabbit antibodies to Der p I were used. The Der f I assay was a combined determination of the two species Df and Dm of the Df group. The rabbit antibodies used (coating as well as conjugated antibody) were anti-Der f I; they were immunoabsorbed on a Dpt-Sepharose column and further affinity purified by acid elution from a Der m I-Sepharose column. The assay was performed according to the method described by Lind [13]. In short, 100-µl dust extracts and dilutions thereof were added to the precoated wells for overnight incubation, followed by repeated washings. After a 1-h incubation with enzyme conjugated antibody and repeated washings, substrate (hydrogen peroxide/orthophenyleneamine) was added to each well, and reaction was carried out for 15 min in the dark. The absorption at 492 nm (Titertek Multiskan MCC 340, Flow Laboratories, Ricksmansworth, Hertfordshire, UK) was read 5 min after addition of 1 mol/l of sulphuric acid. Standard response curves were constructed from reference antigen solutions of each species with major allergen concentrations in the range of 1.6 to 400 ng/ml (internal standards of ALK, the Der p I standard related to National Institute of Biological Standards and Control 82/518). Results were expressed as nanograms per gram of dust. Assay sensitivity was 5 ng/ml or 15 ng/gm of dust.

Prevalence of House Dust Mites

The concentrations of mite allergen Der p I and Der f I in mattress dust samples varied greatly, as did the total amount and the distribution of Dpt and Df. The

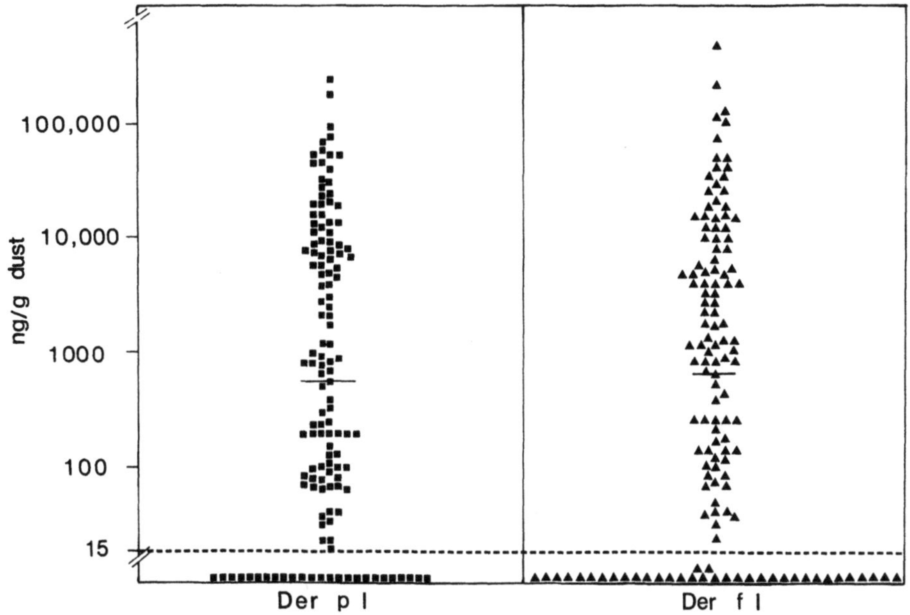

Fig. 1. Concentrations of Der pI and Der fI in 133 mattress dust samples

ranges for Der pI were between undetectable (<15 ng/g of dust) and 210000 ng/g, for Der fI between undetectable and 500000 ng/g (Fig. 1). Atopic and nonatopic subjects were exposed to comparable allergen concentrations. For atopic children the median value was 600 ng/g of Der pI and 675 ng/g of Der f I, for nonatopic children 400 ng/G od Der p I and 450 ng/gml of Der fI. In only 12 dust samples (10 atopic and 2 nonatopic subjects) were we not able to detect either Der pI or Der fI. Fifteen mattresses contained Der fI only (11 atopic and 4 nonatopic subjects), whereas 24 samples had only Der pI (20 atopic and 4 nonatopic subjects). Although there was a similar prevalence of Dpt and Df in the houses participating in the study, in approximately 70% of the individual apartments, one species was clearly dominating, that is, levels of one species tenfold or more higher than the other. We were unable to find any correlation between Der pI and Der fI ($r_s = -0.06$).

We compared the results of Der pI and Der fI analysis with a commercially available guanine test, which was evaluated with a test strip according to the colar intensity reaction. There was a good correlation between the results of the two methods ($r_s = 0.7$), however, the reliability of the guanine test seemed not to be sufficient since the guanine test is less sensitive than the house dust mite ELISA [15].

Seasonal Variations in Allergen Concentrations

In order to measure seasonal variations of mite allergen exposure, we collected mattress dust samples monthly in 13 homes over a period of 1 year. Mite allergen levels were significantly lower from January to June than from July to December ($p < 0.05$), which was mostly due to Der pI variations. Only in six of the studied homes could seasonal variations in mite allergen concentrations according to seasonal variations in outdoor humidity be observed. In seven homes mite allergen exposure stayed constant and seemed to depend only on indoor climate factors [16].

Dose-Response Relationship Between Allergen Exposure and Sensitization

Atopic children with significant (≥2000 ng/g < 10000 ng/g) or high (≥10000 ng/g) amounts of Der pI and the sum of Der pI plus Der fI, respectively, were found to have significantly higher serum IgE antibodies to Dpt ($p < 0.0005$ / $p < 0.0001$, respectively) than patients with very low (< 400 ng/g) concentrations of Der pI plus Der fI (Fig. 2). Similar results could be observed

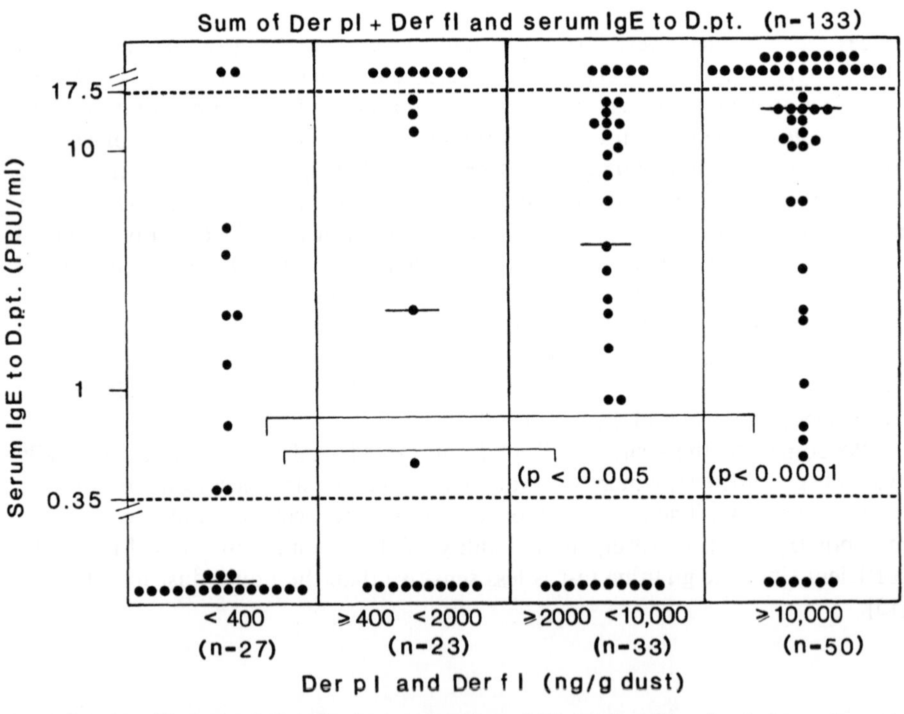

Fig. 2. Mite-specific serum. IgE antibody concentrations of 133 atopic children in relation to domestic mite allergen exposure (some of Der pI + Der fI)

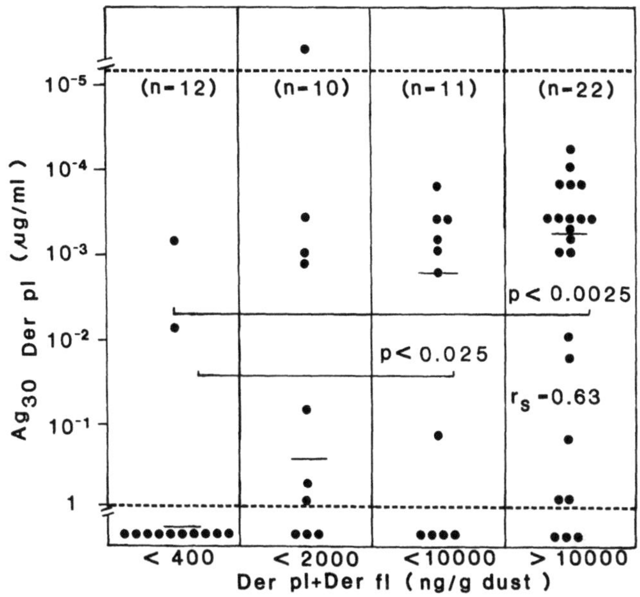

Fig. 3. Leukocyte sensitivity to Der pI and mite allergen (Der pI + Der fI) exposure. *Ag 30 Der pI* represents the allergen concentration necessary for 30% histamine release

for serum IgE antibodies to Df and for Der pI allergen exposure alone and serum IgE to Dpt and Df, respectively [14].

Washed leukocytes from 55 atopic subjects and 14 nonatopic controls were incubated with serial dilutions of Der pI (10^{-6} to 1 µg/ml). After the patients were grouped according to their Der pI and Der fI exposure into four dust classes, HR data revealed 86% of highly exposed children (sum of Der pI plus Der fI ≥ 10000 ng/g of dust) demonstrated positive HR to Der pI compared to 17% in the group with very low exposure (sum of Der pI plus Der fI < 400 ng/g of dust; Fig. 3).

Among all atopic patients there was a positive correlation between basophil sensitivity to Der pI and allergen exposure to Der pI ($r_s = 0.7$; $p < 0.0001$).

From our data, a risk ratio for the risk of exposure for the development of IgE antibodies and positive HR to Der pI in different mite allergen exposure groups was calculated. Comparing atopic subjects with very low house dust mite exposure with highly exposed atopic subjects, the risk is sevenfold to elevenfold higher for atopic subjects with significant and high mite allergen exposure to develop serum IgE to house dust mites and 19- to 32-fold higher to release histamine from sensitized basophils.

Elimination Procedures

Many mite elimination procedures have been suggested in the past, which are now being studied using the new allergen assays. Acaricides as well as allergen denaturing reagents are currently on the market.

We evaluated the short-term efficacy of benzyl benzoate in a double-blind placebo-controlled study. Houses were selected which contained at least 2000 ng/g dust mite allergen. Benzyl benzoate or placebo was applied to mattresses and carpets on day 0 and 10, and dust samples were collected after 30 and 60 days.

Using this protocol our data indicate that short-term efficacy of benzyl benzoate compared to placebo is marginal [17]. Therefore long-term studies are necessary, utilizing different application methods and reagents. Besides efficacy, allergen elimination and reagents should prove to be safe, not influencing, for example, bronchial hyperreactivity of atopic or asthmatic patients.

References

1. Smith TF, Kelly LB, Heyman PW, Wilkins SR, Platts-Mills TAE (1985) Natural exposure and serum antibodies to house dust mite of mite-allergic children with asthma in Atlanta. J Allergy Clin Immunol 76:782–788
2. Korsgaard J (1983) Mite asthma and residency: a case-control study on the impact of exposure to house dust mites in dwellings. Am Rev Respir Dis 128:231
3. Wharton GW (1976) House dust mites. J Med Entomol 12:557
4. Schwartz B, Lind P, Lowenstein H (1987) Level of indoor allergens in dust from homes of allergic and non-allergic individuals. Int Arch Allergy Appl Immunol 82:447–449
5. Dowse GK, Turner KJ, Stewart GA, Alpers MP, Woolcock AJ (1985) The association between *Dermatophagoides* mites and increasing prevalence of asthma in village communities within the Papua New Guinea highlands. J Allergy Clin Immunol 75:75
6. Van Bronswijk JEMH, Sinha RN (1971) Pyroglyphid mites (Acari) and house dust allergy: a review. J Allergy 47:31–52
7. Chapman MD, Platts-Mills TAE (1980) Purification and characterization of the major allergen from *Dermatophagoides pteronyssinus* antigen P1. J Immunol 125:587
8. Lind P (1985) Purification and partial characterization of two major allergens from the house dust mite *Dermatophagoides pteronyssinus*. J Allergy Clin Immunol 76:753
9. Tovey ER, Chapman MD, Platts-Mills TAE (1981) Mite faeces are a major source of house dust allergens. Nature 289:592–593
10. Chapman MD, Heyman PW, Platts-Mills TAE (1987) Epitope mapping of two major inhalent allergens, Der p I and Der f I, from mites of the genus *Dermatophagoides*. J Immunol 39:1479–1484
11. Horn N, Lind P (1987) Selection and characterization of monoclonal antibodies against a major allergen in *Dermatophagoides pteronyssinus*: species-specific and common epitopes in three *Dermatophagoides* species. Int Arch Allergy Appl Immunol 83:404
12. Platts-Mills TAE, Heyman PW, Chapman MD, Hayden ML, Wilkins SR (1986) Cross-reacting and species-specific determinants on a major allergen from *Dermatophagoides pteronyssinus* and *D. farinae*: development of a radioimmunoassay for antigen P1 equivalent in house dust and dust mite extracts. Allergy Clin Immunol 78:398–407
13. Lind P (1986) Enzyme-linked immunosorbent assay for determination of major excrement allergens of house dust mite species *D. pteronyssinus*, *D. farinae*, and *D. microceras*. Allergy 41:442
14. Lau S, Falkenhorst G, Weber A, Werthmann I, Lind P, Büttner-Götz P, Wahn U (1989) High mite-allergen exposure increases the risk of sensitization in atopic children and young adults. J Allergy Clin Immunol 84:718–725

15. Lau S, Rusche A, Weber A, Werthmann I, Büttner-Götz P, Wahn U (1990) Quantification of house dust mite allergens – comparison of ELISA and guanine test. Allergologie 13:12–15
16. Lau S, Weber A, Wertmann I, Wahn U (1990) Seasonal variations in house dust mite allergens – significance for atopic children. Monatsschr Kinderheilkd 138:58–61
17. Lau S, Rusche A, Weber AK, Büttner-Götz P, Wahn U (1990) Short term effect of solidified benzyl benzoate on mite allergen concentrations in house dust. J Allergy Clin Immunol (in press)

House Dust Mites and Protective Measures – A Study on Solidified Benzyl Benzoate

S. Lau-Schadendorf[1], A.F. Rusche[2], B. Ehnert[2], and U. Wahn[1]

[1] Kinder- und Poliklinik (KAVH), Universitätsklinikum Rudolf Virchow, Standort Charlottenburg, Heubnerweg 6, W-1000 Berlin 19, Federal Republic of Germany
[2] Kinderabteilung, Krankenhaus Zehlendorf-Heckeshorn, Zum Heckeshorn 32, W-1000 Berlin 39, Federal Republic of Germany

Introduction

House dust mites of the genus *Dermatophagoides* and their major allergens are of great importance in the development of allergic airway disease and atopic dermatitis [1–4]. In recent years, a dose-response relationship between mite allergen exposure and sensitization to house dust mite could be shown for atopic individuals. A concentration of about 2000 ng of major allergen, i.e., Der p I and Der f I/g, dust turned out to be a threshold concentration above which the risk of specific sensitization was significantly increased for atopic patients [5].

In Europe mite allergen concentrations of *Dermatophagoides* are frequently found to be >10000 ng/g dust [3–7]. To decrease the risk of sensitization for atopics one has to demand that mite and mite allergen reducing measures eliminate at least 90%–99% of mite allergen in order to reduce mite allergen contents below a concentration of 2000 ng/g dust.

There have been several approaches to reduce mites and mite allergen levels. Vacuum cleaning and removal of carpets and soft furnishings often have not achieved sufficient results [8–10]. Different chemicals have been examined for their acaricidal effects, such as lindane [11], pirimiphos-methyl [12], and others. Mite reducing effects of liquid nitrogen [13] and benzyl benzoate [14] have been reported.

Furthermore, tannic acid has been shown to denature mite allergens [15]. Finally, vinyl covered bedding casings can reduce the mite allergen content on the surface of patients' beds [16].

We investigated the short-term effect of solidified benzyl benzoate containing foam and powder, applied to mite infested mattresses and carpets, in a randomized, double-blind, placebo controlled study. Major allergens of *Dermatophagoides pteronyssinus* and *farinae*, Der p I and Der f I, were measured.

Material and Methods

Dust Collection and Application of Benzyl Benzoate

We included 22 homes with significant mite allergen concentrations in mattress dust samples (≥2000 ng Der p I and Der f I/g dust) in our study. Each home was visited four times (days 0, 10, 30, 60) by the same person. Dust samples were collected from the mattress and carpet of the child's room, always using the same vacuum cleaner (800 W) and new, disposable, paper dust bags. Vacuuming time was 5 min. Dust samples were kept at 4 °C until analysis. Mattresses and carpets were treated either with solidified benzyl benzoate ($n = 11$) or placebo ($n = 11$) in a double-blind fashion on days 0 and 10. Foam was used on mattresses (60 g/m^2, 2.6% benzyl benzoate) and powder on carpets (60 g/m^2, 5% benzyl benzoate). After 4 h, residues were removed by vacuuming. The benzyl benzoate-containing product (Acarosan, Werner and Mertz, Mainz, Federal Republic of Germany) is supposed to not only kill mites, but also to agglomerate mite allergen which can then be removed by vacuuming.

Dust Extraction

Dust extracts were produced by agitation for 3 h at room temperature 1:5 (w/v) in 0.125 *M* ammonium hydrogen carbonate containing 0.1% sodium azide. After centrifugation the supernatants were filtered and could be stored at −20 °C.

House Dust Mite ELISA

Precoated polystyrene microtiter plates and reagents for sandwich-type ELISA were obtained (ALK, Copenhagen, Denmark). For assay of Der p I, plates coated with monoclonal, non-cross-reacting antibodies [17, 18] and horse radish peroxidase-conjugated, species specific rabbit antibodies to Der p I were used. For assay of Der f I immunoabsorbed, affinity purified rabbit antibodies were used. The assay sensitivity was 15 ng/g of dust.

Statistics

Wilcoxon's matched pairs signed rank test and Mann-Whitney U-Wilcoxon-test were used. Statistical significance was assumed at $p < 0.05$.

Results

There was a significant reduction of mite allergen on mattresses and carpets within benzyl benzoate treated and control groups (reduction of 0%–75% on mattresses in both groups, 23%–91% on carpets in the control group, and 46%–86% on carpets in the treated group), but only the reduction of mite allergens on carpets of the treated group was significantly different from the control group on days 30 and 60 ($p < 0.05$). On day 10, the sum of both allergens on mattresses tended to be lower in the treated group, but the difference did not reach statistical significance.

Conclusion

The allergen reducing effect of acaricides or other mite allergen reducing agents should only be investigated in double-blind, placebo controlled studies since participation in a study seems to have a mite allergen reducing effect itself. In our study, the placebo treatment might have had an unexpected effect. The maximum percentage of reduction achieved in some homes of our study was not sufficient to reduce very high mite allergen concentrations to a threshold concentration with a low risk of sensitization (<2000 ng/g dust) for atopic individuals. For long term evaluation of efficacy and safety, further studies are necessary.

References

1. Voorhorst R, Spieksma FThM, Varekamp H, Leupen MJ, Lyklema AW (1967) The house dust mite (Dermatophagoides pteronyssinus) and the allergen it produces: identity with the house dust allergen. J Allergy 39:325–339
2. Rowntree S, Cogswell JJ, Platts-Mills TAE, Mitchell EB (1985) Development of IgE and IgG antibodies to food and inhalent allergens in children at risk of allergic disease. Arch Dis Child 60:727–735
3. Korsgaard J (1983) Mite asthma and residency: a case-control study on the impact of exposure to house dust mites in dwellings. Am Rev Respir Dis 128:231
4. Tuft LA (1949) Importance of inhalant allergens in atopic dermatitis. J Investig Dermatol 12:211
5. Lau S, Falkenhorst G, Weber A, Werthmann I, Lind P, Büttner-Götz P, Wahn U (1989) High mite allergen exposure increases the risk of sensitization in atopic children and young adults. J Allergy and Clin Immunol 84:718–725
6. Schwartz B, Lind P, Lowenstein H (1987) Level of indoor allergens in dust from homes of allergic and non-allergic individuals. Int Archs Allergy Appl Immun 82:447–449
7. Tovey ER, Chapman MD, Wells CW, Platts-Mills TAE (1981) The distribution of dust mite allergen in the houses of patients with asthma. Am Rev Respir Dis 124:630–635
8. Burr ML, Dean BV, Merrett TG, Neale E, St Leger AS, Verrier-Jones ER (1980) Effects of anti-mite measures on children with mitesensitive asthma: a controlled trial. Thorax 35:506–512
9. Korsgaard J (1983) Preventive measures in mite asthma. Allergy 38:93–102
10. Carswell F, Robinson DW, Oliver J, Clark J, Robinson P, Wadsworth J (1982) House dust mites in Bristol. Clin Allergy 12:533–545
11. Heller-Haupt A, Busvine JR (1974) Test of acaricides against house dust mites. J Med Entomol 11:551–558
12. Mitchell EB, Wilkins SR, McCallum Deighton J, Platts-Mills TAE (1985) Reduction of house dust mite allergen levels in the home: use of the acaricide, pirimiphos methyl. Clin Allergy 15:235–240
13. Colloff MJ (1986) Use of liquid nitrogen in the control of house dust mite populations. Clin Allergy 16:41–47
14. Dietemann A, Hoyet C, Bessot JC, de Blay F, Pauli G (1989) Effects of acaricide application on mite allergen levels and on symptoms of Dermatophagoides pteronyssinus (D. pt.) allergic patients. J Allergy Clin Immunol 83:263 (abstract)
15. Green WF (1984) Abolition of allergens by tannic acid. Lancet I:160
16. Walshaw MJ, Evans CC (1986) Allergen avoidance in house dust mite sensitive adult asthma. Quart J Med 226:199–215
17. Lind P (1986) Enzyme-linked immunosorbent assay for determination of major excrement allergens of house dust mite species D. pteronyssinus, D. farinae and D. microceras. Allergy 41:442–451
18. Horn N, Lind P (1987) Selection and characterization of monoclonal antibodies against a major allergen in D. pteronyssinus: species-specific and common epitopes in three Dermatophagoides species. Int Arch Allergy Appl Immunol 83:404–409

Environmental Pollution and Allergy

Environment and Allergy

T. Miyamoto and S. Takafuji

National Sagamihara Hospital and Department of Medicine and Physical Therapy, University of Tokyo, 18–1 Sakuradai, Sagamihara-shi, Kanagawa-ken 228, Japan

Abstract

Allergic rhinitis caused by pollens had been exceedingly rare in Japan before 1950, though the prevalence rate has markedly increased since then. The incidences of allergic rhinitis caused by Japanese cedar pollens were compared in different environments of the same district. It was found that the incidence of allergic rhinitis caused by Japanese cedar pollens was relatively high among residents alongside the intercity main road with heavy automobile traffic, whereas residents in the cedar forest with less traffic manifested lower incidence. Since pollen counts in both areas were almost identical and there were no differences in age and sex distributions of subjects in the two environments, air pollution was considered as a possible enhancing factor.

Sulphur oxides (SO_x), nitrogen oxides (NO_x), carbon monoxide (CO), photochemical oxidant and suspended particulate matter (SPM) are cited as typical air pollutants at present. In Japan, SO_2 and CO have remarkably decreased while photochemical oxidant has a tendency to decrease in spite of occasional transient increases. However, NO_2 and SPM retain the same level and have not yet decreased in the atmosphere.

SPM consists of small particles less than 10 µm, fractions of which can be carried deep into lungs when inhaled SPM originates from various sources such as exhaust particles and soil dusts in the urban districts of Japan.

In our present study, we collected SPM by a high volume air sampler and examined the effect of the collected SPM on the IgE antibody production of mice to ovalbumin (OA). The IgE antibody responses in mice immunized with intranasal administration of ovalbumin (OA) plus SPM at 3-week intervals were higher than responses in the animals immunized with OA alone. When the dose of OA administered as an antigen was 0.25 µg, the time course and magnitude in enhancement by SPM was comparable to those by killed Bordetella pertussis, a common adjuvant. SPM had an enhancing effect on IgE antibody production even in a small dose such as 0.25 µg administered at 3-week intervals. The possibility cannot be excluded that the natural exposure of humans to SPM in the environmental atmosphere may explain the high prevalence rate of allergic rhinitis caused by pollens in polluted districts in Japan.

Allergy and Common Allergens

There are a considerable number of allergic diseases caused by environmental allergens. Bronchial asthma, which is induced by various environmental allergens, is the most common. The most frequent cause of bronchial asthma in Japan is house dust.

House dust is a mixture of various materials, such as fibers, animal hairs, molds, bacilli, remnants of food, etc. It is well-recognized that the house dust mite is the most important allergen contained in house dust. In fact 1 g of house dust powder in Japan contains 40–2000 mites, and 36 species of house dust mite have been found. Among them, the *Dermatophagoides* family is thought to be the most significant, although some cross-allergenicity exists among mite families. The number of midges has increased a great deal recently. These have also been found to be an important allergen in Japan. As in other countries pollens of trees, grasses, and weeds are common allergens. Among them, Japanese cedar pollen is the most significant and more than 10% of the Japanese population suffer from cedar pollen allergy. Molds such as *Aspergillus*, *Penicillium*, *Alternaria*, *Cladosporium*, and *Candida* are also allergenic.

Unique Allergens in Japan

In addition to the common allergens, there are some allergens which are unique to Japan. One of them, for instance, is silk. Although the production of silk has decreased significantly since World War II, there are still many individuals who develop asthma when exposed to the silkworm or its products. There is also a high incidence of asthma among oyster shuckers. Inhalation of sea squirts, marine animals that grow on oyster shells, and their body juice, which is scattered in the air when the shell is cracked by the workers, also induces asthma. In addition, asthma is found in workers exposed to the powder of konjak (*Amorphophallus rivieri*), which is used to produce a jellylike food. Mushroom workers may develop asthma from the inhalation of mushroom spores.

Hypersensitivity Pneumonitis

Hypersensitivity pneumonitis is another allergic disease caused by environmental allergens, and more and more cases have been recognized in Japan. It occurs as the result of an immunologic reaction producing systemic symptoms, such as cough, dyspnea, fever, chills, myalgia, and malaise, resembling an acute systemic viral or bacterial infection. In a typical case chest X-rays may show fine nodular densities and peripheral infiltrations suggestive of interstitial and alveolar involvement. A few examples of hypersensitivity pneumonitis caused by environmental allergens are farmer's lung, humidifier's lung, and bird fancier's lung.

Blood samples were studied for the detection of precipitins and antibodies using a radioimmunoassay against bird serum. Some 60% of the asymptomatic breeders and 30% of the nonbreeders showed a positive precipitation reaction. IgG, IgA, and IgM antibodies were detected in 38%, 19%, and 8%, respectively, of the asymptomatic breeders. IgE antibodies were not detected in any of the breeders, while IgG antibodies were not detected in nonbreeders. The titer of IgG antibodies correlated with the numbers of budgerigars kept. Much higher titers of IgG, IgA, and IgM antibodies were detected in symptomatic breeders than in asymptomatic breeders. Cases of bird fancier's lung will probably be seen more frequently in Japan since bird keeping is now becoming quite common.

Recently, humidifiers have been commonly used in office buildings and private homes. Consequently more cases of humidifier's lung are being reported.

Summer Type Hypersensitivity Pneumonitis

A unique type of hypersensitivity pneumonitis has been reported in Japan. Symptoms usually occur during the summer and improve a great deal in the hospital but worsen after returning home. All the patient's sera have high titers of an antibody against *Trichosporon cutaneum*; most of them also have positive provocation tests against *Trichosporon* antigen. From these results, it has been postulated that *Trichosporon* – usually found in old and wooden houses – is the most likely cause of this type of pneumonitis.

Suspended Particles and Allergy

Before the end of World War II, cases of pollinosis either did not exist or were quite rare in Japan. In recent years, however, the incidence of pollinosis has increased dramatically. Among these, Japanese cedar pollinosis is the most common in Japan; it was first reported in 1964. It is, however, unreasonable to presume that the amount of airborne pollen is now higher and thus accounts for the striking increase in pollinosis in Japan, as Japanese cedar has been grown throughout Japan for many years. The pollination period of Japanese cedar is usually in March and April, and over 90% of the pollen during this period is Japanese cedar. In 1974, the incidence of pollinosis due to Japanese cedar pollen was less than 3.8%, but it rose to 5.8% in 1977 and 9.4% in 1981. This figure continues to increase and is now over 10%. Consequently, we have carried out prevalence studies of Japanese cedar pollinosis in order to determine the incidence of pollinosis in different areas of Nikko where there are abundant Japanese cedar trees [1]. The sample population was subdivided into five groups according to environmental differences:

1. Those living within 200 miles from intercity roads which are densely lined with old cedar trees and where traffic is heavy all day long
2. Those living in or near cedar forests
3. Those living in or near cedar forests but where automobile traffic is much less

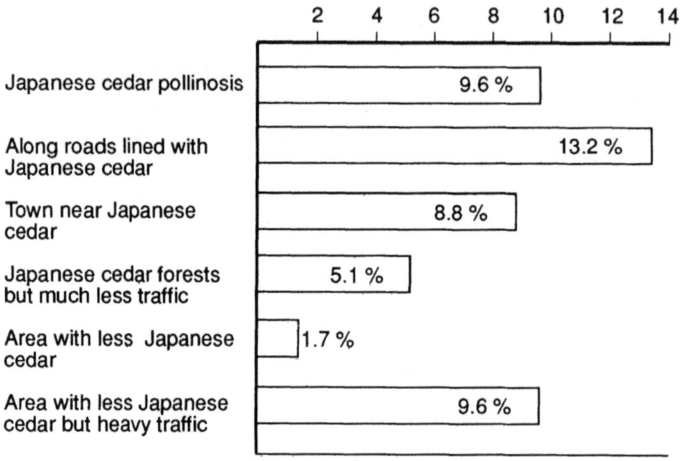

Fig. 1. Prevalence of Japanese cedar pollinosis in different environments in the same area

4. Those living in mountain areas with almost no cedar
5. Those living in towns where Japanese cedar is much less common but automobile traffic is heavy.

As shown in Fig. 1, among people living in areas where Japanese cedar pollen is not so heavy, the incidence of pollinosis is high if the area is heavily congested with traffic. Moreover, another study showed that the prevalence rate of allergic rhinitis among school children in districts with high levels of automobile exhaust was markedly higher than in less polluted districts. In Japan, not only the incidence of allergic rhinitis, but also that of bronchial asthma has increased three-to fourfold during the last 30 years. The incidence of asthma was higher along main roads where automobile traffic is heavy. These findings suggest that automobile exhaust is a possible cause of the higher incidence of allergic diseases.

The number of diesel cars in Japan has increased rapidly, from 20000 in 1951 to 7600000 in 1988; the total number of automobiles was 53000000 in 1988. The amount of diesel exhaust is said to be more than 100 times that of other cars. The number of cars continues to increase dramatically, and automobile exhaust has thus become one of the major causes of air pollution in Japanese urban districts. Sulphor oxides (SO_x), nitrogen oxides (NO_x), carbon monoxide (CO), photochemical oxidants, and suspended particulate matter (SPM) are cited as typical air pollutants of the modern era. In Japan, SO_2 and CO have remarkably decreased in the atmosphere; photochemical oxidants have also tended to decrease in spite of short-term increases. NO_2 and SPM had decreased markedly but have remained unchanged recently.

Diesel exhaust particles were collected, and 0.25 or 2.5 μg of ovalbumin (OA) mixed with 25 μg of diesel exhaust particles was injected repeatedly intraperitoneally into mice (Fig. 2). IgE production was enhanced compared to OA alone [2]. This was confirmed by several additional experiments. Therefore, we exam-

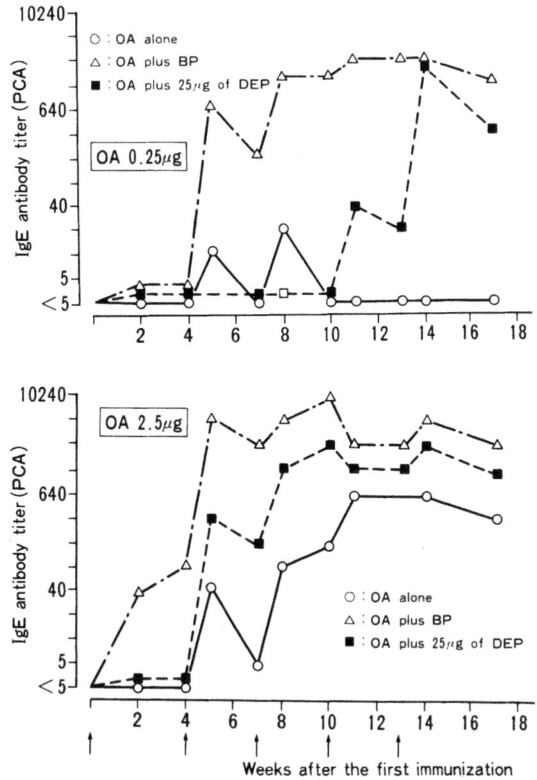

Fig. 2. Anti-OA IgE antibody response. *OA*, ovalbumin; *BP*, Bordetella pertussis; *DEP*, diesel exhaust particles; *PCA*, passive cutaneous anaphylaxis

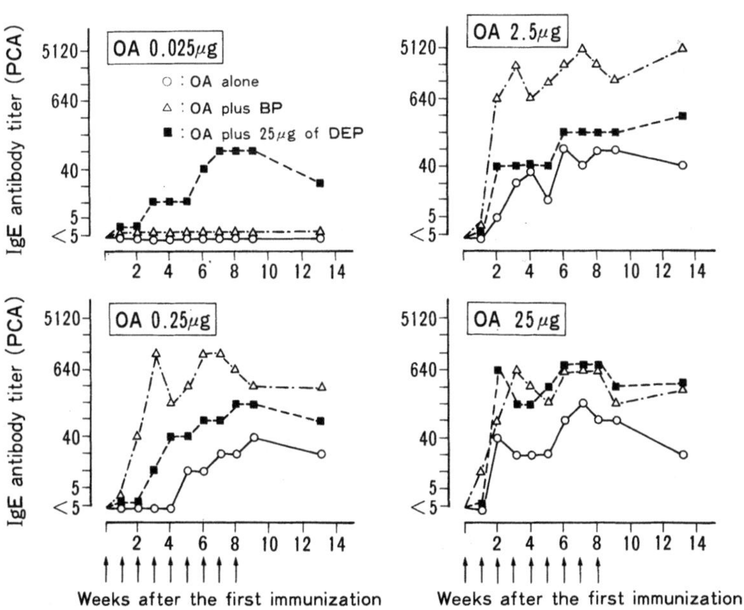

Fig. 3. Anti-OA IgE antibody responses (see Fig. 2)

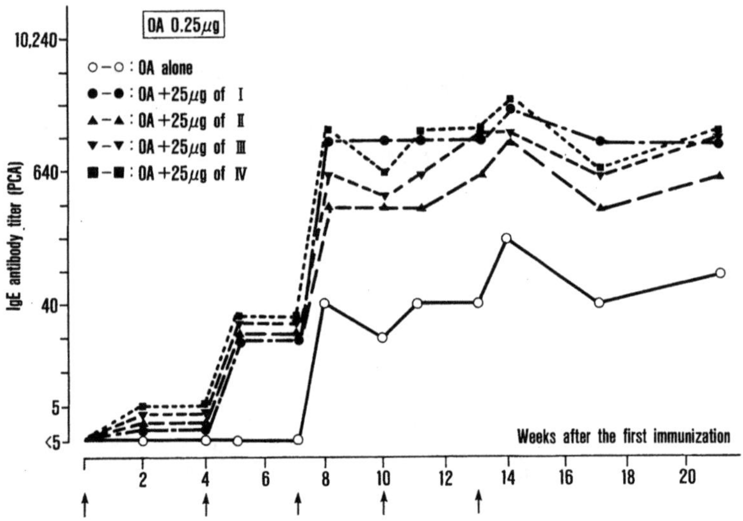

Fig. 4. Anti-OA IgE antibody response. A dose of 0.25 μg OA alone or OA mixed with 25 μg of four different sizes of particles. *I*, ≥7 μm; *II*, 3.3–7 μm; *III*, 2.0–3.3 μm; *IV*, <2.0 μm

ined the adjuvant activity of diesel exhaust particles inoculated by the intranasal route, i.e., the natural route of entry.

Groups of mice were inoculated intranasally once every week on nine occasions with 0.025, 0.25, 2.5, or 25 μg of OA alone or mixed with either *Bordetella pertussis* (BP) or 25 μg of diesel exhaust particles [3]. The magnitude of the anti-OA IgE response in mice immunized with OA plus 25 μg of diesel exhaust particles was greater than in mice immunized with OA without adjuvant throughout a 17-week period. The magnitude of the response was, however, less than that in mice immunized with OA plus BP ($p<0.01$) (Fig. 3).

Further studies confirmed that the diesel exhaust particles had an enhancing effect, even at the small dose of 1 μg inoculated intranasally.

Since diesel exhaust particles have an adjuvant effect, we wondered whether particles suspended in the atmosphere had adjuvant activity for IgE production [4]. Suspended particles were collected in four groups according to their size by a high volume air sampler: 7.0 μm and larger (group I); 3.3–7.0 μm (group II); 2.0–3.3 μm (group III); and less than 2.0 μm (group IV). The particles consisted mainly of carbon, calcium sulphate, quartz, calcite, rock salt, mica, chlorite, cristobalite, and feldspat. The larger the particle size, the more quartz, calcite, and rock salt. The smaller the particle size, the more carbon and calcium sulphate. There was almost no difference in the quantity of mica, chlorite, cristobalite, or feldspat, between large and small particles. The carbon content of the samples was 14.4%, 14.6%, 21.5% and 37.3% according to size.

The 0.25 μg dose of OA alone or OA mixed with 25 μg of four different sizes of particles in 25 μg of borate buffer saline (BBS) were administered directly as nasal drops to five groups of mice and boosted four times. The anti-OA IgE response in mice immunized with OA mixed with particles was greater than that of

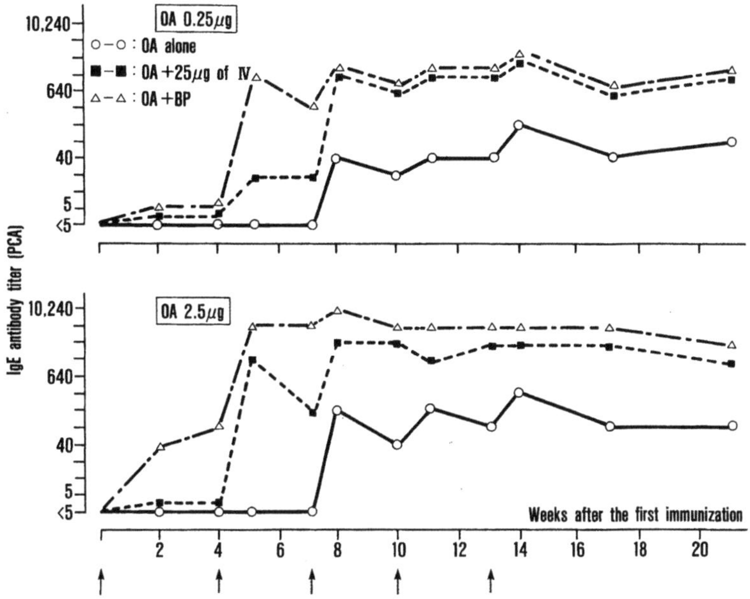

Fig. 5. Anti-OA IgE antibody response. OA was mixed with 25 μg of small (*IV*) particles

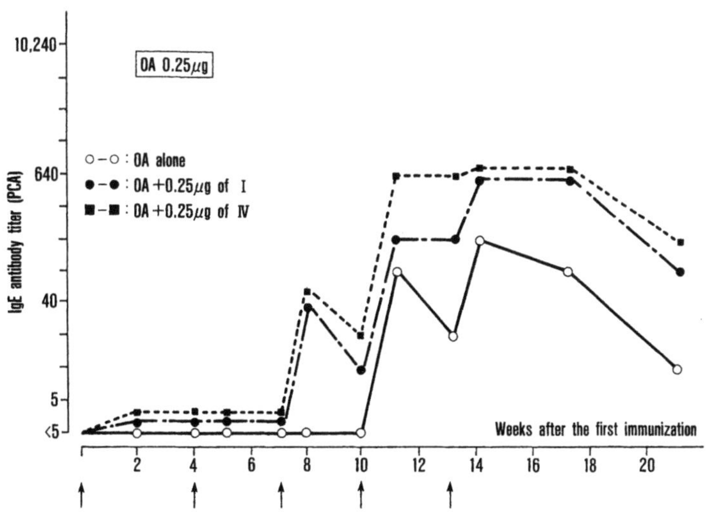

Fig. 6. Anti-OA IgE antibody response. OA was mixed with 0.25 μg of large (*I*) or small (*IV*) particles

mice immunized with OA alone throughout the 21-week period following the first immunization. There were no significant differences in the IgE response in mice immunized with OA and different size of particles (Fig. 4).

Figure 5 illustrates the anti-OA IgE response to 0.25 or 2.5 μg of OA without adjuvant or mixed with either 25 μg of small particles or BP. Anti-OA IgE production was greater in response to OA and particles than to OA alone.

Figure 6 illustrates the anti-OA IgE response to intranasal administration of 0.25 μg of OA alone, OA mixed with 0.25 μg of large particles, or OA with the same dose of small particles. Particles had an enhancing effect on anti-OA IgE production, even at the smallest dose. There was no significant difference in the adjuvant activity between large and small suspended particles, however.

From these results, it was postulated that floating particles may be contributing to the recent increase in allergic disease.

References

1. Ishizaki T, Koizumi K, Ikemori R, Ishiyama Y, Kushibiki E (1987) Studies of prevalence of Japanese cedar pollinosis among the residents in a densely cultivated area. Ann Allergy 58:265–270
2. Muranaka M, Suzuki S, Koizumi K, Takafuji S, Miyamoto T, Ikemori R, Tokiwa H (1986) Adjuvant activity of diesel-exhaust particulates for the production of IgE antibody in mice. J Allergy Clin Immunol 77:616–623
3. Takafuji S, Suzuki S, Koizumi K, Tadokoro K, Miyamoto T, Ikemori R, Muranaka M (1987) Diesel-exhaust particulates inoculated by the intranasal route have an adjuvant activity for IgE production in mice. J Allergy Clin Immunol 79:639–645
4. Takafuji S, Suzuki S, Koizumi K, Tadokoro K, Ohashi H, Muranaka M, Miyamoto T (1989) Enhancing effect of suspended particulate matter on the IgE antibody production in mice. Int Arch Allergy Appl Immunol 90:1–7

Allergens and Pollutants in the Air – A Complex Interaction

H. Behrendt[1], K.H. Friedrich[1], E. Kainka-Stänicke[1], U. Darsow[1], W.M. Becker[2], and R. Tomingas[1]

[1]Medical Institute of Environmental Hygiene at the Heinrich-Heine-University, Auf'm Hennekamp 50, W-4000 Düsseldorf, Federal Republic of Germany
[2]Research Institute Borstel, W-2061 Borstel, Federal Republic of Germany

Abstract

Air pollution is supposed to enhance the risk of allergy. Investigations of the influence of environmental pollutants on allergic inflammatory reactions are therefore of increasing importance. Pollen grains which are the major source or outdoor aeroallergens are said to probably express an altered allergenicity when emitted into a polluted air. We investigated the behavior of pollen grains which had been collected from four differently polluted regions in North Rhine-Westphalia, FRG. Samples were taken with Burkhard traps and/or high volume samplers. In addition, native grass pollen have been exposed to extracts of airborne particulate matter in vitro in a dose- and time-dependent manner. The samples were further processed for scanning and transmission electron microscopy as well as for determination of protein content and release using IEF and SDS-PAGE immunoblot techniques.

The results obtained show that (1) there is an overall higher concentration of pollen grains in polluted urban areas than in rural regions, independent of weather conditions; (2) emission peaks of SO_2, NO_2/NO_x or atmospheric fine dust, but not of O_3, usually precede peaks of high pollen concentrations; (3) pollen grains collected from highly polluted regions are significantly more contaminated with agglomerations of airborne particulates, and the intensity of pollen/particle binding depends on amount and composition of organic compounds adsorbed to the particle; and (4) incubation of purified grass pollen with extracts of atmospheric fine dust results in dose- and time-dependent alterations of structural pollen integrity and of protein release, probably leading to altered allergenicity.

The results indicate that there is a complex interaction between pollen grains and air pollutants, not only with respect to daily emission peaks but also through direct binding of particulate matter to the pollen surface. Therefore, dust-laden pollen grains from heavily polluted areas can induce cytotoxic and mutagenic reactions in addition to sensitization. This fact has to be taken into account when assessing influences of air pollution on allergic inflammatory response.

Introduction

Investigations on the interaction between airborne pollutants and respiratory allergies have mainly been focused on induction of allergic sensitization and/or allergic symptoms. There is some evidence today that air pollution may be responsible for the increase in pollen allergies and asthma in highly polluted areas [7, 14, 23]. Additionally, irritant gases [6, 11, 13, 15] and/or diesel exhaust particles [21] have been shown to express both adjuvant activity for sensitization against common allergens and enhancing effects on allergic symptoms in sensitized individuals.

One has to keep in mind, however, that pollen are carriers not only of allergens but also pollutants when released into a polluted atmosphere [8]. Pollen grains accumulate heavy metals, i.e., lead and cadmium, but also nitrate and sulphur [3]. The amount of sulphur per pollen dry weight has been proposed to be a bioindicator for burden of the atmosphere with SO_2 and other sulphuric compounds [12].

The question to be answered is whether air pollutants are able to alter/impair structure and function of the pollen itself, thereby modulating allergen formation and release.

In this report the complex interaction between allergenic pollen and pollutants in the air is demonstrated. The first part deals with pollen concentrations in differently polluted areas of North Rhine-Westphalia, FRG in relation to emission data of pollutants, as indicated by various emission measurement techniques. It will be shown that even at this particular level there is some explanation for enhanced sensitization rates in individuals living within a polluted atmosphere. The second part demonstrates the direct interaction between pollen and airborne particulate matter in dust samples which had been collected from differently polluted areas using high volume samplers. In the third part we present in vitro effects of extracts of airborne particulate matter on purified grass pollen, as determined by electron microscopy as well as by immunoblotting techniques using sodium dodecyl sulphate polyacrylamide gel electrophoresis (SDS-PAGE) and isoelectric focusing (IEF), in order to identify allergen release.

Concentration of Pollen in Rural and Urban Areas and Influence of Air Pollution

Pollen grains are normally emitted during the early morning under appropriate conditions. They reach higher atmospheric zones during the heat of the day, and when cooling down they sediment in late afternoon. Since sedimentation depends on decrease of temperature and convection streams, and since in large cities with high air pollution temperature remains high even overnight, high pollen counts are detected in the evening within the cities – Düsseldorf, Cologne (Fig. 1) – whereas at the country side – Borken/Westphalia (Fig. 1) – the pollen peak in the early morning [10]. The total number of pollen is also higher in the polluted regions than in the less polluted reference area (see Table 1).

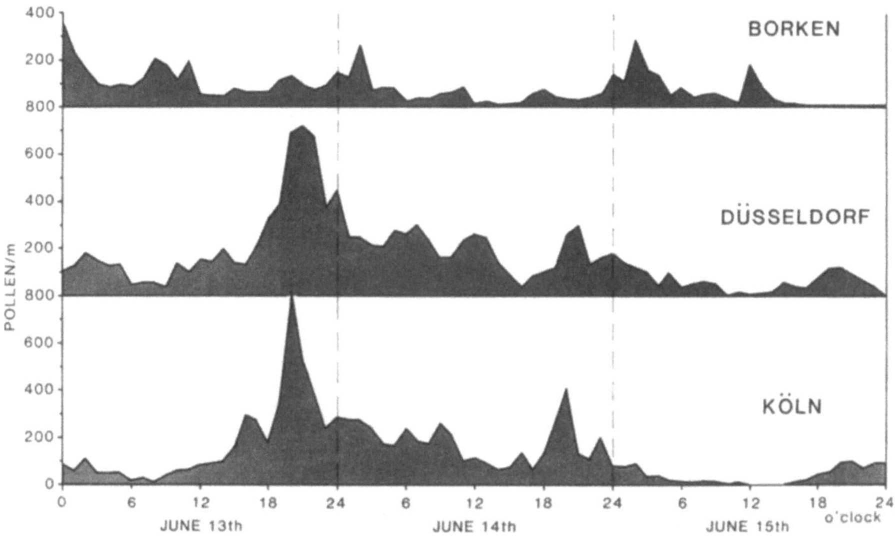

Fig. 1. Diurnal variations of grass pollen concentrations in a rural area (Borken/Westphalia, FRG) and in two cities (Düsseldorf and Cologne) with different air pollution

Table 1. Peak concentrations of total pollen and of birch pollen during birch pollen season 1988. Comparison between differently polluted areas in North Rhine-Westphalia.

Area	Total pollen/m³			Birch pollen/m³		
	16.–20. 4. 1988	Peak 1 16. 4.	Peak 2 19. 4.	16.–20. 4. 1988	Peak 1 16. 4.	Peak 2 19. 4.
Düsseldorf (Reisholz)	5294	864	1798	3797	482	1484
Cologne (Neumarkt)	3051	831	1027	2288	652	734
Borken (City Center)	2342	256	1099	1490	96	841

There is an overall increase in the concentration of birch pollen from 3797 pollen/m^3 in 1988 to 4619 pollen/m^3 in 1989 and to 7520 pollen/m^3 in 1990. The number of days with birch pollen counts over 100 pollen/m^3 also increased between 1988 and 1990, and the beginning of birch pollen season shifted from mid-April in 1988 to end of March in 1990 (Fig. 2).

Figure 3 demonstrates the relationship between pollen concentrations and air pollutants in the center of Cologne, which is highly polluted by combustion products. It represents a characteristic example for the situation present in polluted regions in North Rhine-Westphalia: high emission peaks of NO_x, but also of SO_2 and of atmospheric fine dust, can be measured at times of low pollen concentrations. The pollen count peaks later, when the primary pollutants are already decreasing. High pollen emissions are, however, accompanied by an increase in the secondary pollutant ozone as a result of photochemical reactions. The simulta-

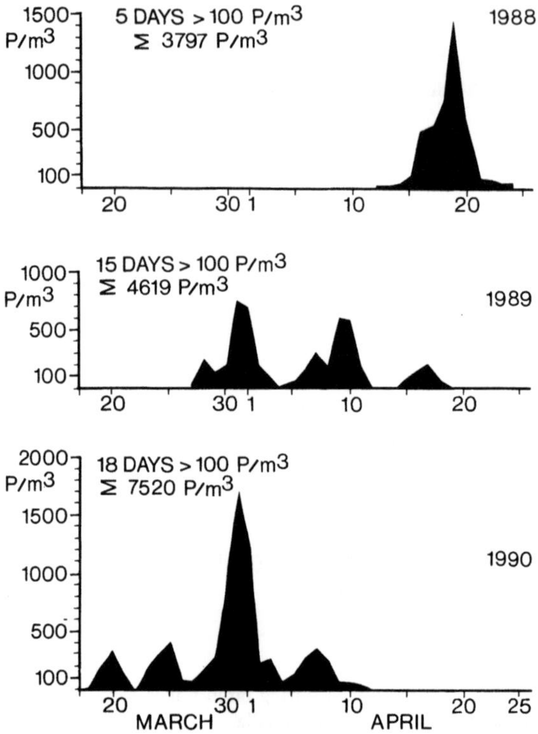

Fig. 2. Concentration of birch pollen (*P*) during the pollen seasons 1988–1990 in Düsseldorf, FRG

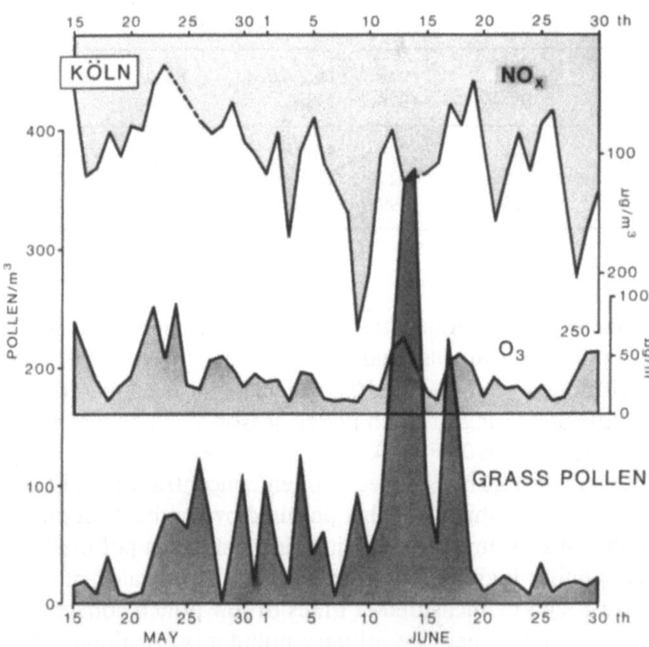

Fig. 3. Relationship between concentration of NO_x, O_3 and grass pollen in the center of cologne, FRG. Data are given as mean values per day

neous increase and decrease of levels of pollen and ozone has recently been observed by Gassner et al. [4].

With respect to allergy, in highly polluted regions a situation within the atmosphere may therefore be found which promotes/favors sensitization. This situation is similiar to one produced under controlled conditions in laboratories in order to induce specific IgE antibodies in experimental animals via the inhalative route. The observed phenomenon may also be an additional factor in explaining enhanced rates of pollen allergies within industrialized regions with high air pollution.

Agglomeration of Airborne Particulate Matter on Pollen Surfaces

In order to study the interaction between pollen and particulate pollutants, atmospheric fine dust – cut off point <7 μm aerodynamic diameter – has been collected during various summer periods from two differently polluted regions using high volume samplers (HVS 150, Ströhlein Comp., Kaarst, FRG). Dust samples

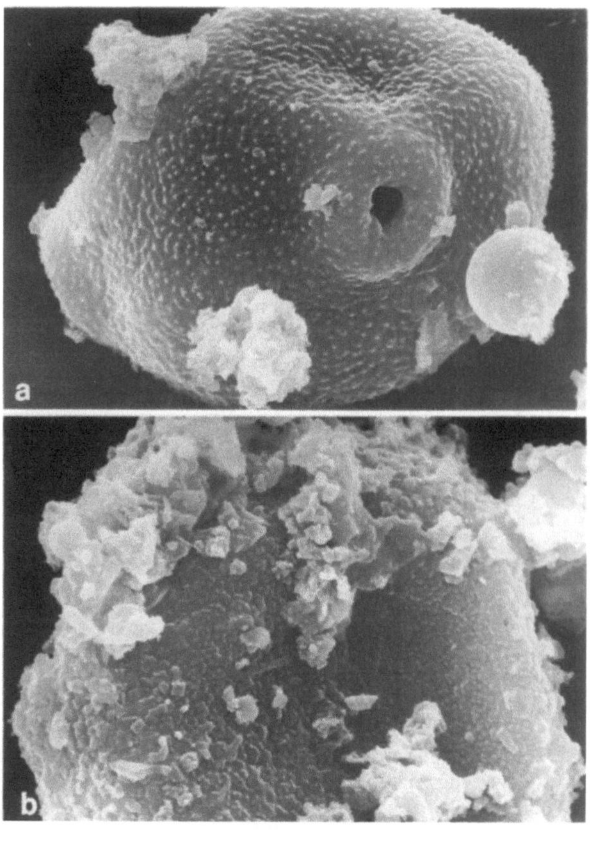

Fig. 4a, b. Scanning electron micrographs of a birch pollen (**a**) and of part of a grass pollen (**b**) exhibiting agglomeration of airborne particles onto their surface. Note that very small particles are present in addition to aggregates. Magnification: × 4700 (**a**), × 5300 (**b**)

were subsequently analyzed by light and electron microscopy, and the degree of dust agglomeration onto pollen surfaces was determined by semiquantitative methods under the light microscope.

Results obtained by light microscopy indicate that pollen in dust samples from Duisburg, one of the most polluted regions in the German Rhine-Ruhr area, show a marked degree of particle agglomeration on their surfaces (see Fig. 5). Particle agglomeration is less frequent and almost negligible in dust samples collected in Düsseldorf [8]. This observation tends to be true for all types of pollen investigated, i.e., birch, grasses, mugwort and common nettle, as well as for spores, i.e., *Cladosporium* and *Alternaria* [9]. The effect of dust agglomeration to pollen surfaces can also be observed in tape preparations deriving from conventional Burkhard traps collecting pollen in Duisburg but not in Düsseldorf.

Dust-coated pollen are most obvious on scanning electron micrographs (Fig. 4A, B), indicating heteromorphy of the particles attached to pollen surfaces. These particles are always below 5 μm in diameter. They may either be aggregated (Fig. 4A) or display microfibers of various length and size. In addition, very small, round, or polygonally shaped particles in the submicronic range can be observed (Fig. 4A, B). Using X-ray microanalysis they have been recognized to belong to the organic particle fraction. Figure 5 summarizes semiquantitative data about pollen-particle interaction and confirms the higher degree of agglomeration in the dust of Duisburg (>75% of particles are of class 3 and class 4 agglomeration) than in dust samples collected in Düsseldorf. In the latter 80% of particles have been recognized as class 2 agglomerated particles.

In order to find out wether dust composition is responsible for particle attachment to pollen grains, dust analysis has been performed. As is shown in Table 2,

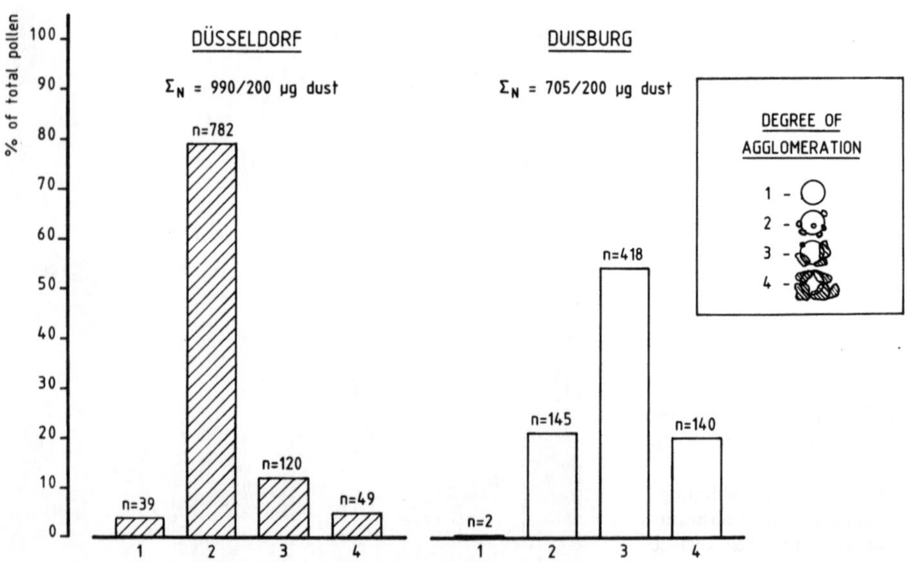

Fig. 5. Effect of airborne particulate matter on the degree of agglomeration of pollen grains from two differently industrialized urban areas in the Federal Republic of Germany (Collection time: 1.4–30.9.1986)

Table 2. Characterization of airborne particulate matter collected from two differently industrialized urban areas in western Germany (collection time: 1. 4. – 30. 9. 86).

Dust		Duisburg	Düsseldorf
pH		5.8	5.1
Total dust concentration (μg/m³)		70	64
Total fiber content/m³		33×10^3	31×10^3
Asbestos fibers/m³		2900	1180
X-ray microanalysis (% particles)			
Mg		0.65	0.12
Al		19.69	22.79
Si		66.36	70.59
S		1.83	0.61
Cr		0.39	0.25
Mn		0.52	0
Fe		23.34	10.78
Zn		0.13	0.12
Pb		0.26	0.37
Organic compounds			
Benzo(a)pyrene	μg/g	32.7	11.2
	(μg/m³)	(2.3)	(0.7)

there are no marked differences between the two dust samples with respect to pH values, to total dust concentration or to mineralogical particle composition as determined by X-ray microanalysis. There are, however, striking differences in the amount of lipophilic organic substances adsorbed to the particles. For example, benzo(a)pyrene concentrations is three times higher in Duisburg than in Düsseldorf (Table 2). Benzo(a)pyrene is at least one of the main combustion products in the steel and fuel industry, the latter being virtually absent in Düsseldorf.

From these observations it can be concluded that the amount and the chemical composition of organic substances adsorbed to airborne particles are responsible for their attachment to the pollen surface.

Effect of Extracts of Airborne Particulate Matter on Grass Pollen *Dactylis glomerata* In Vitro

More than 700 organic substances are known to be adsorbed to airborne particles [18]. These particle-adsorbed organic substances mainly belong to the group of polycyclic aromatic hydrocarbons, of phenols and of azaheterocyclic compounds. They have been shown to induce cytotoxix, mutagenic, carcinogenic, and allergotoxic effects on mammalian cells in vitro [3, 19].

We investigated the effect of organic extracts of airborne particulate matter on purified grass pollen *Dactylis glomerata* using morphological as well as immunochemical methods.

By electron microscopy, grass pollen display an exine, an intine, and a cytoplasm containing regularly arranged organelles. At higher magnification, the ex-

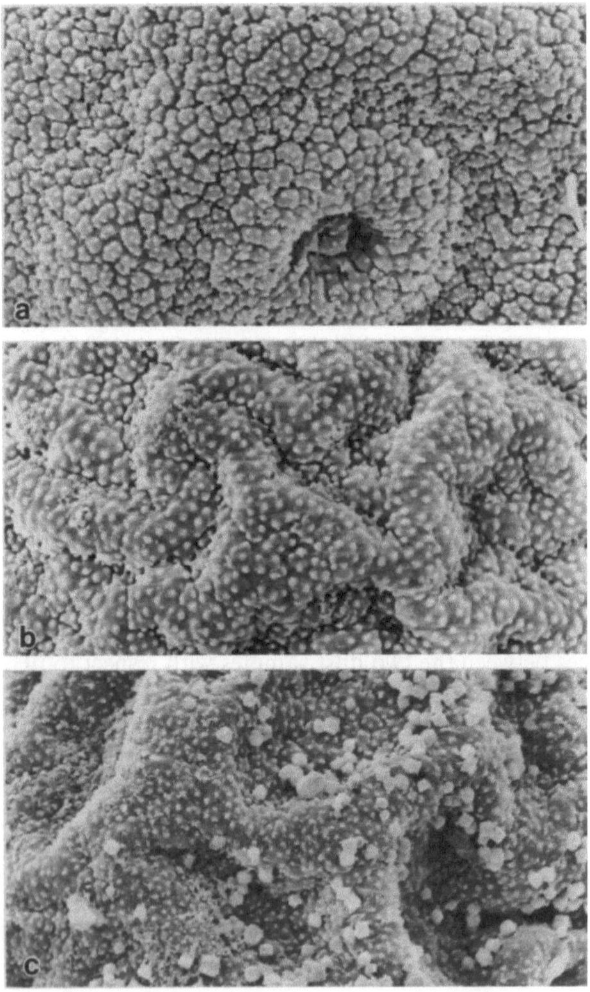

Fig. 6a–c. Scanning electron micrographs of grass pollen surfaces. **a** Control; **b** after a 2-h incubation period with ammonium carbonate buffer; **c** after incubation with aqueous extract of airborne particulate matter. note the submicronic particles appearing on the exine. Magnification: × 6000 (**a**), × 7100 (**b**), × 5500 (**c**)

ine exhibits a typical substructure on scanning electron microscopy (Fig. 6A) and on transmission electron microscopy microchannels through which the intine is connected with the extracellular millieu.

If pollen are stimulated to release allergenic proteins in vitro in a dose- and time-dependent manner (Fig. 7, column 1), they undergo morphological changes already seen on scanning electron microscopy (Fig. 6B). On transmission electron microscopy, there is a reduction of electron density as well as lamellation on the intine. Clusters of granular matrix appear outside the exine just on top of a microchannel. Fusion of cytoplasmic granules and exposure of granular matrices to the intine is a common phenomenon in ammonium carbonate-stimulated grass pollen (Fig. 8A) and indicates that thc cytoplasmic proteins do contribute to release.

Similar morphological results can also be found after incubation of grass pollen with organic extracts of airborne particulate matter, i.e., plaque formation

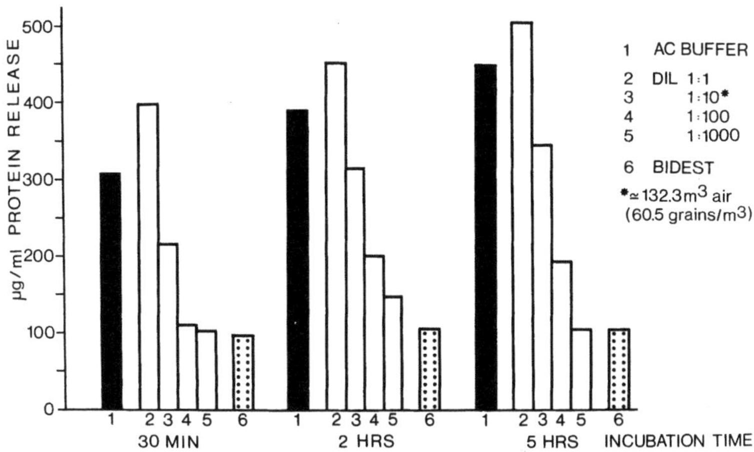

Fig. 7. *Dactylis glomerata*. Time- and dose-dependent effect of total aqueous extract of airborne particulate matter (GEX-w) from a heavily industrialized Rhine-Ruhr area on protein release

outside the exine and exocytosis of cytoplasmic granules (Fig. 8B). In contrast to ammonium carbonate buffer-stimulated grass pollen, however, pollen treated with organic extracts of atmospheric fine dust do not show invasion of exocytosed granules into the intine which then exhibits now sort of dense membranaceous structures (Fig. 8B). The partial activation of grass pollen through organic extracts is also evidenced by measurement of protein release and immunoblotting techniques: the highly active organic extract from dust collected during a smog episode in 1985 releases a small but substantial amount of proteins (11.8% of total protein content), but not the extract prepared from dust collected during a 2-week summer period (1.7% of total protein). Both organic extracts, however, induce an additional 15% increase of protein release when dust-loaded pollen are subsequently exposed to ammonium carbonate buffer.

From these experiments it can be concluded that organic substances adsorbed to airborne particles are not only responsible for the attachment of particles to pollen surfaces but also preactivate the coated pollen and produce an enhanced release of proteins upon appropriate stimuli.

There are not only organic substances adsorbed to airborne particles but also heavy metals, i.e., cadmium, lead, nickel, mercury, chromium, manganese, and bromium (R. Tomingas and H. Behrendt, manuscript in preparation). These metals are usually found within the aqueous phase of airborne particulate matter, as is true for several organic substances of low molecular weight (carbonic acids, phenols, aldehydes; R. Tomingas and H. Berendt, manuscript in preparation). In order to test the effect of aqueous extracts of airborne particulate matter on pollen, purified grass pollen *Dactylis glomerata* were incubated with various concentrations of aqueous extract under isotonic conditions. As is indicated in Fig. 7, the aqueous extract releases pollen proteins in a dose- and time-dependent manner. For example, an extract prepared from atmospheric fine dust which is present in an air volume of 132.3 m^3 releases up to 300 µg/ml protein from purified

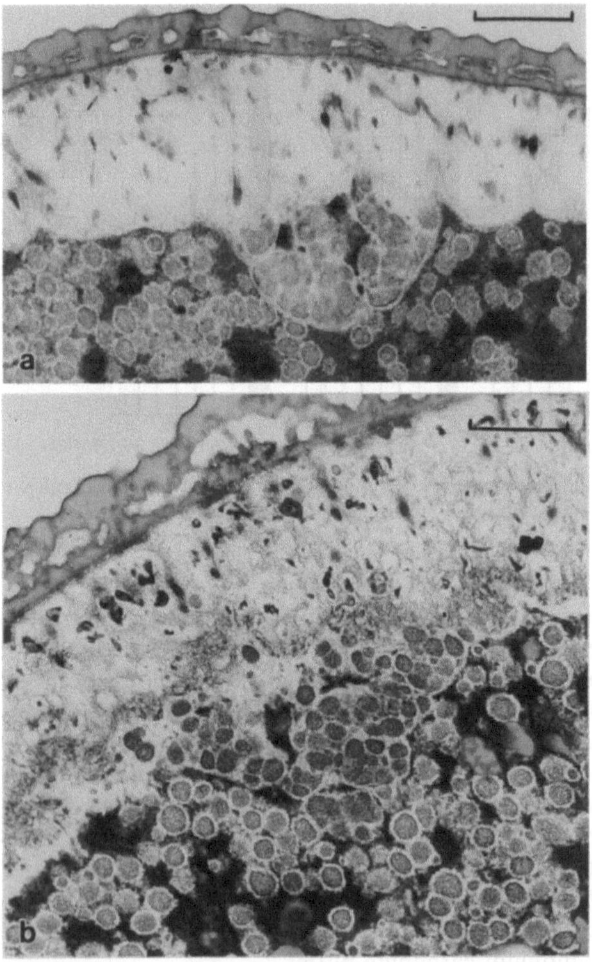

Fig. 8a, b. Transmission electron micrographs of parts of grass pollen *Dactylis glomerata* after incubation with either ammonium carbonate buffer, pH 8.3 (**a**) or with organic smog extract (**b**). Note "degranulation" and release of cytoplasmic proteins into the intine. Magnification: × 20000. *Bar*, 1 μm

grass pollen of a calculated amount of 60.5 grains per m^3 of air (Fig. 8), a concentration which also occurs during the grass pollen season.

The aqueous extract also induces release of allergenic proteins from *Dactylis glomerata*. This is evidenced by performing SDS-PAGE immunoblotting and probing the blot with pool serum of grass pollen allergic patients: an altered pattern of proteins is visible. There is a dose-dependent shift in intensity of IgE binding reactivity to the lower molecular weight site [2]. Recently, alterations of allergenicity of certain airborne pollen grains due to some gaseous atmospheric pollutants have also been observed by Ruffin et al. [16, 17].

Using scanning electron microscopy, grass pollen which had been treated with aqueous extract of airborne particulate matter consequently display morphological alterations similiar to those observed after forced allergen release induced by ammonium carbonate buffer (Fig. 6C). Additionally, small polygonal particles appear on the pollen surface (Fig. 6C). These particles are smaller than 1 μm in diameter. They therefore belong to the submicronic fraction of particulates. They are similiar to those seen on the surface of pollen which had been collected in regions highly polluted with combustion products (Fig. 4A, B).

From these experiments it can be concluded that chemical substances which are present in the aqueous phase of airborne particles (1) release allergenic proteins with altered IgE binding reactivity and (2) contribute to the formation of allergen aerosols in the submicronic range under the influence of appropriate weather conditions.

The results obtained provide an explanation for the mode of generation of allergens carried by atmospheric aerosols previously observed by others [1, 5, 20].

Conclusions

In highly polluted regions airborne pollen grains do not only carry allergens but also pollutants. There is a complex interaction between pollen and pollutants in the air, not only with respect to the dynamics of emission peaks – which in turn may favor sensitization – but also with respect to direct contact between airborne particles and pollen surfaces. This interaction leads to local pollen preactivation, to modulation of allergen release, to generation of allergenic aerosols within moist atmospheres, and to adsorption of pollen proteins to airborne particles.

References

1. Agarwal MK, Swanson MC, Reed CE, Yunginger JW (1984) Airborne ragweed allergens: association with various particle sizes and short ragweed plant parts. J Allergy Clin Immunol 74: 687–693
2. Becker WM, Darsow U, Behrendt H (1990) Effect of extracts of airborne particulated matter on grass pollen *Dactylis glomerata*: allergen release and morphology. Allergologie 13:434
3. Behrendt H, Fischer I, Winzer A, Tomingas R, Friedrichs KH (1990) Histamine-releasing activity of airborne particulated matter. Allergologie 13:441
4. Gassner M, Peeters AG, Primault B (1987) Relation von meteorologischen Gegebenheiten mit Pollen- und Luftschadstoffimmissionen, insbesondere Ozon, im Rheintal. Bull Méd Suisses 68:1079–1082
5. Habenicht HA, Burge HA, Muilenberg ML, Solomon WR (1984) Allergen carriage by atmospheric aerosol. II. Ragweed-pollen determinants in submicronic atmospheric fractions. J Allergy Clin Immunol 74:64–67
6. Holt PG, Britten D, Sedgwick JD (1986) Suppression of IgE responses by antigen inhalation: studies on the role of genetic and environmental factors. Immunology 60:97–102
7. Ishizaki T, Koizumi K, Ikemori R, Ishiyama Y, Kushibiki E (1987) Studies of prevalence of Japanese cedar pollinosis among the residents in a densely cultivated area. Ann Allergy 58:265–270
8. Kainka-Stänicke E, Behrendt H, Friedrichs KH, Tomingas R (1988) Morphological alterations of pollen and spores induced by airborne pollutants: observations from two differently polluted areas in West Germany. Allergy 43:Suppl 7, 57
9. Kainka-Stänicke E, Behrendt H, Friedrichs KH, Tomingas R (1989) Surface alterations of pollen and spores by particulate air pollutants. J Hyg Environm Med 188:516
10. Kainka-Stänicke E, Behrendt H, Friedrichs KH, Tomingas R (1990) Mögliche Einflüsse von Luftverunreinigungen, Klima und Urbanität auf allergische Rhinitis. Allergologie 13:67

11. Matsumara Y (1970) The effects of ozone, nitrogen dioxide, and sulphur dioxide on the experimentally induced allergic respiratory disorder in guinea pigs. Am Rev Respir Dis 102:430–447
12. Noll KE, Khalili E (1988) Dry deposition of sulfate associated with pollen. Atmospheric Environment 22:601–604
13. Oberbarnscheidt J, Stiller-Winkler R, Krämer U, Dolgner R, Behrendt H (1990) Untersuchungen zum Einfluß von Luftschadstoffen auf die Sensibilisierung und den Immunstatus 6jähriger Kinder. Allergologie 13:316–317
14. Osebold JW, Gershwin LJ, Zee YC (1980) Studies on the enhancement of allergic lung sensitization by inhalation of ozone and sulphuric acid aerosol. J Environ Pathol Toxicol Oncol 3:221–234
15. Riedel F, Krämer M, Scheibenbogen C, Rieger CHL (1988) Effects of SO_2 exposure on allergic sensitization in the guinea pigs. J Allergy Clin Immunol 82:527–534
16. Ruffin J, Williams D, Banerjee U, Pinnix K (1983) The effects of some environmental gaseous pollutants on pollen-wall proteins of certain airborne pollen grains. Grana 22:171–175
17. Ruffin J, Evans V, Banerjee S, Banerjee UC (1984) A preliminary study of the allergenicity of red oak *Quercus rubra* pollen extract after contamination with some common atmospheric pollutant (e.g. NO_2, SO_2 and CO). J Palynol 20:17–30
18. Schlipköter HW, Abel J, Behrendt H, Dehnen W, Gleichmann E, Seemayer N, Wiegand H (1986) Zelluläre und molekularbiologische Aspekte in der Umwelttoxikologie. Zbl Bakt Hyg B 182: 431–448
19. Seemayer NH, Hadnagy W, Behrendt H, Tomingas R (1988) Indicators of potential health risks by airborne particulates: cytotoxic, mutagenic and carcinogenic effects on mammalian cells in vitro. In: Seemayer NH, Hadnagy W (eds) Environmental hygiene. Springer, Berlin Heidelberg New York, pp 54–59
20. Spieksma FTM, Kranmps JA, Nikkels AH, Plomp A, Koerten HK (1990) Detection of pollen allergen on micronic airborne particulates. Allergologie 13:433
21. Takafuji S, Suzuki S, Koizumi K, Tadocoro K, Miyamoto T, Ikemori R, Muranaka M (1987) Diesel-exhaust particulates inoculated by the intranasal route have an adjuvant activity for IgE production in mice. J Allergy Clin Immunol 79:639–645
22. Wolters JHB, Martens MJM (1987) Effects of air pollutants on pollen. Botanical Rev 53:372–414
23. Yoshida K, Oshima H, Imai M (1966) Air pollution and asthma in Yokkaichi. Arch Environ Health 13:763–768

Platinum Salt Asthma*

G. Schultze-Werninghaus, R. Merget, and W. Zachgo

Klinikum der Johann Wolfgang Goethe-Universität, Zentrum der Inneren Medizin, Abteilung für Pneumologie, Theodor-Stern-Kai 7, W-6000 Frankfurt/Main 70, Federal Republic of Germany

Abstract

Platinum salt allergies have been almost exclusively restricted to workers in platinum refineries in the past. A more recent source of platinum salt exposure is the increasing number of catalyst factories. There has been some concern about allergic diseases in the general population due the increasing use of platinum catalysts in cars to reduce air pollution. However, there have been no convincing data to prove this assumption. Allergic reactions to metallic platinum (e.g., jewellery) are unknown. Subjects exposed to platinum salts develop symptoms of an immediate type allergy, including rhinitis, conjunctivitis, and/or asthma, often associated with dermatitis/urticaria, varying between 15 days and several years after exposure. The sensitization index (i.e., the rate of subjects with symptoms) may exceed 50%. The high prevalence of respiratory symptoms in platinum refineries demands preventive measures. The legal concentration limits do not prevent an unacceptable rate of asthma cases. Medical history is unequivocal in most cases. To confirm the anamnestic data, skin prick tests, which are a simple and reliable tool, may be performed. Stepwise testing from an initial dilution of $10^{-8}\,M$ $(PtCl_6)^{2-}$ is employed in order to avoid anaphylactic side effects. Bronchial provocation tests with platinum salts may cause severe side effects by overdose of the agent. An initial dilution until $10^{-10}\,M$ $(PtCl_6)^{2-}$ may be necessary. The reactions may be of the immediate or dual type. The sensitivity of bronchial provocation tests is higher than that of skin prick tests. They are specific; atopic or normal controls do not react to platinum salt inhalation. The immune mechanism is not yet fully understood. It is postulated that platinum salts act as haptens by changing the molecular structures of certain human proteins, rendering them immunogens or allergens, and also by changing nonimmunogenic surface structures of cell membranes into allergenic epitopes. The excessive allergen-inducing activity of $(PtCl_6)^{2-}$ might be due to the reaction with free carbonyl or amino groups and/or particularly with sulphhydryl or methionine side chains. The "immunogenic" activity of platinum salts is related to the number of chlorine ligands of the compounds. An allergic mechanism is suggested by a number of observations: (a) latency between first exposure and first symptoms, (b) no reactions in a pro-

* Parts of this work were supported by Degussa, Frankfurt/Main, FRG.

portion of exposed subjects, (c) reactions to minimum amounts of $(PtCl_6)^{2-}$ after "sensitization", (d) experimentally induced sensitization in monkeys, (e) specific skin test in exposed symptomatic subjects. Passive transfer of skin test reactivity from "sensitized" subject to primates and nontoxic histamine release from basophils was demonstrated by several groups including our own. Several investigators demonstrated higher "platinum salt-specific" IgE by modified RAST in exposed asthmatic subjects compared with exposed healthy subjects or nonexposed controls. However, in vitro techniques are of a relatively poor specificity; results can be correlated to total IgE concentrations.

Introduction

Metal salts, such as nickel and chromium compounds, are common low molecular weight allergens. The most frequent manifestation of metal salt allergy is contact dermatitis, both in the general population (e.g., nickel dermatitis) and in certain occupations (e.g., chromate eczema in masons). In contrast, metal salt-induced diseases of the respiratory tract are relatively rare and are confined to occupational situations. Asthmatic symptoms have been reported after inhalation of aluminium, boron, chromium, cobalt, nickel, platinum, and vanadium compounds [18, 26].

Platinum salts are a relatively common cause of metal salt induced respiratory tract symptoms. Apart from earlier reports of toxic effects [10], allergic symptoms were described as early as 1911 by Karasek and Karasek [12] in subjects who were exposed to platinum paper in the photochemical industry.

Which platinum salts might act as allergens (or, more probably, as haptens) is still unknown. Several groups have tried to unravel the mechanisms of action of platinum salts in allergic symptoms, such as conjunctivitis, rhinitis, and asthma; among them, particularly Prof. J. Pepys and his co-workers [6, 7, 17, 20, 21]. Our own experience with platinum salt asthma began around 1975, when we were able to demonstrate quantitative histamine release in a "sensitized" subject and passive transfer of platinum salt allergy to monkeys [24]. Since then we have had the opportunity to investigate a larger number of workers from platinum refineries [5, 14] and in a car catalyst factory.

Epidemiology

Platinum salt allergies are almost exclusively restricted to workers in platinum refineries, where metallic platinum is refined from ore or recycled from industrial waste, e.g., exhausted catalysts (Table 1). Various platinum salts may result from these chemical procedures, one of the most important compounds being platinum hexachloride $(PtCl_6)^{2-}$, which is the most common cause of platinum salt asthma.

Exposed subjects develop symptoms rather frequently. The sensitization index (i.e., the rate of symptoms among all exposed subjects) may, under certain condi-

Table 1. Relative uses of platinum in various industries. (From [4]).

Industry	Total use (%)
Automotive	51
Electrical	13
Petroleum refining	10
Chemical	9
Ceramic, glass	3
Jewelry, arts	3
Dentistry	2
Other	8

tions, exceed 50% [22]. The prevalence of platinum salt-induced symptoms has not changed very much since the first survey in 1945 by Hunter and co-workers, despite the introduction of exposure limits (0.002 mg Pt/m^3 in the Federal Republic of Germany and other countries). In our cross-sectional investigations we determined a prevalence of platinum salt induced allergic symptoms of about 20% in workers in two refineries [5, 14], the frequency of symptoms being significantly correlated with the degree of exposure to platinum salts at different workplaces.

Whether a familial or individual history of atopy might predispose an increased risk of platinum salt allergy is unclear. While earlier authors thought so [19, 22], this could not be confirmed in larger surveys [8]. In our own studies we found only a weak trend towards a higher proportion of symptomatic workers who also had a family incidence of allergy compared to those who had no historical links with such illness [14].

It has recently been reported that smokers are at increased risk (relative risk: 5.05) of sensitization by platinum salts [27]. Own data from a recent cross-sectional study in a catalyst factory confirm this finding (Merget et al., in prep.). That irritants may enhance sensitizations to platinum salts was also described in a monkey model, using ozone as the chemical irritant [3].

There has been some concern about allergic diseases in the general population due to the increasing use of platinum catalysts in cars to reduce air pollution. To date, there have been no convincing data to prove this assumption. On the contrary, it was thought unlikely that catalytic devices from cars could cause platinum salt allergies, because allergic reactions to metallic platinum (e.g., jewellery) are unknown. In recent years, however, it could be demonstrated that automobile catalytic converters release significant quantities of platinum into the roadside environment [11]. In this study, dust samples collected from plants contained 0.7 ppm platinum. Furthermore, it has been estimated that 10% of the released platinum consists of soluble platinum salts, thereby increasing the risk that reactive platinum compounds may concentrate in roadside soil and water systems. Therefore, further investigations in this field are urgently needed.

Symptoms

Between 15 days and several years [14] after exposure, symptoms of an immediate type allergy, such as rhinitis, conjunctivitis, and/or asthma, often associated with dermatitis/urticaria, may be seen in exposed workers. Symptoms usually are progressive and they may become irreversible, underlining the importance of early removal of the worker from the work place. Symptoms suggestive of other immunological conditions, such as chronic dermatitis (eczema), are infrequent.

Diagnostic Procedures

Medical history is unequivocal in most cases. Doubts about the causal relationship between work place and disease may be investigated, if either nonoccupational allergy is a concomitant causal factor or if the worker does not provide proper information due to ignorance or fear of losing his job [14]. To confirm the anamnestic data, skin tests, which are a simple and reliable tool, may be performed. The skin prick test is recommended due to its simplicity and low risk of unwanted side effects. Stepwise testing from an initial dilution of 10^{-8} *M* $(PtCl_6)^{2-}$ is employed in order to avoid anaphylactic side effects, which have been observed during skin tests [9]. The dose response curve is relatively flat (Fig. 1). Results from skin prick tests are highly specific (100%) and sufficiently sensitive (80%–90%) [6, 14, 16, 20].

Bronchial provocation tests with platinum salts may be performed. They require a considerable familiarity with this procedure, as severe side effects may be caused by an overdose of the agent. An initial dilution until 10^{-10} *M* $(PtCl_6)^{2-}$ may be necessary in highly sensitized subjects [13, 20]. The reactions may be of the immediate or dual type, with unexpectedly severe late reactions [15] (Fig. 2).

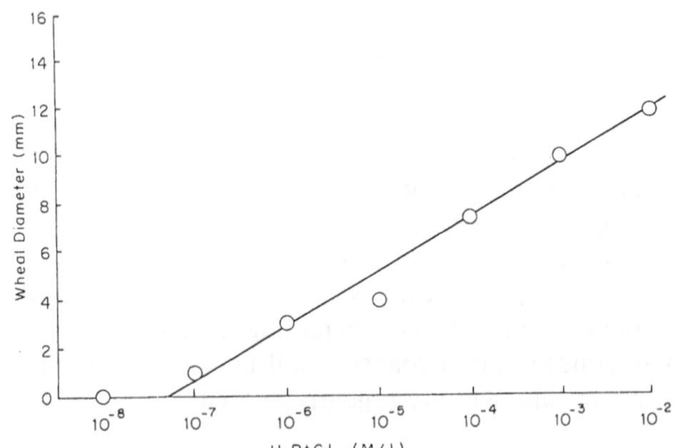

Fig. 1. Skin test with $(PtCl_6)^{2-}$ in 10 subjects; mean concentration-effect curve. Prick test: mean wheal diameter (mm); concentration of platinum salt in *M*

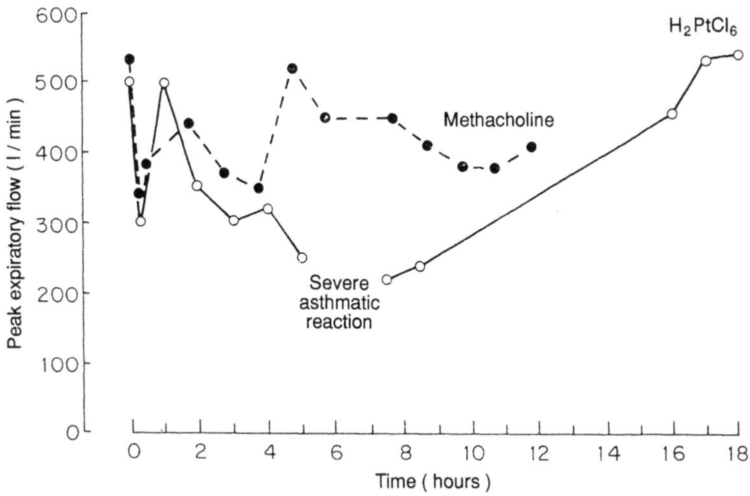

Fig. 2. Peak flow (l/min) after bronchial provocation tests with methacholine (-●-●-●-) and $(PtCl_6)^{2-}$ (-○-○-○-) in one subject. Dual reaction; maximum decreases after 15 min and 5–7 h

It has not been determined whether nonspecific airway reactions may be provoked by bronchial challenge tests with $(PtCl_6)^{2-}$ in humans, as has been seen in primates [1]. We have not been able to induce airway obstruction with $(PtCl_6)^{2-}$ inhalation in normal subjects, but can do so in exposed subjects with negative skin tests and positive history [16]. Therefore we feel that a challenge test is a useful tool under certain circumstances, sensitivity of bronchial challenge tests being higher than that of skin prick tests. As a diagnostic standard, however, we recommend only the allergic history and a skin prick test.

In Vitro Test and Recent Immunological Findings

The immune mechanism is not yet fully understood. It is postulated that platinum salts act as haptens by changing the molecular structures of certain human proteins, rendering them immunogens or allergens, and also by changing nonimmunogenic surface structures of cell membranes into allergenic epitopes. The excessive allergen-inducing activity of $(PtCl_6)^{2-}$ might be due to the reaction with free carbonyl or amino groups and/or particularly with sulphhydryl or methionine side chains. Cleare et al. [6] found that the "immunogenic" activity of platinum salts is related to the number of chlorine ligands of the compound.

It is a matter of debate whether all reactions to platinum salts are of an immunologic nature and are also toxic under certain circumstances. Hardman and Wright [10] observed a toxic reaction to high concentrations of platinum salts in 1896; toxic histamine release from blood cells has been reported in experimental animals [23], and more recently, airways obstruction was demonstrated in monkeys who had never before been exposed to platinum salts [1]. Therefore, nonspecific mediator release seems probable, particularly in concentrations above $>10^{-3}\,M$ [25].

An allergic mechanism, however, is suggested by a number of observations:
1. Latency between start of exposure and first symptoms
2. No reactions in a proportion of exposed subjects
3. Reactions to minimum amounts of $(PtCl_6)^{2-}$ after "sensitization"
4. Experimentally induced sensitization in monkeys [1]
5. Specific skin and bronchial provocation tests in exposed symptomatic subjects [14, 16].

Circumstantial evidence for an IgE-mediated immune mechanism has prompted several groups to develop in vitro systems for the detection of platinum salt-specific IgE. Cleare et al. [6] did not detect signs of IgE-mediated reactions by either the radioallergosorbent test or passive cutaneous anaphylaxis (PCA). Our group was the first to clearly demonstrate passive transfer of skin test reactivity from a highly "sensitized" subject to primates (*Macaca arctoides*) [24], probably due to transfer of IgE, together with positive skin tests and quantitative histamine release from basophils in the "allergic" subject.

Cromwell et al. [7] demonstrated higher "platinum salt specific" IgE in a modified RAST in exposed asthmatic subjects than in exposed healthy subjects or nonexposed controls. Similar findings were reported by other authors, e.g., Biagini et al. [2], using a RAST modification with platinum salt-malic dehydrogenase conjugates coupled to methylcellulose disks, and Murdoch et al. [17], using a RAST modification [6].

In these studies the specifity of RAST reactions was not very high and specific binding rates of the immunoassays were relatively low, thus failing to provide convincing evidence for an IgE-mediated mechanism. A general finding in these studies was, however, that skin test-positive, symptomatic workers had higher mean IgE titers than skin test-negative, asymptomatic controls. Therefore, the available evidence is in favor of an IgE-related mechanism underlying platinum salt-induced symptoms, and the lack of specificity and sensitivity of IgE assays may be due to technical problems with platinum salt in RAST assays.

In recent studies of two platinum refineries [5, 14], we used two in vitro techniques, histamine release from basophils and a modified RAST [28]. These investigations confirmed the low specificity of the in vitro tests and the superiority of the simple skin prick test method.

These results showed that:
1. Total IgE is elevated in most, but not all cases; this has been previously described by Cromwell et al. [7] (Fig. 3).
2. Platinum salt-specific IgE is elevated in exposed asthmatic subjects, as previously demonstrated [2, 7, 21]. However, comparable binding rates are found in controls with elevated total IgE; there is a correlation with the concentration of total IgE (Fig. 3). We concluded that serum IgE binds in a nonspecific manner to platinum salt-solid phase complexes, independently of the modifications of these systems previously used by different groups.
3. Histamine release from leukocyte suspensions (basophils) is consistently positive in a concentration-dependent manner [14, 24], with release characteristics

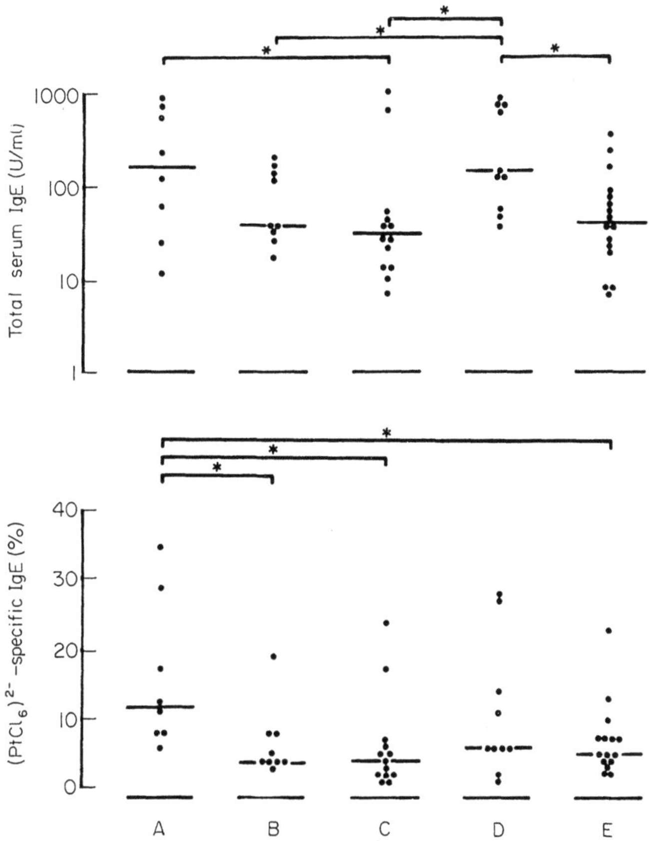

Fig. 3. Total-IgE and platinum salt-specific IgE in platinum salt-exposed subjects. *A*, work-related symptoms; *B*, doubtful work-related symptoms; *C*, no work-related symptoms. Controls with (*D*) or without (*E*) atopic history (*$p<0.05$). (From [14])

of an allergic, but not toxic, mechanism and a maximum release at $10^{-4}-10^{-5}\,M$. The release is calcium dependent and is also present under protein-free conditions [14].

Histamine release with platinum salts is related to the concentration of total IgE (Fig. 4), pointing to a nonspecific, but IgE-related release mechanism. Moreover, there is a close correlation between histamine release by platinum salts and by anti-IgE (Fig. 4). This leads to a platinum salt-induced histamine release in atopic controls who have never been exposed to platinum.

In conclusion, in vitro techniques are of a relatively poor specificity. These observations suggest an IgE-related, nonspecific release mechanism in vitro. It is not known whether these nonspecific, IgE-related mechanisms are also of clinical importance. Should this be the case, atopic subjects would be expected to develop a more rapid onset of "allergic" symptoms than previously healthy subjects. Many observations, including our own, do not support the assumptions. Therefore, the

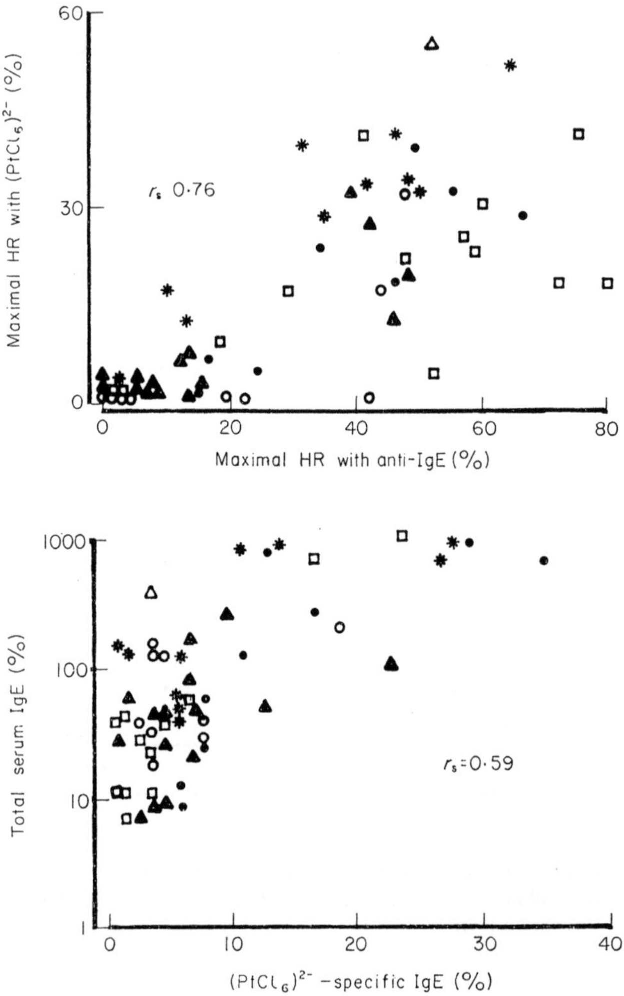

Fig. 4. Correlation of histamine release with $(PtCl_6)^{2-}$ and with anti-IgE. Correlation of total IgE with $(PtCl_6)^{2-}$ Specific IgE. (●) Exposed, allergic; (○) exposed, doubtfully allergic; (□) exposed, healthy; (★) atopic controls; (▲) nonatopic controls. (From [14])

in vitro findings are probably not related to the clinical situation. They may only demonstrate that platinum salts in vitro react with proteins, particularly IgE or IgE-related structures.

Conclusions

Platinum salt-induced airway symptoms are of interest for a number of reasons. First, in occupational medicine, there is a relatively high risk of occupational airway disease, but a lack of criteria for preventive investigations. Second, the small molecular size of the substance and its unknown mechanism of action are of interest to both allergologists and immunologists.

Medical history and quantitative skin prick tests are recommended as diagnostic standards. In vitro tests are of low specificity, due to interference with nonspecific IgE.

The high prevalence of respiratory symptoms in platinum refineries demands preventive measures. The legal exposure limits do not prevent an unacceptable rate of asthma cases. The actual limit (0.002 mg Pt/m^3) is in the range of concentrations that may induce asthmatic symptoms in positive provocation tests! Therefore other measures are necessary:

1. *Preventive medical examinations* which, however, would only avoid a minority of cases ("high risk individuals" with previous atopic symptoms).
2. *Early change of workplace*, e.g., within the company.
3. *Drastic reduction of workers' exposure* to platinum salt aerosols. This is the most important measure to be tackled.
4. *Reduction of the exposure limits* below 0.002 mg Pt/m^3.

Acknowledgement. The authors express their gratitude to all colleagues, students, and technicians who have been engaged in these studies, with invaluable contributions by Mrs. B. Aulbach, Mrs. E.-M. Bergmann, Dr. U. Bolm-Audorff, Dr. R. Breitstadt, Dr. A.-H. Bury, Dr. W. Friedrich, Dr. E. Gonsior, Dr. Androniki Roesch, Dr. O.-H. Wilhelms, and others.

References

1. Biagini RE, Moormann WJ, Smith RJ, Lewis TR, Bernstein IL (1983) Pulmonary hyperreactivity in cynomolgus monkeys from nose-only inhalation exposure to disodium hexachloroplatinate Na_2PtCl_6. Toxicol Appl Pharmacol 69:377–384
2. Biagini RE, Bernstein IL, Gallagher JS, Moorman WJ, Brooks S, Camm PH (1985) The diversity of reagin immune responses to platinum and palladium metallic salts. J Allergy Clin Immunol 76:794–802
3. Biagini RE, Moorman J, Lewis TR, Bernstein L (1986) Ozone enhancement of platinum asthma in a primate model. Am Rev Respir Dis 134:719–725
4. Boggs PB (1985) Platinum allergy. Cutis 35:318–320
5. Bolm-Audorff U, Bienfait H-G, Burkhard J, Bury A-H, Merget R, Pressel G, Schultze-Werninghaus G (1990) Respiratory allergy in chemical workers exposed to platinum salts. In: Sakurai H et al. (eds) Occupational Epidemiology. Elsevier, Amsterdam, pp 157–160
6. Cleare MJ, Hughes EG, Jacoby B, Pepys J (1976) Immediate (type I) allergic responses to platinum compounds. Clin Allergy 6:183–195
7. Cromwell O, Pepys J, Parish WE, Hughes EG (1979) Specific IgE antibodies to platinum salts in sensitized workers. Clin Allergy 9:109–117
8. Dally MB, Hunter JV, Hughes HG, Stewart M, Newman-Taylor AJ (1980) Hypersensitivity to platinum salts: a population study. Am Rev Respir Dis 121:A230
9. Freedman SO, Krupey J (1968) Respiratory allergy caused by platinum salts. J Allergy 42:233–237
10. Hardman RS, Wright CH (1896) A case of poisoning by chloroplatinate of potassium. Brit med J 1:529
11. Hodge VF, Stallard MO (1986) Platinum and palladium in roadside dust. Environ Sci Technol 20:1058–1060

12. Karasek SR, Karasek M (1911) The use of platinum paper. Report of Illinois State Commission of Occupational Diseases, p 97
13. Merget R, Schultze-Werninghaus G, Zachgo W, Zerfass G (1985) Platinsalzallergie – Vergleich von in vitro und in vivo Testverfahren. Prax Klin Pneumologie 39:953–954
14. Merget R, Schultze-Werninghaus G, Muthorst T, Friedrich W, Meier-Sydow J (1988) Asthma due to the complex salts of platinum – a cross sectional survey of workers in a platinum refinery. Clin Allergy 18:569–580
15. Merget R, Schultze-Werninghaus G, Zachgo W, Meier-Sydow J (1988a) Sofort- und Spätreaktionen im inhalativen Provokationstest mit Platinsalzen – eine Falldemonstration. Allergologie 11:196–197
16. Merget R, Zachgo W, Schultze-Werninghaus G, Bergmann E-M, Bolm-Audorff U, Friedrich W, Bury A-H, Meier-Sydow J (1990) Quantitativer Hauttest und inhalativer Provokationstest bei Asthma durch Platinsalze. Pneumonologie 44:226–228
17. Murdoch RD, Pepys J, Hughes EG (1986) IgE antibody responses to platinum group metals: a large scale refinery survey. Br J Ind Med 43:37–43
18. Parkes WR (1982) Occupational lung disorders, 2nd ed. Butterworths, London
19. Parrot J-L, Saindelle A, Ruff F (1969) Platinum and platinosis. Arch Environ Health 19:685–691
20. Pepys J, Pickering CAC, Hughes EG (1972) Asthma due to inhaled chemical agents – complex salts of platinum. Clin Allergy 2:391–396
21. Pepys J, Parish WE, Cromwell O, Hughes EG (1979) Passive transfer in man and the monkey of type I allergy due to heat labile and heat stable antibody to complex salts of platinum. Clin Allergy 9:99–108
22. Roberts AE (1951) Platinosis. Arch Ind Health Occ Hyg 4:549–559
23. Saindelle A, Ruff F (1969) Histamine release by sodium chloroplatinate. Br J Pharmac 35:313–321
24. Schultze-Werninghaus G, Roesch A, Wilhelms O-H, Gonsior E, Meier-Sydow J (1978) Asthma bronchiale durch berufsbedingte Allergie vom Soforttyp gegen Platinsalze. Untersuchungen zur Immunpathologie und arbeitsmedizinische Problematik. Dtsch med Wschr 103:972–975
25. Schultze-Werninghaus G, Zachgo W, Merget R (1985) Dual mechanism of immediate type reactions in occupational asthma to platinum salt. Ann Allergy 55:265
26. Schultze-Werninghaus G (1986) Asthma bronchiale durch Metallsalze. Allergologie 9:479–486
27. Venables KM, Dally MB, Nunn AJ, Stevens JF, Stephens R, Farrer N, Hunter JV, Stewart M, Hughes EG, Newman Taylor AJ (1989) Smoking and occupational allergy in workers in a platinum refinery. Brit Med J 299:939–942
28. Zachgo W, Merget R, Schultze-Werninghaus G (1985) Bestimmungsverfahren für spezifisches Immunglobulin E gegen niedermolekulare Substanzen (Platinsalze). Atemw-Lungenkrkh 11:267–268

Induction of Mediator Generation in Human Inflammatory Cells by Polychlorinated Biphenyls

M. Raulf and W. König

Institut Medizinische Mikrobiologie und Immunologie, AG Infektabwehrmechanismen, Ruhr-Universität Bochum, Universitätsstrasse, 150 MA 01/240, W-4630 Bochum 1, Federal Republic of Germany

Abstract

Environmental agents of various origin interfere with the functional activity of the immune system and may activate immunological and nonimmunological responses. A variety of environmental agents are not necessarily cytotoxic; but some of them induce allergic or pseudo-allergic reactions with the subsequent release of inflammatory mediators. Some of these are of low molecular weight, e.g., histamine, prostaglandins, leukotrienes, and platelet-activating factor (PAF). Others, e.g., cytokines and growth and differentiation factors are of high molecular weight. Mast cells also express mRNA for granulocyte macrophage colony-stimulating factor (GM-CSF) and interleukin-4 (Il-4) and may thus interfere with the growth of inflammatory cells and class switching. In this regard Il-4, Il-6, and CD23 are involved in IgE regulation. As to hypersensitivity reactions, environmental agents may either activate inflammatory cells directly or induce an IgE response or delayed-type hypersensitivity (DTH) reaction either against the eliciting agent directly or against unrelated factors. The purpose of our study was to elucidate the effects of different environmental agents on cellular responses and inflammatory mediator release. In extension we demonstrated that polychlorinated biphenyls (PCBs) also induce and modulate the generation of lipoxygenase products, such as leukotrienes and hydroxyeicosatetraenoic acids (HETEs), from different human cells (platelets, polymorphonuclear granulocytes, and monocytes) under noncytotoxic conditions. Various PCB congeners were potent inducers of platelet aggregation, serotonin release, and 12-HETE generation. Furthermore, when platelets were incubated with PCBs, the enzymatic steps controlling the metabolism of PAF were modulated. With regard to lymphocyte functions (e.g., proliferation, synthesis of Ig, and expression of CD23 and CD25), the various PCB isomers showed differential effects. A direct relationship between the extent of cell activation and the chlorosubstitution pattern of PCBs exists. Our results clearly emphasize that environmental agents, such as pesticides and PCBs, induce and modulate both mediator release and cytokines involved in acute and chronic inflammatory disease processes.

Introduction

A variety of chemical and environmental agents are able to impair the functional integrity of the immune system. They may influence one or more components and thus interfere with the balanced system of host defense and the ability to resist infection and malignant disease. Environmental agents do not necessarily express cytotoxic functions; but some of them lead to inflammatory, allergic, or pseudo-allergic reactions. Direct contact of inflammatory target cells with the environmental agent may induce the release of mediators as part of a pseudo-allergic reaction [5, 17]. Various cells, e.g., mast cells, neutrophil granulocytes, macrophages, lymphocytes, and platelets, are involved; during activation they are able to generate and/or release a variety of biologically active mediators including cytokines such as granulocyte/macrophage colony-stimulating factor (GM-CSF), and interleukins-1 – 10, as well as low molecular weight factors such as histamine, serotonin, prostaglandins, leukotrienes, and platelet-activating factor (PAF). These mediators modulate additional cellular responses, such as growth and differentiation and the generation and release of further mediators, and also participate in cell-cell interactions.

Previous results have demonstrated that pesticides, such as dieldrin, DDT, heptachlor, and heptachlor epoxide induce histamine release from rat mast cells and human basophils [17] and that the incubation of macrophages with polychlorinated cyclic hydrocarbons (γ-HCH) leads to the release of lipoxygenase products [10].

It was the purpose of our study to elucidate the effects of environmental agents, in particular polychlorinated biphenyls (PCBs), on cellular responses and inflammatory mediator release from different human cells.

Properties of PCBs

Since 1970, PCBs have been recognized as potential environmental and occupational hazards [22]. PCB refers to 209 possible chlorobiphenyl isomers with different numbers of chlorine atoms attached to the basic biphenyl structure [1] (Fig. 1). Commercial PCBs are mixtures of these various isomers. PCBs are stable, fat soluble substances that are poorly excreted from the body. In commercial use they have been employed in capacitors and transformers; as plasticizers in paints, inks, and paper; as hydraulic fluids and as heat transfer fluids. PCBs are poisonously inert chemicals; due to their stability and lipophilicity they accumulate in the environment and within the organism. Biomagnification of PCBs discharged into the environment, coupled with the contamination of food from packaging, containing PCBs, has resulted in over 90% of the general population having detectable levels of PCB in their adipose tissue. Fat levels of PCB are 300 – 400 times higher than serum levels.

In addition to their carcinogenic potential, these compounds also elicit numerous toxic effects including immunosuppression with thymic atrophy, edema, hyperkeratosis, hepatotoxicity, and lethality [9]. In humans, the most characteris-

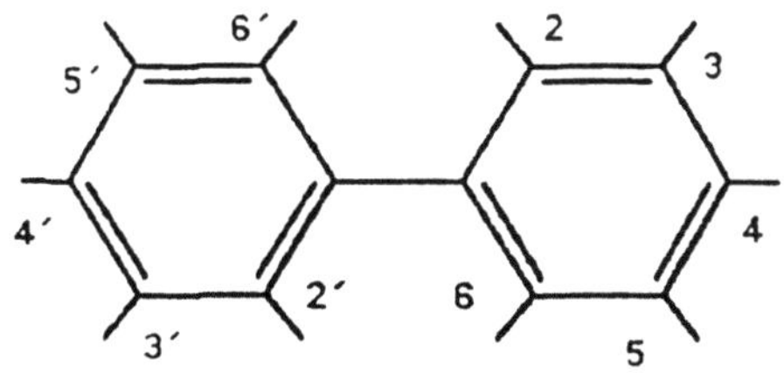

Fig. 1. Basic structure of polychlorinated biphenyls (PCBs)

tic and frequently observed lesion produced by chlorinated aromatic hydrocarbons, such as PCBs, is chloracne.

Studies with single PCB congeners in various systems have indicated a correlation with both the percent chlorine content and the chlorine substitution pattern. Chlorination of PCB congeners in the meta and para position is associated not only with a slow rate of elimination and a tendency to accumulate in tissue, but also with greater toxicity. Accordingly, PCB congeners chlorinated in both the meta and para position (3,3′, 4,4′-TCB and 3,3′, 4,4′, 5,5′-HCB) are among the most potent toxic PCB congeners [12, 19, 20].

In general, the structural characteristics of PCB congeners related to their slow elimination are also positively correlated with binding to the cytosolic "aryl hydrocarbon (AH) receptor", an event which has been postulated to be of critical importance for initiation of the toxic effects of PCBs and other halogenated aromatic compounds. In their planar conformations, PCBs which are strictly aryl hydrocarbon hydrolase (AHH) inducers are isosteric with 2,3,7,8-tetrachlorodibenzo-*p*-dioxin (TCDD).

For our study PCBs were dissolved in methanol and 10 μl of the methanolic solution were added to the cell suspension (700 μl). The following maximal concentrations were tested: 3,3′-DCB, 1 mg/l; 2,4,4′-TCB, 0.085 mg/l; 2,2′,3,3′-TCB, 0.034 mg/l; 3,3′,4,4′-PCB, 0.175 mg/l; 2,2′,4,5,5′-PCB, 0.031 mg/l; and 2,2′,4,4′,5,5′-HCB, 0.088 mg/l. The various concentrations resulted from the different water solubility of the PCBs. The effects of $1-0.1\ \mu M$ of the test compounds were then determined.

Effect of PCBs on Chemiluminescence and Leukotriene Generation in Human Polymorphonuclear Neutrophil Leukocytes

Neutrophils represent the first line of defense against invading microorganisms. In this regard the primary function of the neutrophil is phagocytosis, killing, and digestion of microorganisms. At the inflammatory site, phagocytosis is facilitated by humoral substances and opsonins such as IgG or C3b. Phagocytosis and activation of particular receptors stimulate numerous intracellular events including G protein involvement, calcium mobilization, phosphoinositol, turnover, and protein kinase C activation and lead to oxygen consumption, glycogenolysis, glucose oxidation via the hexose monophosphate shunt, exocytosis of acid hydrolases and

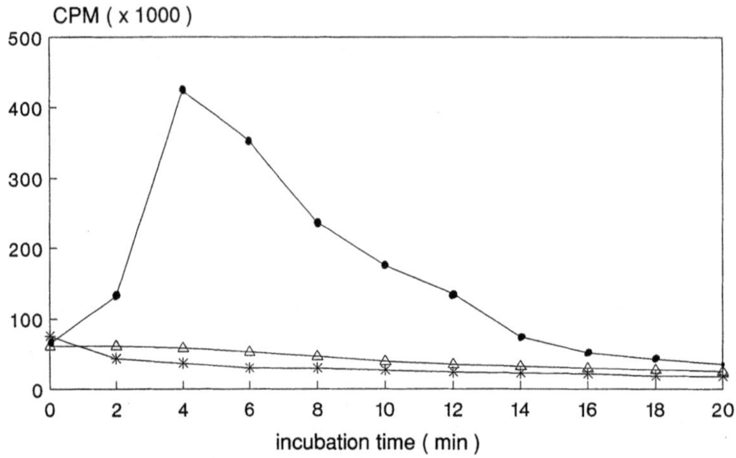

Fig. 2. Effects of PCBs on the luminol-dependent chemiluminescence response of neutrophils. PMNs (1×10^6 in 270 μl phosphate-buffered saline) were incubated in the presence of calcium (1 m*M*), magnesium (0.5 m*M*), and luminol with either the various PCBs (10 μl) or with the same volume of methanol as a control. —△— control; —●— 3,3′,4,4′-TCB; —★— 2,2′,3,3′-TCB

proteases, and generation of lipid mediators. A result of such cell activation is the respiratory burst and generation of oxygen radicals.

To analyze the effects of PCBs on the chemiluminescence response human polymorphonuclear neutrophil leukocytes (PMNs) (1×10^6 in 270 μl buffer) were incubated in the presence of calcium (1 m*M*), magnesium (0.5 m*M*), and luminol with either different PCBs (10 μl) or the same volume of methanol (control). Incubation of the PMNs with 3,3′,4,4′-TCB (0.175 mg/l = 0.6 μ*M*) induced chemiluminescence, with an early maximum response after 4 min of incubation followed by a slow decrease (Fig. 2). The baseline level was reached after 15 min of incubation. The remaining PCB congeners, at various concentrations, or the addition of methanol by itself did not lead to a significant response. Incubation of neutrophils with 3,3′,4,4′-TCB over 5 min significantly reduced the subsequent chemiluminescence induced by opsonized zymosan (2 mg) as compared to the methanol control.

It is well established that upon stimulation granulocytes generate free arachidonic acid from phospholipids: arachidonic acid is predominantly converted into lipoxygenase products, i.e., the biologically active leukotrienes (LTs). The biosynthesis of LTs is initiated in a lipoxygenase type reaction leading to 5-hydroperoxyeicosatetraenoic acid (5-HPETE). This product is the precursor of 5-hydroxyeicosatetraenoic acid (5-HETE) and LTA_4. LTA_4 may be hydrolyzed to LTB_4 or nonenzymatically to other dihydroxy acids. Alternatively, LTA_4 may conjugate with glutathione to produce LTC_4. LTC_4 is transformed to LTD_4 and LTE_4. LTB_4, the major lipoxygenase product of human neutrophils, is a chemotactic and chemokinetic agent for granulocytes, monocytes, and macrophages [2, 11] and affects several functions of human lymphocytes, including enhancement of natural killer cell activities and involvement in T cell activation, by providing regulatory signals [18]. The ω-oxidated LTB_4 metabolites (20-OH-LTB_4 and 20-COOH-LTB_4) have diminished biological activities.

Experiments were then performed to analyze the capability of the various PCB isomers to activate and/or modulate LT generation from human granulocytes. PMNs (1×10^7) were incubated in the presence of calcium and magnesium with the different PCBs (at a wide concentration range) or methanol (as control) over various times at 37 °C. Our data demonstrate that the PCBs alone, in the absence of any additional stimuli, were not sufficient to induce LT generation.

Insignificant amounts of lactate dehydrogenase (less than 5%) were released from the cells under these conditions; the results suggest that the cells remained intact during incubation and stimulation with the indicated PCBs. We then examined the modulatory capacity of PCBs in combination with additional cell stimuli such as opsonized zymosan, the calcium ionophore A23187, and the G protein activator sodium fluoride (NaF) on LT formation in human PMNs. For this purpose cells were incubated simultaneously with opsonized zymosan (2 mg) [16] and the respective PCBs for 30 min at 37 °C. The incubation of opsonized zymosan in the presence of the same volume of methanol instead of PCBs served as control (Fig. 3). Generation of LTs was analyzed by reverse phase high-performance liquid chromatography (RP-HPLC) [10]. The addition of opsonized zymosan and PCBs increased the generation of LTs as compared to the control. A comparison of the different PCBs showed that 3,3′,4,4′-TCB activity exceeded that of the remaining congeners. The other PCBs did not affect LTB_4 formation.

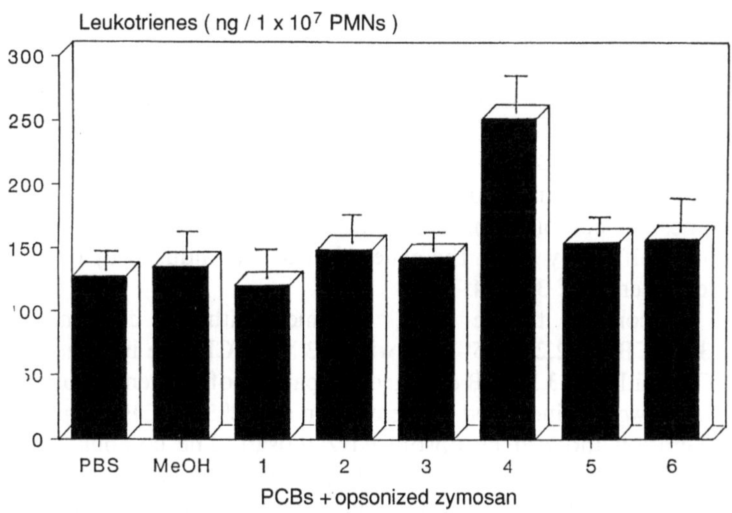

Fig. 3. Incubation of PMNs in the presence of PCBs with opsonized zymosan. PMNs (1×10^7), in the presence of calcium (1 m*M*) and magnesium (0.5 m*M*), were incubated simultaneously with opsonized zymosan (2 mg) and phosphate buffered saline (*PBS*) or the respective PCBs for 30 min at 37 °C. The incubation of opsonized zymosan in the presence of the same volume of methanol instead of PCBs served as a control. Leukotriene generation was measured by RP-HPLC; $n = 3$, mean ± SD. *1* = 3,3′-DCB; *2* = 2,4,4′-TCB; *3* = 2,2′,3,3′-TCB; *4* = 3,3′,4,4′-TCB; *5* = 2,2′,4,5,5′-PCB; *6* = 2,2′,4,4′,5,5′-HCB

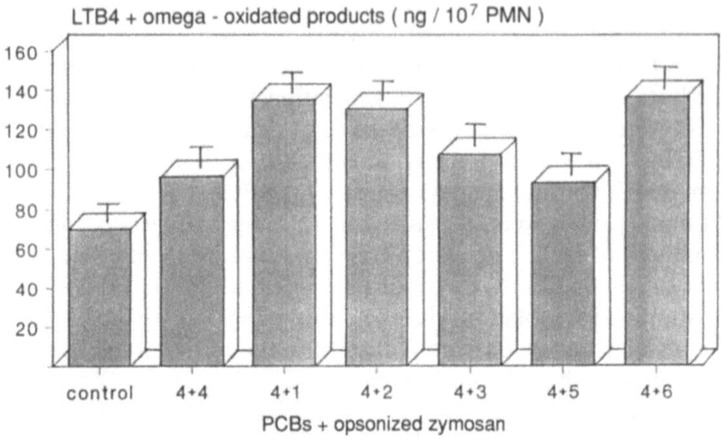

Fig. 4. Combined effects of two different PCBs on leukotriene generation induced by opsonized zymosan. PMNs (1×10^7) were incubated simultaneously with opsonized zymosan (2 mg), 3,3′,4,4′-TCB (4) (10 μl), and the respective PCBs (10 μl) for 30 min at 37 °C. Incubation with opsonized zymosan in the presence of methanol (20 μl) instead of the PCB combination served as a control. Leukotriene generation was measured by RP-HPLC ($n = 3$, mean ± SD). *1* = 3,3′-DCB; *2* = 2,4,4′-TCB; *3* = 2,2′,3,3′-TCB; *4* = 3,3′,4,4′-TCB; *5* = 2,2′,4,5,5′-PCB; *6* = 2,2′,4,4′,5,5′-HCB

Our data clearly demonstrate that pretreatment of PMNs with PCBs, in particular 3,3′,4,4′-TCB, enhances LT generation induced by opsonized zymosan. Our subsequent experiments were then designed to study the combined effects of two different PCBs on LT generation induced by opsonized zymosan. For this purpose PMNs (1×10^7) were incubated simultaneously with opsonized zymosan, 3,3′,4,4′-TCB, or 2,2′,3,3′-TCB and the respective PCBs for 30 min at 37 °C. Incubation of the cells with opsonized zymosan in the presence of methanol instead of the PCB combination served as the control (Fig. 4). Incubation of neutrophils with 3,3′,4,4′-TCB in combination with 3,3′-DCB, 2,3,3′-TCB, or 2,2′,4,4′,5,5′-HCB increased the generation of LTs as compared to incubation with 3,3′,4,4′-TCB alone. The combination of 3,3′,4,4′-TCB with 2,2′,3,3′-TCB or 2,2′,4,5,5′-PCB did not significantly affect the generation of LTs induced by opsonized zymosan in the presence of 3,3′,4,4′-TCB.

In contrast to the effects obtained with the combination of 3,3′-DCB-2,3,3′-TCB, or 2,2′,4,5,5′-PCB with 3,3′,4,4′-TCB, the incubation of the indicated PCBs with 2,2′,3,3′-TCB changed the pattern of LT generation in a different manner. A twofold increased concentration of 2,2′,3,3′-TCB completely suppressed LT generation induced by opsonized zymosan. The combination of 2,2′,3,3′-TCB, 2,4,4′-TCB, and 2,2′,4,4′, 5,5′-HCB enhanced the generation of LTs as compared to the effect of 2,2′,3,3′-TCB alone; in comparison to the control, a reduction was observed. No significant changes were obtained when 2,2′,4,5,5′-PCB and 3,3′-DCB were combined with 2,2′,3,3′-TCB. Only the combination of 2,2′,3,3′-TCB with 3,3′,4,4′-TCB resulted in a significant enhancement of LT generation induced by opsonized zymosan.

In a previous publication [3] we demonstrated that fluoride ions (NaF) are potent stimuli for LT generation from PMNs due to the activation of G proteins.

We then studied the modulatory effect of PCBs on LT generation induced after stimulation with NaF. Addition of NaF and 3,3'-DCB, 2,2',3,3'-TCB, and 3,3',4,4'-TCB had an inhibitory effect on LT generation as compared to NaF stimulation in the absence of PCBs. No significant changes were observed when the remaining PCBs were combined with NaF as a stimulus. Incubation of PMNs with PCBs had no significant effect on LT generation induced by the calcium ionophore A23187 as compared to the methanol control.

The effects described here pertain only to neutrophils. PCBs at the described concentrations did not change LT formation in a human lymphocyte, monocyte, or basophil suspension.

Effect of PCBs on Human Platelets

Platelets play a vital role in hemostasis and thrombosis [7]. They respond to a wide variety of stimuli by changing their shape and releasing their granules (e.g., serotonin). In the presence of calcium ions they aggregate. They also produce and metabolize bioactive mediators such as 12-HETE and PAF.

The purpose of the subsequent experiments was to elucidate the effects of the PCB congeners with regard to different platelet responses [15]. Stimulation of human platelets with thrombin (2.5 U/ml) caused aggregation as recorded by a change in light transmission. A comparable aggregation was observed when platelets were incubated with 3,3',4,4'-TCB. The aggregation peak induced by 3,3',4,4'-TCB reached about 80% of that of thrombin-induced aggregation. The other compounds (3,3'-DCB, 2,2',3,3'-TCB, and 2,2',4,5,5'-PCB) at various concentrations or the addition of methanol (10 μl as control) showed no effects.

Further on, we examined the capacity of PCBs to stimulate the release of serotonin (Fig. 5). Incubation of platelets with PCBs increased the release of serotonin as compared to the control. A comparison of the different PCBs with the other compounds showed that 3,3',4,4'-TCB was a potent, dose-dependent inducer of serotonin release. In addition to the release of serotonin platelets were able to generate and metabolize newly generated mediators, such as the 12-lipoxygenase products (12-HETE) and the platelet-activating factor (PAF).

In order to analyze the metabolism of PAF, platelets (1×10^8) were preincubated for 2 min at 37 °C with [^{3}H]PAF (0.74 kBq); subsequently the various PCBs, the same volume of methanol (as control), or A23187 (5 μ*M*) were added and incubation proceeded for an additional 20 min. Platelets metabolize exogenously added PAF into lyso-PAF and alkyl-acyl-GPC. After 20 min of incubation in the presence of the ionophore more than 75% of the PAF was metabolized and alkyl-acyl-GPC was the main metabolite; only minute amounts of lyso-PAF were detected. Platelets incubated with methanol (10 μl) metabolize 60% of PAF into lyso-PAF (20%) and alkyl-acyl-glycero-3-phosphocholine (GPC) (40%). In contrast, incubation of platelets with PCBs decreased the metabolism of exogenously added [^{3}H]PAF to [^{3}H]lyso-PAF and [^{3}H]alkyl-acyl-GPC. The results thus suggest that the incubation of platelets with PCBs affects the enzymatic steps in-

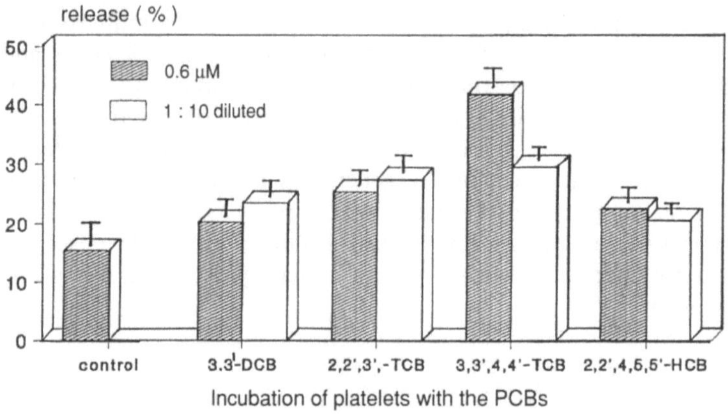

Fig. 5. Effects of PCBs on serotonin release in human platelets. [^{3}H]Serotonin-labeled platelets (1×10^8) were incubated with the indicated PCBs for 20 min at 37 °C. The released amount of serotonin was calculated as a percentage of the total radioactivity present in the supernatant and cell pellet. The data represent the means (±SD) of three independent experiments

volved in the metabolism of PAF; the activities of the enzymes acetylhydrolase and acyltransferase were decreased.

Experiments were then carried out to analyze the effects of PCB incubation on 12-HETE formation in platelets. Platelets are the major source of 12-HETE, which is a potent chemokinetic compound for neutrophils and which may mediate leukocyte diapedesis through the vascular endothelium. Human platelets (1×10^8) were incubated with either the indicated PCBs, a combination of two PCBs, or the same volume of methanol (as control) for 20 min at 37 °C (Fig. 6).

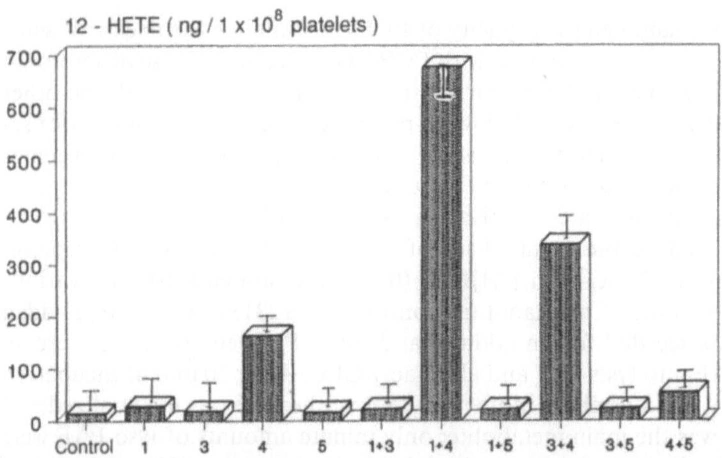

Fig. 6. Effects of PCB incubation on 12-HETE formation in platelets. The cells (1×10^8) were incubated with either the indicated PCBs, a combination of two PCBs, or the same volume of methanol (control) for 20 min at 37 °C. 12-HETE generation was measured by RP-HPLC. The data are expressed as the mean ± SD of three independent experiments. *1* = 3,3′-DCB; *3* = 2,2′,3,3′-TCB; *4* = 3,3′,4,4′-TCB; *5* = 2,2′,4,5,5′-PCB

As is apparent, the generation of 12-HETE was significantly enhanced when the platelets were stimulated with 3,3′,4,4′-TCB. In contrast, 3,3′-DCB, 2,2′,3,3′-TCB, and 2,2′,4,5,5′-PCB were not effective. The combination of 3,3′-DCB or 2,2′,3,3′-TCB with 3,3′,4,4′-TCB resulted in a synergistic effect with regard to 12-HETE generation. Incubation of platelets with 3,3′,4,4′-TCB in combination with 2,2′,4,5,5′-PCB led to less 12-HETE formation than incubation with 3,3′,4,4′-TCB alone. No significant changes were observed when the remaining PCBs were combined and analyzed.

We then studied the modulatory effect of PCBs on 12-HETE generation induced after stimulation with NaF. Platelets were incubated simultaneously with NaF (20 m*M*) and the respective PCBs for 20 min at 37 °C. Incubation of NaF in the presence of the same volume of methanol instead of the PCBs served as a control. Addition of NaF and PCBs had an enhanced effect on 12-HETE generation as compared to NaF stimulation in the absence of PCBs. A synergistic effect was obtained by a combination of NaF and PCBs.

The enhanced 12-HETE generation in the presence of a G protein activator (NaF) and PCBs suggests that more than one signal transduction pathway is apparently involved in 12-HETE generation.

Effects of PCBs on Lymphocyte Functions

In a series of experiments we analyzed the effects of PCBs on lymphocyte responses such as proliferation and CD25 and CD23 expression. When human peripheral blood lymphocytes (PBL) were cultured for 3 days in the presence of PCBs or methanol (control) no significant effects with regard to proliferation were obtained.

Incubation of PBL for 3 days with PCBs in the presence of mitogens such as pokeweed mitogen (PWM), phytohemagglutinin (PHA), or *Staphylococcus aureus* Cowan I (SAC), a B cell-specific mitogen, affected lymphocyte proliferation as compared to the control. 3,3′,4,4′-TCB decreased proliferation and the inhibitory effect was independent of the mitogen used for stimulation (Table 1).

Table 1. Proliferation of peripheral blood lymphocytes in the presence of PCBs.

PCB	PCBs + SAC (1 : 10000)[a] (%)	PCBs + PHA (30 μg/ml)[b] (%)
MeOH (control)	100 ± 4	100 ± 6
3,3′-DCB	106 ± 18	138 ± 31
2,4,4′-TCB	98 ± 14	116 ± 28
2,2,3,3′-TCB	89 ± 23	132 ± 456
3,3′,4,4′-TCB	32 ± 22*	76 ± 15*
2,2′,4,5,5′-PCB	54 ± 57	185 ± 175
2,2′,4,4′,5,5′-HCB	56 ± 46	202 ± 40

SAC, *Staphylococcus aureus* Cowan I; PHA, phytohemaglutinin.
[a] 100% = 2000 – 3000 cpm; $n = 3$, mean ± SD.
[b] 100% = 5000 – 7000 cpm; $n = 3$, mean ± SD.
* Indicates a significant difference as compared to the control.

In subsequent experiments the effects of PCBs on the expression of the T cell-activation marker CD25 (Tac antigen [18]) were determined. In the presence of 3,3′,4,4′-TCB, increased expression of CD25 observed.

Preliminary results with regard to the effect of PCBs on CD23 expression were obtained. The CD23 antigen represents an activation marker which is expressed during the early stages of B cell maturation [8]. It serves as the low affinity receptor for IgE and the low molecular weight B cell growth factor (LMW-BCGF) [4, 6]. CD23 is up-regulated upon stimulation of B cells with cytokines (interleukin-4, interleukin-2) [14]. Our data demonstrate that in the presence of 3,3′,4,4′-TCB the expression of CD23 on PBLs was decreased.

Concluding Remarks

Defined PCBs initiate and/or modulate responses of human blood cells. Incubation of platelets with PCBs decreased the metabolism of exogenously added radiolabeled PAF to lyso-PAF and alkyl-acyl-GPC. The data suggest that incubation of platelets with PCBs modulates the enzymatic steps required for PAF metabolism; the activities of the enzymes acetylhydrolase and acyltransferase were decreased. The PCB congener 3,3′,4,4′-TCB, with chlorosubstitution in two para and two meta positions, is more potent in platelet aggregation, serotonin release and 12-HETE generation than the other PCBs. In combination with these other PCBs, 3,3′,4,4′-TCB showed synergistic effects, such as enhanced formation of 12-HETE, LTB_4 and ω-oxidation products, when 3,3′-DCB and 2,2′,3,3′-TCB were applied simultaneously. The combined incubation of platelets with PCBs and NaF, an activator of G proteins, resulted in synergistic 12-HETE generation as compared to stimulation with NaF or PCBs alone. The simultaneous incubation of PMNs with NaF and 3,3′-DCB, 3,3′,4,4′-TCB, and 2,2′,3,3′-TCB-inhibited LT generation compared to NaF stimulation in the absence of PCBs. PCBs alone, in the absence of any additional stimuli, were not sufficient to induce LT generation. The combination of opsonized zymosan and PCBs increased the generation of LTs. The activity of 3,3′,4,4′-TCB exceeded that of the other congeners in a dose-dependent manner.

Due to the strong lipophilic character of PCBs they interact with cellular membranes, but the precise mechanisms of either PCB-cell interaction of the subsequent stimulation of the signal transduction sequence are unknown. Our data show a direct relationship between the extent of cell stimulation and the chlorosubstitution pattern (3,3′,4,4′-TCB vs 2,2′,4,4′-TCB).

Whether PCBs might be involved in the induction and modulation of pseudoallergic reactions must be clarified in future studies.

References

1. Ballschmitter K, Zell M (1980) Analysis of polychlorinated biphenyls (PCB) by glass capillary gas chromatography: composition of technical Arochlor and Clophen-PCB mixture. Z Anal Chem 302:20–31

2. Bray MA (1986) Leukotrienes in inflammation. Agents Actions 19:87–99
3. Brom C, Köller M, Brom J, König W (1989) Effect of sodium fluoride on the generation of lipoxygenase products from human polymorphonuclear granulocytes, mononuclear cells and platelets – indication for the involvement of G proteins. Immunology 68:240–246
4. Bujanowski-Weber J, Brings B, Knöller I, Pfeil T, König W (1989) Expression of the low affinity receptor for IgE ($Fc_\varepsilon RII$, CD23) and IgE-BF (soluble CD23) release by lymphoblastoid B cell line RPMI 8866 and human peripheral lymphocytes of normal and atopic donors. Immunology 66:505–511
5. Diel F, Neidhardt B, Opree W (1981) Application of rat mast cell incubated as a possible short-time test for sensitizing occupational agents. Int Arch Occup Environ Health 48:369–375
6. Gordon J, Webb AJ, Walker L, Guy GR, Rowe M (1986) Evidence for an association between CD23 and the receptor for a low molecular weight B cell growth factor. Eur J Immunol 16: 1627–1639
7. Kienast J, Arount J, Pfliegler G, Deckmyn H, Hoet B, Vermylen J (1987) Sodium flouride mimics effects of both agonists and antagonists on intact human platelets by simultaneous modulation of phospholipase C and adenylate cyclase activity. Blood 69:859–866
8. Kikutani J, Suemura M, Barsumian EJ, Hardy RR, Kishimoto T (1986) Fc_ε receptor, a specific differentiation marker transiently expressed on mature B cells before isotype switching. J Exp Med 164:1455–1469
9. Kimbrough RD (1987) Human health effects of polychlorinated biphenyls (PCBs) and polybrominated biphenyls (PBBS). Annu Rev Pharmacol Toxicol 27:87–111
10. Knöller J, Schönfeld W, Köller M, Hensler T, König W (1988) Arachidonic acid metabolites from polymorphonuclear leukocytes of healthy donors, severely burned patients and children with cystic fibrosis. Routine monitoring by high-performance liquid chromatography. J Chromatography 427:199–208
11. König W, Schönfeld W, Raulf M, Köller M, Knöller J, Scheffer J, Brom J (1990) The neutrophil and leukotrienes – role in health and disease. Eicosanoids 31:22
12. McKinney JD, Chae K, McConnell EE, Birnbaum LS (1985) Structure-induction versus structure-toxicity relationships for polychlorinated biphenyls and related hydrocarbons. Environ Health Perspect 60:57–68
13. Meade CJ, Harvey J, Boot JR, Turner GA, Bateman PE, Osborne DJ (1984) γ-Hexachlorocyclohexane stimulation of macrophage phospholipid hydrolysis and leukotriene production. Biochem Pharmacol 33:289–293
14. Pfeil T, Fischer A, Bujanowski-Weber J, Luther H, Altmeyer P, König W (1989) Effects of cytokines on spontaneous and allergen induced CD23 expression, CD23 release and Ig(E,G) synthesis from peripheral blood lymphocytes. Immunology 68:37–45
15. Raulf M, König W (1991) In vitro effects of polychlorinated biphenyls on human platelets. Immunology 72:287–291
16. Raulf M, Stüning M, König W (1986) Effect of cations on leukotriene release – requirements for the peptidoleukotrienes (leukotriene C4, D4) by human polymorphonuclear granulocytes. Immunology 58:479–487
17. Rohr U, König W, Selenka F (1985) Influence of pesticides on the release of histamine, chemotactic factors and leukotrienes from rat mast cells and human basophils. Zentralbl Bakteriol Mikrobiol Hyg [B] 181:469–486
18. Rola-Pleszcynski M (1985) Immunoregulation of leukotrienes and other lipoxygenase metabolites. Immunol Today 6:302–307
19. Safe S, Robertson LW, Safe L, Parkinson A, Bandiera S, Sawyer T, Campbell MA (1982) Halogenated biphenyls: molecular toxicology. Can J Physiol Pharmacol 60:1057–1064
20. Safe S, Bandiera S, Sawyer T, Robertson L, Safe L, Parkinson A, Thomas PE, Ryan DE, Reik LM, Levin W, Denomme MA, Fujita T (1985) PCBs: structure-function relationships and mechanism of action. Environ Health Perspect 60:47–56
21. Uchiyama T, Broder S, Waldmann TA (1981) A monoclonal antibody (anti-TAC) reactive with activated and functionally mature human T cells. J Immunol 126:1293–1297
22. Wolff MS, Thorntor J, Fischbein A, Lilis R, Silikoff IJ (1982) Disposition of polychlorinated biphenyls congeners in occupationally exposed persons. Toxicol Appl Pharmacol 62:294–299

The "Clinical Ecology Syndrome" ("Eco-Syndrome"): Psychology or Allergy?

J. Ring[1,2], D. Vieluf[1,2], B. Przybilla[2], G. Gabriel[2], M. von Rad[3], and O. Braun-Falco[2]

[1]Universitäts-Hautklinik und Allergie-Abteilung, Universitäts-Krankenhaus Eppendorf, University of Hamburg, Martinistrasse 52, W-2000 Hamburg 20, Federal Republic of Germany
[2]Dermatologische Klinik und Poliklinik der Ludwig-Maximilians-Universität München, Frauenlobstrasse 9–11, W-8000 München 2, Federal Republic of Germany
[3]Psychosomatische Abteilung des Klinikums rechts der Isar, Technische Universität München, Langerstrasse 13, W-8000 München 80, Federal Republic of Germany

Abstract

In the allergist's practice in past years, an increasing number of patients suffering from polysomatic complaints with a subjective feeling of allergy against environmental noxious agents have been seen. We have suggested as a "working diagnosis" the term clinical ecology syndrome (eco-syndrome) for this group of patients.

Although often clearly evident at the first consultation, the patients usually deny relevant psychosomatic interactions. We examined 30 patients (20 females and 10 males) with this "syndrome", applying intensive allergological investigations including placebo-controlled oral challenge tests with food additives together with careful interdisciplinary investigations (internal medicine, otolaryngology, gynecology, dental medicine as well as psychosomatic medicine). Most of the patients complained of various subjective symptoms (average seven) involving several organ systems (average three). Some 65% of the patients had suffered from atopic diseases themselves and in 77% it was part of the personal and/or family history. Some 60% of the patients showed positive skin prick tests against common food and airborne allergens. In oral provocation procedures 13% were clearly positive to certain foods, 10% to food additives, and 13% to drugs (mostly mild analgesics). In 7% focal infections of clinical relevance for the given complaints were detected and treated successfully. In 60% of the patients psychiatric or psychosomatic disturbances were obvious. When among the numerous diagnoses a list of the major pathophysiological conditions relevant for the given complaints was established, "psychogenic condition" and "allergy" were represented with 60% or 40% respectively; it was found that 47% of the patients suffered mainly from severe psychosomatic disorder, 10% from manifest endogenous psychoses, 33% from allergic or pseudo-allergic reactions, one patient from pension neurosis (3%) and 7% from focal infectious disease.

We conclude from our experience that these very difficult patients need the concentrated efforts of an experienced allergist in an interdisciplinary approach. Exhausting all options, including placebo-controlled provocation tests, the existence of possible hypersensitivity reactions – both allergic and pseudo-allergic in origin – has to be excluded before fruitful cooperation with an experienced psychiatrist or psychologist can be started.

Introduction

Few medical problems of our time are being discussed as emotionally as the connection between environmental pollution and allergy [8, 21, 27, 31, 32, 38, 47, 65, 68, 71, 85, 103, 115]. Often the suspected or proven increase in the prevalence of allergic diseases is regarded without further questioning as a consequence of environmental pollution [4, 10, 25, 46], leading to increasing anxiousness in the population [4]. In the allergist's practice in past years, an increasing number of patients suffering from polysomatic complaints with a subjective feeling of "allergy against environmental noxious agents" have been seen [17, 31, 38, 71, 81, 99, 103].

We have suggested as a "working diagnosis" the term clinical ecology syndrome (eco-syndrome) [84, 87] for this group of patients, since a certain "alternative" movement in medicine calling itself "clinical ecology" uses similar arguments to describe almost any impairment of well-being as an allergy, most commonly against environmental pollutants, preferable in foods [12, 20, 56, 72–74]. According to this theory in particular psychological abnormalities including manifest psychotic diseases are regarded as food allergies.

Many of these patients have frequented special institutes where they have been strongly influenced such that they believe in these ideas even more, i.e., positive reinforcement. Some patients have experienced short-term improvement after such visits, however, followed by long-term deteriorations. Many, almost all, patients have undergone several psychiatric treatments, but deny the diagnosis in this area.

Definition

Our working diagnosis, clinical ecology syndrome (eco-syndrome), comprises patients with polysomatic complaints with suspected "allergy against environmental pollutants" [84, 87].

In many patients routine allergy tests do not yield positive results and patients are referred to a psychiatrist with the remark "no evidence for allergy". They then feel frustrated and misunderstood; a major problem of these patients seems to be the feeling of "not being taken seriously". Similar cases have been reported as environmental illness [103], allergy to the 20th century [4, 17] or total allergy syndrome [64].

In the following the clinical symptomatology and both somatic and psychosomatic findings together with allergological test results obtained in 30 patients with this "syndrome" will be briefly presented. A detailed analysis of these data has been published previously [87].

Clinical Symptoms

The most important clinical characteristics are shown in Table 1. There was a predominance of the female sex with a ratio of 2:1 and a predilection of the age group between the ages of 35 and 50 years. The subjective (Table 2) and objective (Table 3) symptoms comprised various organs and a multitude of different symptoms. The most frequently suspected noxious agents are shown in Table 4.

Many patients had completed an odyssey of visiting various specialists and had undergone many kinds of so-called alternative or parascientific procedures (Table 5).

Table 1. "Clinical Ecology Syndrome" ("Eco-Syndrome"): Clinical data of 30 patients.

Age: 16 – 56 years (median 44 y)		
Sex: 20 f., 10 m.		
Duration of symptoms:	0.3 – 29 years	(median 6 y)
Number of subjective symptoms:	2 – 16	(median 7)
Number of objective symptoms:	0 – 5	(median 1)
Organs involved:	2 – 6	(median 3)
Observation period:	1 – 4 years	

Table 2. Subjective symptoms in 30 patients with "Clinical Ecology Syndrome".

Itch	Nausea	Headache
Burning eyes	Meteorism	Fatigue
Hoarseness	Abdominal pain	Tension
Nasal obstruction	Diarrhoea (suspected)	Vertigo
Dyspnoe	Obstipation	Anxiousness
Joint pain	Back pain	Loss of sleep
Hair loss		Loss of memory
		Difficulties to concentrate
		Paraesthesia
		Psychic alteration

Table 3. Objective symptoms in 30 patients with "Clinical Ecology Syndrome".

Physical:	Abdominal pain on pressure	(20%)
	Renal percussion pain	(7%)
Dermatological:	Allergic contact eczema	7%
	Atopic eczema	7%
	Chronic urticaria	3%
	Relapsing flush	3%
	Acne (papulo pustular)	3%
	Venous ulcer	3%
Laboratory:	Bacteriuria [a]	53%
	Leukocyturia [a]	17%
	ESR elevation [a]	20%
	Leukocytosis	3%
	Liver enzymes elevated	3%

[a] in 1 patient regarded to be relevant for major complaints.

Table 4. Clinical Ecology Syndrome: Most frequently suspected noxious agents.

Car exhaust
Pesticides
Formalin
Preservatives
Organic solvents
Detergents
Electromagnetic irradiation

Table 5. Alternative/parascientific procedures performed in previous history of 30 patients with "Clinical Ecology Syndrome".

Acupuncture
Homeopathy
Auraskopy
Cytotoxic food test
Hair mineral analysis
Radiaesthesia
Autologous urine injection
"Fresh cell" therapy
Detection of underground water or electromagnetic fields
Several, partly extreme diets

Most of the objective signs and symptoms were not considered relevant to the main complaints of the patients except for two patients with focal infection (one with pyelonephritis and one with maxillary osteomyelitis, where symptoms improved dramatically after medical or surgical treatment).

The Role of Allergy

In the genetic background, 57% of the patients had a personal history of atopic disease and 77% had either a personal and/or family history of atopy. In prick and/or intradermal tests with airborne and food allergens 60% of the patients showed positive test results (Table 6). Oral provocation tests (if possible placebo-controlled) revealed positive results in a significant number of patients reacting to foods, food additives or drugs (Table 7).

Psychosomatic Findings

In a detailed psychosomatic evaluation marked alterations were found in almost half of the patients, mostly in the sense of a depressive reaction, but also as manifest endogenous psychoses or other psychopathic conditions.

When among the numerous diagnoses a list of the major pathophysiological conditions relevant for the present complaints was established, it was found that 47% of the patients suffered mainly from severe psychosomatic disorders, 10%

Table 6. Skin test results in 30 patients with "Clinical Ecology Syndrome".

		% positive
Patch test:	Nickel sulfate	13
	Neomycin	7
	$HgCl_2$	3
	Total	23
Prick test:	Foods	33
	(additionally in intradermal test)	10
	House dust mite	30
	Pollen	27
	Animal epithelia	17
	Others	10
	Total	60

Table 7. Results of provocation tests in 30 patients with "Clinical Ecology Syndrome".

		% clearly positive[a]
Oral: Foods	– Fish	7
	– Cows milk	3
	– Potato	3
	– Mint tea	3
	Total	13
Additives:	– Colourings	10
	– So-Benzoate	7
	– $K_2S_2O_5$	7
	Total	10
Drugs:	– Analgesics[b]	13
	– Antibiotics	3
Subcutaneous:	– Local anesthetics	13
Nasal:	– House dust mite	0
Bronchial:	– Wild satin	3

[a] "Placebo background" subtracted.
[b] 2 additional patients (7%), showed weakly positive reactions to benzoates and sulfites.

from manifest endogenous psychoses, one patient from pension-neurosis, 33% from allergic or pseudo-allergic hypersensitivity reactions and 7% from focal infectious disease (Fig. 1).

In Table 8 a typical case report is given.

Interpretation of Allergy Test Results in Patients with Clinical Ecology Syndrome (Eco-Syndrome)

The results of our study have shown that although psychological abnormalities seem to be predominant in these patients, a careful general and allergological investigation had to be performed. In 40% of the patients' somatic pathophysiological conditions were regarded as predominant cause of the present complaints.

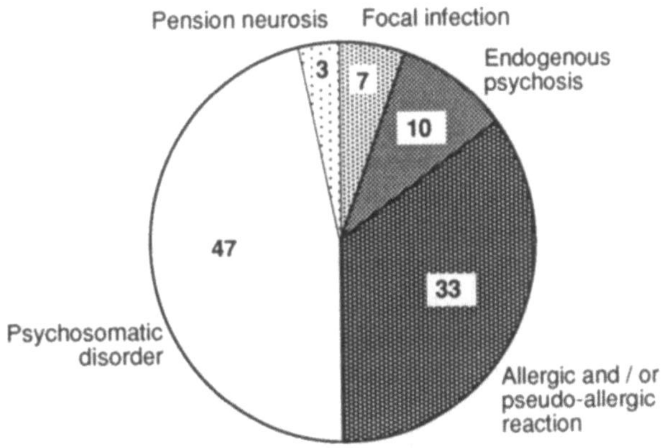

Fig. 1. Final "main" diagnoses (i.e., regarded as relevant for the major present complaints) in 30 patients with "clinical ecology syndrome" ("eco-syndrome")

Table 8. Case report.

Pat. R.S., female, 33 y
For 9 y fatigue, nausea, diarrhoea, hair loss, anxiousness due to "pollutants in food", restricted "bio"-diet. Pollinosis as child
General exam.: n.a.d., Routine lab.: n.a.d.
Skin test: (Prick) nuts + + +, (l.d.) milk + +, no late reactions
RAST: ∅
Oral provocation (foods and additives): fish (doubtful), "Placebo background"
Psychosomatics: Somatized depressive-hysteric neurosis (partner conflict)

Many patients, however, exhibited various pathophysiological patterns including somatic and psychosomatic alterations. Among the patients with predominant psychosomatic disease, not infrequently were positive allergy skin tests or provocation tests seen, especially against drugs.

The Role of Psychosomatic Factors

The high percentage of patients with an atopic diathesis in their personal or family history might explain why the psychosomatic alterations in these patients tend to find their somatic correlate in hypersensitivity reactions. The mechanism of an allergic reaction seems to be more tolerable to these patients than accepting a psychosomatic disease. On the other hand, the influence of psychosomatic interactions upon allergic reactions is wellknown [44, 45, 77, 81, 82, 86, 99, 101].

The most frequent psychosomatic diagnosis in these patients was a depressive reaction, more or less manifest. The patients tended to project the "evil principle" onto their environment rather than to look inside their own lives. Due to increasing pollution and an increasing public awareness of it [10, 17], environmental noxious agents became easily accessible in the patient's own argumentation. Most of these individuals perceive exhaust, pesticides, formaldehyde, detergents, preservatives, ionizing radiation or electromagnetic fields etc. as a threat to their well-being.

In two female patients there was a history of sexual abuse. Similar observations have been reported by J. Selner in Denver (pers. commun.). Furthermore, drug abuse has to be considered very carefully in the differential diagnosis of these patients.

In this context, the actual effect of air pollution on the psychological state of exposed people has to be discussed seriously. It has been reported that increased levels of air pollution can impair reaction time to visual stimuli as well as the ability to concentrate and general well-being [10]. These findings may be explained rather as an indicator of the effects of chronic stress [100] on cognitive functions than as evidence for the neurotoxic effects of pollutants on the central nervous system [10]. Increased air pollution levels, e.g., SO_2 concentrations, can act as a chronic stimulus and stressor leading to subclinical alterations in psychological functions [5, 10, 109].

Critical Remarks to the Ideas of Clinical Ecology

The theories of clinical ecology are not new, but derive from American allergology dating back to the 1920s [14, 26, 88, 89, 92–94]. The most important postulates state that almost any kind of impairment of "feeling well" is an "allergy" against some environmental substance, most commonly against a pollutant chemical, and that especially psychological abnormalities or psychiatric diseases are manifestations of allergic reactions most commonly to foods or chemicals in foods. The proponents of clinical ecology have so far failed to produce convincing evidence for these theories; their books mostly contain anecdotal reports.

The methods used by clinical ecologists seem – when regarded superficially – similar to those used in classical allergology, comprising skin test procedures, in vitro diagnostics and provocation tests. However, in practice and application as well as interpretation of the test results there are serious differences. Skin tests are performed in decreasing concentrations to find the so-called neutralizing dose. Positive skin tests are defined by the increase of wheal formation in a given time after injection of some allergen extract and not by controlled comparison with nonallergic volunteers.

In vitro diagnostics comprise the so-called cytotoxic food test and an IgG food allergy test. The detection of spermidin or cryptopyrrole in blood and urine as well as hair mineral analyses are performed in order to detect "imbalances" in the organism of possible relevance for the psychological abnormalities (code word "orthomolecular psychiatry"). Furthermore, many other so-called "alternative" therapeutic and diagnostic procedures are used also by clinical ecologists. Most of the diagnostic and therapeutic strategies advised or recommended by clinical ecology have been proven either unreliable or inefficient in large-scale controlled studies [2, 13, 16, 19, 32–34, 36, 40, 49, 50, 54, 55, 61, 62, 71, 95, 99, 103].

The hypothesis that environmental chemicals are damaging the human immune system in a way that hypersensitivity reactions against foods and other substances develop was thoroughly investigated by Terr [103] in 50 patients before and after the therapeutic intervention in a clinical ecology institution. Only two patients improved, while the condition of 26 patients remained unchanged; however, 22 patients showed clear-cut deterioration by clinical ecology therapy. There was no significant change in immunological parameters including T-cell counts and function during this period. All patients were suffering from panic fear of chemicals, foods, drugs, and odors.

The fact that the methods of clinical ecology have not shown convincing results should not be regarded as proof that environmental pollution has no role in the development of allergy. There are still a lot of problems in really elucidating these kinds of clinical and pathophysiological conditions. It is possible that certain forms of food hypersensitivity are not yet diagnosable with current methods [29, 37, 39, 40, 52, 59, 60, 104, 107, 110, 111], especially with regard to non-IgE-mediated reactions or some pseudo-allergic reactions with unknown elicitors.

Furthermore, the problem of false-negative tests has to be kept in mind; there can be false-negative provocation tests even when using the protocol of double-blind placebo-controlled food challenge, as shown with the method of intragastral provocation under endoscopic control (IPEC) [76] where strongly positive mucosal reactions in the gastrointestinal tract were observed after food provocation in patients without any subjective or objective general symptoms.

We do not have the tools and reagents necessary to diagnose allergic reactions against small chemicals, with the exception of some drugs and occupational substances such as penicillin or isocyanates etc. [6]. There is a need for hapten-protein conjugates for a whole variety of environmental noxious agents.

Furthermore, not enough is known about the neurotoxicology of many chemicals. Some studies have indeed shown central nervous system changes or migraine after intake of certain foods [23, 24, 42, 58, 64, 66]. Many foods contain vasoactive or psychoactive substances possibly leading to psychological effects in some individuals [1, 3, 15, 96, 112, 113].

Another major problem is the evaluation of the allergotoxicology of chemicals in the environment, namely, the property of certain substances to influence the process of allergic sensitization or reaction [7, 9].

The measurement of the chemicals in the environment, not only the air but also the ground, the food and the drinking water or the textiles etc. [5, 30, 53, 68, 75, 90, 91, 97, 98, 109] is yet another consideration.

Even if detection methods are now sensitive enough to measure low concentrations, still the final question of relevance of the detected chemical concentration for the patient is for most substances not answered.

Therefore it is possible that in some of these patients, even with strong psychosomatic overlap, true hypersensitivity reactions against hitherto unidentified substances are hidden. The problem of the influence of air pollution upon psychological well-being has already been discussed [10].

Environmental Pollution and Allergy

In the past years an increasing amount of evidence has been presented from clinical, epidemiological and experimental studies showing that there is a complex interaction between environmental pollution and allergic inflammatory reactions [9, 21, 48, 51, 65, 67, 75, 79, 81, 109, 114, 115]. Many of the classical pollutants have been shown to exert not only irritant effects but also enhancing activities regarding IgE-mediated sensitization: sulphur dioxide does not only provoke bronchial obstruction in a dose-dependent manner in most of the people with asthma, especially corticoid-dependent asthmatic patients [115], but also can elicit life-threatening anaphylactoid reactions after inhalation or oral administration [80, 83]. In experimental animals SO_2 has been found to enhance IgE-mediated sensitization to protein allergens [79].

Tobacco smoke has equally been found to be associated with increased IgE formation both in humans and in experimental animals [11, 114]. Smoking of the mother during pregnancy was associated with a significantly increased risk of atopic disease in the child in an epidemiological study [48].

Pesticides such as dieldrin, DDT, heptachlorepoxide and biphenyl were shown to induce histamine release from rat mast cells and human basophils in a dose-dependent and calcium-dependent manner; some pesticides also induced leukotriene secretion and platelet aggregation [75].

An epidemiological study from Japan has reported an increasing incidence of allergic rhinitis to Japanese Cedar pollen during the past 30 years; in the same period, SO_2 and CO as well as photochemical oxidant concentrations in the air have decreased. However, suspended particulate matter, most likely from car exhaust, has increased. These exhaust particles have been shown to enhance IgE antibody production of mice to ovalbumin in a dose dependent manner [65, 67].

The interaction of air pollutants and pollen allergens were studied by Behrendt et al. [9] who found an overall higher concentration of pollen counts in polluted areas than in rural regions with a preceding peak of SO_2 and NOX emission in the atmosphere. Pollen collected from highly polluted areas were found to be loaded with pollution particles consisting of anorganic and organic compounds adsorbed to the pollen surface. When pollen was incubated with dust particles from polluted areas, it was activated to release allergenic proteins [9].

In an epidemiological survey in Bavaria, FRG, there was no statistically significant correlation between indoor SO_2 and NOX exposure to prevalence of atopic diseases in children; however, there was a significant dependence of prevalence of atopic diseases from the living area which was not explained by SO_2, NOX and CO levels in the air, but rather suggested other yet unknown environmental factors [47].

These studies clearly show what tremendous efforts in research will have to be taken in order to elucidate the relation between environmental pollutants and allergy. Allergology is the discipline which has been dealing with environmental diseases for over a hundred years, distinguishing by scientific methods between general toxic effects and individual hypersensitivity reactions of various kinds. Regarding the multitude of chemicals – some experts speak of people being subjected to in 63000 substances in industrialized countries – one might be tempted to give up. However, we must remind ourselves of Charles Blackley who – 120 years ago – identified pollen as the cause of hay fever; there were critical opinions expressed those days by individuals who believed that it would never be possible to differentiate between the multitude of different pollens in the air. Yet, we

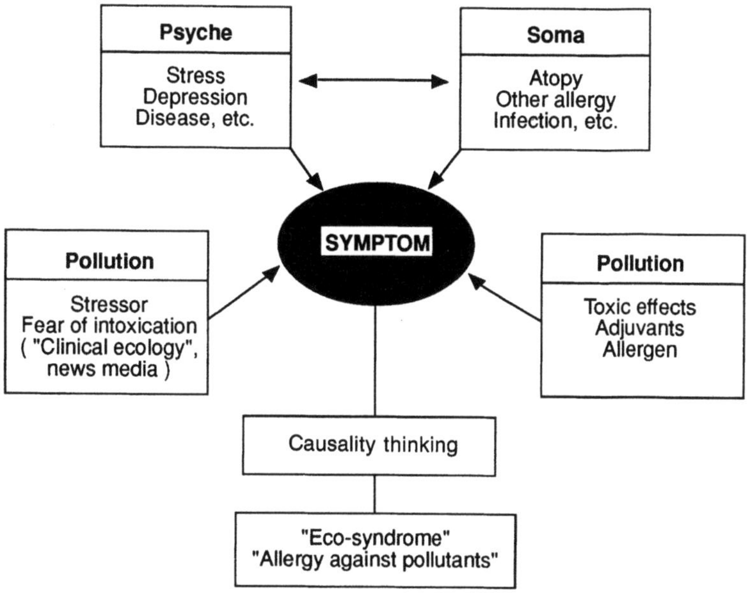

Fig. 2. Hypothetical synopsis of the effects of pollution on both psyche and soma in exposed individuals tending to suffer from allergic reactions

learned that allergology, as a growing science, was very well able to deal with the different kinds of pollen allergens, to the point of clearly describing the molecular characteristics of single pollen allergens. The major task now is to develop the tools and reagents to diagnose and investigate the role of environmental chemicals upon various hypersensitivity reactions.

A synopsis of possible pathophysiological events shows that pollution per se not only represents a somatic phenomenon acting as a possible allergen, adjuvant or toxic-irritant, but also as psychological stressor affecting a person's psychological well-being (Fig. 2). Sensitive individuals might not only react somatically but also be predisposed to increased anxiety reactions which can be further promoted by news media or movements such as clinical ecology. Finally, since human beings like to think in terms of causality, adverse symptoms or impairment of well-being will be regarded as allergy to pollutants.

Practical Recommendations

For the practical management of patients with clinical ecology syndrome (eco-syndrome) a climate of mutual confidence is a prerequisite for success. This has been seriously disturbed in most patients by previous contacts with doctors. Many of these patients are suffering in particular of being classified as psychologically abnormal. We conclude from our experience that these very difficult patients need the concentrated efforts of an experienced allergist in an interdisciplinary approach.

Exhausting all options, including placebo controlled provocation tests, the existence of a possible allergy or pseudo-allergy has to be excluded before fruitful cooperation with an experienced psychiatrist or psychologist can be started.

References

1. Adler G (1981) Current concepts in psychiatry: the physician and the hypochondriacal patient. N Engl J Med 304:1394–1396
2. American Academy of Allergy (1981) Position statement –controversial techniques. J Allergy Clin Immunol 67:333–338
3. Anger WK (1984) Neurobehavioral testing of chemicals: impact on recommended standards. Neurobeh Toxicol Teratol 6:147–153
4. Associated Press (1981) A sealed refuge for people allergic to the 20th century. San Francisco Sunday Examiner and Chronicle, Oct 13, A 10
5. Bach B, Molhave L, Pedersen OF (1987) Human reactions during controlled exposures to low concentrations of formaldehyde – performance tests. In: Seifert B, Esdorn H, Fischer M, Rüden H, Wegner J (eds) Indoor air '87, vol 2., Institute of Water, Soil and Air Hygiene, Berlin, pp 620–624
6. Baur X (1986) Asthma, Alveolitis, Aspergillose, Charakterisierung ursächlicher Allergene. Springer, Berlin Heidelberg New York
7. Behrendt H, Wieczorek M, Wellner S, Winzer A (1988) Effect of some metal ions (Cd^{++}, Pb^{++}, Mu^{++} on mediator release from mast cells in vivo and in vitro. In: Seemayer NH, Hadnagy W (eds) Environmental hygiene, pp 104–110. Springer, Berlin Heidelberg New York
8. Behrendt H (1989) Grundlagen der Allergie und mögliche Angriffspunkte für Umweltchemikalien. Allergologie 12:95–99
9. Behrendt H, Friedrichs KH, Kainka-Stänicke F, Darsow U, Becker W, Tomingas R (1991) Allergens and pollutants in the air – a complex interaction. This volume
10. Bullinger M (1990) Psychological effects of air pollution on healthy residents – a time-series approach. J Environ Psych (in press)
11. Burrows D, Halonen M, Barbee RA, Lebowitz MD (1981) The relationship of serum IgE to cigarette smoking. Am Rev Respir Dis 124:523–525
12. Bell IR (1982) Clinical ecology: a new medical approach to environmental illness. Common Knowledge Press, Bolinas, CA
13. Benson TE, Arkins JA (1976) Cytotoxic testing for food allergy: evaluations of reproducibility and correlation. J Allergy Clin Immunol 58:471
14. Black AP (1959) A new diagnostic method in allergic disease. Pediatrics 17:716–723
15. Boyd EM, Boyd EE (1973) Toxicity of pure foods. CRC Press, Cleveland
16. Breneman JC, Harst A, Heiner D, Leney FL, Morris D, Josephson B (1974) Final report of the food allergy committee of the American College of Allergists on the clinical evaluation of sublingual provocation testing method for diagnosis of food allergy. Ann Allergy 33:164
17. Brodsky CM (1983) Allergic to everything: a medical subculture. Psychosomatics 24:731–742
18. Bryan WTK, Bryan WP (1971) Cytotoxic reactions in the diagnosis of food allergy. Otolaryngol Clin North Am 4:523
19. Crawford LV, Liebermann P, Hart HA, Hale R, Nelson H, Selner J, Wittig H, Postman M, Zietz A (1976) A double-blind study of subcutaneous food testing sponsored by the food committee of the American Academy of Allergy. J Allergy Clin Immunol 57:236
20. Dickey LD (1976) Chemical ecology. Thomas, Springfield
21. Day JH, Thomson G, Evers S, Gerrard J, McCourtie DR, Woodward W (1987) Environmental hypersensitivity – an assessment. J Allergy Clin Immunol 79:236
22. Draper IW (1972) Food testing in allergy: intradermal provocative test vs. deliberate feeding. Arch Otolaryngol 95:169
23. Egger J, Wilson J, Carter CM, Turner MW (1983) Is migraine food allergy? A double-blind controlled trial of oligoantigenic diet treatment. Lancet ii:865–869
24. Egger J, Carter CM, Gurnley D, Graham PH, Soothill J (1985) Controlled trial of oligoantigenic diet treatment in the hyperkinetic syndrome. Lancet i:426–428

25. Enders F, Przybilla B, Ring J, Burg G, Braun-Falco O (1988) Epikutantestung mit einer Standardreihe. Ergebnisse bei 12026 Patienten. Hautarzt 39:779–786
26. Feingold B (1975) Why your child is hyperactive. Random House, New York
27. Fruhmann G (1975) Rauch, Staub und andere umweltbedingte Krankheitsfaktoren für die Entstehung chronisch obstruktiver Atemwegserkrankungen. Therapiewoche 25:4023–4026
28. Fuchs E, Schulz KH (eds) (1988) Manuale allergologicum. Dustri, München-Deisenhofen
29. Gandhi MD, Bahna SL (1985) Skin testing (ST) versus oral challenge (OC) in food sensitivity. J Allergy Clin Immunol 74:400
30. Gebefügi I, Parlar H, Korte F (1979) Occurrence of pentachlorphenol in enclosed environments. Ecotoxicol Environ Safety 3:269–300
31. Golos N, Gobitz FG, Leighton FS (1979) Coping with your allergies. Simon and Schuster, New York
32. Grieco MH (1982) Controversial practices in allergy. J Am Med Assoc 247:3106–3111
33. Hambidge KM (1982) Hair analyses: worthless for vitamins, limited for minerals. Am J Clin Nutr 36:943–949
34. Harley JP, Ray RS, Thomas L, Eichman PL, Mathews CG, Chun R, Cleeland CS, Traisman E (1978) Hyperkinesis and food additives. Testing the Feingold hypothesis. Pediatrics 61:818–828
35. Herman RH, Hagler L (1979) Food intolerance in humans. West J Med 95–116
36. Hirsch S, Kalbfleisch JH, Golbert TM, Josephson BM, McConnell LH, Scanton R, Kniker WT, Fink JN, Murphree J, Cohen SH (1980) Rinkel method, a controlled study. Second Report. J Allergy Clin Immunol 5:192
37. Hofer Th, Wüthrich B (1985) Nahrungsmittelallergien: II. Häufigkeit der Organmanifestationen und der Allergie-auslösenden Nahrungsmittel. Schweiz Med Wochenschr 41:115
38. Holborow P, Berry P (1985) The clinical ecology debate: some issues arising. Bull Br Psychol Soc 38:49
39. Illig L (1977) Moderne Aspekte der Urtikariapathogenese unter besonderer Berücksichtigung des Intoleranz-Phänomens. Hautarzt 28:102–112
40. Jewett DL, Greenberg MR (1985) Placebo responses in intradermal provocation testing with food extracts. J Allergy Clin Immunol 75:205, abstr. 401
41. Kailin EW, Collier R (1971) "Relieving" therapy for antigen exposure. J Am Med Assoc 217:78
42. King DS (1981) Can allergic exposure provoke psychological symptoms? A double-blind test. Biol Psychiatry 16:3–19
43. Kleinhans D, Galinsky T (1982) Zur möglichen Provokation eines Bronchialasthmas und einer Urtikaria durch Natriumdisulfit. Allergologie 5:120–121
44. Kleinsorge H (1964) Allergie – eine psychosomatische Erkrankung? Med Klin 30:59
45. Koblenzer CS (1983) Psychosomatic concepts in dermatology. Arch Dermatol 119:501–512
46. Kunz B, Ring J, Überla K (1989) Frequency of atopic diseases and allergic sensitization in preschool children in different parts of Bavaria. Allergologie 2 [Suppl 1]:44
47. Kunz B, Ring J, Gries A, Überla K (1990) Indoor air concentration of SO^2 and NO_X and frequency of atopic diseases in children. J Allergy Clin Immunol 85:250
48. Kunz B, Ring J, Dirschedl K (1989) Smoking during pregnancy increases risk of atopic diseases in children. J Invest Dermatol 92:465A
49. Lehrman CW (1980) A double-blind study of sublingual provocative food testing: a study of its efficacy. Ann Allergy 45:144–149
50. Lehrman CW (1980) The leukocytic food allergy test: a study of the reliability and reproducibility. Effect of diet and sublingual food drops on this test. Ann Allergy 45:150
51. Levy D, Gent M, Newhouse MT (1977) Relationship between acute respiratory illness and air pollution levels in an industrial city. Am Rev Respir Dis 116:167–173
52. Lessof MH (1983) Clinical reactions to food. Wiley, Chichester
53. Lewtas J (1989) Toxicology of complex mixtures of indoor air pollutants. Am Rev Pharmacol Toxicol 29:415–439
54. Lieberman P, Crawford L, Bjelland J, Connel B, Rice M (1974) Controlled study of the cytotoxic food test. J Am Med Assoc 231:728
55. Lowell FC, Heiner DC (1972) Food allergy cytotoxic diagnostic technique not proven. J Am Med Assoc 220:1624
56. Mackarness R (1976) Not all in the mind. Pan, London

57. McGovern JJ (1983) Food and chemical sensitivity. Clinical and immunologic correlates. Arch Otolaryngol 109:292–297
58. Mansfield LE, Ting S, Haverly RW, Rauls DO, Vaughan TR (1985) Plasma histamine elevation during blind food challenges which provoke migraine. J Allergy Clin Immunol 75:205, abstr. 402
59. May CD, Bock SA (1978) Adverse reactions to food due to hypersensitivity. Clin Science 2:1159–1171
60. May CD, Bock SA (1978) A modern clinical approach to food hypersensitivity. Allergy 33:166–188
61. van Metre TE, Adkinson NF, Lichtenstein IM, Mardiney MR, Norman PS, Rosenberg GL, Sobotka AK, Valentin MD (1980) A comparative study of the effectiveness of the Rinkel method of immunotherapy for ragweed pollen hay fever. J Allergy Clin Immunol 65:288
62. van Metre RT, Adkinson NF, Amodio FJ, Lichtenstein IM, Mardiney MR, Norman PS, Rosenberg GL, Sobotka AK, Valentine MD (1980) A comparative study of the effectiveness of the Rinkel method and the current standard method of immunotherapy for ragweed pollen hay fever. J Allergy Clin Immunol 66:500
63. Miller JB (1972) Food allergy: provocative testing and injection therapy. Thomas, Springfield
64. Mills N (1986) Depression and food intolerance: a single case study. Hum Nutr Appl Nutr 40A:141–145
65. Miyamoto T, Takafuji S (1991) Environmental pollution and allergy. This volume
66. Monro J, Carini C, Brostoff J (1984) Migraine is a food-allergic disease. Lancet ii:719–721
67. Muranaka M, Suzuki S, Koizumi K, Takafuji S, Miyamoto T, Ikemore R, Tokiwa H (1986) Adjuvant activity of diesel-exhaust particulates for the production of IgE antibody in mice. J Allergy Clin Immunol 77:616–623
68. National Research Council, Food Protections Committee (1973) Toxicants occurring naturally in food. National Academy of Science, Washington DC
69. Nixon PGF (1982) "Total allergy syndrome" or fluctuating hypocarbia? Lancet i:516
70. Orehek J, Massari JP, Gaynard P, Grimand P, Charpin J (1984) Effect of short term low level nitrogen dioxide exposure on bronchial sensitivity of asthmatic patients. J Clin Invest 57:301–307
71. Pearson DJ, Rix KJB, Bentley SJ (1983) Food allergy: how much in the mind? A clinical and psychiatric study of suspected food hypersensitivity. Lancet ii:1259–1261
72. Randolph TG (1945) Fatigue and weakness of allergic origin (allergic toxemia) to be differentiated from "nervous fatigue" or neurasthenia. Ann Allergy 3:418–430
73. Randolph TG (1959) Ecologic mental illness – psychiatry exteriorized. J Lab Clin Med 54:936
74. Randolph TG, Moss RW (1980) An alternative approach to allergies. The new field of clinical ecology unravels the environmental causes of mental and physical ills. Lippincott and Cromwell, New York
75. Raulf M, König W (1991) Pesticides and allergy. This volume
76. Reimann HJ, Ring J, Ultsch B, Wendt P (1985) Intragastral provocation under endoscopic control (IPEC) in food allergy. Clin Allergy 15:195–202
77. Reimann HJ (1981) Stress and histamine. In: Ring J, Burg G (eds) New trends in allergy. Springer, Berlin Heidelberg New York, pp 50–57
79. Riedel F, Krämer M, Scheibenbogen C, Rieger CHL (1988) Effects of SO_2 exposure on allergic sensitization in the guinea pig. J Allergy Clin Immunol 82:527–534
80. Ring J, Przybilla B, Steger O, Schwab-Przybilla U (1987) Sulfit-Überempfindlichkeit. Allergologie 10:100–106
81. Ring J (1988) Angewandte Allergologie, 2nd edn. MMV-Vieweg, Munich
82. Ring J (1986) Pseudo-allergic drug reactions. In: Reed C et al (eds) Proceedings of the XIIth international congress of allergology and clinical immunology. Mosby, St. Louis, pp 75–79
83. Ring J (1987) Anaphylaxis and an anaphylactoid reactions. In: Baethmann A, Messmer K (eds) Surgical research: recent concepts and results. Springer, Berlin Heidelberg New York, pp 210–221
84. Ring J (1987) Das "Klinische Ökologie Syndrom": polysomatische Beschwerden durch "Subjektive Allergie gegen Umweltschadstoffe". In: Braun-Falco O, Schill W-B (eds) Fortschritte der praktischen Dermatologie und Venerologie XI. Springer, Berlin Heidelberg New York, pp 434–436
85. Ring J (1987) Luftverschmutzung und allergische Erkrankungen. Muench Med Wochenschr 129:182–185

86. Ring J (1987) Mechanisms of pseudo-allergic reactions to drugs. In: Estabrook RW, Lindenlaub E, Oesch F, de Weck AL (eds) Toxicological and immunological aspects of drug metabolism and environmental chemicals, pp 569–595
87. Ring J, Gabriel G, Vieluf D, Przybilla B (1991) "Das klinische Ökologie Syndrom" ("Öko-Syndrom"): polysomatische Beschwerden bei vermuteter Allergie gegen Umweltschadstoffe. Muench Med Wochenschr 133:50–55
88. Rinkel HJ (1944) Food allergy: the role of food allergy in internal medicine. Ann Allergy 2:115–124
89. Rinkel HJ (1949) Inhalant allergy. Part I: the whealing response of the skin to serial dilution testing. Ann Allergy 7:625–630, 650
90. Römmelt H, Dirnagl K, Schuh A (1988) Principles and methods for control of air pollution in health resorts. In: Seemayer NH, Hadnagy W (eds) Environmental hygiene. pp 201–204 Springer, Berlin Heidelberg New York
91. Rom WN (1983) Environmental and occupational medicine. Little Brown, Boston
92. Rowe AH (1930) Allergic toxemia and migraine due to food allergy. Calif West Med J 33:785
93. Rowe AH (1944) Clinical allergy in the nervous system. J Nerv Ment Dis 99:834–841
94. Rowe AH, Rowe A (1972) Food allergy. Its manifestations and control and the elimination diets. A compendium. Thomas, Springfield
95. Samter M (1972) Sublingual desensitization for allergy not recommended. J Am Med Assoc 215:1210
96. Sapeika N (1969) Food pharmacology. Thomas, Springfield
97. Seifert B, Esdorn H, Fischer M, Rüden H, Wegner J (eds) (1987) Indoor Air '87, vol 1–4. Institute of Water, Soil and Air Hygiene, Berlin
98. Seifert B (1989) Innenraumluftverunreinigungen. Allergologie 3:114–117
99. Selner JC, Staudenmayer H (1986) The relationship of the environment and food to allergic and psychiatric illness. In: Young SH, Rubing JM, Daman HR (eds) Psychobiological aspects of allergic disorders. Praeger, New York
100. Selye H (1976) Stress in health and disease. Butterworth, Boston
101. Speer F (1979) The history of allergy of the nervous system. Thomas, Springfield
102. Staudenmayer H, Lefkowitz MS (1981) Physician-patient psychosocial characteristics influencing medical dicision making. Soc Sci Med 15E:77–81
103. Terr AI (1986) Environmental illness, a clinical review of 50 cases. Arch Intern Med 146: 145–149
104. Thiel C, Fuchs E (1983) Nahrungsintoleranzen durch Fremdstoffe. Muench Med Wochenschr 123:125
105. Walker WA, Isselbacher KJ, Bloch KF (1973) Intestinal uptake of macromolecules: Effect of parenteral immunization. J Immunol 110:221
106. Walsh PF, Dudney CS, Copenhaven ED (1983) Indoor air quality. CRC Press, Boston
107. Werner M (1967) Krankheiten infolge peroraler Allergeninvasion. In: Hansen K, Werner MS (eds) Lehrbuch der klinischen Allergie. Thieme, Stuttgart, p 179
108. Willoughby JW (1974) Serial dilution titration skin tests in inhalant allergy: a clinical quantitative assessment of biologic skin reactivity to allergenic extracts. Otolaryngol Clin North Am 10:579–615
109. Witek TJ Jr, Schachter EN, Tosun T, Leaderer BP, Beck GJ (1986) Controlled human studies on the pulmonary effects of indoor air pollution: experiences with sulfur dioxide and formaldehyde. Environ Int 12:129–135
110. Wüthrich B (1981) Nahrungsmittelallergie. Allergologie 4:320–328
111. Wüthrich B (1983) Allergische und pseudoallergische Reaktionen der Haut durch Arzneimittel und Lebensmitteladditiva. Schweiz Rundsch Med Prax 72:691–699
112. Wurtman RJ (1982) Nutrients that modify brain function. Sci Am 246:50–59
113. Wurtman RJ (1983) Behavioural effects of nutrients. Lancet 2:1145–1147
114. Zetterström O et al. (1985) Increased IgE antibody responses in rats exposed to tobacco smoke. J Allergy Clin Immunol 75:594–598
115. Zweimann B, Slavin RG, Flinberg RJ, Falliers CJ, Aaron TH (1972) Effects of air pollution on asthma: a review. J Allergy Clin Immunol 50:305–314

Prophylaxis and Therapy

Eicosanoid Metabolism and Antiallergic Strategies

T. Ruzicka

Department of Dermatology, Ludwig-Maximilians University, Frauenlobstrasse 9–11, W-8000 München 2, Federal Republic of Germany

Abstract

Eicosanoids are a class of compounds derived from arachidonic (eicosatetraenoic) acid. Prostaglandins are formed by the enzyme cyclooxygenase, whereas various leukotrienes and the mono-HETEs are generated mainly by 5- and 12-lipoxygenases. Cyclooxygenase is inhibited by NSAIDs, whereas glucocorticosteroids block the formation of all eicosanoids by inhibiting the release of arachidonic acid from phospholipids via phospholipase A_2. Eicosanoids exert proinflammatory and immunoregulatory actions by their effects on blood vessels and inflammatory cells; they also act in growth regulation of epithelia. In atopic eczema and other inflammatory dermatoses, highly elevated concentrations of LTB_4 and 12-HETE were measured in lesional skin. This may be due to enhanced releasability of eicosanoids, as was demonstrated by us upon immunological stimulation of peripheral blood leukocytes. Chronic administration of these lipoxygenase-derived eicosanoids in skin results in leukocytoclastic vasculitis and epidermal hyperplasia, which may be suppressed by PGE_2, suggesting a tissue protective role of this mediator in skin. LTs and HETEs are chemotactic for fibroblasts and epidermal cells suggesting, in addition to their pathogenetic action in inflammation, a physiological role in cutaneous wound repair. The chemotactic effects are mediated by specific receptors. Recently, we could demonstrate the presence of specific high-affinity receptors for 12(S)-HETE on human epidermal cells. Pharmacologic interventions into eicosanoid metabolism may prove useful in inflammatory dermatoses and allergic disorders. They are possible are various levels: substrate competition, e.g., by eicosapentaenoic acid; inhibition of phospholipases, e.g., by glucocorticoids; specific inhibition of cyclooxygenase and lipoxygenases; receptor antagonism at the LTB_4 (leukocytes) or 12-HETE (epidermal cells) receptor. In addition, treatment with prostaglandin analogs may exert antiinflammatory effects.

Eicosanoids – Metabolic Pathways and Biological Actions

Eicosanoids are a class of compounds derived from arachidonic (eicosatetraenoic) acid. They are generated by the action of specific enzymes leading to the formation of terminal metabolites [1, 2]. Prostaglandins (PG) E_2, D_2, $F_{2\alpha}$, prostacyclin and thromboxane are formed by the enzyme cyclooxygenase; the 5-lipoxygenase enzyme leads to the production of 5-hydroxyeicosatetraenoic acid (5-HETE), and the leukotrienes (LT) B_4, LTC_4 and LTD_4. The 12-lipoxygenase enzyme generate 12-HETE. Cyclooxygenase is blocked by the inhibitory action of nonsteroidal antiinflammatory drugs (NSAIDs) [3], whereas glucocorticosteroids block the formation of all eicosanoids by inhibiting the release of arachidonic acid from phospholipids via phospholipase A_2 [4].

The interest in eicosanoid metabolism and pharmacology results from their biological effects. They exert proinflammatory and immunoregulatory action by influencing microvascular [5] and various functions of leukocytes [6]. In addition, they may act as growth factors in epithelia.

A further hint for the involvement of eicosanoids in inflammatory and/or allergic skin diseases is the demonstration of highly elevated cutaneous levels of the lipoxygenase metabolites LTB_4 and 12-HETE. This has been demonstrated in atopic [7] and allergic [8] contact eczema as well as in psoriasis [7, 9, 10–12]. In atopic eczema patients, enhanced releasability of eicosanoids is operative in peripheral blood leukocytes which may contribute to the enhanced tissue concentrations [13]. Inflammatory infiltration of the skin in atopic eczema is probably due to elevated concentrations of chemotactic mediators rather than to altered responsiveness of inflammatory cells to chemotactic stimuli, since leukocytes of atopic individuals display normal numbers and affinity of their LTB_4 receptors [14].

Repeated intradermal injection of LTB_4 and 12-HETE leads to epidermal hyperplasia and a dense cellular infiltration in the dermis bearing strong similarities to the histological picture of leukocytoclastic vasculitis [15]. Thus, in the wide clinical range of cutaneous and systemic diseases characterized by histological changes of leukocytoclastic vasculitis, eicosanoids may be operative as well. It should be kept in mind, however, that eicosanoids may not only exert harmful, proinflammatory effects, but also beneficial, antiinflammatory ones, and also may possess physiological functions in tissues. There is evidence pointing along these lines.

Prostaglandins such as PGE_2 or PGD_2 formed in large amounts by the immunocompetent Langerhans cells [16] and also by mast cells [17] may exert antiinflammatory effects by inhibiting various leukocyte functions such as chemotaxis, cytotoxicity, release of lysosomal enzymes or inflammatory mediators etc. Thus, they potentiate the acute vascular phase of the inflammatory reaction by their effects on microvessels, but act as switch-off signals during the chronic, tissue destructive, cellular phase of inflammation. This has been demonstrated directly in skin by the tissue-protective effect of PGE_2 on LTB_4-induced inflammatory reaction [15]. Thus, inhibition of PG synthesis may prove to be a double-edged sword. In fact, in inflammatory skin diseases, inhibitors of prostaglandin synthesis are hardly ever therapeutically useful. On the contrary, they may exacerbate or provoke a wide range of dermatoses.

A physiological function of eicosanoids in wound repair is suggested by the chemotactic effects of various lipoxygenase products on fibroblasts and keratinocytes [18].

Eicosanoid Receptors

The effects of eicosanoids are mediated via specific receptors. We recently identified and characterized a specific high-affinity receptor for 12-HETE, the main product of arachidonic acid in skin, on human epidermal cells [19, 20]. The receptor mediates keratinocyte chemotaxis, but is not involved in growth promotion. The receptor shows dramatic upregulation by γ-interferon [21] and downregulation by 12-HETE [20]. It is markedly inhibited by the antipsoriatic agent dithranol (L. Kemeny, E. Gross, P. Arenberger, T. Ruzicka, manuscript in preparation) and UV-B (L. Kemeny et al., in preparation), and is dramatically altered in psoriasis (P. Arenberger et al., in preparation).

Pharmacological Interventions in Eicosanoid Metabolism

Pharmacological interventions in eicosanoid metabolism may prove useful in inflammatory dermatoses and allergic disorders. Particular attention has been paid to the extremely common skin diseases atopic eczema [22] and psoriasis. Pharmacological manipulations are possible at various levels: substrate competition, e.g., by eicosapentaenoic acid; inhibition of phospholipases by glucocorticosteroids or phospholipase-inhibiting proteins such as lipocortin; specific or dual inhibition of cyclooxygenase and lipoxygenase enzymes; antagonism at the leukocyte LTB_4 receptor or epidermal 12-HETE receptor. Finally, the antiinflammatory action of prostaglandins [15] may prove therapeutically useful.

Eicosanoids Metabolism and Antiallergic Strategies – Perspectives

In designing antiallergic strategies by pharmacological manipulations of arachidonic acid metabolism, it must be kept in mind that eicosanoids not only exert proinflammatory properties, but sometimes also antiinflammatory ones. In addition, they most probably are not only pathogenic agents, but must possess some physiological functions as well.

Pharmacological interventions into arachidonic acid metabolism will therefore lead to hardly predictable net effects. Thus, development of molecular tools for probing the pharmacological effects of eicosanoids in skin is necessary, and only through carefully designed experiments can it be determined whether an antagonist or enzyme inhibitor of the eicosanoid cascade will yield the desired clinical effect.

References

1. Needleman P, Turk J, Jakschik BA, Morrison AB, Lefkowitz JN (1986) Arachidonic acid metabolism. Annu Rev Biochem 55:69
2. Ford-Hutchinson AW (1990) Arachidonic acid metabolism: enzymatic pathways. In: Ruzicka T (ed) Eicosanoids and the skin. CRC Press, Boca Raton, pp 3–22
3. Vane J, Botting R (1987) Inflammation and the mechanism of action of anti-inflammatory drugs. Faseb J 1:89
4. Hong SL, Levine L (1976) Inhibition of arachidonic acid release from cells as the biochemical action of anti-inflammatory corticosteroids. Proc Natl Acad Sci USA 73:1730–1734
5. Bisgaard H (1990) Effects of eicosanoids on microcirculation in the skin. In: Ruzicka T (ed) Eicosanoids and the skin. CRC Press, Boca Raton, pp 157–167
6. Rosenbeck T, Czarnetzki BM (1990) Chemotactic effects of eicosanoids and their role in the pathophysiology of inflammatory dermatoses. In: Ruzicka T (ed) Eicosanoids and the skin. CRC Press, Boca Raton, pp 127–148
7. Ruzicka T, Simmet T, Peskar BA, Ring J (1986) Skin levels of arachidonic acid-derived inflammatory mediators and histamine in atopic dermatitis and psoriasis. J Invest Dermatol 86:105–108
8. Barr RM, Brain S, Camp RDR, Cilliers J, Greaves MW, Mallet AI, Michel K (1984) Levels of arachidonic acid and its metabolites in the skin in human allergic and irritant contact dermatitis. Br J Dermatol 111:23–28
9. Hammarström S, Hamberg S, Samuelsson B, Duell E, Stawiski M, Voorhees JJ (1975) Increased concentrations of nonesterified arachidonic acid, 12L-hydroxy-5,8,10,14-eicosatetraenoic acid, prostaglandin E_2, and prostaglandin F_{2alpha}, in epidermis of psoriasis. Proc Natl Acad Sci USA 72:5130
10. Grabbe J, Czarnetzki MB, Rosenbach T, Mardin M (1984) Identification of chemotactic lipoxygenase products of arachidonic metabolism in psoriatic skin. J Invest Dermatol 82:477
11. Camp RDR, Mallet AI, Woollard PM, Brain SD, Kobza A, Greaves MW (1983) The identification of hydroxy fatty acids in psoriatic skin. Prostaglandins 26:431
12. Kragballe K, Fisher GJ, Voorhees JJ (1990) Eicosanoids, phosphoinositides, and the pathophysiology of psoriasis. In: Ruzicka T (ed) Eicosanoids and the skin. CRC Press, Boca Raton, pp 67–78
13. Ruzicka T, Ring J (1987) Enhanced releasability of prostaglandin E_2 and leukotrienes B_4 and C_4 from leukocytes of patients with atopic eczema. Acta Derm Venereol (Stockh) 67:469–475
14. Meier F, Gross E, Klotz K-N, Ruzicka T (1989) Leukotriene B_4 receptors on neutrophils in patients with psoriasis and atopic eczema. Skin Pharmacol 2:61–67
15. Ruzicka T, Burg G (1987) Effects of chronic intracutaneous administration of arachidonic acid and its metabolites. Induction of leukocytoclastic vasculitis by leukotriene B_4 and 12-hydroxyeicosatetraenoic acid and its prevention by prostaglandin E_2. J Invest Dermatol 88:120
16. Ruzicka T, Auböck J (1987) Arachidonic acid metabolism in guinea pig Langerhans cells: studies on cyclooxygenase and lipoxygenase pathways. J Immunol 138:539–543
17. Ikai K, Imamura S (1988) Prostaglandin D_2 in the skin. Int J Dermatol 27:141–149
18. Hein R, Rieger G, Ruzicka T, Krieg T (1990) Effects of eicosanoids on human fibroblast chemotaxis. In: Ruzicka T (ed) Eicosanoids and the skin. CRC Press, Boca Raton, pp 149–155
19. Gross E, Ruzicka T, von Restorff B, Stolz W, Klotz KN (1990) High affinity binding and lack of growth promoting activity of 12-HETE in a human epidermal cell line. J Invest Dermatol 94:446
20. Gross E, Ruzicka T (1991) Epidermal eicosanoid receptors. In: Mukhtar H (ed) Pharmacology of the skin. CRC Press, Boca Raton (in press)
21. Süss R, Arenberger P, Gross E, Ruzicka T (1991) Regulation of 12(S)-HETE binding sites in human epidermal cells by interferon gamma. Exp Cell Res 191:204–208
22. Ruzicka T (1991) Inflammatory mediators in atopic eczema. In: Ruzicka T, Ring J, Przybilla B (eds) Handbook of atopic eczema. Springer, Berlin Heidelberg New York Tokyo (in press)

Development of New Antiasthmatic Drugs from Traditional Medicine?

W. Dorsch[1] and H. Wagner[2]

[1]Children's Hospital of the Johannes Gutenberg University, Department of Allergology and Pneumology, Langenbeckstrasse 1, W-6500 Mainz, Federal Republic of Germany
[2]Institute of Pharmaceutical Biology of the Ludwig Maximilian University, Karlstrasse 27, W-8000 Munich 2, Federal Republic of Germany

Abstract

Several plants are used in traditional medicine in the treatment of bronchial asthma. We are trying to identify the active compound(s) and their mode of action.

As *chemical methods* we use different chromatographic methods, high and middle pressure liquid chromatography, elementary analysis, UV, mass, proton and carbon magnetic resonance spectroscopy. Whole plant extracts, fractionated extracts and pure compounds were tested by the following pharmacological test systems: cyclooxygenase and lipoxygenase pathway of arachidonic acid metabolism, bronchial obstruction of guinea pigs after inhalation of allergens, platelet-activating factor (PAF), histamine or acetylcholine, PAF-induced bronchial hyperreactivity of guinea pigs, histamine release, chemoluminescence and chemotaxis of human polymorphonuclear leukocytes as well as thromboxane biosynthesis of human platelets.

As active compounds in onion extracts thiosulphinates and cepaenes could be identified. They exert a wide spectrum of pharmacological activities both in vitro and in vivo.

Tetragalloyl quinic acid from *Galphimia glauca* suppressed allergen- and PAF-induced bronchial obstruction, PAF-induced bronchial hyperreactivity (5 mg/kg orally) in vivo, and thromboxane biosynthesis in vitro.

Hitherto unknown alkaloids from *Adhatoda vasica* showed pronounced protection against allergen-induced bronchial obstruction in guinea pigs (10 mg/ml aerosol).

Androsin from *Picrorhiza kurroca* prevented allergen- and PAF-induced bronchial obstruction and bronchial hyperreactivity in vivo (10 mg/kg, orally). Histamine release in vitro was inhibited by other compounds of the plant extract yet to be identified.

Pharmacological effects of plant extracts and pure compounds in humans are under investigation.

Introduction

Bronchial asthma is a disease not only of modern times. People have been trying to treat this difficult disease for years and we learned from their experience. Five thousand years ago in China extracts from Ma Huang (*Ephedra vulgaris*) were recommended for the treatment of asthma [1, 2]. Instead of ephedrine, we now use *betasympathomimetics*, which are highly bronchoselective and act directly. Tea, the source of *theophyllin* and other xanthine derivatives, comes from China, too. In Europe 500 years ago individuals suffering from asthma inhaled the smoke of atropa belladonna leaves and related plants [3]; now we use synthetic *anticholinergics*. The development of *disodium cromoglycate* was initiated by the discovery of the antiasthmatic properties of khellin, the active agent of an Egyptian plant named *Ammi visnaga* [4].

The Egyptian *Papyrus Ebers* describes the use of onions in a lot of major and minor disorders [5]. In 1983 we reported on the antiasthmatic and antiinflammatory properties of onion extracts. Recently we identified thiosulphinate and cepaene as active compounds [6–19].

Table 1. Chemical-analytical methods used in the bioguided identification of active compounds in plant extracts.

Chemical methods
Silicagel column chromatography
Sephadex column chromatography
High pressure liquid chromatography
Middle pressure liquid chromatography
Elementary analysis
Ultraviolet-infrared spectroscopy
Mass-spectroscopy
[^{1}H] and [^{14}C] magnetic resonance spectroscopy
Two-dimensional magnetic resonance imaging, correlated spectroscopy, nuclear overhauser effect
X-ray spectroscopy

Table 2. Pharmacological test methods used for the identification of active compounds and their mode of action in plant extracts.

Pharmacological test systems
In vitro
– Cyclooxygenase pathway of arachidonic acid metabolism
– Lipoxygenase pathway of arachidonic acid metabolism
– Histamine release of human polymorphonuclear leukocytes
– Chemoluminescence of human polymorphonuclear leukocytes
– Chemotaxis of human polymorphonuclear leukocytes
– Thromboxane biosynthesis of human platelets
In vivo (experimental animals)
– Allergen-induced bronchial obstruction in guinea pig
– PAF-induced bronchial obstruction in guinea pigs
– Histamine-induced bronchial obstruction in guinea pigs
– Acetylcholine-induced bronchial obstruction in guinea pigs
– PAF-induced bronchial hyperreactivity in guinea pigs
In vivo (human volunteers)
– Anti IgE-induced dual skin reactions
– (Bronchial obstruction after allergen inhalation)

PAF, platelet-activating factor.

Many plants or plant extracts are used in different countries for the treatment of bronchial asthma. We are trying to identify chemically well defined compounds in these plants with antiasthmatic and/or antiinflammatory activities. For this purpose we can use a battery of different chemical and pharmacological methods (Tables 1, 2). In this paper we report briefly on the results of our investigations on *Allium cepa* (onions), *Galphimia glauca*, *Adhatoda vasica* and *Picrorhiza kurrooa*.

Material and Methods

Plants

The plants were purchased from Indian drug companies or collected from botanists in the USA and South America. Specimens of all drugs are deposed in the herbarium of the Institute of Pharmaceutical Biology, Munich.

Chemical Methods

Fractionation of the extracts was performed partly by classical solvent extraction and silica gel or sephadex column chromatography using various solvent systems or by application of middle and high pressure liquid chromatographic (HPLC) procedures. The structures of the isolated compounds were elucidated by ultraviolet, infrared, proton, carbon and mass spectroscopy with all modern variants, i.e. two-dimensional magnetic resonance imaging (MRI) correlated spectroscopy (COSY) and nuclear overhauser effect (NOE) experiments. In some cases X-ray spectroscopy was used.

Pharmacological Methods

In Vitro Experiments

5-Lipoxygenase Activity of Porcine Leucocytes. A suspension of porcine leukocytes in phosphate buffer was incubated with calcium chloride, eicosatetraenoic acid, genuine plant extracts, their fractions and pure compounds, calcium ionophore A23187 and [1-^{14}C]arachidonic acid for 5 min at 37 °C. The reaction was stopped by the addition of formic acid. Arachidonic acid and its metabolites were extracted by ethylacetate. Separation and quantification was performed by reversed-phase HPLC using an acetonitrile/water gradient system. The labeled compounds were detected and quantified by measurement of radioactivity (details in [11, 31]).

Cyclooxygenase Activity of Sheep Vesicular Glands. Cyclooxygenase activity of sheep seminal vesicle microsomes (isolated according to Nugteren and Hazelhof) was tested by the method of Kuhl et al. [20]: 8 μg protein in 2.0 ml tris-HCl buffer (pH 8.0), 1 m*M* reduced glutathione, 1 m*M* epinephrine bitartrate and 0.05 m*M* NaEDTA were incubated for 5 min at 20 °C with different concentrations of the test material (1 to 100 μ*M*) in ethanol (final concentration: 2.5%) or ethanol for control. The reaction was started by adding 0.1 μCi [1-^{14}C]arachidonic acid at 37 °C. After 20 min the reaction was stopped by 525 μl ice-cold 1% formic acid. Arachidonic acid and its labeled metabolites were extracted with ethylacetate, separated by reversed-phase HPLC (acetonitrile/water/0.1% 1 N H_3PO_4, 11 min 36% acetonitrile, then 15 min 80% acetonitrile), detected by radioactivity-monitoring (Berthold, radioactivity monitor LB 503) and quantified by peak areas. Results will be given as percent inhibition of prostangladin E biosynthesis.

Chemotaxis of Human Polymorphonuclear Leukocytes. Venous blood was taken from healthy adult volunteers who denied any drug intake for at least 4 weeks and heparinized. Neutrophilic granulocytes were isolated by density separation (Ficoll Hypaque). The cells were washed and mixed with fetal calf serum in a 4:1 ratio (cell count: 1000 cells/μl; purity: 94.5±5.9%). Chemotaxis under agarose was tested according to Nelson [21]. Agarose gels in tissue culture dishes (60×15 mm) were prepared from agarose, fetal calf serum, Medium solution (Flow Laboratories) and adjusted to pH 7.4. Three concentric circuits of each five wells (diameter: 3 mm) were cut in the solidified gel. The wells of the internal circuit were each filled with 10 μl of the medium alone (control for spontaneous migration). The external punches were filled with the chemotactic peptide f-methionine-leucine-phenylalanin (f-MLP).

The five wells of the intermediate circuit contained 10000 cells incubated with different concentrations of the extracts or agents tested. Spontaneous and f-MLP-induced migration of the cells was estimated by a graduated microscope (for details see [17–21]).

Platelet Activating Factor-Induced Chemoluminescence of Human Polymorphonuclear Leukocytes. As a nonspecific sign of cell activation superoxide production was measured. Human polymorphonuclear leukocytes were incubated at 37 °C with the test material or its solvent, cytochalasin B and luminol. The reaction was started by the addition of platelet-activating factor (PAF) and followed up over 10 min (Bioluminat LB9505, Beckmann, USA; software by Berthold, FRG – details in [11]).

Histamine Release from Human Polymorphonuclear Cells. Venous blood was taken from atopic donors. Peripheral leukocytes were isolated by dextrane sedimentation and preincubated with 4 different concentrations and the solvent of the test substances. Ten minutes later the cells were challenged with rabbit anti-human IgE antibodies, anaphylatoxin $C_{5\alpha}$, calcium ionophore or saline. Thirty minutes later the reaction was stopped. Histamine in the supernatant was measured spectrofluorometrically [22], the results being expressed as percentage of maximal release by perchloric acid corrected for spontaneous release without stimulation.

Thromboxane Biosynthesis of Human Platelet-Rich Plasma. Citrated plasma was harvested from atopic volunteers. Platelet-rich plasma (PRP) was adjusted at

90000 platelets per milliliter in phosphate-buffered saline. PRP 1 ml was incubated for 3 min in duplicate with different concentrations of the test material and control solutions. The PRP was stimulated with 1 and 10 IU thrombin. After 15 min the reaction was stopped by adding ice-cold methanol. Thromboxane in the supernatant was determined by radioimmunoassay (RIA) in triplicate corrected by recovery rates (80% – 100%) according to the method of Siess et al. [23].

In Vivo/Animal Experiments

Inhalation Challenge of Guinea Pigs with Allergen, Platelet-Activating Factor, Histamine and/or Acetylcholine. Spontaneously breathing animals were set in a two-chamber body plethysmograph, the chambers separated by a water-filled rubber cuff around the head of the animal. Volume changes in both chambers were measured by pressure transducers. The degree of bronchial obstruction was estimated by the parameter "compressed air." This technique has been shown to be about tenfold as sensitive as other invasive methods [24].

All tests were performed according to a randomized crossover protocol: groups of 8 – 20 animals were divided into two subgroups and treated either with the test material or control solutions. Three or four days later the tests were repeated: animals which previously received active compounds were given control solutions and vice versa. (Each animal received the plant extract, fraction or compound to be tested or its solvent once.)

Ovalbumin, histamine hydrochloride and acetylcholine was dissolved in saline (1:99, 1:999, 1:99 w/v), PAF first in ethanol and then in saline containing 0.25% bovine serum albumin, yielding a final concentration of 1 μg PAF/ml. Ovalbumin, PAF, histamine and acetylcholine were given as aerosol nebulized ultrasonically.

The effect of plant extracts or compounds on PAF-induced hyperreactivity was tested by the sequential inhalation of histamine, PAF, and histamine: a group of animals was divided into two subgroups; both subgroups inhaled histamine at a dose provoking an intermediate bronchial obstruction. One hour later one group received the substances to be tested, the other group received the vehicle alone. Both groups were challenged later by the sequential inhalation of PAF and histamine: first 1 μg PAF and 60 min later the same histamine dose given before. The second histamine challenge provokes in control animals usually asthmatic reactions three times as severe as the first one (details in [15]).

In Vivo Experiments in Human Volunteers

Immediate and Late Skin Reactions After Reverse Anaphylaxis. Immediate and late cutaneous reactions were induced in healthy adult volunteers who denied any drug intake for at least 4 weeks by the intracutaneous injection of 20 and/or 200 IU rabbit anti-human IgE antibodies into the volar side of their forearms. Test and control solutions (50 μl) were injected simultaneously. The diameters of wheals and flares were measured 10 and 20 min later; the diameters of late cutaneous reactions (redness) were read hourly up to 8 h. Edema formation in late skin reactions were measured by a skin calliper [6] in recent investigations by ultrasound.

Immediate and Late Bronchial Obstruction After Allergen Inhalation. Systemic administration of test compounds to asthmatic patients can be performed, of course, only after extensive toxicologic and pharmacologic examinations. Therefore pilot studies were performed only with ethanolic onion juice and onion capsules.

Adult volunteers suffering from allergic bronchial asthma entered the study after informed consent. They were challenged by the inhalation of their antigen according to the rules of the German Society of Research in Allergology and Immunology [25]. Bronchial obstruction was measured by whole body plethysmography and, in most cases, spirometry (flow volume diagrams). The test were repeated 4 weeks later after pretreatment with either ethanolic onion juice of onion capsules.

Statistics

All figures show mean and standard deviation (SD). The statistical significance of difference was estimated using Student's *t* test for unpaired data. In addition, the inhibitory activity of the test material was estimated by comparing maximal values after control (solvent) treatment (100%) with maximal values after active treatment (x%). The degree of percent inhibition was calculated for each test separately and will be given as mean ± SD. The statistical significance of percent inhibition was estimated by Student's *t* test and the Wilcoxon test for paired data.

Results and Discussion

Onions

As reported earlier, cepaenes and thiosulfinates have been identified as biologically active compounds in onion juice. These compounds are not present in the intact bulb. They are synthestized from sulfur-containing amino acids by, for example, squeezing or slicing. Zwiebelanes seem to be a by-product of onion chemistry without pronouned pharmacological properties (Fig. 1).

Cepaenes and thiosulphinates exert a wide range of pharmacological effects both in vitro and in vivo (Tables 3–5).

Cepaenes, hitherto unknown compounds, are by far the most active inhibitors of the lipoxygenase pathway of arachidonic acid metabolism found in plants or plant extracts up to now. The effects on cyclooxygenase are less pronounced [11–13, 16]. Platelet function and thromboxane biosynthesis has been shown to be reduced [11, 12]. Infiltrating cells play a major role in the pathogenesis of in-

Table 3. Effects of thiosulphinates either isolated from onion extracts or synthesized on mediator systems and cell functions in vitro.

	Histamine release	LTB4-biosynthesis	LTC4-biosynthesis	5-Lipoxygenase	Cyclooxygenase	Thromboxane-biosynthesis	Chemotaxis	Chemoluminescence
Dimethyl-TS*	0	0	0	0	0	↓		↓
Methyl-propyl-TS*+				0	0			
Dipropyl-TS*	↓↓	↓	↓	0	0			↓↓
Diallyl-TS	↓	↓↓	↓↓	↓↓↓	↓↓		↓↓	
Methyl-phenyl-TS				↓↓↓	↓↓		↓	↓↓↓
Phenyl-methyl-TS				↓↓↓	↓↓		↓	
Diphenyl-TS	0	↓↓	↓↓	↓↓↓	↓↓	↓↓	↓↓↓	↓
Methyl-1-propenyl-TS*				↓↓↓	↓↓↓	↓↓		↓↓
Propyl-1-propenyl-TS*				↓↓↓	↓↓↓			↓↓↓

↓↓↓, Reduction by more than 30% at concentrations of 1 μ*M*; ↓↓, at 10 μ*M*; ↓, at 100 μ*M*; *, identified in *Allium cepa* L.; +, isomeres; TS, thiosulphinates.

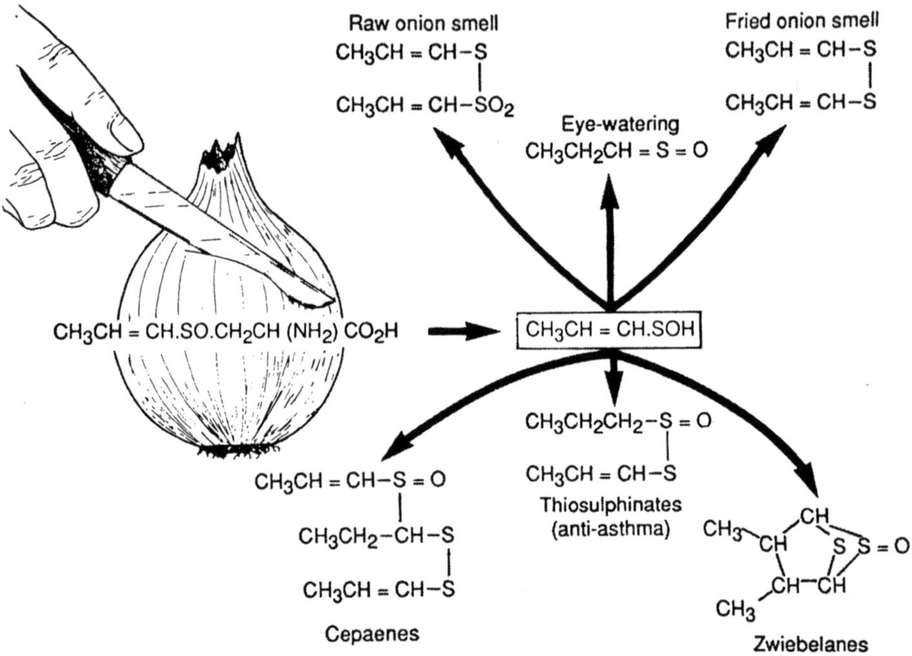

Fig. 1. Chemistry of *Allium cepa* L. (onion) [modified from The New Scientist]

Table 4. Effects of cepaenes isolated from onion extracts on 5-lipoxygenase and cyclooxygenase in vitro.

	5-Lipoxygenase	Cycloxygenase
CS 1	↓↓	↓
CS 2	↓↓↓	↓
CS 3	↓↓	↓
CS 4	↓↓↓	↓

↓↓↓, Reduction by more than 30% at concentrations of 0.25 μ*M*; ↓↓, at 1 μ*M*; ↓, at 2.5 μ*M*; CS, cepaenes.

flammation and bronchial asthma [26]. Cepaenes and thiosulphinates are highly active in inhibiting the chemotaxis of human polymorphonuclear cells [17].

In experimental animals onion extracts, both natural and synthetic thiosulphinates, are able to counteract allergen- and PAF-induced bronchial obstruction as well as PAF-induced bronchial hyperreactivity [12, 15].

In humans, topical onion extracts depress immediate and late allergic skin reactions [6]. Similarly, immediate and late bronchial obstruction after allergen inhalation challenges were markedly suppressed in volunteers after the oral intake of ethanolic onion extract prepared from 200 g of onions [10]. Pharmacological data on pure, i.e., synthetic, compounds are not available as yet. A lot of work, including toxicological studies, has to be done in this field. Ethanolic onion ex-

Table 5. Effect of thiosulphinates on guinea pig bronchial obstruction due to the inhalation of ovalbumin (allergen) and bronchoactive mediators. Histamine- and acetylcholine-induced bronchial obstruction was not altered by TS.

	Allergen	PAF	PAF-induced hyperreactivity
Dimethyl-TS*	↓	↓	
Dipropyl-TS*	0	0	
Diallyl-TS	0	0	
Methyl-phenyl-TS	↓	0	
Phenyl-methyl-TS	0	↓	
Diphenyl-TS	↓	↓↓	↓↓
Methyl-1-propenyl-TS*	↓↓		
Whole onion extract	↓↓	↓↓	

↓↓, Reduction by more than 30% after oral doses of 10 mg/kg; ↓, oral dose of 100 mg/kg; *, identified in *Allium cepa* L.; TS, thiosulphinate; PAF, platelet-activating factor.

tracts can hardly be used in the treatment of asthma; the specific smell would make the patient a social outcast. We are trying to improve onion extracts with regard to smell, stability, and reproducibility of their pharmacologic effects. Presently we have onion capsules which might be suitable for use in patients.

Galphimia glauca

Galphimia glauca (synonym *Thyrallis glauca*), abundant in Middle and South America, is prescribed from medicine men of some tribes in the rain forest of

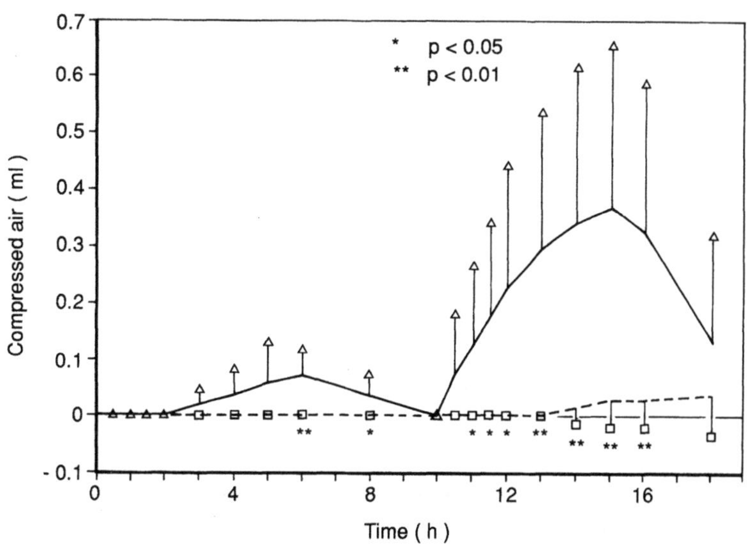

Fig. 2. Prevention of allergen (ovalbumin)-induced bronchial obstruction in 10 guinea pigs by the oral intake of 1 ml *Galphimia glauca* extract 12 h prior to the inhalation challenge (0 and 10 min). *Solid line*, control; *broken line*, *Galphimia*

South America against allergies. The plant was collected by Dr. W. Schwabe during a plant excursion through Brazil and brought to Germany. Preliminary studies on patients with pollinosis were promising [27, 28], but no information was available as yet on active compounds and their mode of action. We observed that the

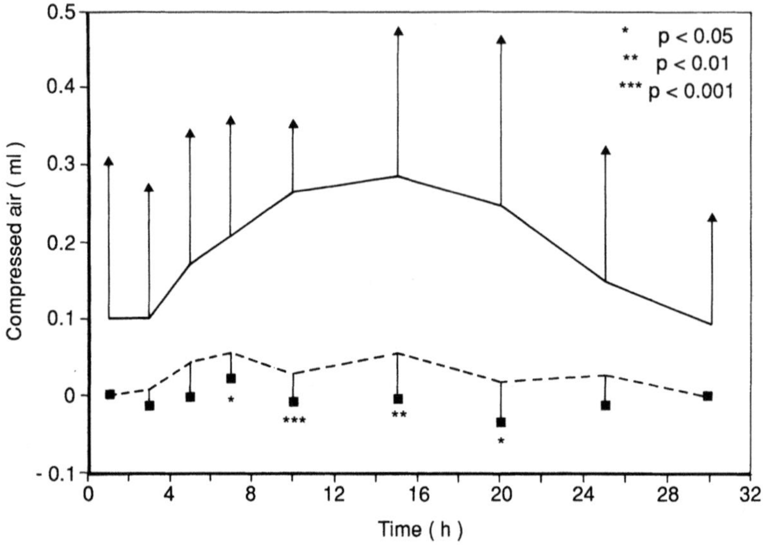

Fig. 3. Prevention of PAF-induced bronchial obstruction in 10 guinea pigs by the oral intake of 1 ml *Galphimia glauca* extract 12 h prior to the inhalation challenge. *Solid line*, control; *broken line*, *Galphimia*

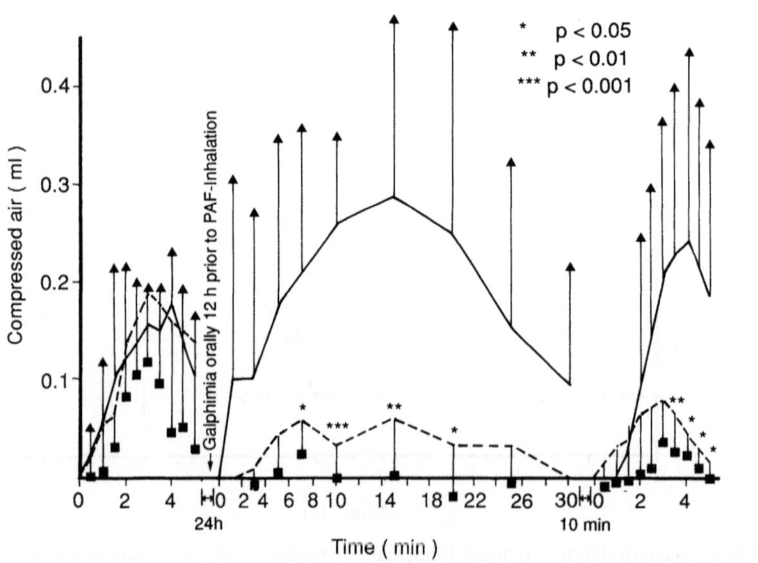

Fig. 4. Prevention of PAF-induced bronchial hyperreactivity in 10 guinea pigs by the oral intake of 1 ml *Galphimia glauca* extract 12 h prior to the inhalation of histamine, PAF, and histamine

oral intake of 1 ml extract protect guinea pigs against allergen- and PAF-induced bronchial obstruction (Figs. 2, 3). This effect persists up to 4 days after one single dose [29, 30]. The PAF-induced bronchial hyperreactivity can be prevented, too (Fig. 4).

A great number of experiments have been performed in order to identify the active compounds. The results will be described elsewhere in detail [29, 31]. We found tetragalloyl quinic acid to be the most active substance followed by methyl gallate (Figs. 5–8). Quercetin and gallic acid, also present in the active extracts, were less active (percent inhibition of PAF-induced bronchial obstruction by 53% and 37%, respectively). It seems of special interest that only the oral route of administration worked. Neither the histamine- nor the acetylcholine-induced bronchial obstruction was affected by *Galphimia glauca* or its active compounds. In vitro, inhibition of histamine release from human polymorphonuclear leukocytes and adenoidal mast cells was observed [32]. The chemotaxis of human polymorphonuclear leukocytes was not affected.

Many data are available on other biological effects of methyl gallate and related compounds. They are potent radical scavengers and used in food and cosmetics as antioxidants [33, 34]. A radical scavenger of similar structure has been shown previously to be highly effective in preventing bronchial obstruction in guinea pigs [24]. Gallic acid and its derivatives may be suitable for the treatment of viral and bacterial infections [35, 36].

We are in the process of testing these compounds for antiasthmatic effects in humans.

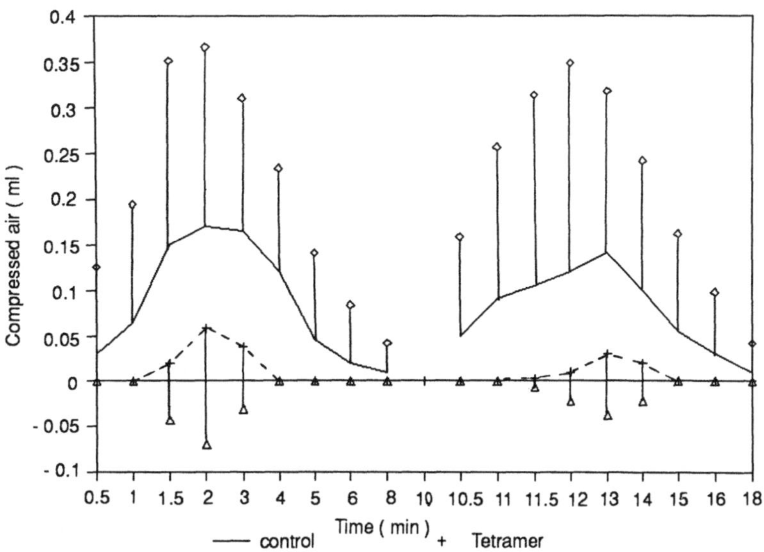

Fig. 5. Prevention of allergen (ovalbumin)-induced bronchial obstruction in 10 guinea pigs by the oral intake of 5 mg/kg tetragalloyl quinic acid 2 h prior to the inhalation challenge (0 and 10 min; percent inhibition of bronchial obstruction: 87% ± 22%, 67% ± 71%). *Solid line*, control; *broken line*, tetragalloyl quinoic acid

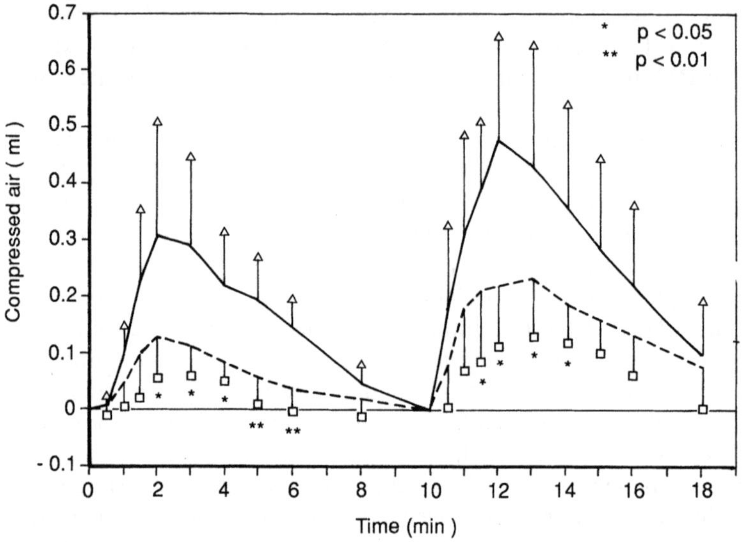

Fig. 7. Prevention of PAF-induced bronchial obstruction in 10 guinea pigs by the oral intake of 45 mg/kg methylgallate 12 h prior to the inhalation of PAF (percent inhibition of bronchial obstruction: 65%). *Solid line*, control; *broken line*, methylgallate

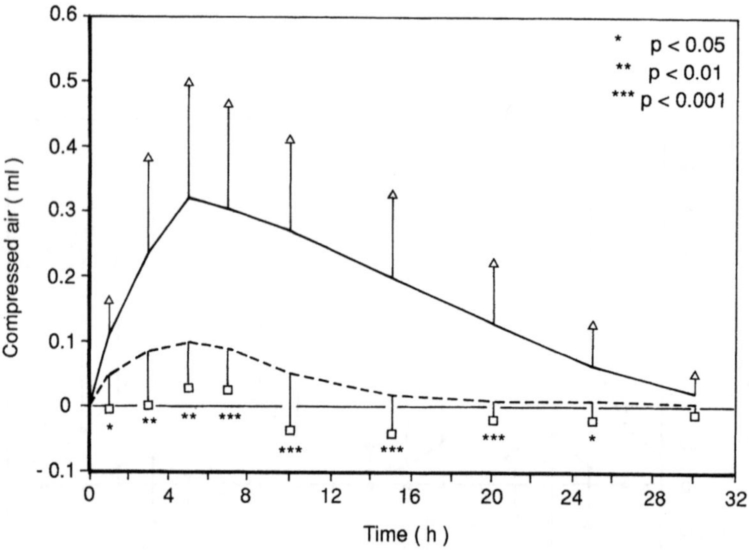

Fig. 6. Prevention of allergen (ovalbumin)-induced bronchial obstruction in 10 guinea pigs by the oral intake of 45 mg/kg methylgallate 12 h prior to the inhalation challenge (0 and 10 min; percent inhibition of bronchial obstruction, 43%). *Solid line*, control; *broken line*, methylgallate

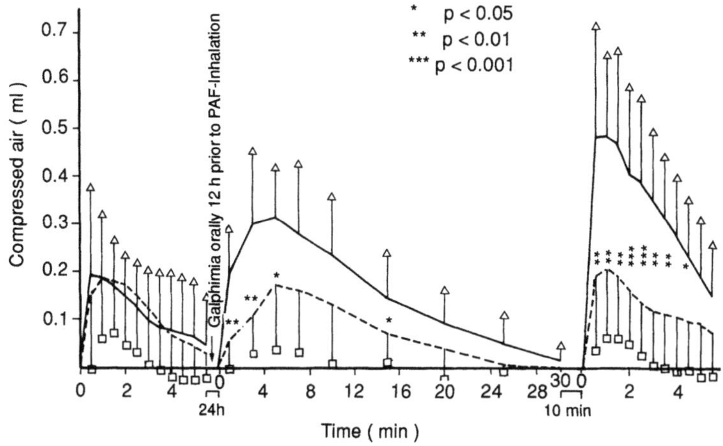

Fig. 8. Prevention of PAF-induced bronchial hyperreactivity in 10 guinea pigs by the oral intake of 45 mg/kg methylgallate 12 h prior to the inhalation of histamine, PAF, and histamine (percent inhibition of bronchial obstruction: 45% and 57%, respectively). *Solid line*, control; *broken line*, methylgallate

Adhatoda vasica

Extracts from *Adhatoda vasica* leaves are widely used in India to treat cough, bronchitis, and bronchial asthma. In none of several investigations has the active principle been identified [37–42]. There are some in vitro data on the broncho-

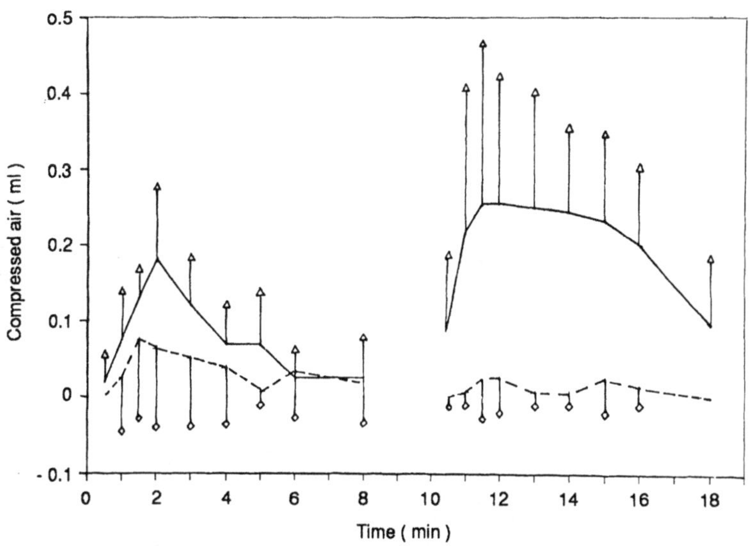

Fig. 9. Prevention of allergen (ovalbumin)-induced bronchial obstruction in eight guinea pigs by the inhalation (90 s) of 6 mg/ml whole plant extract from *Adhatoda vasica* 10 min prior to the first ovalbumin inhalation (0 and 10 min; percent inhibition of bronchial obstruction: 56.2%, 76.8%). *Solid line*, control; *broken line*, *Adhatoda vasica*

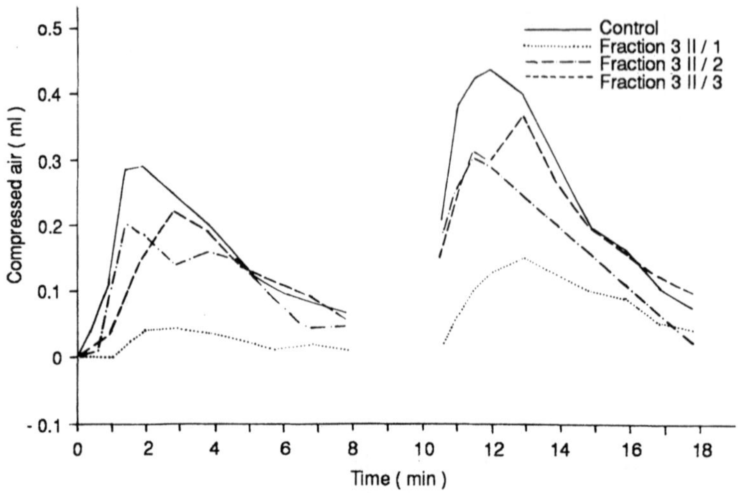

Fig. 10. Effect of different fractions from *Adhatoda vasica* on allergen (ovalbumin)-induced bronchial obstruction of at least 10 guinea pigs in each group. Fraction 3 II 1. (10 mg/ml aerosol) contained alkaloids, fraction 3 II 2. (20 mg/ml aerosol) astringents and fraction 3 II 3. (10 mg/ml aerosol) flavonoids. Only the alkaloid fraction showed pronounced effects

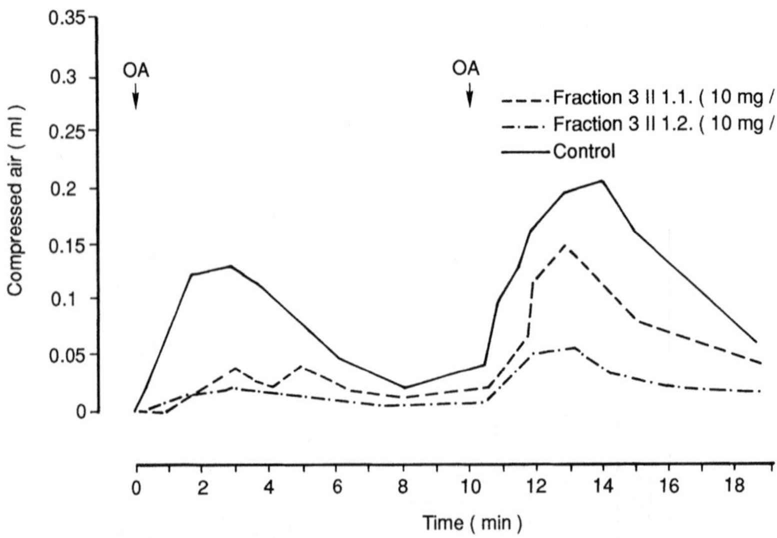

Fig. 11. Prevention of allergen (ovalbumin, *OA*)-induced bronchial obstruction in 12 guinea pigs by the inhalation (90 s) of 10 mg/ml subfraction 3 II 1.1. and 3 II 1.2. of *Adhatoda vasica* 20 min prior to the first OA inhalation. Fraction 3 II 1.1 contained vasicinon and vasicin and was less active (percent inhibition of bronchial obstruction: 62% and 41%) than fraction 3 II 1.2. containing other alkaloids (percent inhibition of bronchial obstruction: 58% and 66%)

lytic activity of vasicinon, but this alkaloid becomes rapidly converted into the bronchoconstrictive alkaloid vasicin.

At first we were unable to detect any pronounced protective effect of the plant extract. Using improved extraction methods, however, we could demonstrate marked protection against allergen-induced bronchial obstruction (Fig. 9). Sequential fractionation of this extract led to the discovery of alkaloids other than vasicinon/vasicin as active compounds (Figs. 10, 11). They will be identified, synthestized and tested in future studies.

Picrorhiza kurrooa

Picrorhiza kurrooa, a small herb with tuberous roots, grows in the Himalayan area at altitudes of 3000–5000 m. It is mainly used in Ayurvedic medicine to treat liver and lung diseases, but also in the treatment of chronic dysentery and other complaints. Controlled trials in different arthritic conditions showed marked improvement in the clinical symptoms [42, 43]. *Picrorhiza kurrooa* root powder was found to inhibit histamine release from guinea pig lung tissue and to enhance the bronchodilator effects of sympathomimetic amines [44, 45]. The active compounds have not been identified as yet. Previous phytochemical investigations demonstrated the presence of iridoid glycosides and phenol glycosides [46, 47].

All substances were extracted from the roots of the plant using the Soxhlet extractor and the following solvents: hexane, chloroform, ethylacetate and methanol. The methanol extract was divided into a water-soluble and a butanol-soluble subfraction. Neither altered histamine release from human polymorphonuclear leukocytes or PAF-induced bronchial obstruction in guinea pigs. The chloroform

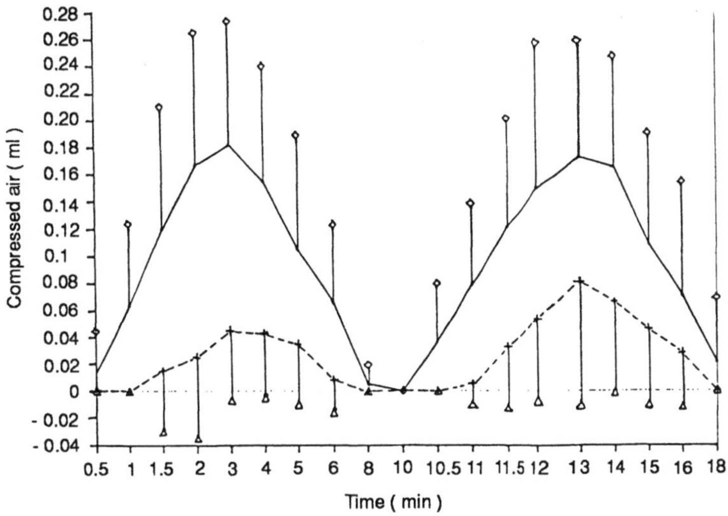

Fig. 12. Prevention of allergen (ovalbumin)-induced bronchial obstruction in 10 guinea pigs by the oral intake of 100 mg/kg ethyl acetate fraction of powdered *Picrorhiza kurrooa* roots 1 h prior to the inhalation challenge (0 and 10 min). *Solid line*, control; *broken line*, EtOAc fraction of *Picrorhiza kurrooa*

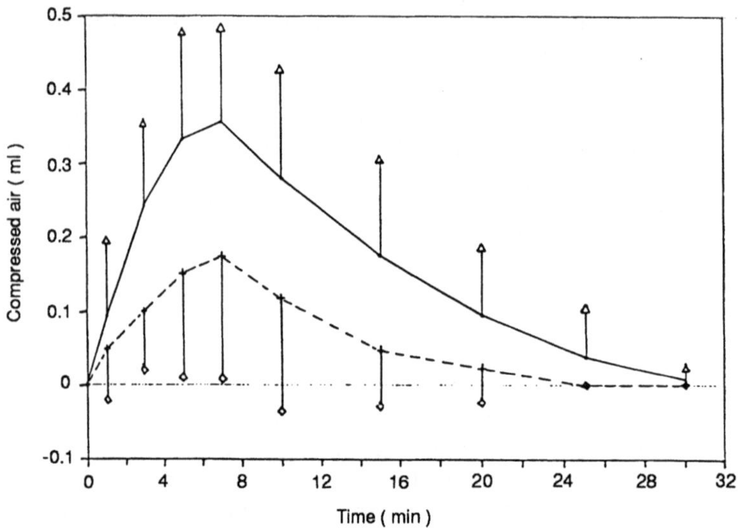

Fig. 13. Prevention of PAF-induced bronchial obstruction in 10 guinea pigs by the oral intake of 100 mg/kg ethyl acetate fraction of powdered *Picrorhiza kurrooa* roots 1 h prior to the inhalation challenge. *Solid line*, control; *broken line*, EtOAc fraction of *Picrorhiza kurrooa*

and ethyl acetate fractions in contrast demonstrated significant effects. Both fractions showed nearly identical chromatographic characteristics. Further investigations were performed therefore on the ethyl acetate fraction. We observed marked inhibitory effects on the PAF- and allergen-induced bronchial obstruction of guinea pigs (Figs. 12, 13). The ethyl acetate fraction was divided by Sephadex LH20 chromatography into two subfractions (11–17 and 18–29). The former contained cucurbitacinglycosids and was found inactive, similar to its major component, the cucurbitacinglycosid Cuc3 (25-acetoxy-2-beta-D-glucosyloxy-3,16,20-trihydroxy-19-norlanosta-5,23-diene-22-one). The active fraction [18–29] was divided into the inactive subfraction PIC containing Pikrosid II, minecosids, veronicosid and feruloylctalpol and the active subfraction Pic 1 and androsin. Pic 1 did not alter the allergen-induced bronchial obstruction in guinea pigs. Androsin, in contrast, demonstrated significant inhibitory effects on bronchial reactions to the inhalation of allergen and PAF (Figs. 14–16). Apocynine, the aglykon of androsin, and acetophenons of similar chemical structure are pharmacologically even more active.

Conclusion

In the past, traditional medicine has stimulated the development of new therapeutic principles, including drugs for the treatment of bronchial asthma such as betasympathomimetics, anticholinergics, xanthine derivatives and cromolyn sodium. We hope that similar methods will be successful in the future and will im-

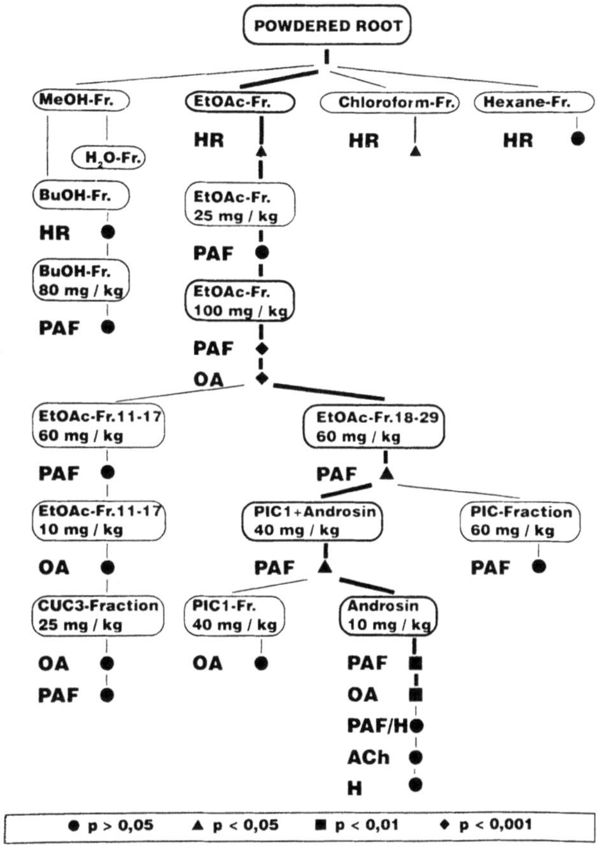

Fig. 14. Identification of the active compound in *Picrorhiza kurrooa*.
HR, histamine release from human polymorphonuclear leukocytes;
OA, allergen induced (ovalbumin) bronchial obstruction in guinea pigs;
PAF, PAF-induced bronchial obstruction in guinea pigs; *PAF/H*, PAF-induced bronchial hyperreactivity in guinea pigs;
H, histamine-induced bronchial obstruction in guinea pigs;
Ach, Acetylcholine-induced bronchial obstruction

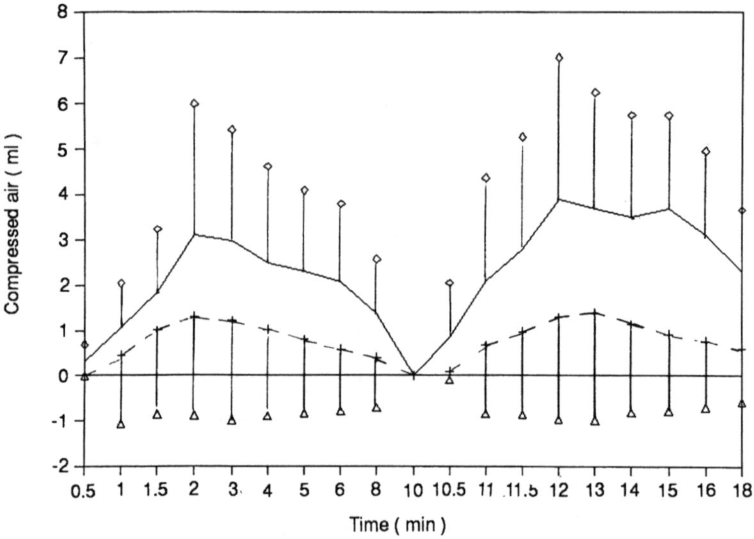

Fig. 15. Prevention of allergen-induced bronchial obstruction in 10 guinea pigs by the oral intake of 10 mg/kg androsin 1 h prior to the inhalation of ovalbumin (0 and 10 min; percent inhibition of bronchial obstruction: 57% and 71%, respectively). *Solid line*, control; *broken line*, androsin

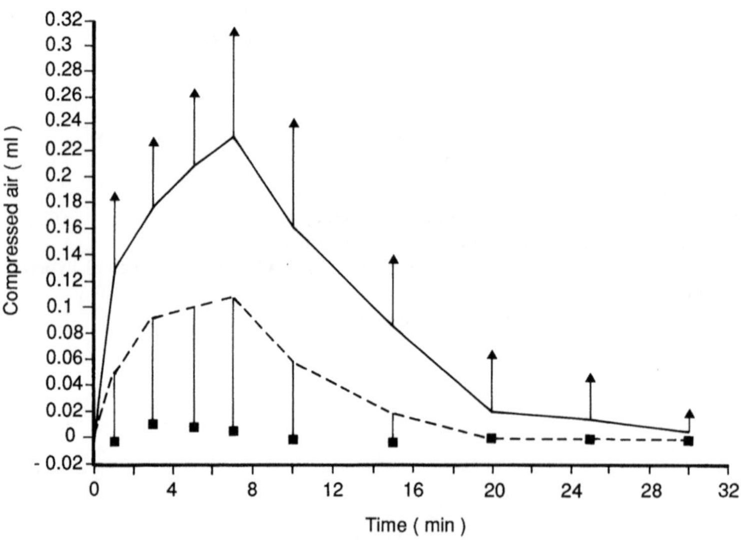

Fig. 16. Prevention of PAF-induced bronchial obstruction in 10 guinea pigs by the oral intake of 10 mg/kg androsin 1 h prior to the inhalation of PAF (percent inhibition of bronchial obstruction: 58.5%). *Solid line*, control; *broken line*, androsin

prove the possibilities of treating bronchial asthma and allergic and inflammatory disorders.

References

1. Kuo-chün S, Oshou-hsün C (1958) Sheng-yao-hsüeh ("pharmacognosy"). Peking, p 254–260
2. Schramm G (1960) Zur Frühgeschichte der chinesischen Droge Ma-huang (Herba Ephedrae). Pharm Ztg 105:972–973
3. Eiden W (1990) Atropin: Erlebnisse eines Wirkstoffmoleküls. Pharm Ztg 135:2145–2154
4. Uhlenbrook K, Mulli K, Schmied O (1953) Khellin. 1. Mitt Beitrag zur Pharmakologie der Inhaltsstoffe der Ammi visnaga. Arzneimittelforsch 3:130–133
5. Joachim H (1890) Papyros Ebers. Reimer, Berlin
6. Dorsch W, Ring J (1984) Suppression of immediate and late cutaneous allergic skin reactions by alcoholic onion extract applied topically. Allergy 39:43–49
7. Dorsch W, Weber J (1984) Prevention of allergen-induced bronchial obstruction by crude alcoholic onion extract. Agents Actions 14:626–629
8. Dorsch W, Adam O, Weber J, Ziegeltrum T (1985) Antiasthmatic effects of onion extracts – detection of benzyl- and other isothiocyanates (mustard oils) as antiasthmatic compounds of plant origin. Eur J Pharmacol 107:17–24
9. Dorsch W, Ettl M, Hein G, Scheftner P, Weber J, Bayer T, Wagner H (1987) Antiasthmatic effects of onions – inhibition of PAF-induced bronchial obstruction by onion oils. Int Arch Allergy Appl Immunol 82:535–536
10. Dorsch W, Adelmann-Grill B, Bayer T, Ettl M, Hein G, Jaggy H, Ring J, Scheftner P, Schneider T, Wagner H (1987) Zwiebelextrakte als Asthma-Therapeutika? Allergologie 10:316–324
11. Bayer T (1988) Neue schwefelhaltige Inhaltsstoffe aus *Allium cepa* L. mit antiasthmatischer und antiallergischer Wirkung. Thesis, Ludwig Maximilian University, Munich
12. Dorsch W, Wagner H, Bayer T, Fessler B, Hein G, Ring J, Scheftner P, Sieber W, Strasser T, Weiss E (1988) Antiasthmatic effects of onions – alk(en)ylsulfinothioic acid alk(en)ylesters inhibit histamine release, leukotriene and thromboxane biosynthesis in vitro and counteract PAF- and allergen-induced bronchial obstruction in vivo. Biochem Pharmacol 37:4479–4485
13. Bayer T, Wagner H, Wray V, Dorsch W (1988) New inhibitors of cyclooxygenase and 5-lipoxygenase from lipophilic onion extracts. Lancet 15:906
14. Dorsch W, Wagner H, Bayer T (1989) Asthmaschutzwirkung von Zwiebelinhaltsstoffen – Wirkprofil von Thiosulfinaten. Allergologie 12:388–396
15. Dorsch W, Scharff J, Bayer T, Wagner H (1989) Antiasthmatic effects of onions – prevention of PAF-induced bronchial obstruction to histamine in guinea pigs by diphenylthiosulfinate. Int Arch Allergy Appl Immunol 88:229–230
16. Wagner H, Dorsch W, Bayer T, Breu W, Willer F (1990) Antiasthmatic effects of onions – inhibition of 5-lipoxygenase and cycloxygenase in vitro by thiosulfinates and "cepaenes". Prostaglandins, Leukot Essent Fatty Acids 39:59–62
17. Dorsch W, Schneider E, Bayer T, Breu W, Wagner H (1990) Antiinflammatory effects of onions – inhibition of chemotaxis of human polymorphonuclear leukocytes by thiosulfinates and cepaenes. Int Arch Allergy Appl Immunol 92:39–42
18. Bayer T, Wagner H, Block E, Grisoni S, Zhao SH, Nesmelyi A (1989) Zwiebelanes: novel biologically active 2,3-dimethyl-5,6-dithiobicyclo (2.1.1) hexane 5-oxides from onion. J Am Chem Soc 111:3085–3086
19. Bayer T, Seligmann O, Wray V, Wagner H (1989) Novel biologically active thiosulphinates and alpha-sulphinyldisulfides from allium cepa. Phytochemistry 28:783–789
20. Kuhl P, Shiloh H, Jha H, Muraski U, Zilliken F (1984) 6,7,4-Trihydroxyisoflavan: a potent and selective inhibitor of 5-lipoxygenase in human and porcine peripheral blood leukocytes. Prostaglandins 28:783–789
21. Nelson RD (1975) Chemotaxis under agarose. J Immunol 115:1650–1660
22. Ring J, O'Connor R (1979) In vitro histamine and serotonin release studies in atopic dermatitis. Int Arch Allergy Appl Immunol 58:322–330
23. Siess W, Roth P, Weber PC (1981) Stimulated platelet aggregation, thromboxane B2 formation and platelet sensitivity to prostacyclin: a critical evaluation. Thromb Haemost 45:204–209

24. Dorsch W, Waldherr U, Rosmanith J (1981) Continuous recording of intrapulmonary "compressed air" as a sensitive noninvasive method of measuring bronchial obstruction in guinea pigs. Pflügers Arch 391:236–241
25. Gonsior E (ed) (1984) Richtlinien für die Durchführung von bronchialen Provokationen mit Allergenen und pharmakodynamischen Substanzen bei obstructiven Atemwegskrankheiten. Allergologie 7:238–242
26. Gleich J, Dorsch W (1990) The late phase allergic reaction. Summary and conclusion. In: Dorsch W (ed) The late phase allergic reaction, chap 52. CRC, Boca Raton (Handbook)
27. Martinez M (1969) Las plantas medicinales de Mexico. Botas, Mexico, p 402
28. Schwabe W (1980) Übersicht über neuere Arzneipflanzen. Allg Homöop Ztg 225:217–229
29. Bittinger M (1991) Asthmaprotektive Wirkung von *Galphimia glauca* L. Identifikation von Wirksubstanzen und Wirkmechanismen. Thesis, Johannes Gutenberg University, Mainz
30. Wagner H, Dorsch W, Bittinger M, Koch S (1989) Long lasting antiasthmatic effects of extracts from *Galphimia glauca.* Allergologie 12:139
31. Dorsch W, Bittinger M, Kaas A, Dumoulin S, Kreher B, Wagner H (1991) Antiasthmatic effects of galphimia glauca – gallic acid and related compounds prevent allergen- and PAF-induced bronchial obstruction as well as bronchial hyperactivity in guinea pigs. Int Arch Allergy Appl Immunol (to be published)
32. Bent S, Wagner H, Dorsch W, Schmutzler W (to be published) Zwiebel- und *Galphimia glauca* Extrakt hemmen die ConA induzierte Histaminfreisetzung aus humanen adenoiden Mastzellen. Workshop of the German Society for Research in Allergology and Immunology, Mainz, spring 1990. Allergologie
33. Forgo T, Büchi J (1970) Synthese, physikalisch-chemische Eigenschaften und antioxydative Wirkung einiger Gallussäure-ester. Pharm Acta Helv 45:207–226
34. Römpp H (1986) Römpps Chemielexikon. Thieme, Stuttgart, p 1939
35. Boyd I, Beveridge EG (1981) Antimicrobial activity of some alkyl esters of gallic acid (3,4,5-trihydroxybenzoic acid) against *E. coli* NCTC 5933 with particular reference to *n*-propyl-gallate. Microbios 30:73–85
36. Kane CJM, Menna JH, Yeh YC (1988) Methyl gallate, methyl13,4,5-trihydroxybenzoate is a potent and highly specific inhibitor of herpes simplex virus in vitro. I. Purification and characterisation of methylgallate from *Sapium sebiferum.* Biosci Rep 8:85–94
37. Bhat VS, Nanavati DD, Mardikar BR (1978) Adhatoda vasica nees – an ayurvedic medicinal plant. Indian Drugs 15:62–66
38. Bhalla HL, Nimbkar AY (1982) Preformulation studies. III. Vasicinone, a bronchodilatory alkaloid from *Adhatoda vasica nees* (absorption, potency and toxicity studies). Drug Dev Indian Pharm 8:833–846
39. Jain MP, Sharma VK (1982) Phytochemical investigation of roots of *Adhatoda vasica.* Planta Med 46:250–258
40. Thapa BB (1985) Pharmacognostical and chromatographic studies on *Adhatoda vasica.* J Nepalese Animals 12:21–26
41. Grampp V, Koch S, Wagner H, Dorsch W (1989) New antiasthmatic alcaloids from *Adhatoda vasica.* Allergologie 12:125
42. Langer JG, Gupta OP, Atal CK (1981) Clinical trials on *Picrorhiza kurroa* as an immunoregulator. Indian Pharmacol 13:98–103
43. Mogre K, Vora K, Sheth UK (1981) Effect of *Picrorhiza kurroa* and *Eclipta alba* on Na^+ K^+ ATPase in hepatic injury by hepatotoxic agents. Indian J Pharmac 13:253–259
44. Mahajani SS, Kulkarni RD (1977) Effect of disodium cromoglycate and *Picrorhiza kurroa* root powder on sensitivity of guinea pigs to histamine and sympathicomimetic amines. Int Arch Allergy Appl Immunol 53:137–144
45. Mahajani SS, Kulkarni RD (1979) Induction of resistance to isoprenaline in guinea pigs and its modulation by disodium cromoglycate, *Picrorhiza kurroa* and indometacin. Aspects Allergy Appl Immunol 12:205–215
46. Stuppner H, Wagner H (1989) Minor iridoid and phenol glycosides of *Picrorhiza kurrooa.* Planta Med 55:467–469
47. Dorsch W, Wagner H, Stuppner H, Demoulin S, Gropp M (to be published) Asthmaschutzwirkung von *Picrorhiza kurroa.* Identifikation von Wirksubstanz und Wirkmechanismen. Workshop of the German Society for Research in Allergology and Immunology, Mainz, spring 1990. Allergologie

Ultraviolet Light and Suppression of Epidermal Immune Response

T.A. Luger[1,3], T. Schwarz[2,3], A. Urbanski[3], J. Krutmann[4], A. Köck[3], and E. Schauer[3]

[1]Department of Dermatology, University Münster, Von-Esmarch-Strasse 56, W-4400 Münster, Federal Republic of Germany
[2]Department of Dermatology, Hospital Vienna-Lainz, Wolkersbergenstrasse 1, 1130 Vienna, Austria
[3]Department of Dermatology II, Ludwig Boltzmann Institut, Laboratory of Cell Biology, University of Vienna, Alserstrasse 4, 1090 Vienna, Austria
[4]Department of Dermatology, University Freiburg, Hauptstrasse 7, W-7800 Freiburg, Federal Republic of Germany

Abstract

There is clear evidence that the keratinocyte does not only represent a mechanical barrier to the outside, but is a fully immunocompetent cell endowed with the capacity to release various immunomodulating cytokines such as interleukin (IL) 1, IL3, IL6, IL8, tumor necrosis factor α, colony stimulating factors (CFS) and several growth factors. The constitutive production of these mediators by keratinocytes both in vivo and in vitro is low, however, can be significantly enhanced by stimuli such as tumor promoters or endotoxin. In addition, ultraviolet (UV)-light has turned out to be one of the most potent inducers of cytokine synthesis and release. Accordingly UV exposure results in an increased production of interleukins, TNF, CSF and growth factors by epidermal cells. The secretion of these cytokines causes local immunologic and inflammatory reactions following UV-irradiation. These factors, however, also may enter the circulation thus being responsible for systemic effects. UV-light also induces keratinocytes to release immunosuppressive factors such as epidermal cell suppressor factor (ECSF), epidermal cell-contra IL1 (EC-contra IL1), transforming growth factor β and a recently characterized specific IL1 receptor antagonist (IL1ra). Furthermore, upon stimulation with UV-irradiation keratinocytes produce α-melanocyte stimulating hormone (MSHα), a cleavage product of the protein proopiomelanocortin (POMC). MSHα has been shown to block IL1 activity and a contact hypersensitivity reaction. The production of such immunoinhibitors may play an essential role during UV-induced immunosuppression.

Introduction

Exposure to ultraviolet (UV) irradiation is known to contribute not only to the development of skin cancer, but also to cause local and systemic immunosuppression [10]. Accordingly, following exposure of mice to UV light, cutaneous application of contact allergens, such as dinitrofluorobenzene (DNFB), to UV-irradiated skin produced only a minimal contact hypersensitivity (CHS) response. Administration of DNFB to an unexposed site resulted in a normal CHS reaction [26]. The induction of this unresponsiveness correlated with both a diminished number and morphologic and functional alterations of Langerhans' cells at the site of UV exposure. Moreover, it was demonstrated that this suppression was associated with the induction of hapten-specific suppressor cells [5].

UV irradiation also may cause systemic immunosuppression. Accordingly, UV exposure of animals followed by application of DNFB to a UV-protected skin area resulted in suppression of CHS induction [6] and was associated with the generation of antigen-specific T suppressor cells [3]. In contrast to the local suppression of CHS, the systemic form does not correlate with morphologic alterations of Langerhans' cells [17]. Although the pathogenesis is not clear yet, the finding of an abnormal response to an antigen applied at a distant non-UV-exposed skin area may be explained by the induction of a soluble circulating mediator produced in the skin upon UV exposure [11]. In the following, findings concerning the UV-induced production of immunoinhibiting mediators by epidermal cells will be briefly discussed.

UV-Induced Immunosuppressive Cytokines

Keratinocytes are a well-known source of a variety of immunostimulating cytokines including interleukins (IL-1, IL-3, IL-6, IL-8), tumor necrosis factors (TNFs), and colony-stimulating factors (CSFs) [16]. Moreover, it has been demonstrated that the synthesis and release of these cytokines by epidermal cells is affected by UV light [20]. However, another important effect of UV light is the induction of local and systemic immunosuppression [6, 11]. Since keratinocytes are the main target of UV-B light and exhibit immunosecretory capacities, they have to be considered as a primary source of inhibitory mediators which may enter the circulation and cause systemic immune suppression. Accordingly, it has been demonstrated that i. v. injection of supernatants derived from UV-treated murine epidermal cells resulted in the inability to induce CHS to potent sensitizing agents in the recipient animals [21]. Therefore, upon UV irradiation murine epidermal cells in culture release an immunosuppressing factor which blocks the induction of CHS. This factor is referred to as epidermal cell suppressor factor (EC-SF) and is not detectable in supernatants of unirradiated keratinocytes. EC-SF has a molecular mass of approximately 20–50 kDa and, according to its biochemical characteristics, it is distinct from other epidermal, cell derived, immunoinhibiting factors, such as eicosanoids and urocanic acid, a soluble compound located in the corneal layer of the epidermis which may be a photoreceptor for immunosuppression [3, 21]. However, EC-SF might be related to other epidermal cell-derived suppressor factors blocking delayed-type hypersensitivity [7] and inducing antigen-specific T suppressor cells [27].

It recently has been discovered that, following UV exposure, murine epidermal cells in culture release a cytokine which blocks the biological activities of IL-1 (Schwarz et al. 1987). This IL-1 inhibitor, EC-contra-IL-1, has a molecular mass similar to EC-SF and blocks both natural and recombinant IL-1 in a dose-dependent manner [22]. EC-contra-IL-1 seems to inhibit IL-1 specifically, as it does not suppress IL-2 or IL-3 activity and does not block spontaneous cell proliferation, thus excluding a toxic effect.

Similar to EC-SF, EC-contra-IL-1 is not constitutively produced by keratinocytes. The release has to be induced by UV exposure or by stimulation with the tumor promotor phorbol myristate acetate (PMA) [22]. Recently, an IL-1 inhibitor with similar characteristics has been detected in the sera of total body UV exposed mice, suggesting that the production of EC-contra-IL-1 is not only an in vitro phenomenon [23]. This circulating factor was not found in irradiated animals and maximum levels appeared between 12 and 24 h after UV exposure. These observations support the view that epidermal cells, upon UV irradiation, release EC-contra-IL-1 which may enter the circulation and perhaps cause systemic immunosuppression.

EC-contra-IL-1 recently has also been detected in human cell lines. This mediator was isolated and partially purified from either UV exposed or tumor promotor treated human epidermoid carcinoma cell lines [28]. Human EC-contra-IL-1 shares obvious biological and biochemical similarities with the murine IL-1 inhibitor (Table 1). According to its biochemical characteristics, human EC-contra-IL-1 also appears to be distinct from a recently cloned monocyte derived IL-1 receptor antagonist (IL-1ra) [4].

IL-1 and IL-6 may function as signals provided by accessory cells in augmenting T cell activation [12]. Accordingly, human EC-contra-IL-1 was shown to down regulate human T cell activation in an accessory cell dependent system by specifically blocking accessory cell derived IL-1 activity; IL-6 activity remained unaffected [13]. These studies reveal a novel mechanism by which UV irradiation, in addition to its previously defined direct effects on human accessory cells, may modulate human accessory cell activity in an indirect manner via the induction of suppressor factors such as EC-contra-IL-1 [14].

The in vivo functions of these inhibitors are not yet clear; however, they may represent part of a physiological feedback mechanism down-regulating IL-1 activity after its excessive release. Although there are some similarities between these different IL-1 inhibitors, including EC-contra-IL-1 and EC-SF, only further purification, sequencing, and gene cloning will reveal whether they are identical or

Table 1. Human epidermal cell contra-IL-1.

Source	Keratinocytes, epidermoid carcinoma cell lines (A431, KB)	
Stimulant	UV irradiation, phorbol myristate acetate	
Biochemical characteristics		
Moleuclar mass		40 kDa
pI		9
Biological activities	Blocks the biological activity of natural and recombinant IL-1α, IL-1β	

distinct cytokines released by keratinocytes. Moreover, it remains to be clarified whether these mediators are new factors or well-known immunomodulators with so far undescribed capacities [15].

Another keratinocyte derived cytokine with recently discovered immunosuppressive properties is transforming growth factor-beta (TGF-β) [1, 29]. TGF-β, previously characterized as a 25 kDa protein consisting of 5 subtypes (TGF-β_{1-5}) regulates cell growth, differentiation, and extracellular matrix production [24]. Moreover, TGF-β blocks the activities of several immunomodulating cytokines inducing IL-1, IL-2, and CSF and thus may down-regulate immunologic and inflammatory reactions. Accordingly, TGF-β has turned out to be responsible for a variety of immunosuppressive activities previously described under various names. A glioblastoma derived suppressor factor inhibiting IL-1 and IL-2 activity showed homology to TGF-β_2 [31]. Furthermore, a keratinocyte derived factor suppressing mixed lymphocyte reactions, keratinocyte lymphocyte inhibitory factor (KLIF), exhibited partial homology to TGF-β [19]. Although TGF-β has been demonstrated to be a potent inhibitor of IL-1 activity, EC-contra-IL-1 seems to be unrelated to TGF-β since its activity could not be blocked by antibodies directed against TGF-β. EC-contra-IL-1 also does not interfere with IL-2 activity [28].

UV-Mediated Production of Immunosuppressive Neuroendocrine Hormones

There is increasing evidence for a link between the neuroendocrine and immune systems [2]. Accordingly, it has been demonstrated that cytokines such as IL-1 and IL-6 may stimulate the release of corticotropin releasing factor (CRF) in the hypothalamus [18], and IL-2 stimulates the release of adrenocorticotropin (ACTH) in the pituitary gland [30]. Pituitary gland derived hormones, such as α-melanocyte stimulating hormone (α-MSH), ACTH, or β-endorphin, may also modulate certain immune functions. Accordingly, α-MSH has been shown to inhibit some biological activities of IL-1 and TNF-α. Moreover, α-MSH is able to block the induction of a CHS reaction and to suppress the expression of class I major histocompatibility antigens [2, 8].

α-MSH is a cleavage product of the protein proopiomelanocortin (POMC), which also represents the precursor of ACTH and β-endorphin [2]. Immunoreactive α-MSH was found in human skin [25]; thus, it was determined whether keratinocytes in culture could produce α-MSH. Using a commercially available radioimmunoassay it was demonstrated that both normal human keratinocytes and an epidermoid carcinoma cell line are able to produce α-MSH [9]. In addition, epidermal cell derived α-MSH exhibited biological activity as detected in the tyrosinase assay. Moreover, treatment of epidermal cells with PMA or UV light resulted in a significant stimulation of epidermal cell α-MSH production (Table 2). In order to investigate whether epidermal cells are able to synthesize the α-MSH precursor, POMC northern blot analysis was performed using a POMC cDNA probe. Keratinocytes constitutively expressed POMC specific mRNA, which was further up-regulated upon treatment with PMA or UV light [9]. These

Table 2. α-MSH production by human epidermoid carcinoma cells.

Stimulus	α-MSH (pg/ml) mean $\pm$ SE
0	39 ± 6
PMA (10 ng/ml)	104 ± 17
UV-B (100 J/m^2)	62 ± 10

A431 cells (1×10^6/ml) were either left untreated or stimulated with PMA or UV-B light. After a 48 h incubation supernatants were tested for α-MSH using an α-MSH radioimmunoassay.

findings indicate that keratinocytes are able to synthesize and release α-MSH and that UV irradiation is a potent stimulus of α-MSH production by epidermal cells. Thus, UV light, by inducing α-MSH, may not only regulate melanin production in the skin but, through the immunoinhibiting capacities of α-MSH, may also be involved in the down-regulation of immune responses.

Conclusion

The finding that epidermal cells, in particular keratinocytes, exhibit the capacity to release both inhibitory cytokines and neuroendocrine hormones with immunosuppressive capacities further supports the concept of the epidermis as an immunologic organ. It demonstrates that keratinocytes not only may initiate the immune response by providing immunoenhancing mediators, but also may turn down ongoing inflammatory and immunologic reactions via the production of suppressor factors. The capacity to release agonistic and antagonistic factors, such as IL-1 and contra-IL-1, however, might not be unique to keratinocytes but common to all immunosecretory cells. Consequently, immunosuppressive situations may originate from keratinocytes. This seems to be true for UV induced immunosuppression, as UV mediated release of immunosuppressive factors by keratinocytes may at least partly explain local and, in particular, systemic immunosuppressive states following UV exposure. However, the mechanisms leading either to the release of stimulating or suppressing factors after UV exposure remain to be determined.

References

1. Akhurst RJ, Fee F, Balmain A (1988) Localized production of TGF-β mRNA in tumour promotor-stimulated mouse epidermis. Nature 331:363–366
2. Bateman A, Singh A, Kral T, Solomon S (1989) The immune hypothalamic pituitary adrenal axis. Endocr Rev 10:92–112
3. DeFabo EC, Noonan FP (1983) Mechanism of immune suppression by ultraviolet irradiation in vivo. I. Evidence for the existence of an unique photoreceptor in skin and its role in photoimmunology. J Exp Med 157:84–89

4. Eisenberg SP, Evans RJ, Arend WP, Verderber E, Brewert MT, Hannum CH, Thompson RC (1990) Primary structure and functional expression from complementary DNA of a human interleukin-1 receptor antagonist. Nature 343:341–346
5. Elmets CA, Bergstresser PR, Tigellar RE, Wood PJ, Streilein JW (1983) Analysis of the mechanism of unresponsiveness produced by haptens painted on skin exposed to low dose ultraviolet radiation. J Exp Med 158:781–794
6. Jessup M, Hanna N, Plaszynski E, Kripke ML (1978) Mechanisms of depressed reactivity to dinitrochlorobenzene and ultraviolet-induced tumors during ultraviolet carcinogenesis in Balb/c mice. Cell Immunol 39:105–111
7. Kim TA, Golden P, Ullrich SE, Kripke ML (1990) Immunosuppression by factors released from UV-irradiated epidermal cells: selective effects on the generation of contact and delayed hypersensitivity after exposure to UVA or UVB radiation. J Invest Dermatol 94:26–32
8. Köck A, Schauer E, Schwarz T, Luger TA (1991) Human keratinocytes synthesize and release neuropeptides such as α-MSH and ACTH. In: Meltzer M. and Mantovani A (eds) International Conference on Leukocyte Biology. Wiley Sons Inc (in press)
9. Köck A, Schauer E, Schwarz T, Luger TA (1990) MSH-α and ACTH production by human keratinocytes: a link between the neuronal and the immune system. J Invest Dermatol 94:543
10. Kripke ML (1986) Immunology and photocarcinogenesis. J Am Acad Dermatol 14:149–156
11. Kripke ML, Morison WL (1986) Studies on the mechanism of systemic suppression of contact hypersensitivity by ultraviolet B radiation. Photodermatology 3:4–11
12. Krutmann J, Schwarz T, Kirnbauer R, Urbanski A, Luger TA (1988) Modulation of OKT3-induced activation of human T-lymphocytes by interleukin-6 and epidermal cell derived contra-interleukin-1. J Invest Dermatol 91:382
13. Krutmann J, Schwarz T, Kirnbauer R, Urbanski A, Luger TA (1990) Epidermal cell-contra-interleukin-1 inhibits human accessory cell function by specifically blocking IL-1 activity. Photochem Photobiol 52:783–788
14. Krutmann J, Wallis RS, Kahn IU, Zhang F, Koehler KA, Rich EA, Jacobson K, Ellner JJ, Elmets CA (1990) The cell membrane is a major locus for ultraviolet-B-induced alterations in accessory cells. J Clin Invest 85:1529–1536
15. Larrick JW (1989) Native interleukin-1 inhibitors. Immunol Today 10:61–65
16. Luger TA, Schwarz T (1991) Epidermal cell derived secretory regulins. In: Schuler G (ed) Epidermal Langerhans' cells. CRC, Boca Raton, pp 217–251
17. Morison WL, Bucana C, Kripke ML (1984) Systemic suppression of contact hypersensitivity by UVB radiation is unrelated to the UV-induced alterations in the morphology and number of Langerhans' cells. Immunology 52:299–306
18. Naitoh Y, Fukata J, Tominaga T, Nakai Y, Tami S, Mori K, Imura H (1988) Interleukin-6 stimulates the secretion of adrenocorticotropic hormone in conscious freely moving rats. Biochem Biophys Res Commun 155:1459–1465
19. Nickoloff BJ, Mitra RS (1988) Transforming growth factor-beta is a keratinocyte-derived lymphocyte inhibitory factor. J Invest Dermatol 90:592–596
20. Schwarz T, Luger TA (1989) Effect of UV irradiation in epidermal cell cytokine production. J Photochem Photobiol 4:1–13
21. Schwarz T, Urbanska A, Gschnait F, Luger TA (1986) Inhibition of the induction of contact hypersensitivity by a UV-mediated epidermal cytokine. J Invest Dermatol 87:289–295
22. Schwarz T, Urbanska A, Gschnait F, Luger TA (1987) UV-irradiated epidermal cells produce a specific inhibitor of interleukin-1 activity. J Immunol 138:1457–1463
23. Schwarz T, Urbanski A, Kirnbauer R, Köck A, Gschnait F, Luger TA (1988) Detection of a specific inhibitor of interleukin-1 in sera of UVB-treated mice. J Invest Dermatol 91:536–540
24. Sporn MB, Roberts AB, Wakefield LM, deCrombrugghe B (1987) Some recent advances in the chemistry and biology of transforming growth factor-beta. J Cell Biol 105:1039–1045
25. Thody AJ, Ridley K, Penny RJ, Chalmers R, Fisher C, Shuster S (1983) MSH peptides are present in mammalian skin. Peptides 4:813–816
26. Toews GB, Bergstresser PR, Streilein JW (1980) Epidermal Langerhans cell density determines whether contact hypersensitivity or unresponsiveness follows skin painting with DNFB. J Immunol 124:445–450
27. Ullrich SE (1988) Induction of suppressor cells by a factor released by UV-irradiated epidermal cells. Fed Proc 47:a1680

28. Urbanski A, Schwarz T, Schneider FJ, Adolf G, Luger TA (1989) Release of an inhibitor of IL-1 activity by human epidermoid carcinoma cells. J Invest Dermatol 92:536
29. Wahl SM, Hunt DA, Wong HL, Dougherty S, McCartney-Francis N, Wahl LM, Ellingsworth L, Schmidt JA, Hall G, Roberts AB, Sporn MB (1988) Transforming growth factor-β is a potent immunosuppressive agent that inhibits IL-1 dependent lymphocyte proliferation. J Immunol 140:3026–3031
30. Woloski BMRNJ, Smith EM, Meyer WJ III, Fuller GM, Blalock JE (1985) Corticotropin-releasing activity of monokines. Science 230:1035–1038
31. Wrann M, Bodmer S, deMartin R, Siepl C, Hofer-Warbinek R, Frei K, Hofer E, Fontana A (1987) T-cell suppressor factor from human glioblastoma cells is a 12.5 kD protein closely related to transforming growth factor-beta. Eur Mol Biol Organ J 6:163–168

New Trends in Allergy Therapy

A. L. de Weck

Institute of Clinical Immunology, Inselspital, 3010 Bern, Switzerland

Abstract

New approaches to allergy therapy are often a mixture of new molecular possibilities with old theoretical concepts. I shall deal in this lecture exclusively with IgE-mediated allergies.

A first goal may be the prevention of sensitization, either by avoidance of exposure to allergens, a theme dealt with by other speakers, of interference with IgE synthesis and/or functions. Various types of antibodies (allergen-specific IgG or IgA antibodies, anti-idiotypic antibodies, anti-isotypic, i.e. anti-IgE antibodies) have been shown to interfere with allergic reactions in various ways and their potential applications in therapy shall be discussed. Other factors interfering with IgE synthesis, such as IgE-binding factors, soluble CD23 fragments or lymphokines such as interleukin-4 and interferon gamma have been most discussed lately. Potential applications of this new knowledge to therapy of allergic diseases may take various focus, which will be reviewed.

Another approach consists in preventing IgE to fulfil some of its pathophysiological functions, such as binding to effector cells. Advances in IgE molecular biology have there paved some new ways.

Finally, how to prevent an already sensitized individual to manifest his IgE-mediated symptoms? Much can be gained from studying experiments of nature, such as the spontaneous decline of allergic reactivity with aging. Priming of effector cells (basophils and mast cells, monocytes, eosinophils) by various lymphokines (IL-3, GM-CSF, IL-5) for effective mediator release is the cellular phenomenon probably responsible for hyperreactivity at the tissue level, a key feature of allergic diseases. This line of research has opened a whole range of new therapeutic approaches and also a better understanding of the mechanisms of action of some of the old and new anti-allergic drugs.

In view of all this approaches based on pharmacological antagonists of inflammatory mediators (e.g. anti-histamines), although still quite successful and widely used in practice, need reevaluation. A number of the new antihistamines appear to be successful because they are not strictly antagonists of histamine binding to the receptors, as originally thought.

Table 1. Possible approaches for therapy of IgE mediated diseases.

Interference with the sensitization process
Isotypic down-regulating of IgE formation
Allergen-specific down-regulation of IgE synthesis
Interference in the balance T help vs T suppression of IgE formation
Interference with IL-4/interferon-γ balance
Interference with the development of effector cells
Down-regulation of differentiation to mast cells/basophils
Target elimination of mast cells/basophils
Interference with the function of effector cells
Interference with IgE receptors/IgE binding
Interference with mediator formation (e.g., arachidonic acid metabolites)
Down-regulation of mediator release ("releasability")
Down-regulation of cytokine induced priming of effector cells for efficient mediator release and/or formation
Interference with secondary cell (eosinophils, monocytes, neutrophils, platelets) functions
Antagonists of pharmacological mediator's effects
Antihistamine
Leukotrine antagonists
Platelet activating factor antagonists
Chemotactic factors antagonists

Introduction

New approaches to allergy therapy are often a mixture of new molecular possibilities based on old theoretical concepts. This lecture will deal exclusively with IgE mediated allergies. The research director of a large pharmaceutical company looking for new drugs and opportunities in the field of allergy would probably make a list of potential products or projects according to the categories indicated in Table 1.

Prevention of Sensitization

A first goal might be the prevention of sensitization, either by avoidance of exposure to allergens (a theme dealt with at this symposium by other speakers) or by interference with IgE synthesis and/or functions.

Current concepts about the regulation of IgE synthesis have been reviewed by Dr. Ishizaka at this meeting and by others recently [15, 16, 19]. With an increasing list of mechanisms and factors which have been implicated in one way or another in the regulation of IgE synthesis [4, 5] (Table 2), a picture of increasing complexity emerges, and the various pieces of the puzzle do not yet appear to fit together perfectly. The complexity of possible pathways increasing or suppressing IgE responses makes it somehow doubtful that interference with the one or the other of the identified IgE regulating factors will ever lead to effective control and manipulation of the IgE immune response in vivo. Indeed, many of the so-called IgE

Table 2. Factors implicated in the regulation of IgE synthesis.

IgE binding factors of cellular origin (fragments of low affinity FC_{ε} receptors: sCD23)
IgE binding factors of T cell origin; enhancing or suppressing IgE according to their degree of glycosylation (Ishizaka)
Glycosylation enhancing or inhibiting factors
Allergen specific T cell enhancing or suppressing factors
Interleukin-4
Interferons γ and α
Cellular contact/interaction molecules
Auto anti-IgE antibodies

Table 3. Effects of IL-4 on IgE regulation.

Induction of de novo synthesis of IgE in peripheral blood mononuclear cell suspensions from normal patients in vitro
Enhancement of spontaneous IgE synthesis in vitro by peripheral blood mononuclear cell suspensions of atopic patients
Anti-IL-4 antibodies abolish IL-4 induced or enhanced IgE synthesis but do not affect the spontaneous, ongoing IgE synthesis in vitro
Anti-IL-4 suppresses primary IgE responses and decreases the secondary/ongoing IgE responses in vivo. Other factors are also involved
Interferons γ and α antagonize the IL-4 effect

regulating factors have been identified in more or less artificial in vitro cell culture systems but have not yet really been shown to play a role in vivo.

Recently, however, a new and more direct molecular biological approach has opened up which will be worth exploring. In the fall of 1988, Dr. Q. Gang in our laboratory, with the help of Dr. Honjo [14], who provided IgE cDNA probes, started to investigate the expression of IgE mRNA in human peripheral blood cells following various types of stimulation and including the induction of IgE synthesis by interleukin-4 (IL-4). The IgE inducing or enhancing effects of IL-4 on cell cultures have been by now extensively described [1] (Table 3), and IL-4 has also been shown to play an important role in IgE synthesis in vivo. The purpose of our investigations was first to establish which types of lymphocyte stimulation would lead to the expression of IgE mRNA and, using in situ hybridization techniques, to determine the type and number of B cells actually synthesizing IgE. Current assays based on immunofluorescent determination of IgE molecules on B lymphocytes, which may be passively transferred, or on plaque assays [9] do not obligatorily reflect actual synthesis by a given cell.

Somewhat to our surprise, the IL-4 induced expression of IgE mRNA, in a mixed population of peripheral blood mononuclear cells, was much more intense and affected more cells than was expected from the relatively low amounts of synthesized IgE detected in such culture supernatants. Closer analysis of the mRNAs expressed following IL-4 induction revealed the successive occurrence of two types of IgE mRNA, a relatively small IgE RNA transcript of 1.7 kb, followed later by the appearance of a larger RNA moiety of 2.2 kb [17]. A follow-up of IgE synthesis in culture revealed that the small IgE mRNA occurs within hours after IL-4

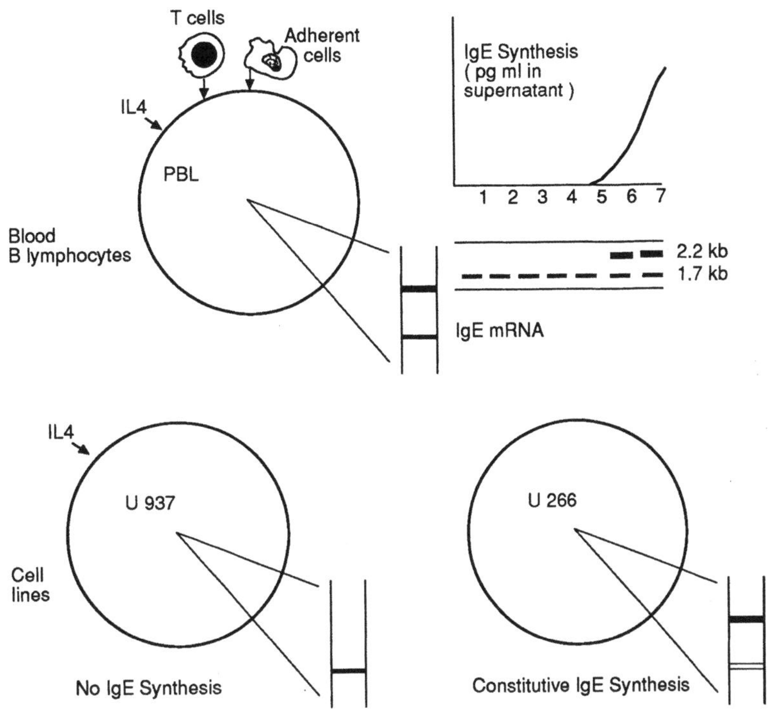

Fig. 1. Expression of IgE mRNA and IgE synthesis in response to IL-4 and other cellular factors. Human peripheral blood B lymphocytes express rapidly, within 24 hours, a short 1.7 kb IgE mRNA. Culture in the presence of T lymphocytes and adherent cells leads, within a few days, to the expression of a longer 2.2 kb IgE mRNA and to the appearance of synthesized IgE in the culture supernatant. Myeloma cells (U 266) constitutively producing IgE express spontaneously both mRNA moieties. IL-4 is also capable of inducing the shorter 1.7 kb mRNA in cell types (e. g., U 937) which do not synthesize IgE

stimulation, while the larger 2.2 kb IgE mRNA moiety only appears around the fourth day of culture, at a time when increased IgE levels also appear in the culture supernatant (Fig. 1). By contrast, the myeloid cell line U-266, which spontaneously synthesizes IgE without an additional requirement for stimulation and/or addition of IL-4, constitutively expresses both IgE mRNA moieties. Addition of IL-4 to other cell line cultures, such as the myeloid cell lines U937 and HL-60, which have no B cell characteristics and are not known to produce IgE, resulted in the expression of the short 1.7 kb IgE mRNA only. No IgE protein, however, could be identified in the supernatants of such cell cultures.

All results, which will appear in detail elsewhere [17], were therefore consistent with the hypothesis that the expression of the 1.7 kb mRNA is due to IL-4 stimulation but by itself does not suffice to induce the expression of the larger 2.2 kb IgE mRNA transcript, which is then associated with IgE synthesis. In collaboration with the group of J. de Vries at the DNAX Institute, in Palo Alto, these observations were soon confirmed and considerably extended [8]. Cloning of the short 1.7 kb mRNA was performed, and the results were consistent with the interpretation that the short IgE mRNA is a sterile germline transcript, similar to those described for other immunoglobulins in mice [11].

As clearly indicated by these experiments, IL-4 stimulation and the ensuing expression of the short IgE mRNA are required prerequisites for IgE synthesis but do not suffice to induce it. What is the nature of the second signal(s) required for the expression of the larger IgE mRNA associated with IgE synthesis? Results of de Vries' group [8] and Romagnani's group [18, 19] suggest that close contact of some T cell clone to the B cell is required, both for IgE synthesis and for the expression of the large IgE mRNA moiety. Suggestions that other lymphokines, such as IL-5 [15] or IL-6 [16], help in IgE synthesis should lead to investigations of their effects on IgE mRNA expression. Indeed, the process of passing from the expression of the short to the large IgE mRNA transcript may prove to be the crucial step amenable to down-regulation of IgE synthesis. Investigations along these lines are in progress.

Various types of antibodies, such as allergen specific IgG or IgA antibodies, anti-idiotypic antibodies, and anti-isotypic, i.e., anti-IgE antibodies, have been shown to interfere with allergic reactions in several ways. Of special interest to us recently have been the anti-IgE autoantibodies, which have been shown to be frequently present both in allergic and in nonallergic individuals [2, 13]. Such antibodies may interfere with IgE determinations, as performed in a number of commercial tests [20]; they also appear to have different functional capacities, according to their fine specificity for epitopes of the IgE Fc fragment. In clinical terms, these IgG anti-IgE seem to play a role in several processes, such as the development and detection of IgE in atopic newborns (IgG anti-IgE transmitted from the mother) [7], in hyposensitized patients [10], and in asthma, in which IgG anti-IgE complexes may also be found in apparently nonatopic patients [13].

Interference with Mast Cell Sensitization

Better knowledge of the factors required for final differentiation of basophils and mast cells, as reported by T. Ishizaka, may also lead to some new approaches to down-regulation of mast cell production and/or function.

Now that the structure of the high affinity receptor for IgE has been elucidated [12] and large amounts of IgE fragments or IgE-related peptides may become available, prevention of IgE binding to mast cells may become a practical possibility.

Interference with Effector Cells

As also discussed by Dahinden [3] at this meeting, priming of effector cells, such as basophils and eosinophils, by cytokines is of paramount importance in maximizing mediator release by basophils and/or eosinophils. Under the influence of IL-3, granulocyte/macrophage colony-stimulating factor (GM-CSF), or IL-5, human basophils become much more responsive to a variety of stimuli and basophil agonists [3]. This priming phenomenon appears closely related to the phenomenon of variable "releasability", in which hyperreactivity at the cellular level is probably the source of tissue hyperreactivity, as defined clinically in terms of tissue or organ hypersensitivity.

It is striking that IL-3, GM-CSF, and IL-4, although having apparently different specific receptors on hemopoietic cells, share the same priming function for basophil agonists and mediator release. Since their effects are identical and not additive, it may be rewarding to look for a common mechanism of action. Selective interference with the priming mechanism might by an elegant means to prevent allergic reactions. It is likely, however, that priming is also required in management of other inflammatory reactions and immunological defenses.

Antagonists of Allergy Mediators

The bulk of anti-allergic drugs used at the present time are still anti-mediator drugs, e.g., antihistamines.

There is a limitation to the development of useful new drugs following this approach, since the great heterogeneity of the mediators involved reduces the expectations assigned to a single drug. Simultaneous manipulation of several pathways by one drug (e.g., steroids) remains the exception, but a combination of various mediator antagonists might become an important contribution to therapy.

Within the framework of drug development and in the study of pathophysiological mechanisms, in vitro models are most frequently used, but the crucial test for any new anti-allergic drug is whether it influences the allergic reaction in vivo. It therefore becomes essential to develop adequate procedures to measure drug effects in the allergic patient in vivo. For immediate-type reactions, measurement of the wheal and erythema diameters induced in the skin by allergens or histamine is relatively easy. Measurement of the crucial late phase reactions, on the other hand, is relatively difficult. Assessment of temperature changes by telethermography during the late phase reaction [6] has recently provided a new tool for the quantitative evaluation of anti-allergic drugs.

In summary, increased knowledge about the pathophysiological mechanisms of allergic reactions has opened up new ways and approaches to develop anti-allergic strategies. There is no doubt that several of these approaches will be explored during the coming years.

References

1. Berton MT, Uhr JW, Vitetta ES (1989) Synthesis of germ line γ_1 immunoglobulin heavy chain transcripts in resting B cells: induction by interleukin 4 and inhibition by interferon γ. Proc Natl Acad Sci USA 86:2829
2. Carini C, Fratrazzi C, Barbato M (1988) IgG autoantibody to IgE in atopic patients. Ann Allergy 60:48–53

3. Dahinden CA, Kurimoto Y, de Weck AL, Lindley I, Dewald B, Baggiolini M (1989) The neutrophil-activating peptide NAF/NAP-1 induces histamine and leukotriene release by interleukin 3-primed basophils. J Exp Med 170:1787–1792
4. Delespesse G, Hofstetter H, Sarfati M (1989) Low affinity receptor for IgE (Fc ERII, CD23) and its soluble fragments. Int Arch Allergy Appl Immunol 90:41–44
5. Delespesse G, Sarfati M, Hofstetter H (1989) Human IgE-binding factors. Immunol Today 10:159–164
6. de Weck AL, Glück U, Derer T (1990) Thermographic analysis of allergic reactions in the skin. ACI News 2:7–11
7. de Weck AL, Derer M, Stadler BM, Bättig M, Hunziker U, Hess S, Seger RA (1990) Simple and rapid determination of low level IgE and IgE complexes in cord blood sera by an immunodot strip (submitted)
8. Gauchat JF, Lebman DA, Coffman RL, Gascan H, de Vries JE (1990) Structure and expression of germline ε transcripts in human B cells induced by IL-4 to switch to IgE production. J Exp Med 172(2):463–473
9. Heusser C, Wagner K, Brinkmann V, Severinson E, Blaser K (1989) Establishment of a memory in vitro murine IgE response to benzylpenicillin and its resistance to suppression by anti-IL-4 antibody. Int Arch Allergy Appl Immunol 90:45–50
10. Loidolt D, Vassella CC, de Weck AL, Stadler BM (1990) Anti-IgE antibodies in hyposensitized patients (submitted)
11. Lutzker S, Alt FW (1988) Structure and expression of germ line immunoglobulin γ_{2b} transcripts. Mol Cell Biol 8:1849
12. Metzger H (1988) Molecular aspects of receptors and binding factors for IgE. Adv Immunol 43:277–312
13. Nawaka Y, Koike T, Yanagisawa T, Iwamoto I, Haya T, Yoshida S, Tomioka H (1984) Anti-IgE autoantibody in patients with bronchial asthma. Clin Exp Immunol 58:348–356
14. Nishiada Y, Miki T, Hisajima H, Honjo T (1982) Cloning of human immunoglobulin ε chain genes: evidence for multiple C_ε genes. Proc Natl Acad Sci USA 79:3833
15. Pène J, Chrétien F, Rousset F, Brière F, Bonnefoy JY, de Vries JE (1989) Modulation of IL-4 induced human IgE production in vitro by IFN γ and IL-5; the role of soluble CD23 (s-CD23). J Cell Biochem 39:253
16. Pène J (1989) Regulation role of cytokines and CD23 in the human IgE antibody synthesis. Int Arch Allergy Appl Immunol 90:32–40
17. Qui G, Vogel M, Gauchat JF, Mandallaz MM, de Weck AL, Stadler BM (1990) Human IgE mRNA expression by peripheral blood lymphocytes stimulated with interleukin 4 and pokeweed mitogen. Eur J Immunol (in press)
18. Romagnani S, Maggi E, Del Prete GF (1983) IgE synthesis in vitro induced by T cell factors from patients with elevated serum IgE levels. Clin Exp Immunol 52:85–88
19. Romagnani S, Del Prete GF, Maggi E (1987) Activation through CD_3 molecules leads a number of T cell clones to induce IgE synthesis in vitro by B cells from allergic and non allergic individuals. J Immunol 138:1744–1749
20. Vassella CC, de Weck AL, Stadler BM (1990) Natural anti-IgE auto-antibodies interfere with diagnostic IgE determination. Clin Exp Allergy 20:295–303

Index of Authors

Subject Index

MIX
Papier aus verantwortungsvollen Quellen
Paper from responsible sources
FSC® C105338

If you have any concerns about our products,
you can contact us on
ProductSafety@springernature.com

In case Publisher is established outside the EU,
the EU authorized representative is:
Springer Nature Customer Service Center GmbH
Europaplatz 3, 69115 Heidelberg, Germany

Printed by Libri Plureos GmbH
in Hamburg, Germany